MANAGING BREEDS FOR A SECURE FUTURE

Strategies for Breeders and Breed Associations

Third Edition

MANAGING BREEDS FOR A SECURE FUTURE

Strategies for Breeders and Breed Associations

Third Edition

D. Phillip Sponenberg
Jeannette Beranger
Alison M. Martin
Charlene R. Couch

Virginia-Maryland College of Veterinary Medicine,
Virginia Polytechnic Institute and State University

The Livestock Conservancy

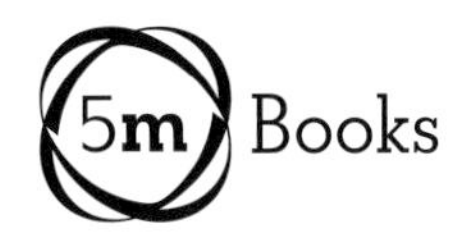

First published 2022

Published by
5M Books Ltd,
Lings, Great Easton,
Essex CM6 2HH, UK,
Tel: +44 (0)330 1333 580
www.5mbooks.com

A Catalogue record for this book is available from the British Library

ISBN 9781789181647
eISBN 9781789181869
DOI 10.52517.9781789181807

Book layout by Cheshire Typesetting Ltd, Cuddington, Cheshire
Printed by Bell & Bain Ltd, Glasgow
Photos by the authors unless otherwise indicated

Contents

Preface

This book was developed over several decades, during which it has seen multiple editions. Many people have had a role in assuring that the material could actually see the light of day. Fred Horak deserves great credit for first pushing this compilation of ideas and approaches into being. Without his gentle but persistent prodding the first edition of this book would have never been written. Many other individuals have subsequently joined Fred to help spur on the development of the ideas presented here and make the coverage of the issues more complete and inclusive. Pat Johnston stands out for pushing for the inclusion of material providing specific details on how to accomplish rescues of especially rare populations. This was one of the main reasons for updating the book with this new edition.

The staff of The Livestock Conservancy has been especially helpful over the years in refining the thinking concerning breeds and their importance to the agricultural landscape. This work would have never been possible without the inputs of the many dedicated and talented people that have staffed The Livestock Conservancy for the past four decades: Chuck Bassett, Margie Bender, Jeannette Beranger, Don Bixby, Michelle Brane, Carolyn Christman, Charlene Couch, Rhyne Cureton, Eric Hallman, Laurie Heize, Libby Henson, Anneke Jakes, Cindra Kerscher, Alison Martin, Don Schrider, Ches Stewart, Brittany Sweeney, Angelique Thompson, and Ryan Walker. Brian Choquet worked diligently to greatly improve many of the figures throughout the book. Margie Bender will always stand out as gently but persistently insisting on clear explanations for inherently complicated biological and political phenomena. Her persistence always helped to refine and focus thinking, and has become a pervasive attitude throughout the culture of The Livestock Conservancy. This approach has shaped an institutional mode of work that has assured success over decades and has also garnered international acceptance and appreciation.

It is especially rewarding to have seen the mission of The Livestock Conservancy make unimpeded progress over many years, even though individuals might cycle in and out. Despite these changes in staff, a consistent presence over time has been key. This is the essential core of successful breed management, and ideally also characterizes breed conservation organizations. Success very much depends on the continuity of commitment to the long-term mission. While each individual in turn takes up the responsibility, it is only if the torch is passed along from individual to individual that breed management and survival can be truly successful in the long term. The Livestock Conservancy has been pivotal in reversing the trend of breed erosion in the USA, and a great debt of gratitude is owed to all of The Livestock Conservancy's members and friends that have been involved in this important work.

As the work of breed conservation has matured, it has expanded outward to involve many international partners that have greatly aided and refined the approaches outlined in this book. It is gratifying to see these same approaches lead to success across the globe. While the general strategies presented here have been developed in a North American setting, they have also been part of an ongoing and ever-increasing international movement to assure breed survival and appreciation around the world. Adapting the approaches to various cultural settings has at times been challenging because each has its own set of unique relationships between people and animals. However, these adaptations have helped to refine the focus on the key elements of managing animal populations for meaningful and successful outcomes. These have allowed for conservation efforts that resonate across various geographic regions and cultural settings. Latin American and Iberian colleagues from the *Red CONBIAND* have been especially helpful in this regard.

The capable and dedicated staff at 5m deserve great credit for the effective and pleasant manner by which they transform manuscripts into attractive finished books. They make the entire process enjoyable and rewarding. Their concern for producing readable and inviting books has been a key part of producing this final work.

While many friends and partners have helped to spur this book into being, all weaknesses and errors are ours alone.

CHAPTER 1

Introduction

... while the right tools can never promise success; the wrong tools can ensure failure.
(Lee Druthman)

This book explains strategies that can assure long-term survival for breeds of livestock, poultry, and dogs. Failures in breed conservation are easy to recognize because numbers tell nearly the whole story: they either fall drastically or the breed becomes extinct. In contrast, lasting success for breed management is subtle because it involves much more than the number of animals in a breed. Long-term successful breed management must be based on multiple factors. These include biological aspects, consistent market demand, and the important and sometimes politically charged role of breed associations as the main advocates for breeds today. Success requires that breeders stay engaged and committed to assuring that a breed has both a strong, healthy population structure and high numbers of animals.

Breeds are fascinating entities. They depend on individual breeders for their continuing existence. Although breeders may come and go, each of them is important and has the potential to make positive contributions to the breed. Individual dedicated breeders can make contributions that endure for decades. One wise breeder noted, "Each year a little better. You only get 30 chances to get it right!" The "30 chances" refers to the usual number of years available for most breeders to work with their stock in a breeding program. This book attempts to provide the knowledge needed to increase the odds of "getting it right" so that the breed itself can benefit from the breeder's contributions.

The thoughts presented in this book result from pondering and discussing many thorny issues over decades of working with livestock breed conservation. Nearly all of this work has been undertaken with The Livestock Conservancy (Figure 1.1), previously known as the American Livestock Breeds Conservancy (ALBC), which was founded in 1977 as the American Minor Breeds Conservancy (AMBC). The Livestock Conservancy has emerged as a globally respected source of information about rare breeds. It is also a trusted source for procedures and practices used in effective breed conservation, largely because of its close attention to the three main factors described above: breed biology, market demand, and

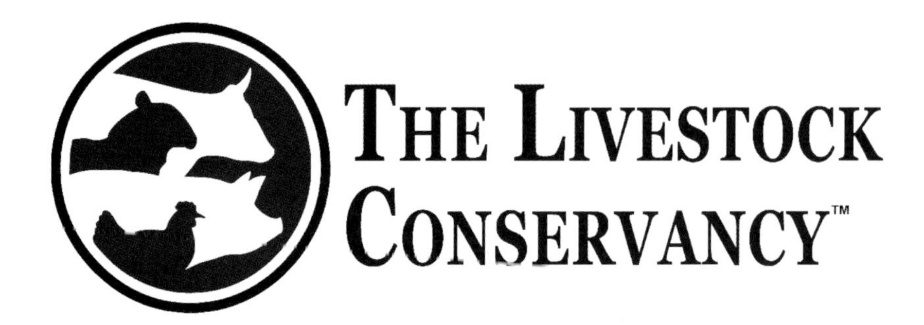

Figure 1.1 The Livestock Conservancy has developed successful protocols for breed conservation and rescue.

the political dynamics among breeders, including interactions between breeders and breed associations.

Individuals, and groups of breeders, have repeatedly alerted The Livestock Conservancy to situations for which clear-headed responses were necessary to assure the survival of important genetic resources. Responding to those challenges and needs over decades has generated strategies that have been distilled to a successful general approach that assures breed survival and utility across a wide variety of situations. The most successful strategies are based on sound biological principles while also being practical. Even the best theoretical approach is doomed to failure if it cannot be achieved in field situations or on the farm. While each breed has unique challenges and needs, they all have a great deal in common. Certain broad strategies can be used with success for nearly all of them.

1.1 How to Use This Book

This book delves into a wide array of topics that surround breed conservation. The book is organized to lead readers step-by-step through a series of topics that develop a deep understanding of what breeds are, how they function genetically, and their cultural setting as they interact with human caretakers.

The information is broken down into several general sections. In each of these, the flow of information begins with general theoretical fundamentals. The fundamentals are then fleshed out with specific examples or experiences to demonstrate their practical application. Finally, specific strategies for moving forward are suggested. A deep understanding of the basic biological aspects of breed function leads to conservation success because breeders can base specific decisions on a sound guiding framework that includes goals and a basic and consistent philosophy. While each strategy for success is tailored specifically for each breed, as well as for its breeder community, key central concepts cut across breed and species boundaries to make powerful generalizations possible.

The early chapters guide readers through the biology of breeds, how they developed, how they function, and why they are important. This includes a detailed discussion of just what "breed" means, how breeds form, and how they function as genetic resources. Gene flow into and out of breeds is also covered in this material. The book then focuses on issues surrounding the definition of specific breeds and how to decide which animals should be included, as well as those that should be excluded. The next chapter discusses the role of breed standards in maintaining breeds and educating breeders, and explains what breed standards are and how they can function either constructively or destructively in maintaining a viable breed population.

The next group of chapters includes the more theoretical issues of breeding strategies, such as inbreeding and outbreeding, and how they affect populations. Important aspects of animal selection are discussed in detail, including the effects of selection based on breeding animals for show and the role of performance testing. These aspects are then put together in practical suggestions for managing breeding strategies and effective ways of pairing animals for secure progress. This includes both traditional as well as modern statistical approaches. This is followed by a discussion of the role of assisted reproductive techniques and the role of cryopreservation of semen and embryos in breed management. A few chapters then delve into how to analyze the population structure of a breed, including various ways used to evaluate the genetic health of a breed. This explains the roles of both pedigree evaluation as well as the useful contributions that DNA technology can provide.

The general background established by the initial chapters is followed by chapters that offer general suggestions for using that material to maintain breeds. This delves into some very specific breeding strategies, including specific templates or recipes. This section also details the genetic consequences of various breeding strategies. Understanding the principles of long-term breed maintenance prepares the reader for the chapters that discuss rescuing the genetic integrity of highly endangered populations containing only a few animals. Rescue is first addressed on a general level and then fleshed out with specific examples to help breeders who are faced with similar situations in their own breeds or herds.

The next chapters focus on non-biological factors involved in breed management. These include market demand for the breed and its products, along with the complex political and cultural aspects of breed maintenance. The pivotal role of breed associations receives detailed coverage. Success in the management of these non-biological aspects is essential for breed survival, and failure assures the collapse of a breed. A final short chapter deals with breeder responsibilities, because dedicated, informed, and capable breeders are essential to the long-term success of any breed.

The book includes many figures and photographs. The attributions are included in the legend for each figure. Most of these were provided by D.P. Sponenberg and J. Beranger, and attributions to these are designated simply as "DPS" or "JB."

A specific note on nomenclature in this book is warranted. Populations of various species of animals are known by different terms: herds of cattle, horses, goats, and swine, flocks of sheep, ducks, chickens, and turkeys, gaggles of geese, and packs of dogs. Throughout this work the usual word chosen is "herd," although this is meant to be inclusive of all species while at the same time avoiding the distracting repetition of "herd/flock/gaggle/pack" when describing groups of animals. Regardless of what a group of animals is called, they all face the same challenges in genetic management, and the same overarching truths can be used in the management of breeds of all species.

The first step along this journey is to explore the details of what is meant by "breed."

1.2 What Is a Breed?

Breeds are the way that domesticated species are divided into genetically distinct and useful subgroups. Breeds are similar to the subspecies classification that is applied to different populations within species of wild animals, although breeds do have many important distinctions from subspecies. Both breeds (domestic) and subspecies (wild) are groups of animals that have significant, distinctive, and reproducible similarities that set them apart from other animals of the same species.

While the term "breed" is frequently bandied about, it is in fact very difficult to define it in a meaningful and consistent way. Difficulty arises because two major factors affect breeds and their function. One factor is the biological aspect that results from the role of a breed within its species. The other factor includes both cultural and political aspects that arise from the important interactions of breeds as they function in human culture and under human management (Figure 1.2). As the biological and cultural aspects meet and interact, they can take the definition of "breed" to different extremes.

The least restrictive definition is that a breed is a "group of animals with a fence around it." This implies that breeds have some degree of identity and isolation, whether genetic or cultural. Juliet Clutton-Brock, in *A Natural History of Domesticated Mammals* (1999), has

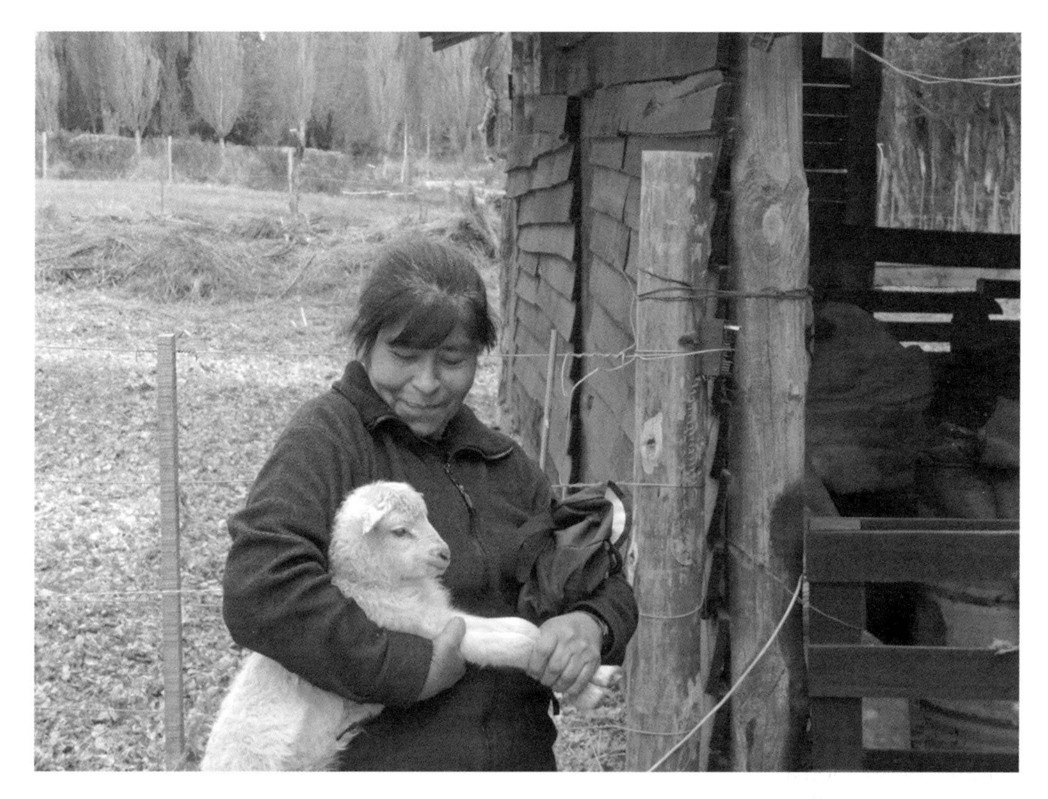

Figure 1.2 Linca sheep survive in Argentine Patagonia and are highly valued by the Mapuche community for their unique fiber and exquisite environmental adaptation. Both sheep and people benefit from this partnership. Photo by DPS.

articulated a biologically based definition of "breed" which asserts that a breed is a group of animals that is consistent enough in type to be readily recognized and logically grouped together, and that when mated within the group reproduces the same type. This definition very ably gets to the core of the biological aspect of the breed concept: breeds are consistent and predictable genetic entities. The status of breeds as genetic resources is a consequence of the fact that breeds breed true. Despite the strength of this definition, it gets a bit fuzzy around the edges in some situations. Still, it is a practical and useful guiding principle for understanding breeds, their importance, and their management.

Another very different definition of "breed" is also widely accepted. By this definition, a "breed" is any animal population that is deemed to be a breed by the governmental authorities in its region of occurrence. This definition is culturally based rather than biologically based. Most breeds by the previous definition would be included under this second definition, even though the second definition is very loose and inclusive. It is derived more from political expediency than from biological principles. By this definition, a breed is anything that breeders say it is. This definition governs the organization of animal breeding in many countries. Under this mindset, some genetically variable populations are included as breeds along with other more genetically distinct breeds. The biologically based definition is much stricter, but is also more useful for conservation purposes because it targets identification of those populations most likely to make significant contributions to biodiversity.

The Food and Agricultural Organization (FAO) of the United Nations uses a definition that is based in biology but that also includes important cultural influences:

> A breed is either a subspecific group of domestic livestock with definable and identifiable external characteristics that enable it to be separated by visual appraisal from other similarly defined groups within the same species, and/or a group for which geographical and/or cultural separation from phenotypically similar groups has led to acceptance of its separate identity. For the purposes of the FAO guidelines, a breed is a subspecific group of domestic livestock with a common history whose members are treated in a common manner with respect to genetic management.

This definition, in most cases, captures both the genetic and cultural components in a constructive and useful way. To be useful and practical, any definition of "breed" must consider the biological aspects of breeds without ignoring the complicated cultural trappings that arise as breeds interact with the people that use them. This definition, based mainly on genetics but also informed by cultural influences, is employed throughout this book when "breed" is used.

If the idea of "breed" is viewed through the lens of practicality, then "functional breed" is a useful concept. Viewed this way, a breed is a specific genetic resource that is shaped by influences that are exerted on the animal population. These influences include the natural environment as well as human management and selection pressures. Functional breeds do not exist in isolation away from these influences.

Secure breeds all require a foundation of sound genetic management, cultural appreciation, and use. Secure breeds can be thought of as resting on a three-legged stool, as shown in Figure 1.3, that is based on:

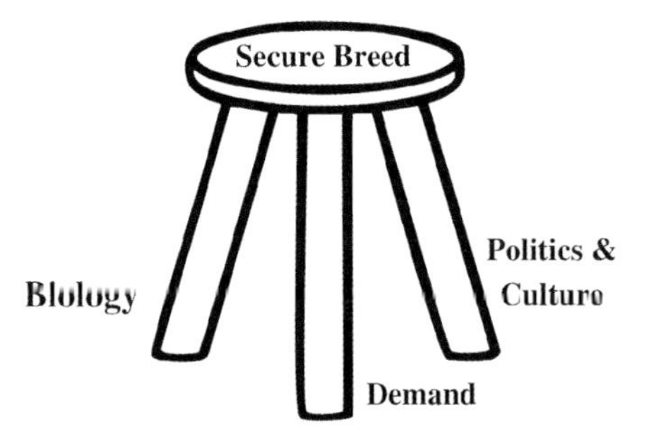

Figure 1.3 Successful breeds are like a three-legged stool that rests securely on biology, demand, and the politics and culture that surround the breed.
Figure by DPS.

- biological issues related to population genetics and dynamics
- demand for the breed and its products
- cultural and political aspects of managing and using a breed.

The complex interaction between all three aspects must be addressed to ensure successful breed management for breed security. The biological issues are intricate and tricky, but are at least superficially a little easier to tackle than the other two because biological management usually involves fewer decision-makers. Despite the relative simplicity of decision-making, biological issues remain a common source of potential failure in breed management. The absence of successful biological management precludes the success of the other dimensions.

Demand for the breed underlies the practicality of keeping the breed around at all. Demand is complicated because it involves many individual actors, many of whom are outside of the breeder community but still have important influences on it. Breeds that lack demand can indeed be maintained, but this tends to be more along the lines of a museum oddity or a cultural relic than as a productive component of a system involving animals, humans, and their interactions with one another.

The cultural aspects of breed management can be daunting at times. These usually are limited to the breeder community, but that community is broad indeed. Multiple participants are involved, each with an independent viewpoint, along with attitudes and approaches that can sometimes make unified action and agreement difficult to achieve.

Each breed is unique, each situation is distinct. The variability, though challenging, is the very core of the reason that breed conservation and management are so important. Fortunately, each of the three main dimensions that contributes to breed security are affected by a few basic principles that help to tilt the balance toward successful outcomes. These few principles weave their way through most situations in most breeds. Understanding them helps to successfully address nearly every situation.

1.3 Genetic Character of Breeds

Breeds serve human needs well because they are readily identifiable genetic packages, and each package is reasonably repeatable among members of the breed. Repeatability serves to make breeds predictable, and this is their main importance whether as agriculturally productive animals or as dogs destined for work, pleasure, or companionship. The animals of a breed are much more than a random assortment of individual genetic variants of different utility to humanity. They are instead a complete package of specific genetic variants that is largely unique to that breed. The whole package tends to repeat throughout the members of the breed, and ideally it persists down through the generations. Individual animals of the breed come and go as the generations proceed. Each individual has its own unique genome, although it shares much of this with other members of its breed. Each animal can contribute in its own turn to the long-term predictability and uniformity of the breed.

An important aspect of the genetic character of breeds concerns the idea of "purebred breeds." Opinions differ on this concept, and some observers now reject the idea of complete breed purity or purebred breeding. This is partly because many breeds have relatively recent and mixed origins, although it remains true that several are indeed ancient and unmixed. Despite a recent origin for some breeds, it is still useful to reflect that those breeds (and bloodlines within those breeds) derive a great deal of their utility from having a sufficient level of genetic uniformity to allow their function to be predictable. This relative uniformity has come from mating animals within the same population to one another. Uniformity tends to be completely lost when animals are mated to animals outside of that population.

While the edges around the concept of "purebred breeding" can get quite blurry, it remains important as a loose concept that guides effective genetic resource conservation. This book therefore uses the terms "purebred" and "purebred breeding," while also recognizing that these concepts might not be absolutely accurate in every situation. This concept, as used here, refers to a deliberate attempt to remain true to a breed's history of foundation, isolation, and selection in order to achieve the ideal balance between uniformity and variability. Importantly, "breed" and "purebred" are used here to reflect the inherent biological character of a population of animals as a genetic resource. These terms are not dependent on the existence or function of a registry or association. Basically, an animal should be considered as a member of a breed because of its genetic character, regardless of its registration status. Breeds pre-date associations and registries, not the other way around. The role and mission of associations and registries should be to prioritize this concept rather than to impose arbitrary restrictions on it.

Predictability is the key strength of "purebred breeding," despite the fact that absolute purity is not entirely accurate and is also not desirable for a host of biological reasons. Somewhere between "completely uniform" and "completely variable" is a zone where breeds reside and remain productive and useful. Most breeds are more toward the "uniform" end of the spectrum rather than the "variable" end. While this is true, it is often the case that the "variability" aspect is the important one for breed security, while not ignoring the "uniformity" aspect that confers utility to populations (Figure 1.4).

The definitions of "breed" that are biologically based are the ones that best serve conservation purposes. Many collections of animals are designated as "breeds" but fall far short of genetic breed status if the biological definition is used. These are usually groups of animals that exhibit a superficial feature in common. For instance, spotting on Pinto horses can appear in many genetically different types of horses, from miniature to draft. Likewise, a physically similar body type can mask great genetic diversity, such as occurs in

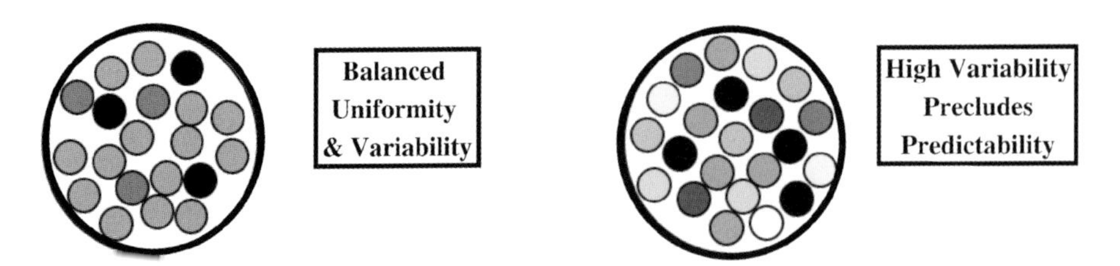

Figure 1.4 Breeds benefit from a balance of genetic uniformity and genetic variability. Figure by DPS.

some Warmblood horse breeds. These looser definitions of breeds do indeed serve as useful designations for breeders interested in animals with certain characteristics, but the genetic variability of these populations decreases their predictability in reproducing that same type. This precludes their usefulness in a conservation sense.

The entire genetic package of a breed is based on a specific combination of genetic variants. The package, as a whole, is much more fundamental to the significance of breeds than the individual genetic variants are, however unique or interesting some of those may be. The philosophy of breeds as packages of genetic combinations, and not just repositories for single genes, leads to the holistic conclusion that entire breeds, rather than just the individual component genes of individual animals, need to be conserved. Breeds must be maintained as intact genetic packages to ensure their continued or potential use in service to humans. This philosophy is useful in guiding conservation and management strategies. Viewing this topic from the breed level is different than viewing it from the level of individual genes or individual animals. Approaching conservation of populations from the breed level brings both individual genes and animals into a broader context that supports breed maintenance and strength.

While breeds are repeatable genetic packages, they also must contain the genetic variation needed for ongoing selection and viability. The tension between the desirability of genetic uniformity and the need for genetic variation gives animal breeders a space in which to work and contribute to meaningful breed conservation. Most animal populations fall somewhere along a continuum from very uniform and predictable genetic packages to completely variable and unpredictable genetic packages. Exactly where to draw the line between genetic "breed" and "non breed" is somewhat arbitrary and frequently controversial. The concept that some culturally defined breeds fall outside of the realm of genetically defined breeds is important. Ignoring this fact can result in conservation efforts being squandered on populations that have little to offer as genetic resources. Only breeds that qualify by the genetic criterion are useful as predictable genetic resources. It is these breeds that should be especially targeted for wise long-term management and conservation.

The genetic management of breeds for a secure future is inherently tricky. Breeders must consider the breed as the unit of interest, more than the individual animals within the breed. That can sound like nonsense, because it is obvious that breeds are made up of individual animals. However, when breeders start to consider the function and future of their herd, or their breed, then the role of the individual animals starts to take on a slightly different character. This shift in thinking views each animal as a component of the whole and allows decision-making to reframe the role of individual animals for the survival and success of the breed.

1.4 Why Breeds Are Important

Breeds in their amazing variation are fascinating in their own right as biological entities. Breeds also have profoundly important roles in maintaining global biodiversity. This role becomes increasingly important due to obvious threats such as changes in climate and emergence of diseases. More subtle threats to breeds, such as the increasing homogenization of world cultures and the urbanization of human populations, are of equal if not greater importance. The practical significance of breeds springs largely from their unique roles in partnership with people. Global homogenization of culture erases these distinctions.

Breeds exist only in domesticated species, and not in wild ones. For most species, the role of breeds in agricultural settings is the main basis for their importance. Dogs, importantly, are valued for a wider range of contributions that include many non-agricultural functions but that are nonetheless vital to assuring that humans have enjoyable and dignified lives. Domesticated species occupy unique biological spaces where both natural and human influences meet. As human populations have exploded over the centuries, agricultural environments have increasingly expanded and diversified and are now large and pivotal components of the global ecosystem. Ensuring that these environments function sustainably is critically important to the future of the earth and its human and nonhuman inhabitants. While livestock are an obvious component of these systems, dogs and other animal partners also have vital roles in the successful function of these systems. Effective management of breeds helps assure that all of these systems can continue to function in positive ways.

Breeds function in a wide variety of agricultural and cultural environments. The roles that different breeds play in these environments are of profound importance. Breeds are shaped by their interaction with their environment. This interaction shapes the breed's genetic character, which is essential to its function. Breeds serve as the primary reservoirs of the genetic diversity within most domesticated species of animals. Half of the biodiversity of most of these species is shared across breeds, while the other half is unshared and is instead contained only within single breeds. Therefore, any loss of breed results in loss of genetic diversity as the species loses the genetic information that is unique to that breed. Figure 1.5 illustrates the genetic diversity in the breeds that make up a domesticated species, and the ways these either overlap or do not overlap.

For example, the Leicester Longwool sheep breed is adapted to wet lowland conditions, while the Merino breed is adapted to dry grasslands (Figure 1.6). These two breeds vary from one another in a host of genetic differences that separate them by wool type, disease resistance, forage use, reproduction, and behavior. Many of the variants within one of these breeds are simply lacking in the other, so to lose one choice or the other through breed extinction would drastically reduce options for future sheep breeders.

The importance of breeds within domesticated species can hardly be overstated. This is especially true for those species, such as cattle and horses, whose wild progenitors are now extinct. Cattle and horses are now uniquely agricultural rather than wild, and consequently

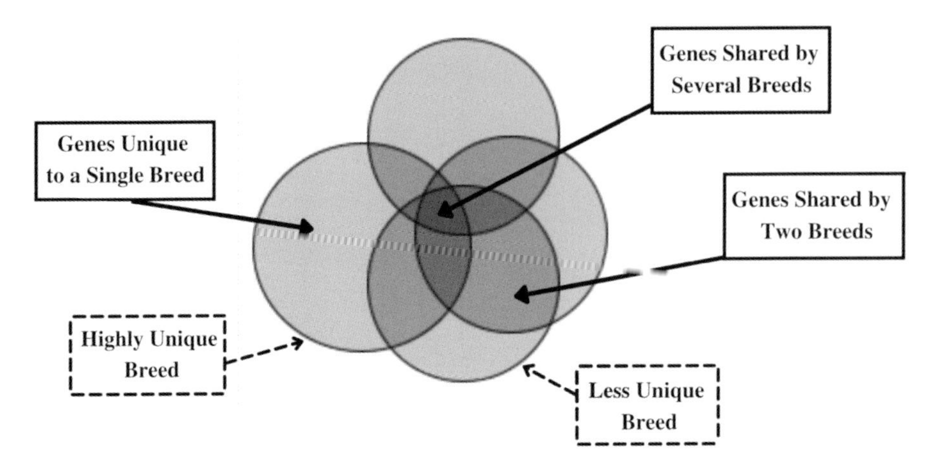

Figure 1.5 The genetic diversity in livestock species is contained in breeds. The circles represent different breeds with the genetic components of each. Some genes are shared among the different breeds. These are in the portions of the circles that overlap. Some genes are unique to only single breeds, and reside in portions that do not overlap. Figure by DPS.

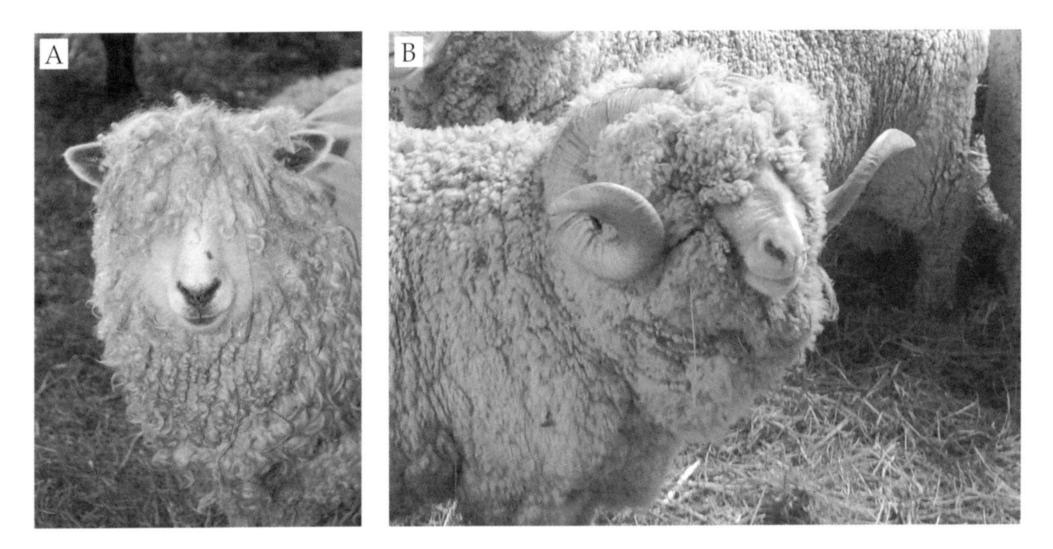

Figure 1.6 The Leicester Longwool (A) and the Merino (B) are two breeds of sheep that are distinct from one another by looks, production, behavior, and environmental adaptation. This is the key to the importance of breeds – no single breed fits all situations. Photo A by Gail Groot, Sunrise Valley Farm. Photo B by DPS.

the various breeds embody the entire genetic diversity of these species. To lose this diversity is to assure that unique components of global biodiversity are lost forever because it is now impossible to return to the wild ancestors of these species for their genetic material. Effective management of breeds is essential to managing the biodiversity of all domesticated species. This issue will only grow in importance as globalization increasingly shrinks the world and its choices.

While the issues of genetic diversity are obvious for domestic species that are extinct in the wild, they are also important for many other species because the domesticated component of the species came from a limited sample of the wild species long ago. Wild Bactrian camels, for example, have little in common with the domesticated sort, and domesticated dogs now share little with today's wolves. In both of these domesticated species the specific wild ancestor is extinct, so that the domesticated ones are now cousins with the wild species rather than lineal descendants.

Agricultural environments have been vital in sustaining human life and cultural development for over 10,000 years. Dogs have contributed to human survival for even longer. As agriculture has expanded around the globe, it has had an increasingly large effect on the overall global ecosystem. Agriculture is the base from which humans dramatically increased in number and became the major determinant of global ecology. Throughout most of human history, agriculture has been viewed as a necessary contributor to human sustenance and has been highly valued in that role. Agriculture has had great and lasting success in those regions where it was viewed as a sustainable and renewable system to be carefully stewarded.

In contrast, mainstream modern thinking, and indeed some thinking long past, has viewed agriculture as an extractive and exploitative endeavor, similar to mining. This mode of thought quickly leads to non-sustainable systems, which cannot continue to remain productive over multiple centuries without massive inputs from outside the agricultural system itself. Fortunately, agricultural thinking has begun to return to a more renewable and sustainable mindset. It is within that mode of thinking that breed diversity best functions and flourishes. Understanding the relationship of breeds to varied agricultural settings is key to appreciating and fostering the performance and survival of a wide variety of breeds.

Breeds of livestock are important components of any renewable and sustainable agricultural system. The breeds are diverse and each functions best in a specific environment and under a specific management strategy. The fit of each breed into a specific environment and specific production goals underscores the value of breed diversity. Any breeds that are removed from their production environments lose much of their powerful contribution to human endeavor and relevance, especially if they are kept only as interesting relics by dedicated hobbyists. They also lose much of their genetic makeup due to changes in selection pressures. Genetic characteristics are likewise lost when multiple breeds within a species are selected to function equally across all environments for a single production goal. This results in loss of the genetic distinctiveness that originally contributed to their agricultural role in a specific setting.

The tendency to homogenize animals across various breeds is especially true of dogs, as the original purpose of many breeds is increasingly changed to their role as companion animals. Despite this trend, many dog breeds do continue with their historic roles. For example, Cur dogs (Figure 1.7) have been an important part of farming life for many generations in the Southeastern USA. While the overall appearance of these dogs is similar, Curs are divided into a wide variety of individual breeds. Each Cur breed is associated with the region where it developed. The Catahoula hails from Louisiana, Mountain Cur from Ohio to Tennessee, the Blue Lacey Cur from Texas, and others come from yet further regions. Curs are widely regarded as tough, rugged, high-energy work dogs that can tackle

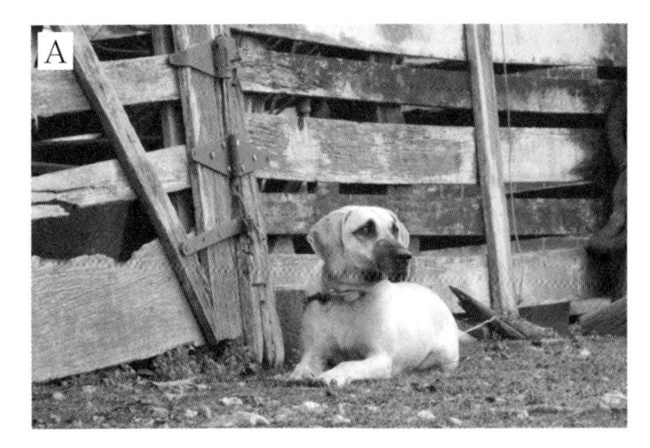

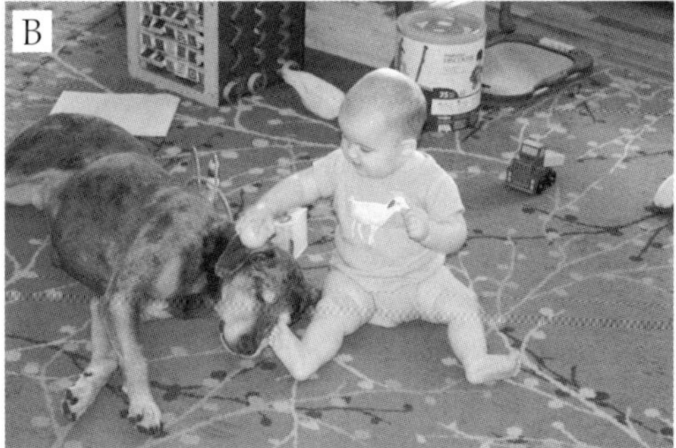

Figure 1.7 Curs are increasingly moving from the farmyard to the living room, and with that move come changes in the selection imposed on these dogs. This Black Mouth Cur (A) is an essential partner in managing cattle in Mississippi, while the Catahoula Cur (B) enjoys being a safe and reliable house pet. Photo A by JB, B by Julie Cecere.

Table 1.1 Genotype by environment interactions can change how breeds A, B, and C rank in productivity.

	Environment 1	Environment 2	Environment 3
Top producer	A	B	C
Medium producer	B	A	B
Lowest producer	C	C	A

just about any job: herding, hunting, and guarding property. As Curs become increasingly popular as companion animals that are incorporated into family life, they are often no longer selected for the same tough qualities that make them superb working dogs that help to manage cattle and hogs on open ranges. Breeders need to be careful to ensure that the traditional working abilities and the mental character of these dogs are conserved. Their versatile working ability was developed over several generations and could easily be lost.

Breeds function in their environments, and maintaining a close relationship to the environment is key to maintaining breed diversity. Each breed best fits a specific environment. The interactions of the genotype with the environment can have powerful influence on the overall productive potential of animals. These interactions can be great enough to change breed rankings in production levels depending on the environments involved, as demonstrated in Table 1.1. This means that the top-ranking breed in one environment might be lower down in the ranking in a different environment. Environment can never be ignored when considering a breed's productive potential.

1.5 Sustaining Breeds over Time

Breeds can indeed be successfully sustained as viable biological entities over long periods of time, but this takes forethought and wise action. A major factor in successful breed prosperity is the steady demand for the breed, which usually arises because of steady demand for the breed's products or services. In a situation of steady demand, breed rarity is avoided.

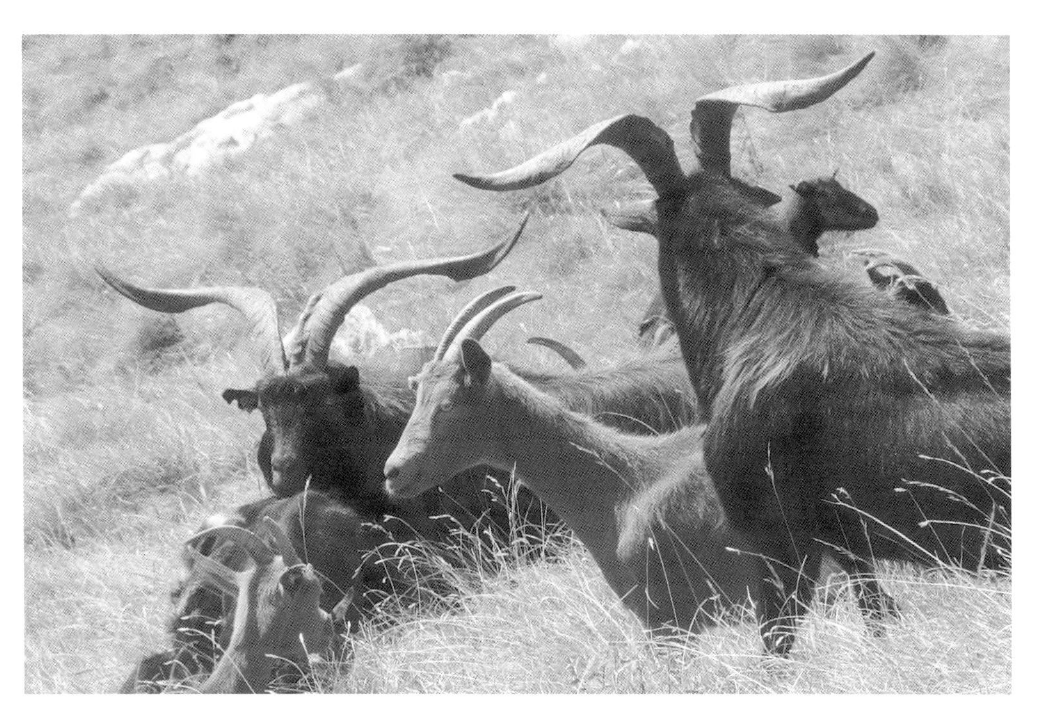

Figure 1.8 The Slovenian Dražnica goat is still called home by words whose meanings are lost in antiquity. Photo by DPS.

The challenge is to organize breeding and promotion so that demand is consistent while also remaining true to the breed's heritage.

Breed-specific production systems can be very important for breed stability and sustainability. Changes in a production system often dictate changes in selection pressures, which result in changes in the genetic makeup of a breed. In the process of change, some genetic information is irretrievably lost. Wise management can help to minimize this loss. More subtle are the effects of sociological changes that accompany changes in production systems. When systems change, so do the cultural trappings that are associated with animal use and maintenance. Much of the vocabulary, procedures, and fine details of animal management are part of a rich culture that is only rarely conveyed in writing. As a result, failure of continuity for even one human generation of caretakers assures that certain cultural practices are lost.

Some examples may seem trivial, but this deep and long relationship between people and their animals is important. In many parts of the United States of America (USA), cattle are called home by shouting "here boss, here bossy," and hogs by "soo-ee." Both of these are Latin, handed down from parent to child, parent to child, for the last 2000 years. The end result is that this may be the only Latin known by some of today's farmers. Similarly, Slovenian goat producers call the goats home from the mountains with a very specific call. Everyone uses it, but the words are from an extinct language, so no one knows what they actually mean! This reflects the deep and abiding interaction of people with their breed resources that covers long centuries (Figure 1.8). Calling animals home is but one small example of how important animal management information can be maintained across generations.

Modern families across the globe commonly, and understandably, leave farming in search of better economic opportunities. Later generations of the same family may then return to agriculture, if only as a hobby or part-time endeavor. While much is saved by this approach, many aspects of the culture and practices of animal production are lost because the intervening non-agricultural generation has failed to provide the continuity that such cultural exchange needs. Even simple details like how to call the cows home can be lost forever if only one generation fails to learn how to do it from the long line of generations that have called them home in the same way for centuries. Such lapses impoverish the richness of the culture of animal production systems.

The threats to the continuity of the cultural aspects of animal production have no easy answers. It is much easier to manage and save the genetics of breeds than it is to save the traditional systems under which they have evolved. It is worth pondering, though, that saving traditional systems will nearly always result in saving the genetic resources (breeds) that they require. In contrast, it is much more difficult to effectively save the intact genetic resources in the absence of the traditional systems responsible for their origin and persistence (Figure 1.9).

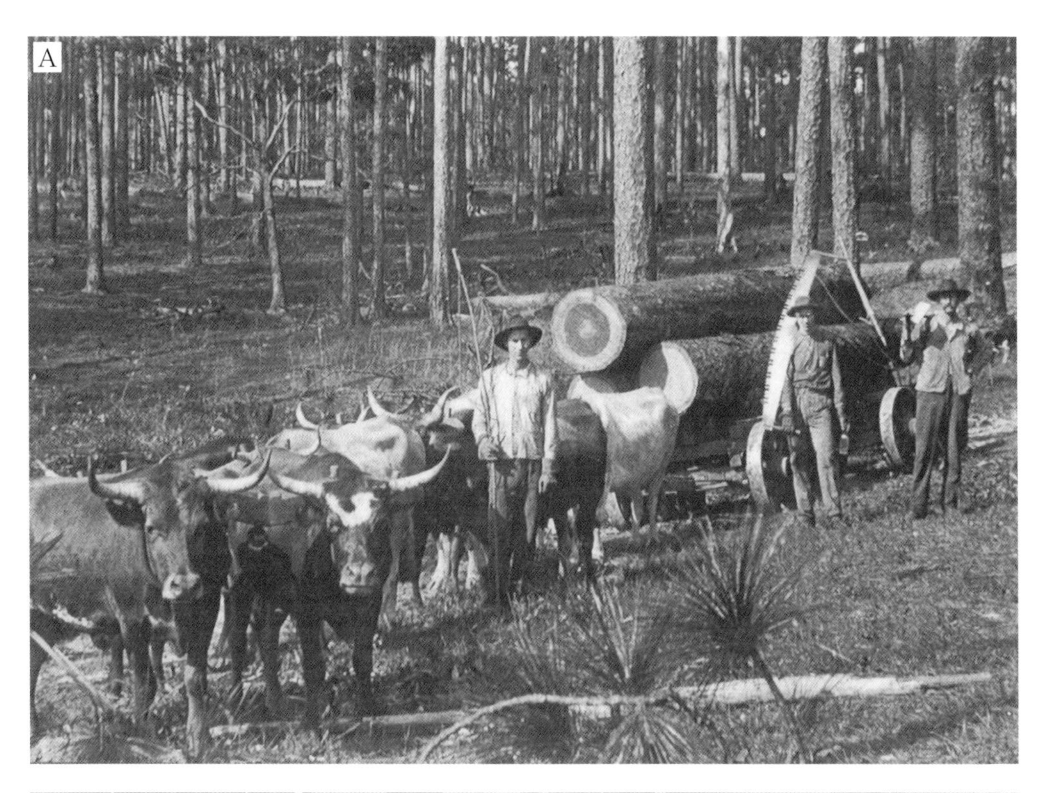

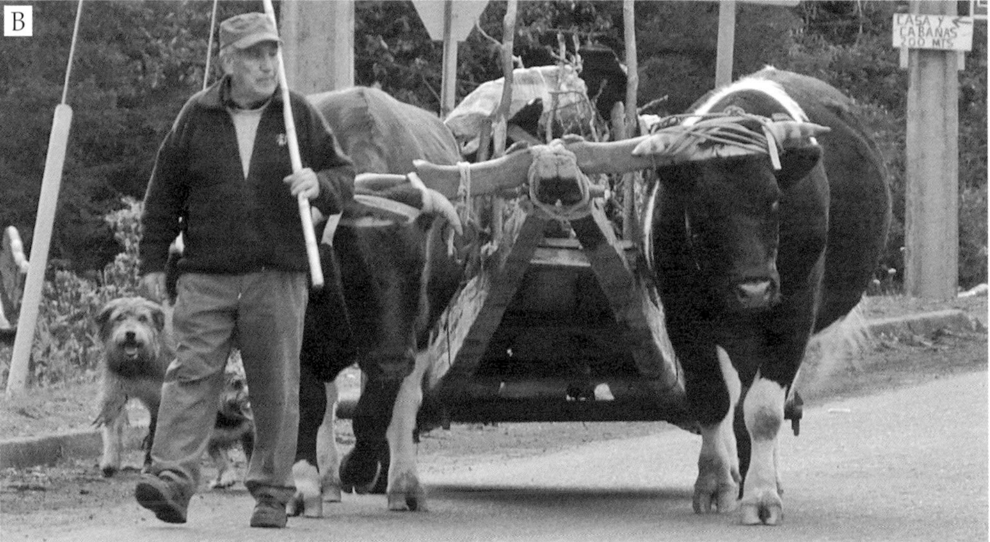

Figure 1.9 The use of oxen has largely faded from modern uses of many breeds (A, Pineywoods oxen from 1907). This has changed the selection goals of the breeders. The strategies for the use of oxen, and even the vocabulary used to control them, have deep regional roots that vary from place to place (B, Overo Negro oxen from Chile). Both North and South America are fortunate in that local ox-driving traditions have never completely vanished, providing continuity for modern ox-drivers. Photo A donated by W.F. Brown, Cowpen Creek Farm. Photo B by DPS.

CHAPTER 2

Breed Basics

2.1 *How Breeds Form*

Breeds vary greatly one from another because each has its own unique combination of history, use, and function. Fortunately, a few general principles hold true across this wide diversity and influence how breeds come into being and how best to guide their management. Breeds are formed by a combination of four main influences: foundation, isolation, natural selection, and human selection (Figure 2.1). The relative importance of each of these varies among breeds, but in nearly all cases all four are involved to some extent.

"Foundation" is the term used for the events at the beginning of a breed population, and includes the specific group of animals involved in starting the breed. Each individual animal in that initial group is referred to as a "founder." The specific character of the foundation varies among general classes of breeds. The foundation of most old, local breeds was almost always an accident of history. The founders just happened to have been the ones originally present in a given area. In contrast, newer and more deliberately formed breeds usually have a foundation that was very carefully chosen to include specific characteristics that were desired in the final breed.

"Isolation" refers to the extent to which the foundation group has avoided the ongoing additions of unrelated animals. Isolation acts to consolidate the genetics of the population and combines with foundation to form a repeatable genetic package. Isolation is essential

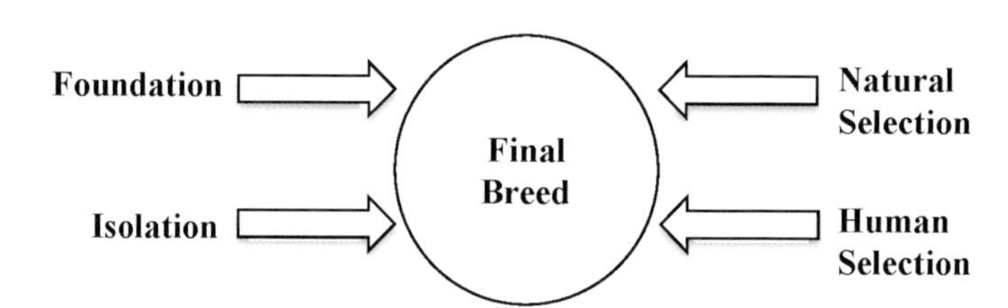

Figure 2.1 The final form of breeds depends on the interaction of foundation, isolation, natural selection, and human selection. Figure by DPS.

in this process because it prevents outside genetic material from disrupting the relative uniformity of the foundation genetic material.

"Selection" refers to the ongoing process of some animals contributing to the next generation, while others do not. Selection has two main aspects: natural and human. Some degree of natural selection is imposed on any population. Some genetic combinations thrive in certain environments, while others fail in those same environments and therefore do not reproduce themselves. Over time, this process shapes the initial genetic material in various ways. Natural selection is more important in compromised or difficult environments than it is in more benign ones, but it can never be completely ignored as a factor that shapes the genetics of animal breed populations.

Selection decisions made by the owners and breeders are also important. This aspect of selection is a very powerful source for the formation of breed genetics. Breed uses vary, and each entails different sorts and degrees of selection by humans. For example, sheep can be selected for different types of wool, a presence or lack of horns, walking ability, growth rate, twinning ability, or milk production (Figure 2.2). Each of these selection pressures ends up taking the population in a different direction. The final product is very different in each case.

These four main factors have functioned over long spans of time to produce the wide array of breeds that exist today. The general pattern over most of the history of human interaction with domesticated animals has been the movement and expansion of each species out from where it was originally domesticated. Human owners essentially took with them a subsample of what was locally available as they settled in new territories. Also, local animals were pressed into use by neighboring people as they began to participate in the interaction of humans and domesticated animals. This expansion process was ongoing, resulting in an ever-expanding number of animal populations (breeds) that radiated and diffused outward from that original domesticated group. Each resulting population differed from the others due to differences in foundation, degree of isolation, natural selection pressures, and human selection practices (Figure 2.3). These differences increased over time as local variants developed, and those in turn diffused outward. The radiation outwards from a central region results in the greatest degree of difference being present between the most peripheral groups.

This process of expansion and the increase in the numbers of types and varieties of animals was the general rule until about 1900. At that point in human history, a dramatic reversal of traditional trajectories took place. Especially by the last half of the 1900s, fewer and fewer breeds were used in a greater number of locations. Local breeds were pushed out and replaced by the few breeds that developed an international and disproportional importance for food production. With the extinction of many breeds, each species lost specific genetic packages, each of which had been developed as a good fit for production goals in a specific environment. This is a dramatic reversal away from the long history during which each agricultural environment developed breed resources tailored specifically to it. The historic trend has now reversed, so that the long process of gradual expansion and differentiation has been replaced by one of contraction and increasing uniformity. The contraction diminishes the close fit of breeds to their environments that characterized the last 10,000 years.

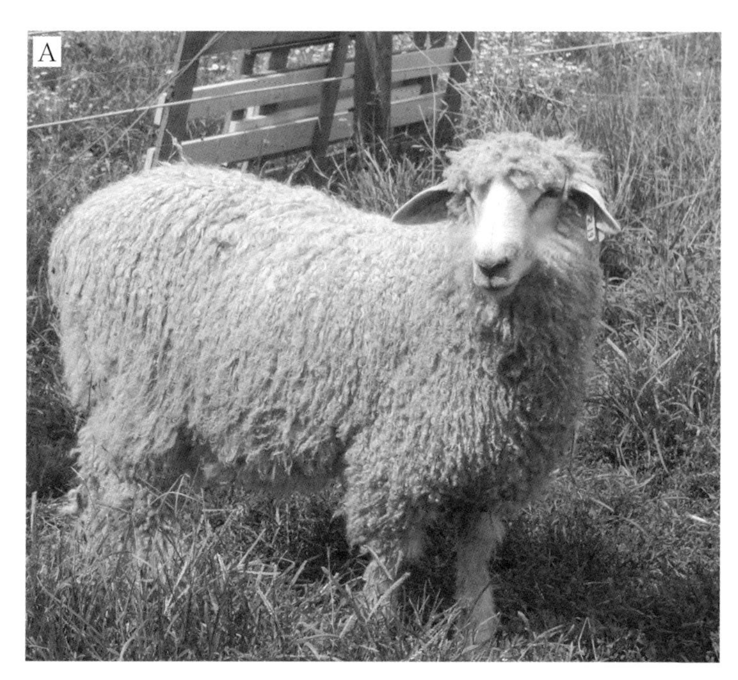

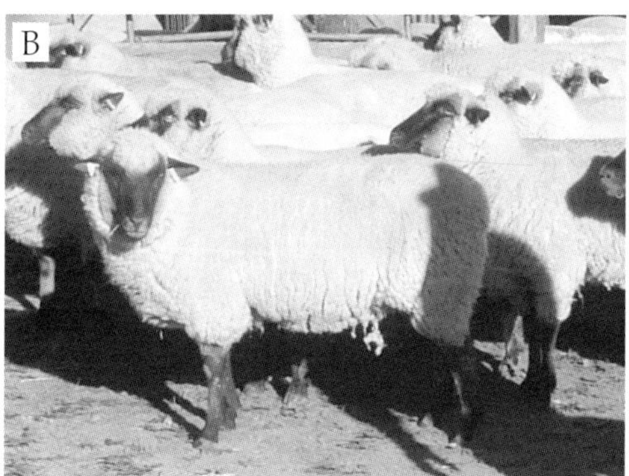

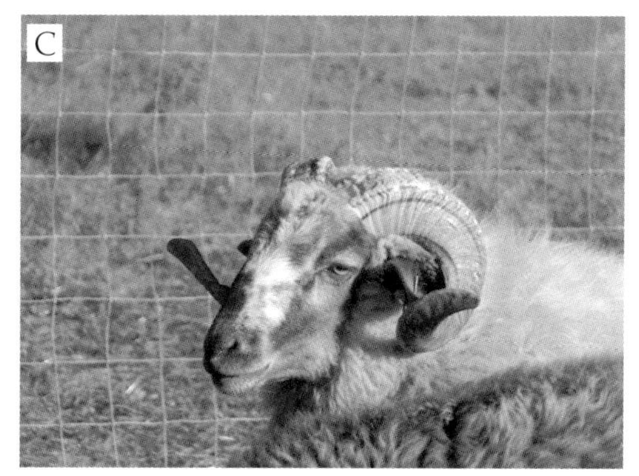

Figure 2.2 Selection decisions of human owners, made over centuries of animal use, result in very different breed packages that are tailored for production in specific environments. These differences are easily seen in breeds today. Lincoln (A), Shropshire (B), and Navajo-Churro (C) sheep each reveal their past interactions with human decisions, as well as the different environments in which these sheep have lived. Photo A by JB, B and C by DPS.

2.2 *Classes of Breeds*

The large group of animal populations that satisfy the biological definition of breed (and some that do not) can be placed into a few major classes. Each general class has a different genetic history, and these differences have important consequences for effective maintenance and conservation. The five major classes of breeds are landraces, standardized breeds, modern "type" or "designer" breeds, industrial strains, and feral populations. Dogs and poultry have other compelling factors that are unique to those species and also need to be discussed. Each of these classifications reflects differences about the attitude of human caretakers toward breeds as genetic packages, and each has something to teach us about breeds, genetic packages, human endeavor, and the interaction between human management decisions and the genetic structure of animal populations.

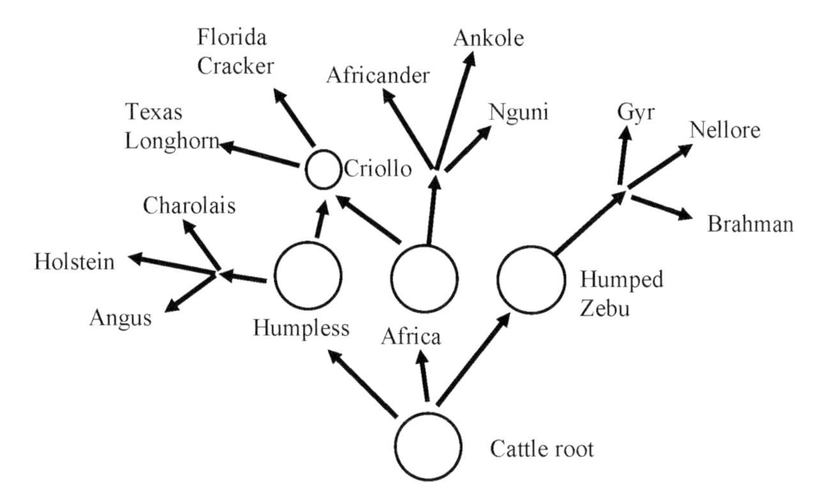

Figure 2.3 Cattle breeds branch out from an early root that divides and subdivides as the pathway goes through major groups of breeds down to individual breeds at the tips of the branches. Figure by DPS.

2.2.1 *Landraces*

Landrace breeds represent an early stage of breed development. "Landrace" is a general term that refers to populations of animals that are isolated to a local area where local production goals and the local physical environment drive selection. The "landrace" designation should not be confused with the specific Landrace swine breed, or with the Finnish Landrace sheep breed that is now known simply as Finnsheep. The landrace concept, as used here, is important as a general pattern for many breeds of all species. Landraces are sometimes called local breeds, natural breeds, or primitive breeds. Many landraces, despite the relative disorganization of their breeding or definition, are in fact highly selected and adapted genetic resources of great utility and importance.

Landraces derive their unique genetic character from the usual combination of foundation, isolation, natural selection, and human selection. The history of most landraces begins with the introduction of animals from some specific source into a specific geographic region with its unique climate, feed resources, topography, and human culture. The foundation of most landraces typically came from whatever animals were conveniently at hand, instead of a careful and comparative investigation into what sorts of foundation might serve best. In most cases this somewhat haphazard (but useful) foundation was followed by isolation from further introduction of genetic material. Most landraces subsequently faced survival pressures imposed by a challenging environment outside of the agricultural mainstream. Founding event, isolation, and natural environmental selection are the three most important factors that determine the overall type and function of landraces (Figure 2.4). All three are important, and all three must be considered when developing effective conservation programs for these unique and useful genetic resources. In contrast, human selection has generally been much less of a driving force in landrace development. Landraces occur in all species, but they are especially few in number in dogs. Those few therefore have great importance for wise conservation.

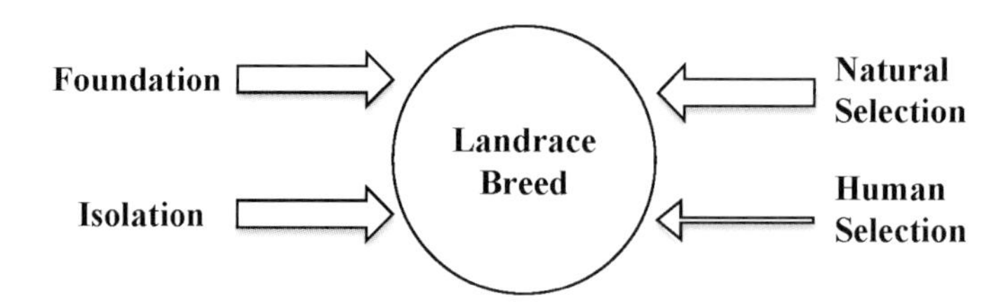

Figure 2.4 Landraces are influenced mostly by foundation, isolation, and natural selection, with human selection having less of an influence. Figure by DPS.

Landraces achieve their genetic consistency and uniqueness by default rather than by design, even though some level of human selection for production goals is typical of most landraces. The foundation of landraces as an accident of history rather than as a careful and deliberate process is especially well illustrated by the family of Criollo cattle breeds of the Americas (Figure 2.5).

Criollo cattle populations were founded by Iberian explorers from cattle brought to the New World from Spain, Portugal, and their Atlantic islands. These cattle were selected by virtue of convenience. They were the closest to the ports of departure in the late 1400s and early 1500s. To these were added cattle from the Canary and Azores Islands with their stronger African influence. Spaniards took fewer than 300 head of these cattle to the Americas, and the Portuguese probably a similar number. Once the cattle hit the Americas, the populations rose rapidly and expanded into a wide range of local environments. These few founder cattle provided the genetic basis for breeds as geographically far-flung as the Texas Longhorn, Florida Cracker, Pineywoods, Romosinuano of Colombia, Criollo of Argentina, and a multitude of breeds in between. All of these breeds are similar by virtue of their close relationship to the original few cattle, which is referred to as the "founder effect." The differences from breed to breed come from centuries of divergent selection, isolated from one another in diverse climates and topographies. The founder package, however, forever constrains the overall range of types that is possible in this important family of breeds. Even today, many individual cattle in nearly all Criollo breeds have such a similar appearance that they could easily be mistaken for cattle of other breeds within the Criollo group.

Following the founding of animal populations, isolation is important for the development of landraces as genetic resources. In contrast, lack of isolation allows for repeated introduction of new genetic variants, resulting in a population that never achieves the genetic consistency expected of a breed. Isolation for most landraces has been due to geographic factors. Relative lack of communication and transportation infrastructure have also been important in the establishment of the genetic isolation typical of many landraces.

The traditional isolation of landraces occurred much more by chance than by deliberate decision. It is increasingly risky to rely on this somewhat casual historic default to isolate landraces. The temptation to crossbreed landraces out of existence is generally more than can be resisted by the caretakers of these genetic resources. Crossbreeding can provide a quick, though temporary, financial return, and can frequently become the strategy for the

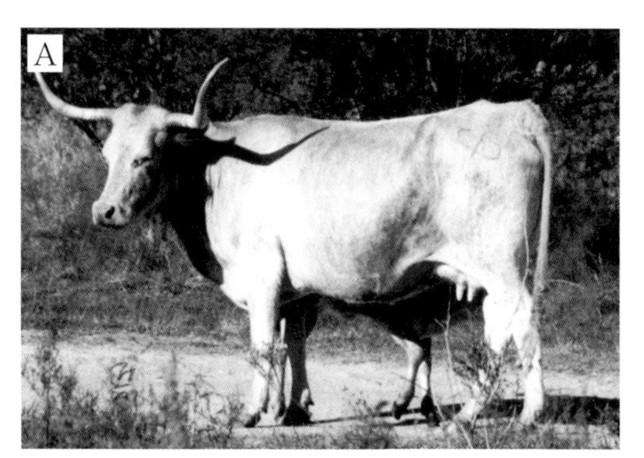

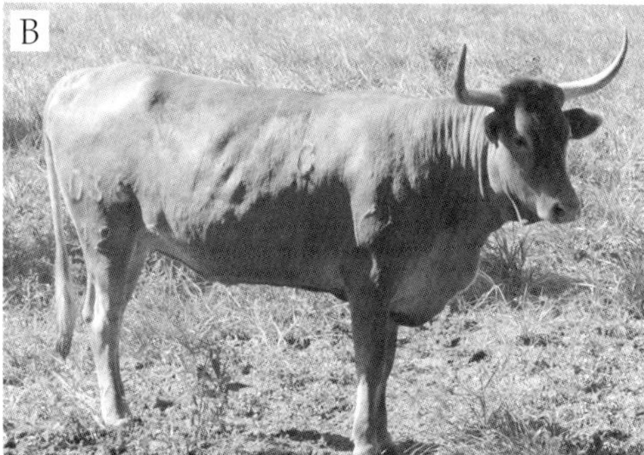

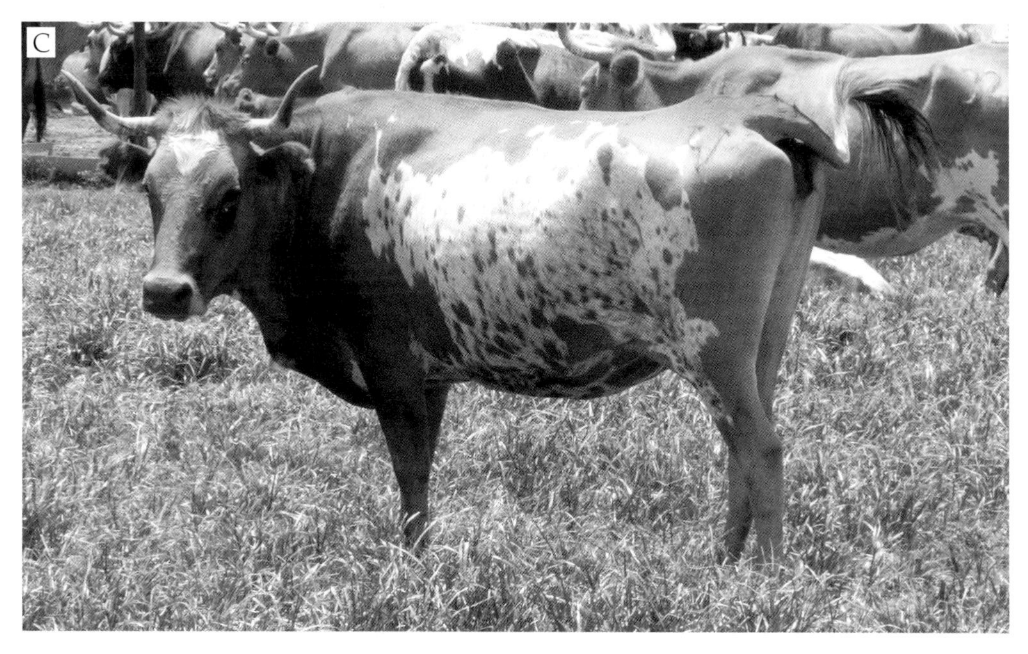

Figure 2.5 The Criollo family of breeds has similar characteristics throughout the Americas. Texas Longhorn (A), Colombian San Martinero (B), and Paraguayan Criollo Pilcomayo (C) cattle show obvious similarities due to their common foundation and despite their long geographic and historic separation. Photos by DPS.

best short-term outcome. Unfortunately, the long-term outcome of such crossbreeding is usually below the productive potential of the original uncrossed landrace. This is usually discovered too late and only after the original landrace is long gone.

Spanish goats demonstrate the complexity of landrace breeds (Figure 2.6). They developed from a foundation of goats brought to the Americas by early Spanish explorers. These goats have had over 400 years to adapt to an environment that is often challenging. This is especially true in the humid Southeast where parasites are a major threat. Newly imported breeds, such as Boer and Kiko, have had much less exposure to this specific environment, and less time to adapt to it. While the larger imported goats may offer short-term profits, the long-term sustainability of goat production favors the local landrace. Local

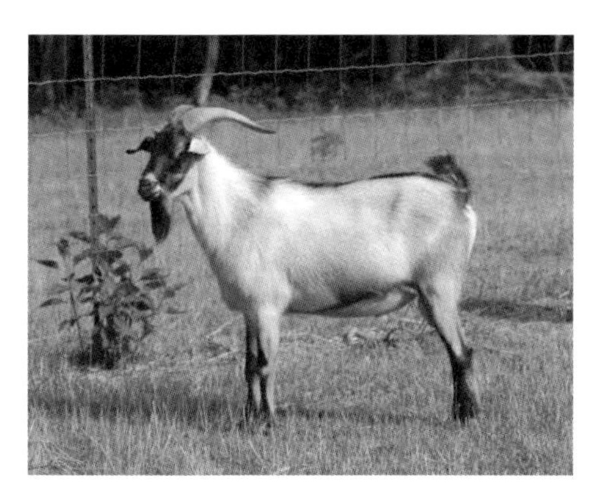

Figure 2.6 Spanish goats in the USA remain true to their landrace roots and also remain well adapted to extensive production conditions. Photo by DPS.

goats typically reproduce over a long lifespan. They also thrive in systems with less input and care when compared to latecomers.

The very cultural setting that once provided for the development and maintenance of landraces is now itself largely gone and can no longer foster the animal genetic resources that it spawned. The biggest hurdle to overcome with landrace conservation is the fact that the cultural and physical space in which they developed has changed dramatically over the last several decades. Isolation that protected them has diminished so that it no longer ensures protection. As long as cultural, geographic, and infrastructural barriers isolated landraces, they were safe in their original habitat and for their original purposes. Homogenization of culture both nationally and internationally has rapidly increased over the last few decades, eroding the unique and peripheral cultural pockets in which landraces long persisted. Conservation must therefore result from carefully crafted intentional efforts rather than from the more casual default of isolation that can no longer be realistically achieved. With decreasing isolation, the uniqueness of many landraces is diminishing, resulting in the loss of many highly adapted and potentially useful genetic packages. Isolation is essential for landraces, as they will otherwise fail to be genetically uniform to the extent necessary for them to serve as useful genetic resources. In addition, some landrace populations have been resettled in new cultural and environmental habitats where historic selection pressures differ from those in their original ranges. Relying on this modified agricultural environment to save landraces is to assure their extinction.

Another large challenge in landrace conservation is that most landraces lack tightly organized breeder organizations. Lack of organization works very well when isolation of the landrace is assured. However, as infrastructure improves and landraces are threatened by outside forces, any non-deliberate isolation fails to function well. At that point, more formal strategies for isolation and organization of landraces must be developed if these genetic resources are to survive.

Examples of radically changed environments include those for both Pineywoods and Texas Longhorn cattle. Both breeds were originally landraces that thrived in vast open-range systems. As society and expectations changed, land became subdivided by fences, and more deliberate mating choices were made. Breed type and breed expectations changed along with irreversible changes in the management and physical environment for both breeds.

The Texas Longhorn went from a wide-ranging adapted animal in extensive systems to one that was more likely to be cared for in a small, carefully tended herd. The selection pressures focused more on looks than on survival. As a result, cattle in the breed became larger, more smoothly conformed, and more dramatically colored than was typical of the cattle in the 1800s when the breed had its widest distribution. Important exceptions to the general rule exist, but the general character of the Texas Longhorn breed has changed much since the 1800s. Conservation-minded breeders are trying to counter this trend by once again emphasizing the original characteristics of the landrace breed.

Pineywoods cattle are at a much earlier stage of modification than Texas Longhorns, due in part to the persistence of the open range for much longer in the Deep South than in Texas. The Pineywoods cattle breeders are much more aware of the potential threat of breed uniformity and loss of variation in the breed, and are likely to succeed in conserving this breed in a form identical to the one that has persisted for centuries. Pineywoods cattle do face drastic changes in the selection environment, as the originally important use for ox production has shifted to one favoring beef production. These changes are nearly unavoidable, but understanding that they do exist can help to conserve the original landrace more effectively.

Tight definition and rigid genetic isolation of landraces also bring with them certain risks. When landraces are consolidated and defined in order to assure conservation, their cultural space quickly changes character away from their original status as local resources that are taken for granted. The transition from peripheral resource to defined resource usually involves taking the animals from a true landrace subsistence system to a more standardized breed in an increasingly production-oriented system. The subtle change in philosophy is not insignificant, for it brings with it the risk that the landrace will become more uniform and more standardized with a loss of rare genetic variants as it makes the transition. Production can replace adaptation as a major goal. This shift in selection pressure can have significant genetic repercussions because adaptation is needed for low maintenance requirements and high survivability.

Landrace conservation has many inherent challenges, not least of which is the very choice of which specific individuals should be included in any landrace during the early phases of conservation. Deciding on where to draw the boundaries around a landrace is not an easy task. Landraces are by their very nature more variable than other classes of breeds. Landraces are characterized by a consistency of biological and adaptation traits, but much less so by uniformity of physical appearance. This superficial variability can lead many observers to dismiss landraces as trivial and unimportant when the reality is just the opposite. They are historically and biologically important genetic resources that are adapted to difficult environments. They are generally productive with few inputs. They excel in survival and adaptation, although generally with less emphasis on high individual levels of production than is typical of the other classes of breeds.

On an international level, the landraces owned by pastoralists highlight and accent many of the problems inherent in landrace definition and conservation. Pastoralists have a single main goal – survival – which largely depends on the survival of their herds. While some pastoral systems may appear to be minimally productive to outside eyes, they are in fact highly organized and tightly and wisely managed in order to minimize the chances of failure. Pastoralist animal populations (breeds) tend to be variable. In many systems, the owners tend to introduce outside animals a bit more frequently than might be considered reasonable to a hard-core breed conservationist. However, just under the surface of what can look chaotic is a system that is carefully preserving genomes that remain productive and that survive in the pastoral system. The introductions are few and the crossbreeding is careful. Crossbreds are carefully tracked to document whether they are in fact superior to what came before in the original landrace. The majority of animals are kept in the original form as a wise insurance policy. Pastoralist herds very much serve as a genetic resource, and one where the most predictable and important trait is survival. To this core is added a certain level of constant and ongoing experimentation, somewhat at the edges, to see if other combinations also might have advantages. The result is a conservative approach at the core with a fascinating peripheral experimental approach at the edges of the population.

2.2.2 *Standardized Breeds*

Standardized breeds are the usual populations that come to mind when the word "breed" is used. Standardized breeds are populations of animals that are enrolled into a herd book, flock book, or stud book. These terms are often used for different species, and in this book "herd book" will be used to cover all three. Standardized breeds are, specifically, mated to conform to a written standard that is usually called a breed standard or a standard of perfection. The standard describes the ideal physical, and in some cases behavioral, type of the breed. The existence of the standard is what gives this group of breeds its name. As a general rule, foundation, isolation, and human selection are the main defining forces that shape standardized breeds. Natural selection is usually much less important (Figure 2.7).

Nearly all standardized breeds descend from earlier landrace populations. Exceptions are those breeds that were developed from new and deliberate combinations of previously standardized breeds. For example, the Columbia sheep breed derived from the Lincoln and Rambouillet breeds, while the Romeldale was formed by blending Rambouillet ewes with highly selected New Zealand Romney rams (Figure 2.8).

The trend toward standardized breeds began once human communication and transportation reached a certain level. The time frame for this development varied from region to region. Improved infrastructure facilitated breeders in getting together to decide on certain parameters that were important to them as they imagined their breed. This

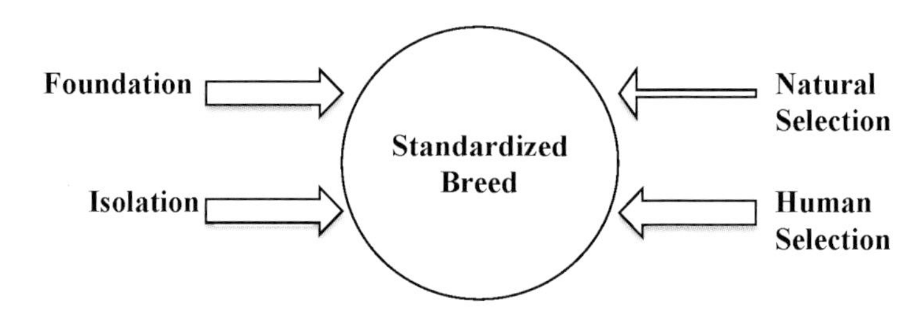

Figure 2.7 Standardized breeds are influenced mostly by foundation, isolation, and human selection, with natural selection having a much less important role. Figure by DPS.

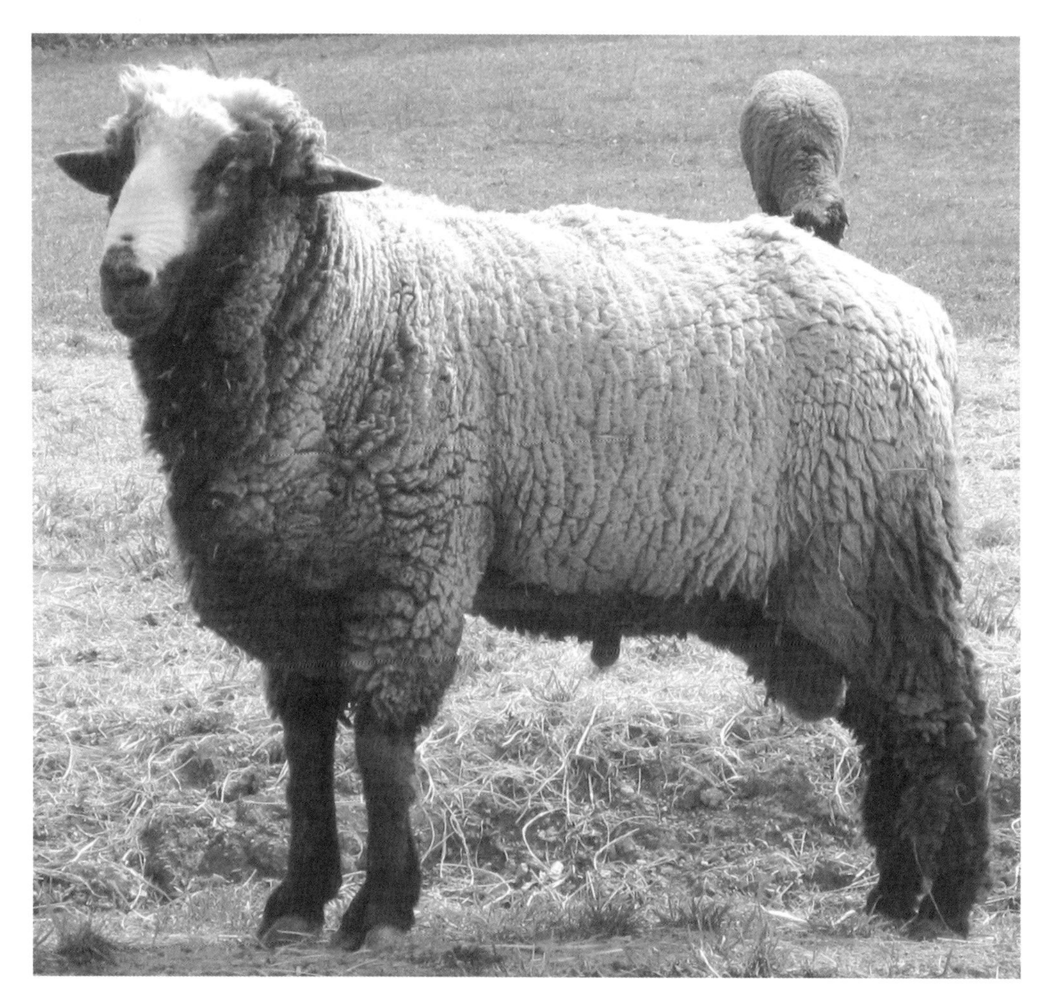

Figure 2.8 The Romeldale breed is a standardized breed derived from a careful blend of Romney and Rambouillet ancestors that were then selected for specific production goals.
Photo by Marie Minnich, Marushka Farm.

process defined what to include and what to exclude in a standardized breed. Eventually, in most standardized breeds, breeders decide to "close" the population, which refers to a rule that only offspring of approved parents (generally those that are themselves registered) can be registered within the breed and accepted as purebred.

As the boundary is drawn around a standardized breed, certain traits can easily be left out. The result is that most standardized breeds have greater physical uniformity than most landraces. Some of this uniformity is relatively trivial, such as horned versus polled, or coat color. As an example, Welsh cattle in the 1800s were a variable landrace group of adapted cattle. As breeders organized and began to define the cattle as a standardized breed, black, which was the most common color, became the only acceptable color. The few red, dun, roan, belted, linebacked, or white individuals nearly drifted to extinction because they were considered outside of the standard breed definition. These and other variants might well have served important functions of adaptation or production but are now lost to the standardized Welsh Black cattle breed. The other colors have been saved only recently after the breeders of these other colors organized a group to save the "Ancient Cattle of Wales." The key concept is that as a breed moves from landrace to standardized status, genetic variation is lost. Effective conservation of both landraces and standardized breeds depends on the recognition of the relative level of variation and the overall philosophy of breed character that each general class of breed brings with it.

Criollo cattle breeds in the Americas reveal that it is almost inevitable to eliminate variation in external traits such as color and horns as landraces become standardized. Many Criollo breeds remain wonderfully polychromatic, reflecting the variation of the original founders centuries ago. Among these are the Texas Longhorn, Florida Cracker, Criollos of Mexico, and Criollo Uruguayo. In contrast, the Criollo Lechero is nearly all uniformly tan, Romosinuano is red and polled, Barroso Salmeco is dun, and Blanco Orejinegro is white with black points. The Criollo Argentino is at an earlier stage of standardization, with increasing frequency of solid-colored, polled cattle at the expense of other colors and cattle with horns.

The breeder associations of many Criollo cattle breeds deliberately restrict external traits such as color and horns (Criollo Lechero, Romosinuano, Barroso Salmeco, Blanco Orejinegro). Even in the absence of such a breed-wide trend, individual breeders often reduce external variability. Traditional Pineywoods cattle breeders tended to each favor a specific color, so that Holt cattle tended to be black and white, Conways red and white, and Griffins a yellow dun. Some breeds simply drift toward lowered variability due to a more general breeder preference that is not imposed by any sorts of rules or regulations, as demonstrated by the Criollo Argentino slowly moving toward being a solid-colored polled breed. Once a breed gains a name and identity, many breeders cannot resist imposing an external uniformity. This follows the common thinking that breeds should be externally uniform, without which a group of animals is not really a breed.

The narrowing of external variation in standardized breeds is easy to see in the sheep-herding dog breeds of the United Kingdom (UK). Working collies long remained a landrace, defined more by behavior than any other trait. They varied in nearly every external characteristic. Haircoats were short, rough, or wirehaired. Colors included black, brown, sable, black and tan, merle, spotted, and nearly white. Some had long tails, some had short tails. The various modern breeds within this group occupy very different spots along the continuum from variable landrace to tightly standardized breed. Border Collies are currently at an early stage of standardization. Most are black and white with moderately feathered coats, but other variants are accepted and still occur, if rarely. Most other breeds in this group went down the path of standardized breeds and focused on a limited array of the original variation. Show Collies lost the brown and solid black colors and the wirehaired coat, leaving only sable, tricolor, and merle, with rough coat and smooth coat varieties. Bearded Collies lost the short hair and rough hair variants, as well as the sable, black and tan, and merle colors, so that now they are all "bearded" long-coated wirehairs in black or brown (Figure 2.9). Few if any breeds now sport the entire range of characteristics found in earlier landrace sheepherding dogs, each descendant breed having been selected for relative uniformity based on a handful of the numerous original options.

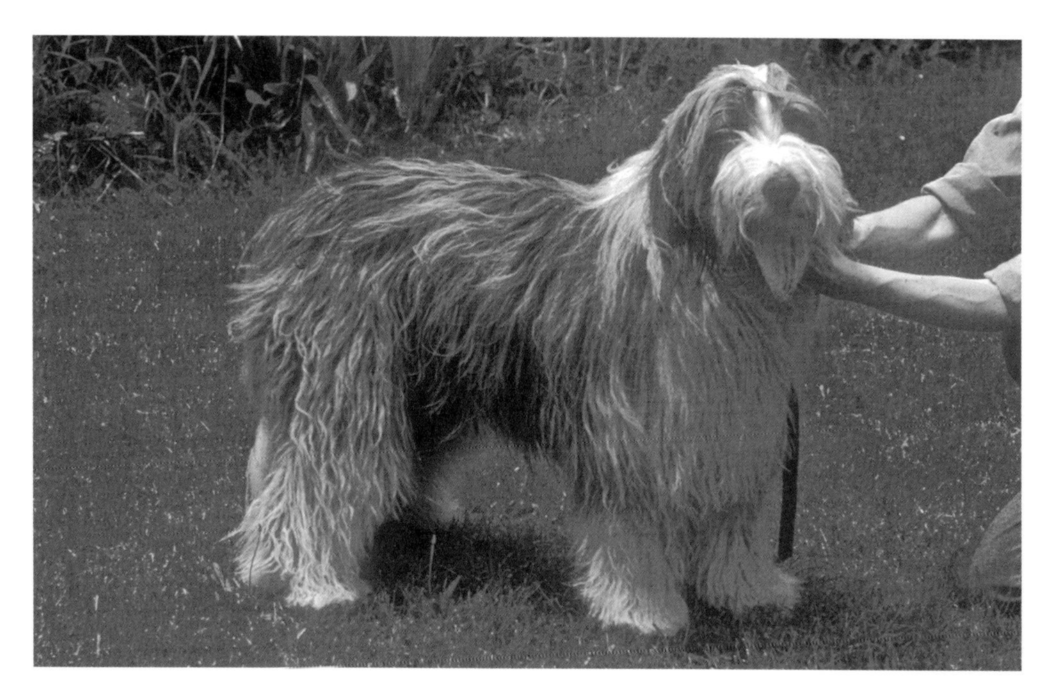

Figure 2.9 Bearded Collie dogs only show a few of the characteristics that were present in earlier landrace working collies. Photo by DPS.

Many standardized breeds are internationally important, and standardization is the basic population management strategy that typifies most international breeds. Standardized breeds are genetically isolated by design. This contrasts to landraces, which can be viewed as genetically isolated more by default, due to their geographically remote settings (at least historically). The Angus cattle breed, for example, is regenerated by matings of parents that are registered. As a result, Angus cattle from whatever country (USA, Scotland, South Africa, Australia, Argentina) are at least potentially part of the same gene pool. The artificial constraint on matings within the breed allows standardized breeds to function as a single gene pool regardless of how geographically separated the individuals of the breed may be.

Some standardized breeds do not have a completely closed population, which can lead some observers to conclude that these are not true genetic breeds (Figure 2.10). In many situations, however, these still do qualify as genetically defined breeds. Quarter Horses, for example, can descend from registered Quarter Horses as well as from crosses with registered Thoroughbreds under specific circumstances. The herd book is "open," but only in one direction, which preserves the ultimate character of the Quarter Horse reasonably well. Likewise, the Paint breed allows parents to be Paint, Quarter Horse, or Thoroughbred, and the Appaloosa breed allows parents to be Appaloosa, Quarter Horse, Thoroughbred, or occasionally Arabian. The end result of these practices is that such breeds are less rigidly defined than those with completely closed herd books. They are generally consistent enough to be reasonably predictable and therefore do indeed qualify as genetically based breeds. Finally, because they all dip into largely the same pool of genetics, they can easily be considered to be a family of breeds of Western Stock Horse type. And, equally importantly,

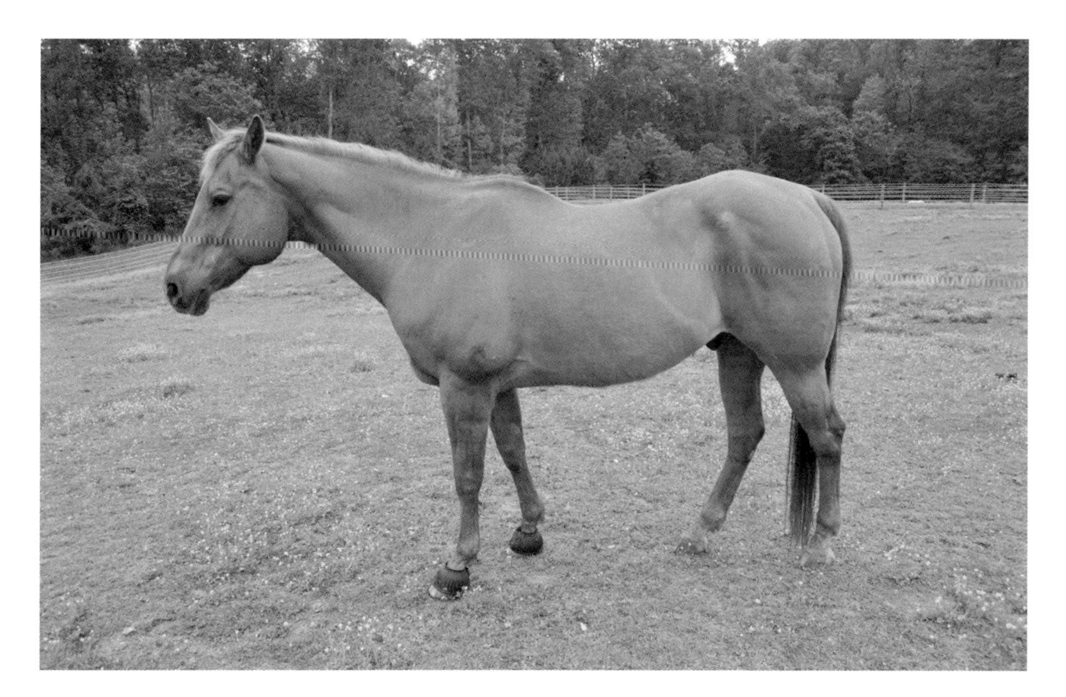

Figure 2.10 Quarter Horses remain a true genetic breed despite continuing to receive occasional outside influences from Thoroughbreds. Photo by JB.

within most of these breeds is a dedicated core of breeders working solely with "foundation" bloodlines. These bloodlines tend to be free from outside breeding, and can be among the most genetically distinctive animals of the breed.

Tightly closed standardized breeds are typical of most species, including cattle, dogs, sheep, and most others. These breeds insist on limiting registration to animals that have two registered parents. The result is that the breed is indeed closed genetically, so that nothing can be introduced except by fraud. This protects the integrity of the breed's genetic package, although it can also be damaging if the package becomes too narrowly constrained such that viability and overall vigor begin to suffer. The negative consequences of rigid closure are beginning to manifest themselves in some horse, cattle, and dog breeds, and the future of the strategy of absolute closure of standardized breeds is now more open to debate than it has been for the last century. Standardized breeds are a relatively recent development. The idea of standardized breeds is only about 200 years old, as contrasted to the backdrop of 10,000 years of agriculture. Strategies for the long-term genetic management of standardized breeds may not yet be fully developed or understood.

2.2.3 Modern "Type" and "Designer" Breeds

In addition to landrace and standardized breeds is a category that is more open than is true of genetically based breeds. These include many of the Warmblood horse breeds, the Pinto horse, and a few other breeds in a number of species. In these "type" breeds, breed character is based more on external type or performance than it is on genetic continuity with any specific and defined breeding population. The result is some very useful animal

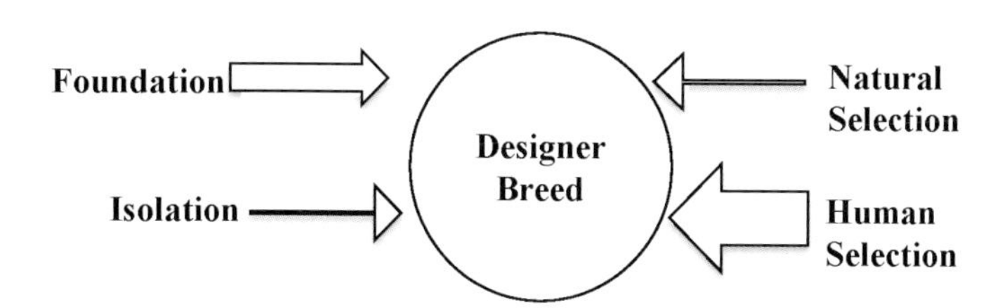

Figure 2.11 Type and designer breeds are greatly influenced by human selection, with less influence from foundation and minimal effect from natural selection or isolation. Figure by DPS.

populations that have only limited genetic consistency and therefore limited predictability in reproducing a specific type. These breeds can be productive, but serve very little utility as genetic resources. They are therefore outside the realm of genetic resource conservation. "Type" and "designer" breeds are minimally influenced by isolation or natural selection, with human selection of founding animals being the main sources of any uniformity. This is illustrated in Figure 2.11.

Breeding practices further confound the neat inclusion of many Warmblood horse breeds into the overall class of modern type breeds. Within many of these breeds is a core of horses that are indeed "purebred" in the narrow genetic sense of having ancestors only of that breed. While these are a small minority in most Warmblood breeds, they reflect the conservatism of traditional breeders and their allegiance to local types and breeding. This core within each of several internationally popular Warmblood breeds conserves the unique portion of what is becoming an increasingly homogenized group of breed resources. Unfortunately, this core and the more numerous outbred portions of the breed usually are labeled as the same breed, so an accurate appreciation of the breed's status can be nearly impossible to ascertain without detailed and prolonged study. This pattern is repeated throughout a few other species, most notably several poultry breeds.

Perhaps the most common examples of breeds in this group are the newer "designer" dog breeds. These usually begin as a cross between two established standardized breeds, and then are further maintained by including ongoing first-generation crosses as well as the results of mating these crosses to one another. "Labradoodles" from a combination of Labrador Retrievers and Poodles are one example. Development of these breeds is usually driven by an attempt to capture a specific phenotype of coat, color, and temperament based on blends of the original breeds. A problem in predictability arises as the generations proceed. The initial crossbred generation is quite uniform, but the generation they produce is highly variable and many off-types can be expected in the progeny well into the future. For that reason they fall outside of the usual definition of breeds as repeatable and predictable genetic packages.

2.2.4 *Industrial Strains*

Industrial strains are usually not characterized as breeds. In most cases these animal populations are very tightly selected lines within a breed, or are stabilized hybrids that descend from initial crosses of a few breeds. The result has been exquisitely productive animals that are highly selected for specific production niches that require high levels of

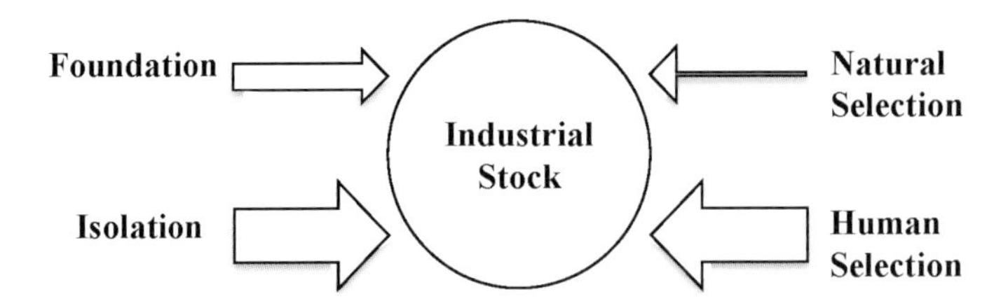

Figure 2.12 Industrial strains result from intense human selection and genetic isolation. Figure by DPS.

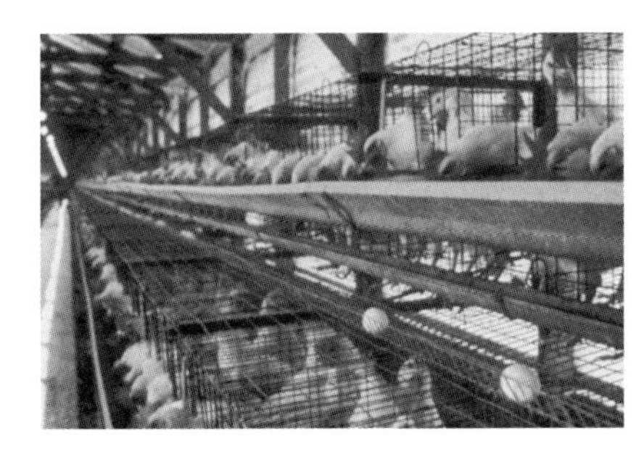

Figure 2.13 Commercial hybrid chickens are exquisitely productive, and are the result of careful and tightly controlled corporate breeding programs. Photo courtesy of Hy-line International.

nutritional, environmental, and housing support. The influences shaping industrial strains are illustrated in Figure 2.12. Industrial strains are scientifically selected, mated, and documented. Industrial strains are successful because they are indeed productive.

Industrial strains are not documented in herd books because they are owned and managed by multinational corporations and are available only through corporate sources. Individual private breeders are not involved, so the documentation of registrations and the like has become superfluous because the seed stock never changes hands. Most broiler and egg-laying chickens, turkeys, and industrial swine are now industrial strains rather than standardized breeds (Figure 2.13). Dairy cattle could also be considered in this class, although these are more widely held and are still reproduced by private individuals. Within dairy cattle breeding, the role of the semen companies serves as a bottleneck through which genetic variation is managed and largely minimized. For dairy cattle breeding, these companies play the role that the multinational corporations have for other industrialized species. The practical result of semen company influence has been a trend toward increasing relatedness among most cattle of any of the dairy breeds. In addition, like other businesses, the companies that control industrial strains tend to merge from time to time. This consolidates the control and marketing of genetic material into fewer and fewer hands.

The control of industrial strains (especially poultry and swine) by large corporations assures that small private breeders have no role to play in their breeding or conservation. They are interesting populations because genetic variability is low and predictability high. Industrial strains can and do become endangered or extinct through corporate decisions, usually after mergers between multinational corporations. Very little, if anything, can be realistically accomplished to reverse that trend, as private breeders simply do not have the resources nor the infrastructure necessary to duplicate the industrial selection environment that maintains these strains.

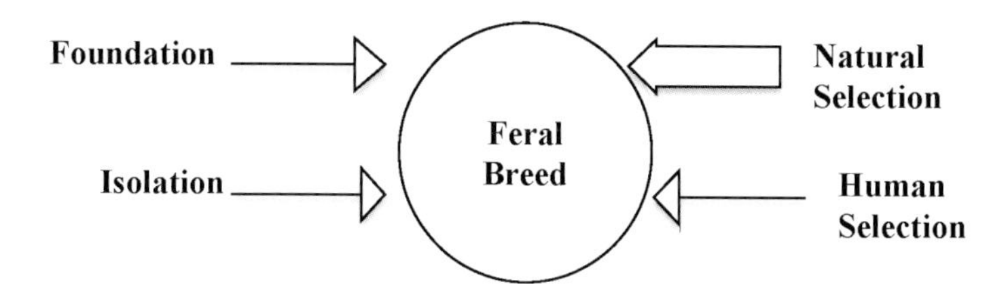

Figure 2.14 Feral populations vary greatly in foundation and isolation, but all have high levels of natural selection along with an absence of human selection. Figure by DPS.

2.2.5 *Feral Populations*

Feral animals are domesticated animals that have escaped domesticated settings and have returned to a free-living state (Figure 2.14). It is a peculiar fact of biology that the truly wild external type and wild genetic components are never fully regained by feral populations, even though some feral animals do indeed approach the wild ancestral type of the species. In some sense "domestication is forever," leaving its imprint even on these animals that have escaped human control.

Feral animals are interesting due to their being returned to a selection environment where nature, rather than humans, decides which ones reproduce and which ones succumb. Distinctive feral populations usually arise from a few founders that then experience isolation for long periods of survival under natural selection. Such populations have much in common with landraces, although nature rather than humans imposes all selection. In contrast to these more distinctive feral populations, most of the modern feral populations have broad genetic variation due to the constant infusion of new recruits from a wide variety of genetic sources. These are therefore unimportant as genetic resources or as targets of conservation.

Only a few feral populations qualify as genetically distinct breeds with limited variability. The few that do qualify are indeed fascinating for their adaptation and survival traits. Examples of these occur for all species: Colonial Spanish horses (specifically Spanish Mustangs), island or isolated populations of goats and sheep (Figure 2.15), Carolina Dogs and dingoes, and swine from a constrained (generally Iberian) origin.

Conservation of genetically distinct feral livestock populations that qualify as breeds is problematic. Most of the populations of conservation interest come from relatively isolated regions. This especially includes islands. On many islands, the feral livestock endanger native flora and fauna, and the usual decision is to favor conservation of the natural resource rather than the introduced one. Conservation of the lineage of feral animals can be accomplished outside of the original environment, but brings with it the very real conundrum that the selection environment is changed from the original, and the genetic result is different than would have been the case in the original feral state, even though the population is based on the same genetic foundation.

Some breeds straddle the boundary between feral and landrace (Figure 2.16). These breeds are raised on extensive ranges with minimal human management. An example of such a practice was used with the Choctaw hog, with the hogs roaming free with minimal intervention. Hogs were occasionally captured for sale, in addition to small numbers kept

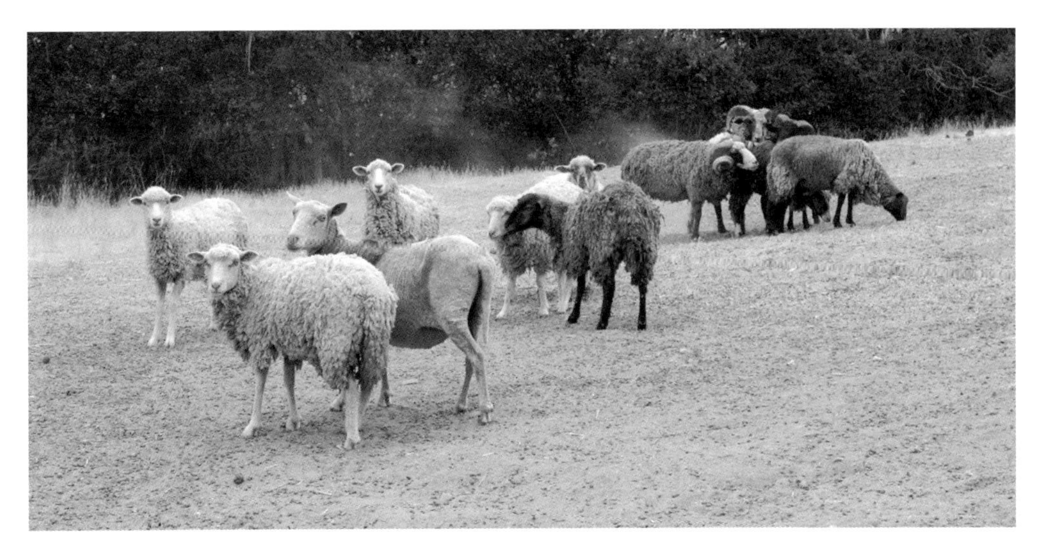

Figure 2.15 The island home of feral Santa Cruz sheep shaped this breed much more than any human influence. Conserving the uniqueness of the island required removal of the sheep, which are fortunately still maintained by private breeders off the island. Photo by JB.

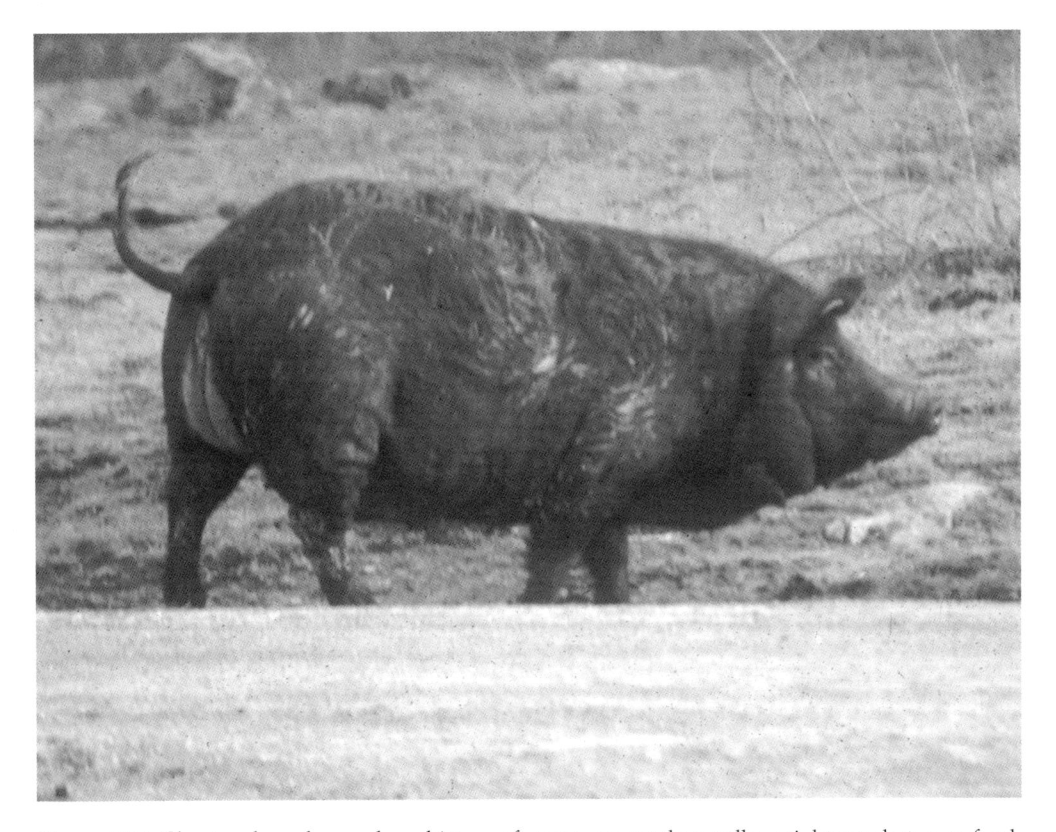

Figure 2.16 Choctaw hogs have a long history of management that walks a tightrope between feral, free-ranging animals, and those more closely managed as homestead hogs. Photo by DPS.

closer to home and managed more closely than their essentially feral brethren. The issue of genetic isolation of such populations has increased in importance as more and more opportunities arise for the introduction of outside genetics for a variety of purposes. For example, the desire for wilder hogs for hunting led to the introduction of wild boar stock into several feral hog populations. Similarly, the late 1800s and early 1900s witnessed the release of coach and other large saddle horse stallions onto the ranges of many feral Colonial Spanish horse populations in the West in order to produce mounts deemed more appropriate for cavalry and other uses. Hawaiian feral sheep populations have had recent introductions of Mouflons for trophy hunting. A close evaluation of candidate feral populations assures that conservation can designate those with a history of isolation as being the most important genetic resources to target.

2.2.6 *Dog Breeds*

Dog breeds deserve special consideration because they have tended to go down a slightly different path than other species. Dogs in Europe went through a process of standardization that quickly left landraces or local breeds behind. These European breeds then spread out over the globe during the era of colonization, so that most of the world's dogs (even mutts!) descend from a standardized, generally European base. The pattern of standardization is so strong in dog breeding that even when landrace breeds from across the world have been imported into Europe, or more recently North America, they have been quickly transformed into standardized breeds. "Gentrification" describes this process of removing a breed from its original setting, maintaining the gene pool intact, but selecting it for different end goals than those that were operating in its original location.

Exceptions do occur, and these allow for the earlier landrace stages of breed development to persist in a few areas. Among these are village dogs, especially from remote areas. Central Africa still boasts the Basenji, and other regional types occur in Africa and elsewhere. Notable examples are Bali, and village dogs in India. No doubt other African and Asian sites still have dogs that pre-date any influence of standardized dogs. Finding such dogs in the Americas has lagged behind the search elsewhere, but these are likely to persist in at least some remote corners. This is especially true of hairless breeds, such as the Xoloitzcuintle and some Peruvian dogs.

In some cases, the local breed persists along with a more gentrified international product. This is true of the Basenji, where the international standardized breed still does occasionally incorporate dogs from the more original landrace setting. As dogs bridge that gap, differences arising from these two underlying philosophies of breeding and breed management can be noted. Past additions of landrace dogs have included at least a few with light yellow eyes, but the standard for the registered Basenji breed favors dark brown eyes. This may seem a trivial difference, but resulted in at least one imported dog being used only minimally for breeding due to falling outside the ideal standard adopted by breeders outside of its Congo homeland.

Feral dogs vary in origin, and this depends on local history. Some are long-term ferals that descend from the earliest domesticated dogs. Included in this group are dingoes, New Guinea Singing Dogs, and Carolina Dogs. Most other modern feral dogs are descended from more recently escaped and randomly mixed standardized breeds. The similar external appearance of the short-term ferals and the long-term ferals does not accurately reveal the underlying genetic differences. Feral dogs rapidly revert to a tan, shorthaired, prick-eared dog with a curled tail. This tends to happen regardless of the original dogs in the mix.

2.2.7 *Poultry Breeds*

Poultry breeds run the gamut of breed types, although standardized breeds predominate and ferals are rare. The general trend for poultry is that the breeds are defined by size and shape, while differences in feather color, feather type, and comb type are used to distinguish varieties within breeds. A few true landraces persist (Icelandic chickens, Cotton Patch geese), and several of the standardized poultry breeds have very old roots in landraces. Most standardized breeds are more recent composites that vary widely in foundation from breed to breed.

Many poultry breeds contain very distinct groups of birds all under the same breed name. Some flocks of birds within most breeds have a long heritage of distinct foundation and isolation, and would be considered genetic breeds by any definition. Others, unfortunately identified under the same breed name, have been crossbred rather recently, while still being exposed to selection to assure that the external phenotype resembles the one that is desired for the breed. Sorting through the details of the exact genetic situation within breeds, varieties, and flocks requires great attention to history and the breeder personalities involved in each setting. The relationships between the various sorts of flocks can be quite complex and tricky to sort through. The varying sorts of genetic populations often are identified by a single breed name, and have a similar enough external phenotype to be nearly indistinguishable by superficial inspection.

While poultry breeds can be confusing, it remains true that the more unique phenotypes do tend to betray unique underlying genotypes. For example, the huge, feather-footed Brahmas and Cochins are indeed genetically distinct from most other breeds. In poultry, the general rule is that the more unique phenotypes cannot experience much introgression from outside the breed without losing their unique appearance. This serves to enforce a degree of genetic isolation on those breeds. In contrast, many breeds are fairly similar in size, shape, and even color. Those breeds are more susceptible to occasional outcrosses by some breeders, even though each breed and variety also has breeders dedicated to the pure genetic resource (Figure 2.17).

2.2.8 *Summary*

The various classes of breeds have profoundly different histories. This is due to the specific combination of founder effect, relative level of genetic isolation, intensity of human selection, and physical environment in which they function. As a general rule, landraces are more genetically variable than standardized breeds, although there are some exceptions. Industrial strains are the least variable of all, but it is important to note that genetic variability and predictability have an inverse relationship. The low variability of industrial strains translates to exquisite predictability. Feral populations include some that are highly variable, and others that are among the most genetically homogeneous of any breed populations. The final result depends on their history of isolation. The modern type-based and designer

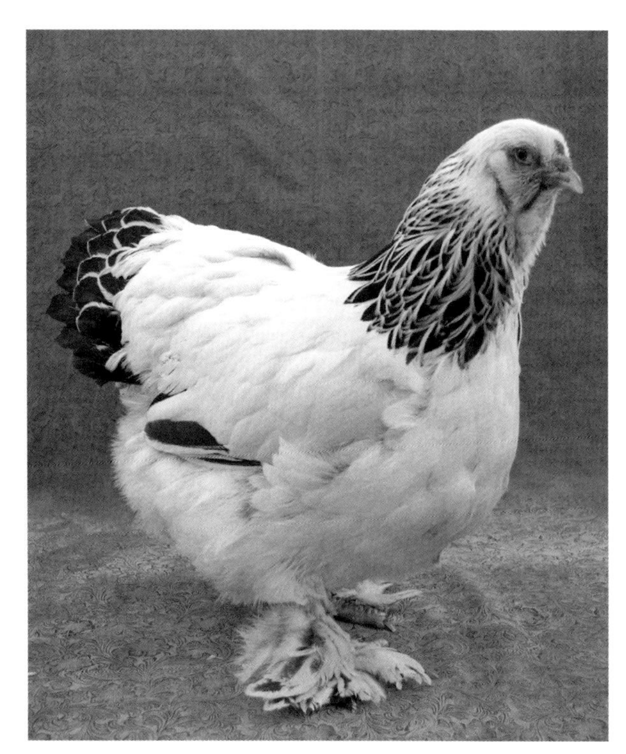

Figure 2.17 Chicken breeds are notoriously difficult to pin down as to the exact degree of genetic isolation used in their maintenance. The genetic package of the more distinctive breeds, such as Brahmas, are protected because their phenotype is easily disrupted by any outcrosses. Photo by JB.

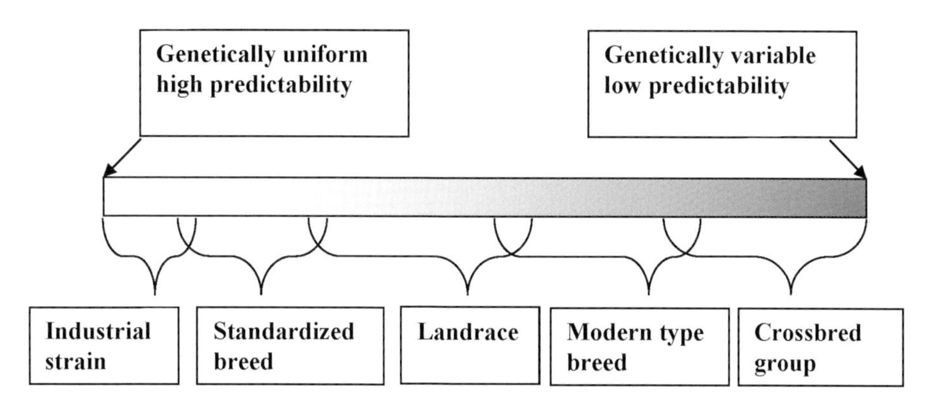

Figure 2.18 Classes of breeds vary in their relative level of genetic uniformity. Figure by DPS.

breeds are usually fairly variable genetically. It is important to understand the relative level of genetic variability of these different classes of breeds, as well as the historical and cultural reasons behind their levels of variation (Figure 2.18). Appreciating the genetic and cultural background of breeds is essential if organizational and breeding strategies are to be successful in conserving them. This book is mostly limited to the active management of standardized breeds and landraces. Private breeders have very little opportunity for action on feral populations or industrial stocks, and the modern type-based and designer breeds generally fall outside the tightest definition of a breed as a genetic resource.

2.3 How Breeds Are Lost

Beginning about 200 years ago, and accelerating dramatically in the last 100 years, the process of breed diversification has reversed, becoming one of increasingly rapid collapse of diversity. This, at least potentially, poses a real risk that future generations will inherit inadequate genetic variation in their livestock to meet their desires and needs.

Breeds are lost, and along with them their genetic diversity, through a wide range of mechanisms. Basically, rare breeds are rare for a reason, and the difficulty is that those reasons vary from breed to breed. At the base of all of these is a lack of production of purebred animals, but countering this challenge requires different strategies depending on the specific threat that is involved. Understanding the basic ways that purebred populations fail to be maintained from generation to generation can help in formulating effective strategies that assure breed survival.

One way that breeds become endangered or extinct is through changing goals for market products. When a breed no longer produces what is desired, then people simply abandon the breed for others. This sounds logical, until it is realized that the market is fickle, and the changes are not consistent over time in a specific set trajectory. For example, over a century ago, a major product from hogs was lard. People worked hard for long hours, and consuming animal fats was a good way to meet their energy needs. Eventually most people became more sedentary, obesity became a problem, and consuming fat was shunned as a way to manage lower caloric intake by humans. This trend is now reversing, as the essential and beneficial roles of fats in human diets are being validated. Fat hogs are seeing a resurgence in interest. What this means is that market demand, by itself, is a poor guarantor of breed security over long periods of time.

As demand changes, selection pressures change. In the example of lard-type hogs transforming to leaner hogs, most breeds changed to fit the demand simply by selecting leaner hogs from within the breed. Through this mechanism breeds stayed intact, at least in name. However, the hog under a specific breed name became very different. This is a subtle loss and has no easy answer because it becomes necessary to classify animals by type as well as by breed.

The issue of various types within a single breed is currently being played out in several sheep breeds and dog breeds. Within many sheep breeds are more traditional types, but also a type that is converging on a "modern show type" that places well in competitive shows. Both are identified by a single breed name, although the show type is not always a good choice for traditional sheep production systems. Show types have achieved such high demand that they bring great economic return to their owners, and this drives a great deal of selection toward that type. Dog breeds, especially working dog breeds, have experienced a similar divergence of a type. One type does well in conformation showing, and another type does well in field trials. In some examples the dogs can barely be recognized as being of a single breed, and the two types are generally maintained in complete genetic isolation one from the other. Beef cattle have also seen selection toward a type that is uniform across breeds, such that it can be difficult to discern breed differences by any signal other than color. And, in many examples, beef cattle have also become black instead of other original colors so that even that hint is now missing.

Introgression from other breeds is also a threat to breed integrity and survival. This is sometimes done fraudulently, but at other times it is done within the rules of the breed association and registry. Sanctioned introgression was used to quickly change the type and function of some cattle breeds, notably the Dairy Shorthorn, Guernsey, and Ayrshire. Within each of these, fortunately, many cattle still lack any introgression. Horse breeds have often used introgression as a strategy to quickly change breed type. The Morgan horse nearly lost its original type through introgression, although many breeders have rigorously maintained older, foundation bloodlines.

Some breeds, among them many Warmblood horse breeds, have combined introgression with selection to change an original heavier cart-horse type into a more modern sport-horse type that is in high demand. The combination of these two strategies has been powerful in driving changes of type and performance. Still, within most of these breeds, especially in Europe, a handful of older conservative breeders still mate their mares to local stallions that are free of introgression from other breeds or regions. In addition, they still select and retain foals of the original multi-use type.

Some breeds have been victims of their own success. These are the breeds that excel in crossbreeding. Especially when the females are in demand, they can be used for crossbred instead of purebred matings. Purebred recruitment can diminish below replacement levels. This pattern has been typical of many adapted breeds, including Criollo cattle breeds throughout the Americas, but also Spanish goats.

Narragansett Pacer horses simply vanished because large numbers of breeders no longer produced them in sufficient numbers to replace the population (Figure 2.19). In early

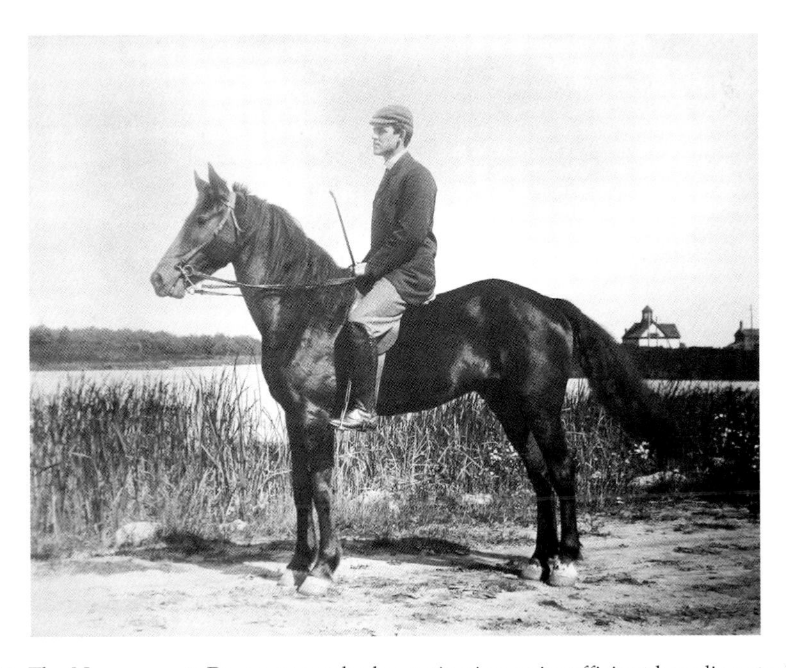

Figure 2.19 The Narragansett Pacer succumbed to extinction as insufficient breeding stock was retained to replace breeding animals lost to export, age, or disease. Ironically, the breed's popularity for crossbreeding was a major factor in its demise. Historic photo.

colonial New England, the Narragansett Pacer of Rhode Island was considered the finest riding animal due to its smooth but quick gait and its stamina. Riders could travel great distances over rough terrain in a shorter period of time on Narragansett Pacers than was possible on any other horse. As better-quality roads were built, the Pacer lost favor to more refined horses of the period. That was coupled with the export of large numbers of Pacers to the plantations of the Southern USA and Caribbean leading to the demise of the breed by the mid-1800s.

In all of these examples, the breed can be considered to be a victim of a loss of a niche to fill. This puts breed extinction in a similar frame as the extinction of wild species. Loss of a place to live and thrive leads to decline and eventual extinction. In the case of breeds, though, this niche is controlled by human action and human choice. This control can be fickle and is sometimes poorly informed or unwise. Because of that, decision-makers need to be clear-headed about long-term goals for the effective maintenance and management of genetic variation that might be needed in the future. Unfortunately, some of the choices that lead to future security may not seem all that logical today, so the safest route is to try to save as wide an array of breeds as possible.

CHAPTER 3

Breeds as Gene Pools: Variability and Predictability

Genetic variability and phenotypic predictability can be viewed as extreme endpoints along a single line. At one end are populations that are completely genetically uniform. These are very predictable, both for their own performance and for the characteristics of their offspring. At the other extreme are populations (almost always crossbred) that are extremely genetically variable and therefore unpredictable as to their own production characteristics, and the overall type and performance of their offspring. The point along this continuum at which populations are useful as predictable genetic packages (breeds) is closer to the genetically uniform end than it is to the genetically variable end. The specific point occupied by a breed along the continuum varies from breed to breed, and also varies broadly across the different general types of breeds.

Breeds serve as genetic resources because they have predictable combinations of genes throughout most of the individuals of that breed. Predictability is vitally important to the usefulness of breeds, and this implies a certain level of genetic consistency. Populations that are highly genetically variable are no longer predictable, which deprives them of the very essence of being a breed in the sense of serving as a genetic resource. Owners choose specific breeds because they are interested in a certain appearance, performance, and behavior. Predictability allows owners to be satisfied with their breed choice.

Tugging at the need for predictability is the need for breeds to be maintained as viable genetic pools in order to assure their continued vitality and vigor. This allows them to survive and serve as genetic resources. Viability requires some level of genetic variability because truly homogeneous populations are not self-sustaining due to declines in reproductive health and overall viability. Populations lose vigor and reproductive fitness if genetic variability becomes too low, which is called inbreeding depression. If breeds are to successfully function as viable populations, as well as genetic resources, they need to have enough variability to be healthy while at the same time having enough consistency to be predictable. Only by balancing these two somewhat opposing forces is it possible to assure that breeds can serve as viable genetic resources.

Breeds are structured along different genetic and population organizational patterns that have consequences for their management as genetic resources. The genetic organization of nearly every breed reflects its past history of management and selection. Fortunately, most of the breeds within either the standardized or landrace classes tend to share patterns, even though the patterns have important differences from one class of breeds to another. Understanding the manner in which a breed is organized genetically is essential if breed management and conservation are to be effective because this helps to find the right balance point between variability and uniformity.

3.1 Standardized Breeds

The most common organizational structure for standardized breeds is a tiered structure with a relatively small bottom tier on which rest larger upper tiers, as illustrated in Figure 3.1. The bottom, smallest portion is called the nucleus, or elite tier, and includes herds that contain the most highly sought animals in the breed. The entire breed rests upon this genetic base. Next up is a larger tier comprising multiplier herds, of somewhat more average quality but still typical representatives of the breed. The top and largest tier is the commercial segment, consisting of herds that are providing animals for final products instead of specifically for purebred breeding replacement.

The tiers within a standardized breed usually interact as a "closed nucleus" system (Figure 3.1). This refers to the general flow of genetic material within the breed. The nucleus tier herds generally produce their own replacements with no introductions from the other levels. This results in little or no gene flow into this portion of the breed from the rest of the breed, but with outflow of breeding animals and their genes from this group to the rest of the breed. The multiplier tier generally buys replacement stock (especially males) from the bottom elite tier, and also saves its own replacement stock, including a relatively few males and a large number of females. The commercial tier usually buys males from the multiplier tier or from the elite nucleus. The overall pattern is a flow of genetic material from the bottom to the top of the structure, but little to no downward flow to affect the base.

Closed nucleus organization is very typical of standardized modern production breeds such as the Angus cattle breed (Figure 3.2). This structure organizes the genetics of the breed to have a relatively small base in the elite herds that supports the larger structure of

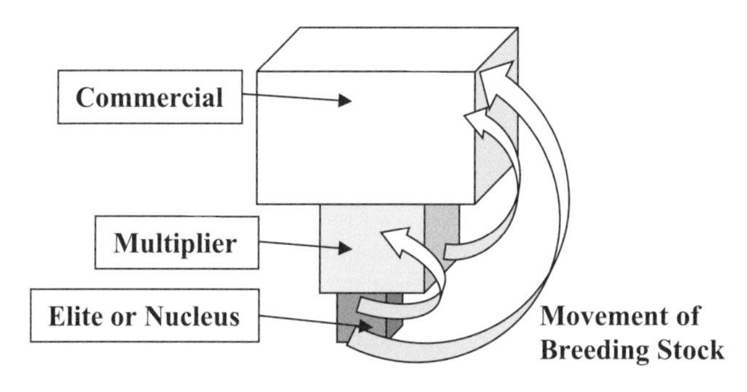

Figure 3.1 The genetic organization of most standardized breeds in a closed nucleus system is arranged in tiers based on genetic material passing only in one direction. Figure by DPS.

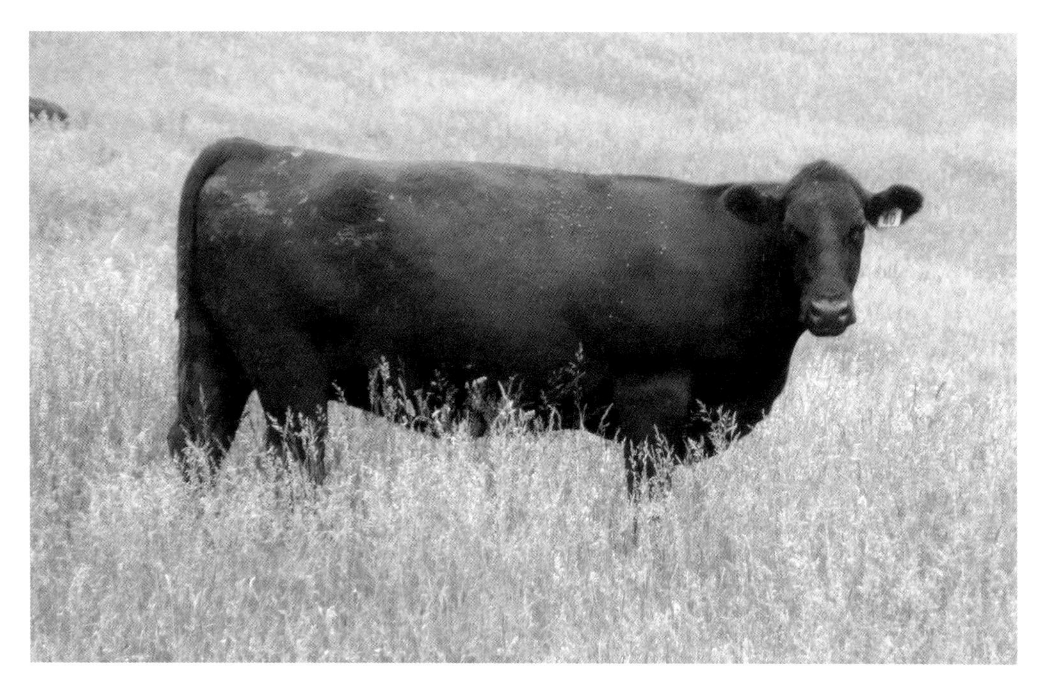

Figure 3.2 The Angus cattle breed has a typical tiered structure common in mainstream commercial production breeds. Photo by DPS.

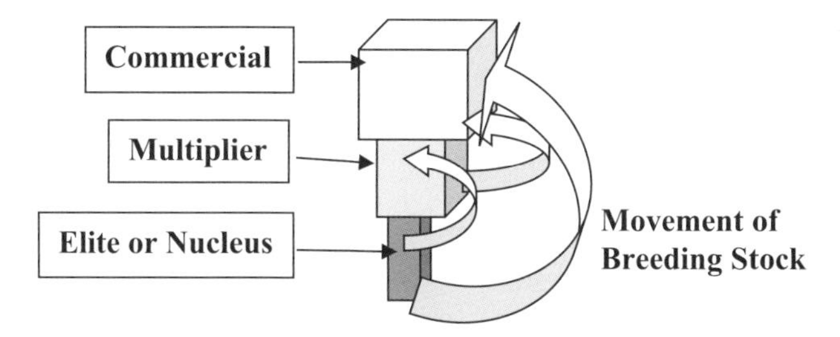

Figure 3.3 After several generations, the closed nucleus breeding system diminishes the greater diversity that is present in Figure 3.1. Figure by DPS.

the overall population. Importantly, as time progresses the genetic variability of the elite nucleus tends to decline, so that the breed rests on a constantly diminishing base. Over several generations, the limited variation of the elite base slowly replaces and reduces the greater diversity of the other tiers (Figure 3.3).

In industrialized breeds, the tiered organization becomes even more extreme because the elite tier is completely closed, while at the same time it is organized to produce huge numbers of animals at the multiplier and commercial tiers. The entire population that results is usually very large, but the genetic base is paradoxically very small. This approach to breeding management provides for the genetic uniformity and predictability that are so desired in commercial industrial stocks. It does this specifically by constraining the population to a very small genetic foundation.

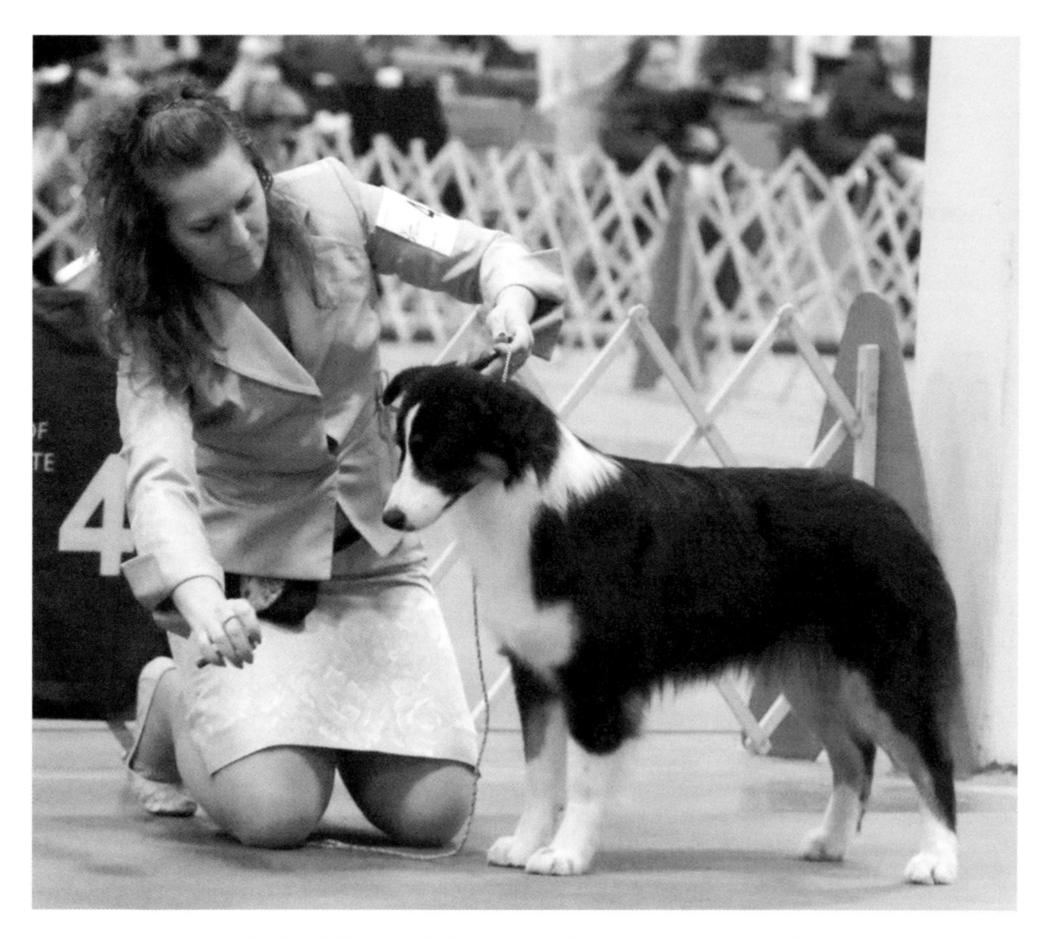

Figure 3.4 Most standardized dog breeds have a tight hierarchy of genetic influence based on show or performance wins. Photo by Julie Cecere.

The most extreme examples of this structure are industrial egg-laying chickens, broiler chickens, and industrial turkeys. Industrial poultry breeding uses specific, highly selected primary strains and crosses these to other similarly inbred primary strains to yield the final production birds. The whole enterprise rests on the narrow genetic base made up of the primary strains. Holstein cattle, while not as extreme an example, have a similarly narrow genetic base. The genetic consolidation in Holsteins is largely a consequence of decisions made by semen companies, and a great deal of genetic narrowing occurs through the use of paternal half-sisters as the dams of widely used bulls.

Most standardized dog breeds also follow breeding practices that use a narrow elite base to heavily influence the breed (Figure 3.4). In this case the elite base is usually show-winning dogs that then go on to be used heavily for reproduction. Following this strategy for even a relatively few generations assures that the original genetic variability of the breed is slowly but surely whittled down.

An alternative organizational model, rarely used, is the "open nucleus" system (Figure 3.5). Males from the elite nucleus are used at both the multiplier and commercial tiers,

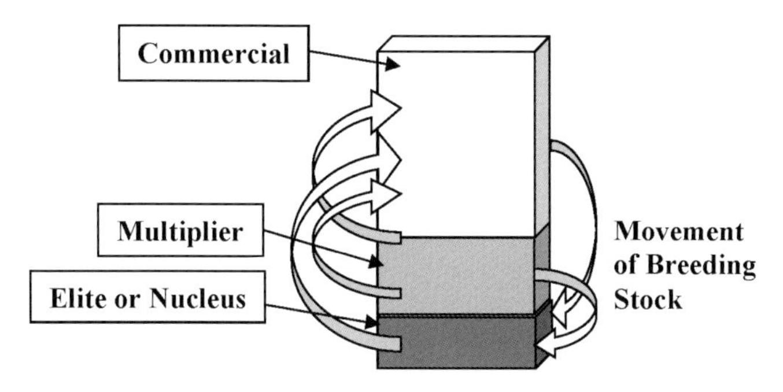

Figure 3.5 An open nucleus system allows genetic material to flow back into the elite or nucleus tier through the use of exceptional female animals from the multiplier and commercial tiers. Figure by DPS.

which is similar to the closed nucleus model. Males from the multiplier tier are used at their own tier as well as the commercial tier, which is again similar to the closed nucleus model. Importantly, though, a small percentage of females with superior performance move down the structure from the commercial and the multiplier tiers to the elite nucleus tier. This may seem to be a subtle and inconsequential shift in strategy, but it provides for much more rapid dissemination of superior genetic combinations throughout the breed than the closed nucleus approach does. Superior animals in the upper tiers have an opportunity to have a wider influence on the breed than is true in the closed nucleus model. This approach broadens the genetic base of the breed.

The open nucleus system has rarely been used in standardized breeds, but has been adopted by some sheep breeding cooperatives in Australia. Each cooperating breeder contributes his elite ewes to a group flock from which all the members can take rams for use in their own flocks. Periodically the best-performing ewes of each cooperating flock are recruited into the elite flock. This strategy succeeds in pulling out the best-performing genomes as they are produced at all levels of the population.

The open nucleus system is also being promoted as a useful strategy for village-based animal breeding in developing countries. It widens farmer participation as well as the supply of animals in programs that target improved production at the local level. It is important to assure that recruitment into the reproducing group is open to all purebred candidates. This can be difficult, but is essential because genetically unique and important animals may reside in compromised situations. Such animals are difficult to encounter in the first place, let alone identify and assure their widespread use. Such animals are of great value to the breed, and their residence in peripheral situations should not preclude their widespread use in reproduction.

3.2 *Landraces*

Landraces usually have a genetic organization that is very distinct from that of standardized breeds, as illustrated in Figure 3.6. Instead of a tall structure with one tier supported by the others, these breeds are much more like a short one- or two-floor building with many

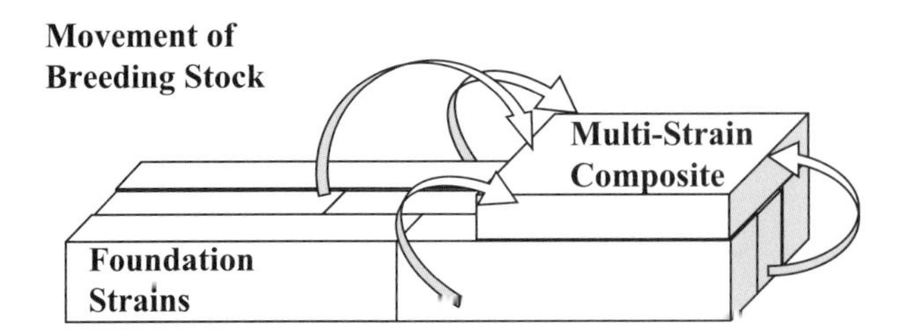

Figure 3.6 The genetic organization of most landraces resembles a short one-floor building made up of distinct foundation strains, with a second floor of composites built from specific combinations of the foundation strains. Figure by DPS.

separate rooms. Each subpopulation (strain or bloodline) within these breeds is variably isolated from the others. In many cases, breeds organized in this manner contain several herds that persist in complete genetic isolation from one another. The genetic similarities in these breeds come from long-standing founder effects and from consistency in the selection environment rather than from the genetic transfers that are usually ongoing among the strains of most standardized breeds. In addition to the foundation strains that are genetically isolated, landraces often also have composites that are built from multiple foundation strains. These composite strains can be imagined as second-floor rooms that lie over several of the first-floor rooms. The composite strains are supported by the genetics of the specific foundation strains that went into the composite.

Pineywoods cattle are an example of a landrace breed with several distinct strains that all interact in different ways (Figure 3.7). Many family breeding herds of Pineywoods have been totally isolated from one another since the early 1900s. These family herds are excellent examples of genetically isolated foundation bloodlines. In addition to these foundation herds are more recently established herds that are based on a composite that includes influences from multiple of these foundation herds. The overall gene flow in this situation is from foundation herds to composite herds, as well as from one composite herd to another. The foundation herds function in nearly total isolation from one another, so that the breed has several distinct and important isolated reservoirs of genetic material rather than the single elite core that is usually the case for standardized breeds. This organizational structure does provide for good maintenance of genetic variation, but the isolated strains are at high risk of loss or extinction due to dispersal or natural disaster.

The persistence of distinct foundation strains assures that genetic diversity is maintained within a breed. Keeping these separate groups intact maintains different lines within the breed. One important consequence is that every animal within the breed has candidate mates that are unrelated, and with which it could produce outbred offspring in the event that such measures are needed to correct inbreeding depression.

The different organizational patterns of breeds have profound consequences for conservation and genetic management. Standardized breeds with a very strictly closed nucleus structure are, at least superficially, the easiest to conserve. In these breeds a reasonable sample of the elite tier is effective in saving most of the genetic variation in the breed. At the other extreme, the "low, broad building" organizational structure of

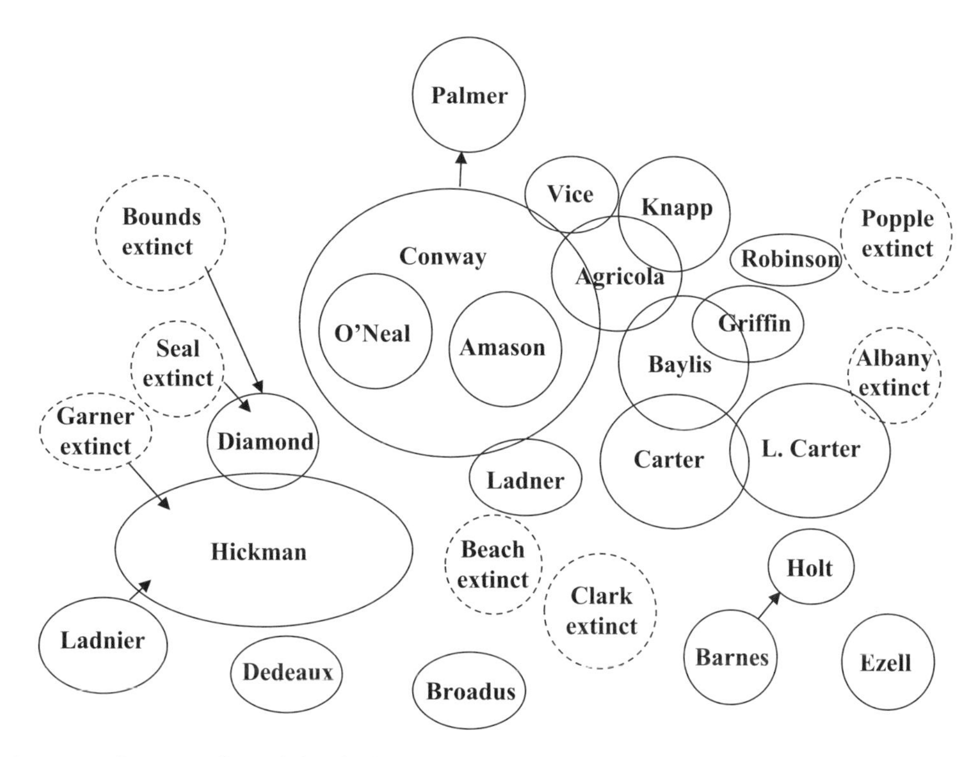

Figure 3.7 Pineywoods cattle herd relationships. Each circle is an old family strain of cattle, generally isolated from the others. Overlapping circles and ovals indicate that strains are related through past exchanges of breeding animals. This organizational pattern results in portions of the breed that are completely unrelated to others, while others are related in various combinations. Figure by DPS.

landraces is much more difficult to conserve, because each and every separate strain should be located and utilized in order to save the entire genetic diversity of the breed. A common misconception in breed conservation programs assumes that the closed nucleus structure with a narrow base is typical of all breeds. The result has been that many important founder strains of landrace populations have been overlooked in conservation work, and several have become extinct.

Gulf Coast sheep have a similar history to that of Pineywoods cattle, but the organizational structure of one group of breeders has recently tended more toward a standardized breed than the Pineywoods structure (Figure 3.8). Some of the distinctive bloodlines that once existed have been lost in the composite of the newly defined population. In addition, the resulting composite is increasingly based on relatively few founding strains rather than a more balanced representation of the variation in the overall landrace. Fortunately, several breeders still maintain isolated and unique strains, and the future genetic health of the breed will depend heavily on breeder decisions regarding these strains and the variability they represent.

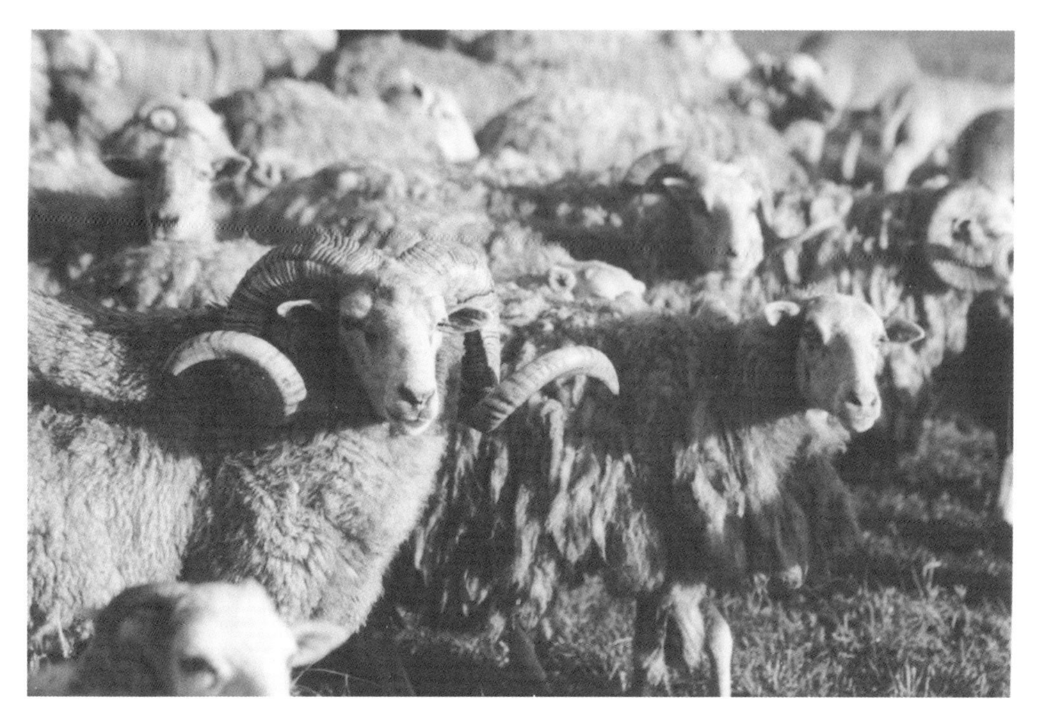

Figure 3.8 Several strains of Gulf Coast sheep have long histories of nearly complete isolation one from another. Photo by DPS.

3.3 Subgroups within a Breed: Bloodlines, Strains, and Varieties

Bloodlines, strains, and varieties are all subgroups within a breed. Each of these can be an important reservoir of variation and genetic diversity. While definitions vary, each of these terms usually designates a subpopulation that has been isolated for several generations (usually four or more) with the consequence that they are somewhat genetically different from other bloodlines. Bloodlines are usually linked to certain breeders or farms, and are usually distinct by both history and genetics. Breeders mold the predictability of bloodlines by combining genetic isolation with individual selection practices.

The degree of distinction of bloodlines can be problematic. It is easily possible to return to the question of "what is a breed?" and the specific degree of genetic distinction that should be included or excluded as a single breed. Some bloodlines could indeed be considered to be their own breeds, although such an approach vastly multiplies the number of breeds that need conservation help. The Livestock Conservancy considers candidate populations as bloodlines of a single breed (rather than each as a distinct breed) if they are more like one another than they are like any other breed. This strategy is especially important in landrace breeds for which several distinct bloodlines are considered to all be members of the same breed instead of a group of cousin breeds. Bloodlines, especially of landraces, are reasonably distinct historically, phenotypically, and genetically, yet remain similar enough to one another that they stand together when compared to other breed resources.

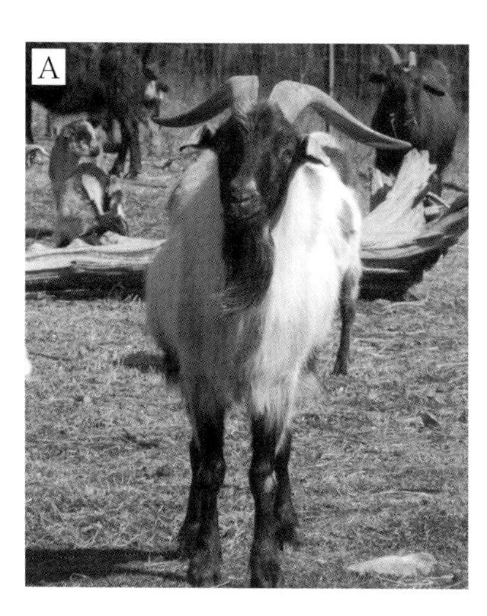

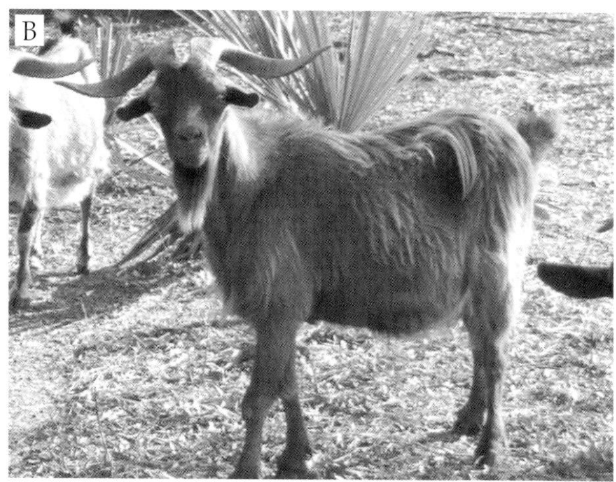

Figure 3.9 Baylis (A) and Low Country (B) Spanish goats share a common original foundation, as well as adaptation to hot, humid conditions, despite having been separated for centuries. Photos by JB.

The Spanish goat is an old landrace breed that has several old bloodlines (Figure 3.9). The breed has been in the Americas ever since the first colonists from Spain arrived in the late 1400s and early 1500s. The goats are hardy and robust, and have adapted to the regions in which the various bloodlines have been isolated for many years. Southeast lines such as Low Country (South Carolina), Jericho (Alabama), and Baylis (Mississippi) tolerate humid subtropical conditions. West Texas lines such as Kensing, Koy, and Bode are more suited to arid regions. Bloodlines from similar environments can be used to good advantage with one another when a boost of genetic variability is needed, so having multiple bloodlines all from a single environment is a boon to the breed and to the breeders.

The bloodlines within a breed can be very important reservoirs of genetic variation, and managing these within the overall breed is important for long-term breed survival. Bloodline conservation can also lead to fads and shifts in popularity of one bloodline over another. Some of these shifting fates may be related to production potential or to breed character, in which case these shifts may be warranted. Many times the popularity of a bloodline is related to the advertising or show ring success of a capable promoter. In those cases, a bloodline can easily swamp a breed with little underlying genetic reason for doing so. In nearly all cases it makes sense for a breed association to work to effectively conserve all of the bloodlines of a breed.

One strategy to avoid is for breeders to all recruit males from a single bloodline. Such a strategy only assures that the genetic diversity of the breed will soon be completely swamped by that one bloodline. Little or nothing of the other bloodlines will survive. While this is an attractive short-term situation for the breeder with the popular line, it is almost invariably bad for the long-term future of the breed. This strategy is all too commonly employed, and quickly takes a breed population to a very constrained closed-nucleus system with all of its inherent challenges.

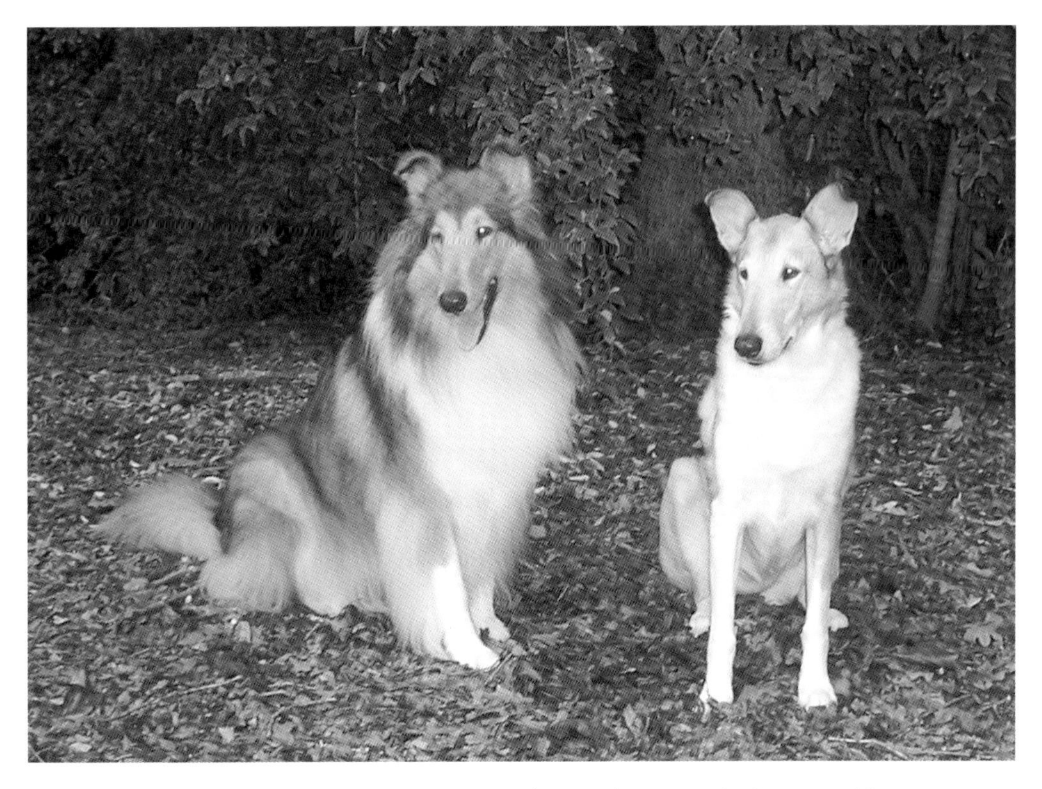

Figure 3.10 Collies have two hair coat varieties, either rough or smooth, determined by a single-gene difference. The two varieties are still from one breed. Photo by Michelle Brane.

Most people use "strain" as a synonym for "bloodline." The use of this term tends to be especially commonly among poultry breeders when describing groups of birds that have been carefully bred and crafted by individual breeders over several generations. Strains usually take on the name of the breeder that crafted them, and many poultry breeds have distinct strains that have been maintained for several decades.

In contrast the term "variety" usually has a specific definition, but this definition varies somewhat from species to species. In most mammalian breeds, "variety" refers to a difference in coat type, color, horns, or some similar attribute that is usually caused by a single-gene change. For example, Collies have two varieties, rough and smooth, and these vary by only a single gene (Figure 3.10).

"Variety" is used in poultry breeding in a manner that is superficially similar to that of mammals, although in reality it often denotes a much more significant genetic difference than is true in mammalian breeds. Poultry breeds are mainly differentiated by relying on phenotype, to which are added issues of geographic origin and purpose. Specific foundation is also involved but usually to a small degree. Many poultry breeds have several varieties. The formal definitions of these are achieved by differences in color, comb type, or feather type. At this point the fine details become important.

Some of the poultry populations designated at the varietal level within a single breed differ from one another by only a single-gene difference. This type of variety can easily

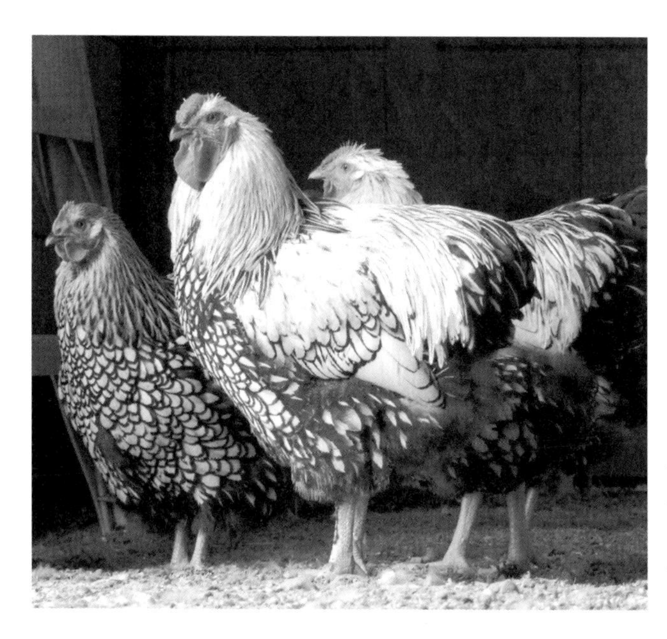

Figure 3.11 The Silver Laced Wyandotte is one of several varieties that are closely related in this breed, in contrast to other varieties with minimal relationship. Photo by JB.

and accurately be considered to be the same basic genetic package except for the one difference. In such populations, "variety" is simply a single-gene variant within a single breed, and the varieties share the same foundation and general history. However, many poultry breeds have varieties within them that have completely different foundations. The different varieties of these breeds, despite their outwardly similar body type, share very little genetically. These sorts of varieties have achieved their similar external phenotype through selection. Varieties of this sort could easily be considered as independent breeds, while those of the first sort are all indeed members of the same breed. Unfortunately the two very different definitions both go under the same name ("variety") so there is no easy way to thread through the nomenclature to get to the biological reality. In poultry breeds, understanding the relationships of varieties within a single breed requires a fairly deep knowledge of the breed and its history.

Examples of varieties that share a common foundation are the various colors of Dorking chickens, along with their varying comb types. In contrast, the three different color varieties of Chantecler chickens each have a very distinct foundation, and consequently share little in common at the genetic level despite their similar appearance. To make matters more confusing, some breeds, such as the Wyandotte (Figure 3.11), have distinctive varieties that originate from a single foundation (Silver Laced, Black, White). Other varieties of Wyandotte have a genetic foundation that is very distinct from these and from each other (Golden Laced, Buff, Partridge, Silver Penciled, Columbian, and Blue).

The relationships of the levels of genetic organization within poultry breeds are therefore very difficult to untangle, and demand a breed-by-breed and variety-by-variety approach to achieve an accurate understanding. Some varieties within some breeds are closely related to one another, others are more distinct. To add yet another layer to the complexity, old strains within varieties are often very distinct. In many breeds certain individual old strains are important components of genetic diversity even though they may be considered superficially similar by virtue of all being members of one single variety. For example, Wishard Bronze turkeys have a long history of isolation from all other turkeys. This strain is more genetically distinct from other bronze turkey strains than several strains of Black turkeys are, because the Black turkey strains are periodically reinvigorated by outcrosses to Bronze turkeys. In this case, despite the obvious superficial differences in the varieties, the differences at the strain level are even more important for breed management. Such a level of detail is notoriously difficult to attain.

Managing the bloodlines, strains, and varieties within a breed is important for long-term maintenance of the genetic variability that is crucial for breed viability. This can be a complicated task, requiring breeders to be informed of the bloodlines within a breed. This deep knowledge base should include the relative popularity and productive potential of the various subunits that occur within breeds.

In the Texas Longhorn breed, several of the eight foundation lines have been crossed so extensively among themselves that they have lost their original genetic distinctiveness. A few others of the original lines are now extinct, and have not contributed to the present-day breed at all. This outcome resulted from a shifting emphasis on certain phenotypic characters, such as color and horn spread, that were present more strongly in some lines than in others. In addition, the breed went through a period that saw an increased tendency to use semen from only a few popular sires. The result is a serviceable breed, but one that is much changed from the original, and even changed from the more recent foundation of today's remnant. Fortunately, conservation-minded breeders in the Cattlemen's Texas Longhorn Registry have been diligent to save as broad a representation of old, pure bloodlines as could be had.

Many breeders plan to have long-term influences in their breeds, and are therefore interested in the steps that go into forming a distinct bloodline, strain, or variety. At the variety level, the formal decision is taken by the multiple-breed organizations such as the American Kennel Club (for dogs) or the American Poultry Association (for poultry). Poultry breeders, especially recently, have become interested in developing a host of new color varieties in several different breeds. These must each meet specific criteria of foundation and must also meet certain numerical requirements at competitive shows. Only after meeting these criteria can a new variety be admitted to the standard. This formal approval process attempts to ensure that new varieties have enough popularity and engagement to persist for long time spans rather than being passing fads.

While varieties, especially of dogs and poultry, have very specific criteria, formal definitions of bloodline do not exist. Defining a bloodline is therefore much more subjective. Exactly when a bloodline is considered to be distinct is open to different interpretations. A few general principles can help, though, and can reflect the idea that a bloodline is reasonably distinct, uniform, and predictable.

Foundation bloodlines are those from which the breed began, and they are therefore the basic units of the breed's original formation. For most long-term standardized breeds, the foundation bloodlines occurred long ago, and since then have been blended to form the present breed. In more recently organized landraces the designation of foundation bloodline should be an ongoing process. For landraces, a useful general principle is to designate as a foundation bloodline those animals that have an origin in a single source that has received

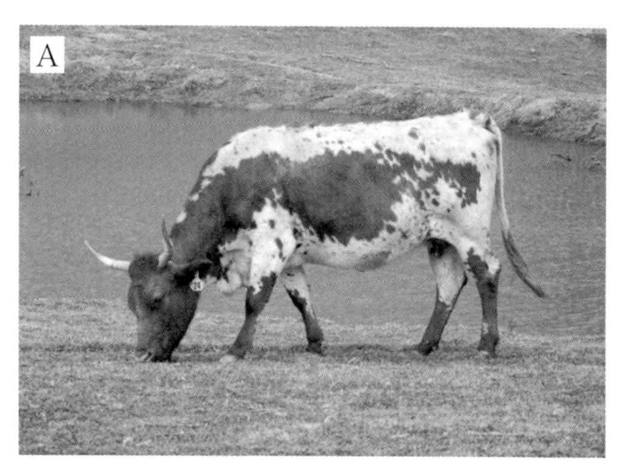

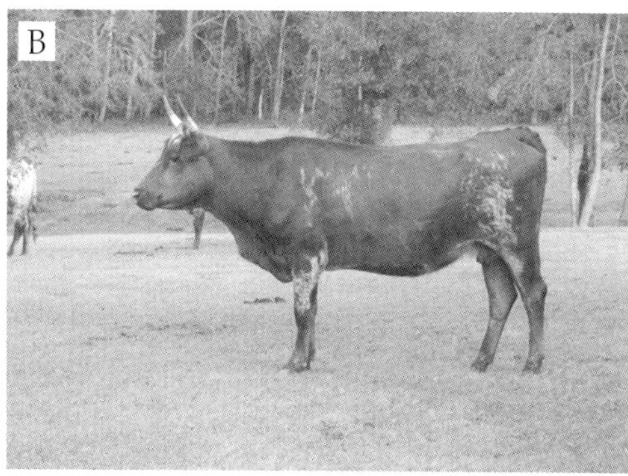

Figure 3.12 Pineywoods cattle benefit from breeders maintaining original foundation strains, such as Conway (A), in addition to blending them for current composite bloodlines, such as Diamond (B). Photo A by JB, B by DPS.

little or no influence from other foundation bloodlines. These are generally old lines owned by families that kept their animals isolated over several generations.

In contrast are the more current bloodlines of any breed, whether standardized or landrace. A tally of current bloodlines can, and should, include foundation bloodlines when these continue to be maintained in isolation by some breeders (Figure 3.12). Another sort of current bloodlines can be formed by breeders blending together foundation or other bloodlines. This generally takes about four generations of isolated breeding within a single population. This threshold can serve as a useful boundary for designation of a breeding group as a formal bloodline. If new animals are constantly introduced, then the breeder is generally unable to reliably "stamp" the animals with a consistent and reproducible type. This, of course, assumes that selection pressures are moderate and consistent. In some herds where selection levels are quite high, a superficial uniformity can be quickly achieved even if genetic uniformity and predictability are somewhat delayed. The breeding of Warmblood horses in Europe serves as an example, where strict performance and inspection procedures assure that the overall phenotype will be achieved well before the underlying genotype is made uniform.

3.4 Gene Flow into and out of Breeds

Genes can and do flow into breeds from outside sources. Crossbreeding to other breeds is the usual source of gene flow. Some flow of genes into pure breeds is inadvertent, but some inflow occurs due to short-term goals and fraud on the part of breeders. Gene flow into breeds, especially if widespread, can easily corrupt and permanently change the breed package to the point that it no longer functions as the original genetic resource it once was.

There are many examples of crossbreeding which have led to loss of breed character. Among these examples is the current convergence of nearly all black-faced sheep breeds in the USA onto a very Suffolk-like frame and head type. A long-time Hampshire sheep breeder interested in pure breeding told the story that in the 1990s he had become disgusted by the fad toward very Suffolk-appearing Hampshires that were winning on the show circuit. At that point he decided to leave the Hampshire breed. But first he did an experiment. He crossed Suffolks to his remaining Hampshires. The first crosses were very close in type to traditional Hampshires, thereby indicating to him that the current fad in "Hampshires" was likely at least 75% Suffolk breeding or more. This crossbreeding, especially if reinforced by show ring success or other market forces, is the death-knell for the genetic uniqueness of breeds. With that loss also goes the true usefulness of the breed, as it quickly becomes a somewhat second-rate copy of a different breed. The fault here lies partly with the breeders involved, but also with the system of showing that rewards animals that inadequately reflect their breed.

The Hampshire sheep example demonstrates that show ring fads that do not place emphasis on distinctive features of a breed type can quickly spell the end of a breed as a purebred genetic resource. Once crossbreds are acknowledged as purebreds within a registry, it is difficult or impossible to regain the genetic package that is so essential to the purebred's ultimate function. The show ring can be particularly damaging to breeds if off-type animals are placed high in the rankings. This provides an incentive for breeders to abandon selection for breed type and can easily lead to introgression of crossbreds into a pure breed (Figure 3.13).

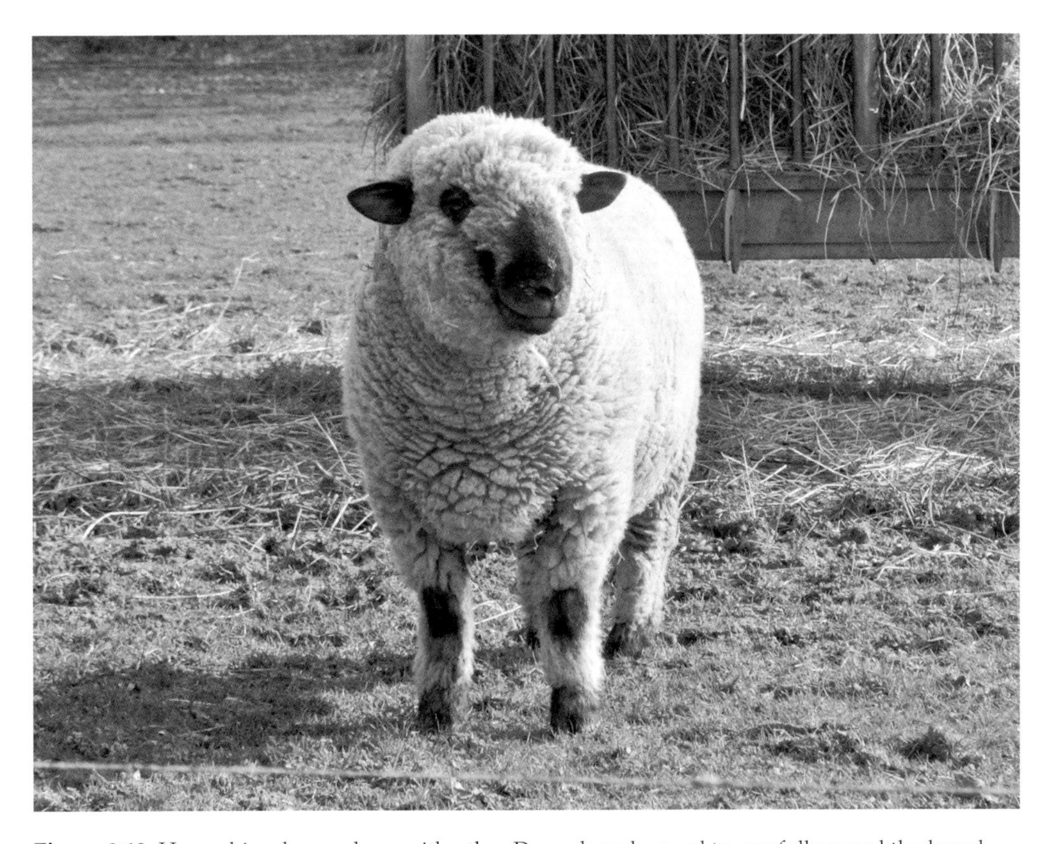

Figure 3.13 Hampshire sheep, along with other Down breeds, need to carefully guard the breed from introgression of the Suffolk that is currently popular in the show ring. This Hampshire shows breed type strongly and clearly, indicating freedom from Suffolk breeding. Photo by JB.

3.4.1 *Upgrading and What It Does*

Upgrading is very distinct from disorganized introgression. In many situations it is a very useful tool for managing breeds. Upgrading is the sequential use of purebred animals over a series of generations to provide a "nearly purebred" result (Figure 3.14). The usual sequence is that a purebred sire is used on females that are not of his breed. These females can either have undocumented ancestry, be crossbred, or be of another breed. The resulting offspring are 50% the pure breed of the sire. The daughters are then mated back to another purebred sire of the breed, providing offspring that are 75% the pure breed. The next generation provides offspring that are 88%; the next is 94%, then 97%, 98%, and finally over 99% and so on. These partbred animals are called "grades" of the pure breed to which they are being sequentially mated. Many breed associations designate a specific percentage at which grade animals can be included as part of the purebred population.

Upgrading has consequences for the genetic integrity of a breed, and also for the breed's numerical strength. These two aspects are distinct, and clear thinking is needed to avoid confusing one aspect with the other. The genetic aspects of upgrading are complicated, and details of those issues follow this introduction. The numerical aspects are usually less important, but have historically been the main drivers of upgrading programs for many breeds imported into the USA.

Upgrading programs were once typical of the European beef cattle breeds that were imported to the USA in the 1970s and 1980s. Breed numbers were low, and imports were

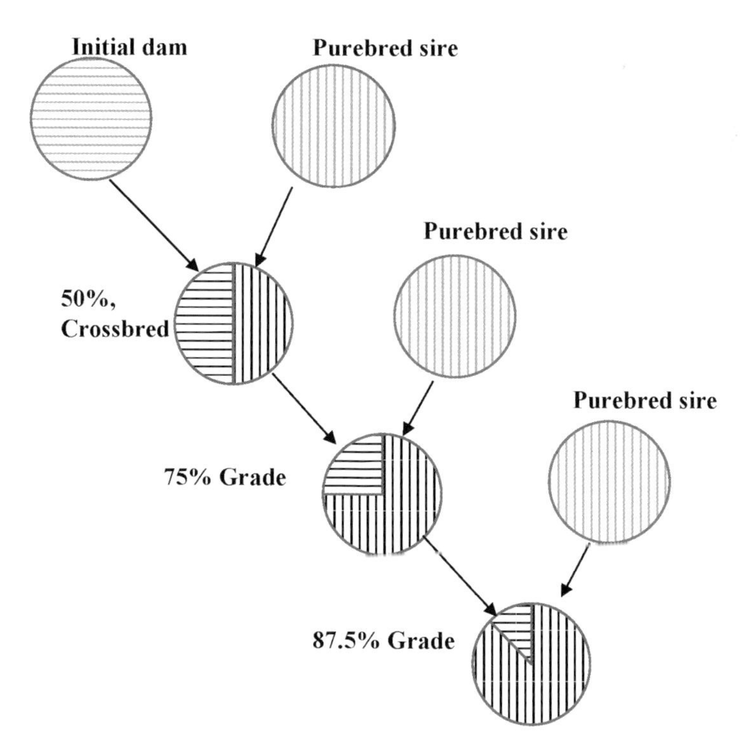

Figure 3.14 The use of a sequence of purebred sires provides for offspring of increasing percentage breeding of the pure breed. This is the essence of upgrading. Figure by DPS.

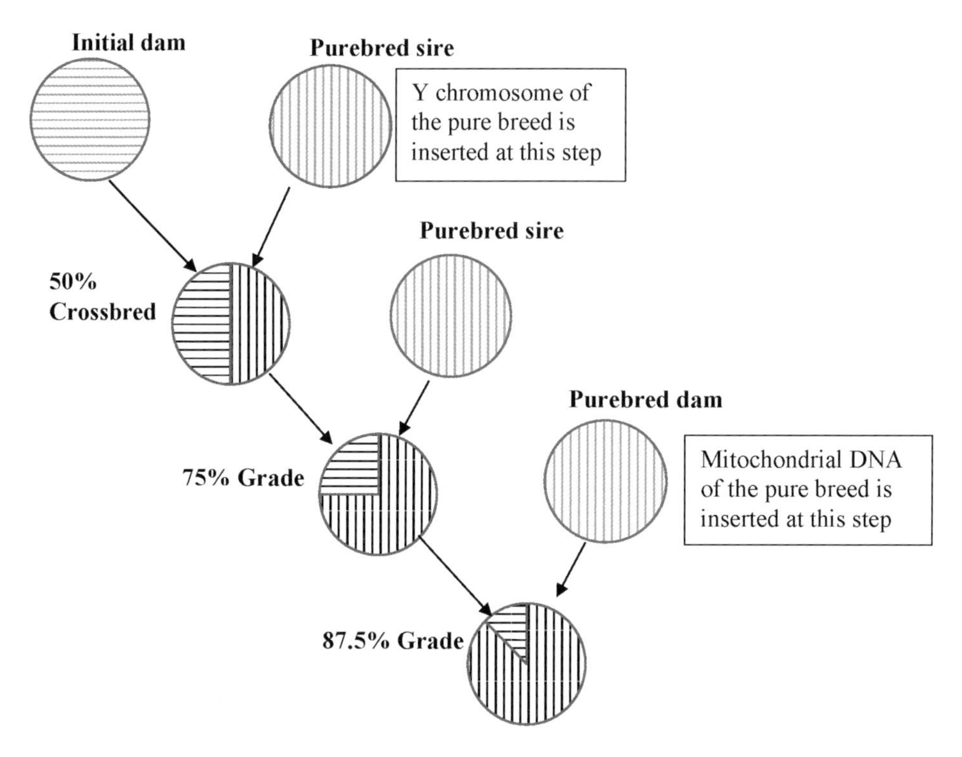

Figure 3.15 It is possible to assure that both the mitochondria (female) and Y chromosome (male) come from the target breed by using both males and females from that breed in upgrading.
Figure by DPS.

expensive. Upgrading was a strategy to increase numbers fairly rapidly, as well as to serve as a main driver for the economic value of purebred bulls used in those upgrading programs. Upgrading programs for Wensleydale, Teeswater, and other recently imported sheep breeds in the USA somewhat follow this early rationale for upgrading programs, although these are based on frozen semen rather than the use of imported rams.

Upgrading in most breeds involves only the use of purebred sires on grade dams. It is also biologically valid, if rarely done, to use purebred dams for this process (Figure 3.15). Due to the unique genetic contributions of females (mitochondrial DNA) it may actually be best for upgrading programs to insist on the use of both purebred males and purebred females in some of the generations to assure that sex-specific (Y chromosomes from males, mitochondria from females), breed-appropriate genetic material has come from the purebred gene pool.

Upgrading has a legitimate and important role in some breeds, but it is generally considered to have little if any benefit to older, long-established standardized breeds. While some old and isolated breeds have little to gain from upgrading, the truth is that upgraded animals can offer many pure breeds a real opportunity for vitality and viability without endangering the breed's genetic heritage. This is only true if the upgrading program is well thought through and well executed. Careful upgrading allows breeds to avoid the problems of a completely closed gene pool with its attendant inevitable inbreeding, while at the same

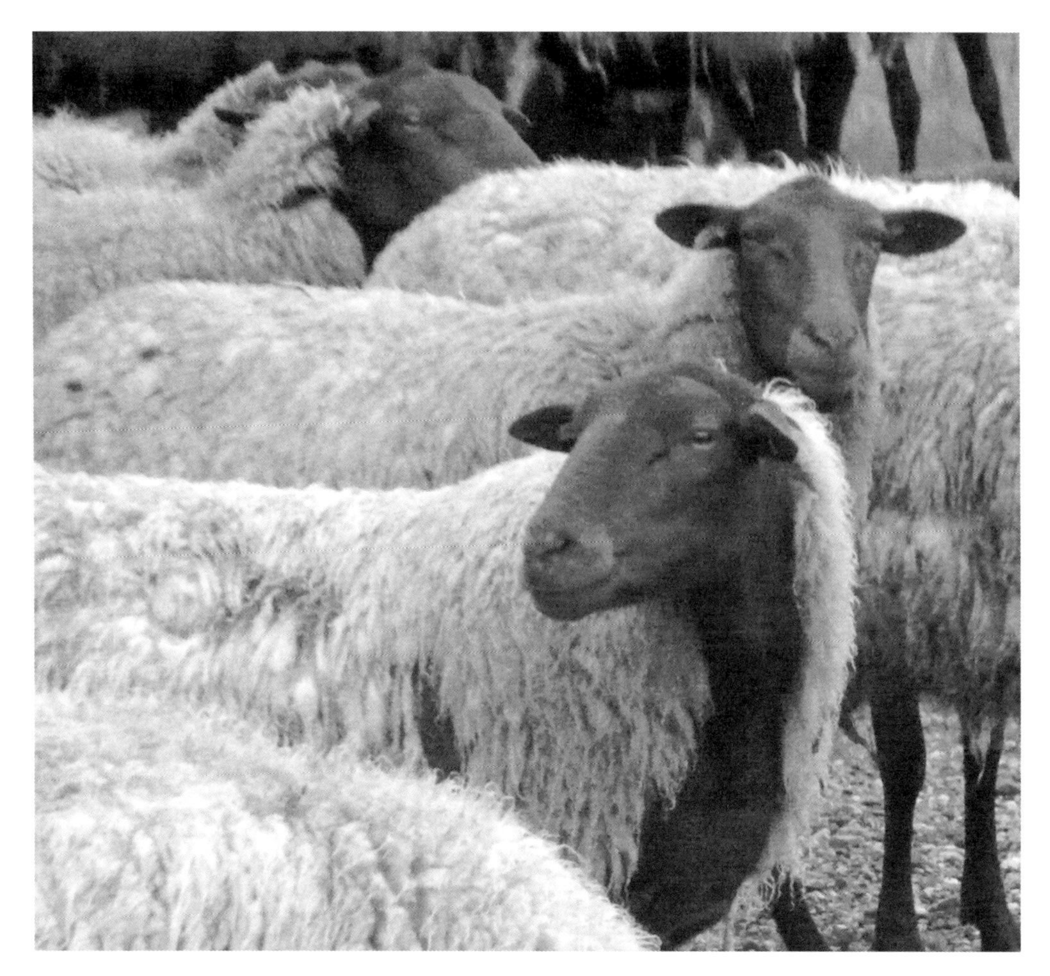

Figure 3.16 Several European breeds, such as Solognot sheep, are managed by routinely allowing upgraded animals into herd books after seven generations of upgrading. This maintains breed integrity while also allowing breeds to be practical and useful, especially when the final generations are inspected for congruence to breed type before acceptance into the purebred registry. Photo by DPS.

time safeguarding the status of breeds as predictable genetic packages. Upgrading is a way to ensure breed survivability over long centuries of purebred breeding. Understanding what upgrading is and how it affects a breed genetically are extremely important issues to breeders of all purebred breeds, whether or not they choose to use this strategy.

Upgrading has been widely used in several livestock species. Upgrading must be managed intelligently or it becomes an avenue for the inclusion of animals into purebred herd books before those animals have acquired the genetic package that makes the breed distinctive and useful (Figure 3.16). Including off-type animals results in corruption of the breed rather than its expansion.

Upgrading has lots of positives, a few negatives, and several facets that make it an interesting biological phenomenon. As a backdrop to the issue of upgrading, it is important to remember the essential character and utility of breeds. Breeds are useful because they are consistent, predictable genetic packages. It is the predictability that is the key to the value of breeds, for without predictability it is impossible to match breed to place, purpose, and system. Any action that conserves breeds as consistent genetic packages tends to be helpful, and likewise anything that detracts from the genetic package is detrimental. Upgrading must always be evaluated in light of this concept.

It is also essential to remember that breeds have cultural importance, and in many instances the dedication of breeders to a purebred breed goes beyond the direct commercial utility of the breed. In the eyes of many breeders, anything except absolute pure breeding pollutes the breed into something else, and these breeders hold that all such strategies are to be avoided. While this thinking is based more in culture than in biology, it is important to recognize this stance as legitimate and sincere.

The key to understanding upgraded animals is that each of them does indeed have at least some potential for including genetic material that is not in the original pure breed. The amount and significance of the outside genetic material are both important. Grades usually begin to resemble the pure breed very closely at levels of 75–87.5% purebred influence. At these levels, however, they still include a good deal of genetic material that is not from the breed in question. It is important to understand that all of this discussion concerns averages. Individual animals could easily be found that are either a lot more or a lot less "pure" or "pure looking." This means that selection toward breed type is especially important in upgrading programs. Upgrading only succeeds if the goal is to add to the pure breed. Upgrading does not succeed if the goal is to change that pure breed into something else, because in that case the outside genetic material will be preferentially retained from generation to generation. For example, black-colored cattle in the USA currently generate a premium in the beef market. As a tactic to maintain market share, some traditionally red-based beef breeds have allowed upgrading in order to introduce the black color. In this example, the upgrading is specifically used to introduce a characteristic alien to the breed, and this raises serious questions about the goal of upgrading. While color may be a superficial example, the overall issue of breed type and purebred breeding must at least be considered.

In some situations, upgrading is accomplished specifically to help solve adverse genetic conditions in purebred breeds. For example, Dalmatian dogs had become genetically uniform for a genetic mutation affecting uric acid metabolism. In an attempt to correct this defect, upgrading from English Pointers was accomplished, tracking the dogs through several generations to assure that the desired allele for normal metabolism could be introduced into the final upgraded animals, and thereby into the breed, without changing the breed character.

At higher levels of grade, which certainly include 97% or anything higher, the influence of outside genetic material is minimal, and the animals perform and reproduce like purebreds. These upgraded animals may have a slight advantage in overall vigor, and in fact do offer breeds a small breath of fresh genetics that can be a great boon to some very rare and potentially inbred breeds. Upgraded animals may add lost productivity, vitality, and vigor to these breeds, while also boosting numbers. If upgrading is wisely managed, the upgraded animals pose minimal threat to the genetic uniqueness of the breed. This reflects the basic truth that breeds are valuable because they are consistent and predictable. Any breeding practice that does not threaten the consistency and predictability of a breed does not threaten its status as a breed, and such breeding practices certainly include prudent upgrading programs.

The 87.5% grades are generally not sufficiently purebred to truly function as genetic members of the breed, while the 97% grades generally are. This leaves in question the intervening generation of 94% animals. Breed associations that allow upgrading do indeed differ on whether 94% animals are sufficiently purebred or not, and the answer to this question has some legitimate leeway when different breeds are considered. These 94% animals are generally "purebred enough" to be considered legitimate breed members.

Acceptance of upgraded animals is often at different levels of grade for males and females because of the potentially broader effect of males on the breed. Some breed associations accept females as "pure" at 87.5%, which may be a bit low for inclusion in the pure breed. As a practical issue, these females (and it is only females accepted at this level) are mated back to purebred sires for the next generation, resulting in 94% offspring (both male and female) that are included in the breed.

Some breeds already have reasonable levels of genetic diversity, and therefore have less need for the boost of the small amount of introduced genetic variation that comes from upgrading. In those breeds it may be wiser to proceed to higher levels of grade before considering the graded animals as purebred. Indeed some populous, productive breeds probably have little if anything to gain from upgrading.

It is important to remember that if a very high level of grade is required (98% for example), then the potential genetic benefits of upgrading will be largely lost to the breed. Additionally, some very tightly constrained old breeds may need more of a boost than what is afforded by introducing only very high grades. There is no single magic cutoff point for the level of grade needed for breed conservation as well as breed vitality. Each situation for each breed must be considered individually, and it is generally unwise for upgraded animals to be allowed to numerically swamp the older, established purebred stock. A possible exception to this rule is situations like the Dalmatian dog where purebreds are homozygous for deleterious alleles and the whole purpose of upgrading is to reverse that situation. One strategy to assure that the original stock is not overwhelmed is to require that all upgraded animals presented as candidates for the purebred herd book pass an inspection and also have a baseline of production characteristics that contribute to the breed's strength without changing its character (Figure 3.17).

Breed purity and upgrading have enormous political overtones in most breed circles. Breed purity is assumed by many breeders to be absolute, inviolate, and ancient. The truth is that the origins of most breeds reach back less than 200 years, while most herd books are even younger. Breed formation was initially a response to a desire for predictable animals of a given type. Most breed origins were fairly broad, so genetic viability was assured. As breed registry books were closed and matings occurred only within the narrowly defined breed, the genetic character of breeds changed from fluid and inclusive to very restricted and closed. Some breeds are now suffering varying degrees of inbreeding depression from being locked down with matings occurring only within the purebred population. Continuing to insist on absolute breed purity may well lead to the demise of at least some

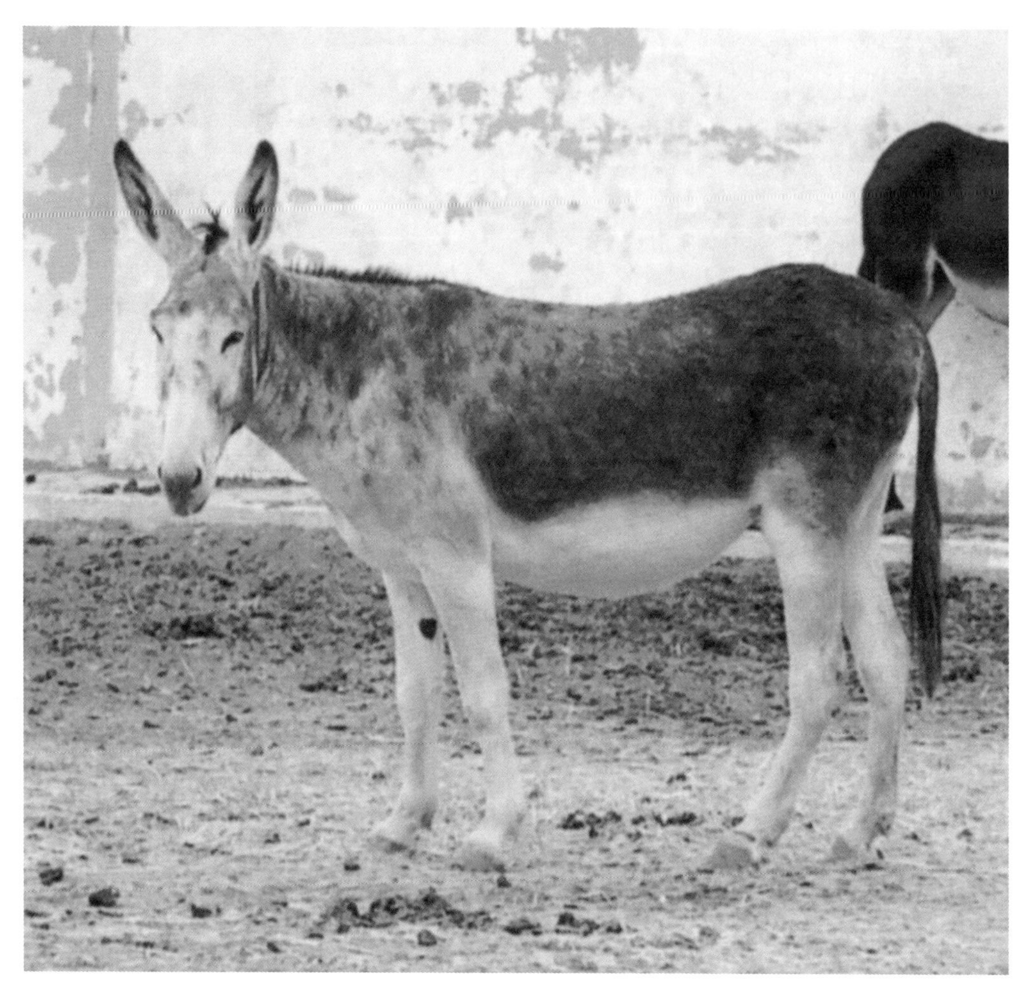

Figure 3.17 Upgrading has helped expand numbers of the distinctive Andalusian donkey, valued in Spain for mule production. Upgraded animals are inspected for their adherence to breed type before they are admitted into the herd book. Photo by DPS.

breeds as they lose their vitality, productive potential, and agricultural relevance. These changes, while initially subtle, result in deviation from original breed type and utility. This has happened in some chicken and heritage turkey varieties. Breeders are now diligent to reverse that trend.

Dairy goat breeding illustrates some of these issues (Figure 3.18). Most dairy goat breed associations in the USA register both purebreds and upgrades, although in separate sections of the herd book. The purebred section registers offspring from matings between only purebred members of the registered breed. Upgrades are registered in a separate section and are designated "American." So a Nubian, for example, is a purebred Nubian, while an American Nubian is an upgraded animal. Breed politics are such that upgraded goats have much less demand as breeding animals when compared to similar purebreds. American goats therefore have lower prices in most markets. Many American upgraded

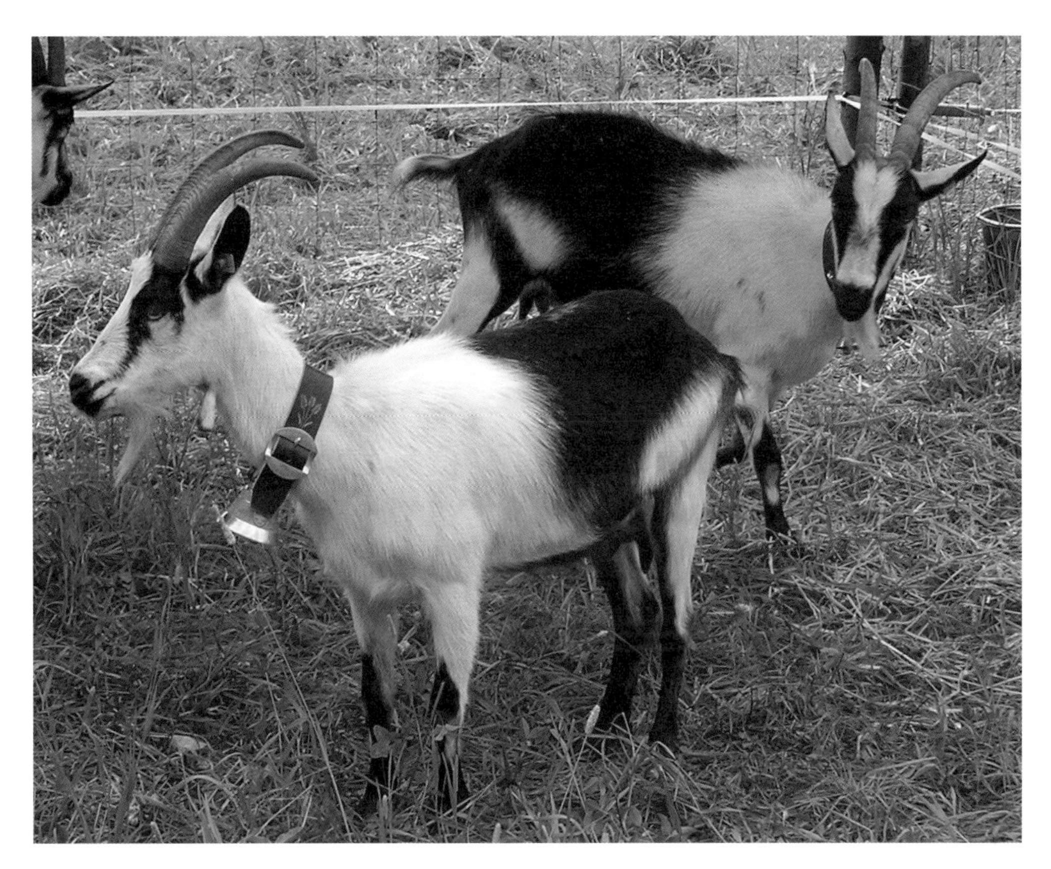

Figure 3.18 Dairy goat registries in the USA carefully identify upgraded goats separately from purebred goats. This goat, in Switzerland, is a similar breed to the Alpine in the USA, but is managed according to European breeding systems. Photo by DPS.

goats outperform their purebred counterparts, so that commercial producers sometimes prefer the American counterpart to the purebred. In this situation, safeguarding the breed resource as a closed genetic pool has, at least sometimes, decreased its utility as a viable commercial entity. This is counter to the original aims of breed development, selection, and use! More rational breed maintenance schemes might involve the inclusion of high grades into the purebred herd book, especially if conformation and production levels exceed the breed average. This would assure the addition of only top-quality animals, would still let the breed "breathe" genetically, and would assure that the upgraded goats do not swamp the breed numerically.

The situation with upgrading in dog breeding is more complicated. Most dog breeds are absolutely and formally closed gene pools, and only a very few dog breeds allow upgrading. Basenji dog breeders have taken a different strategy by allowing in newly imported dogs from the original African landrace foundation stock. This is different than upgrading, because the imported dogs are from the same landrace origin as the Basenjis with long registered pedigrees. These imported Basenji dogs will benefit the breed the most by being directly included into the breed with no breeding restrictions.

Dog breeds tend to be bred in very tightly closed populations, and this has occurred over more generations than is true for many other types of animals. It is therefore likely that certain weaknesses from inbreeding will become more frequent in at least a few of them. It is important for dog breeders to acknowledge this, and to begin a discussion of potential remedies. For most dog breeds, there are other breeds that are close "cousins" that come from a similar foundation and serve similar functions. For example, there are several retriever breeds that are reasonably similar to one another. Likewise, many livestock guardian dogs have a superficial phenotypic similarity and breeds from neighboring regions likewise have historic genetic links. In these cases, an initial outcross followed by a set number of upgrading generations may help to restore vitality to breeds without losing their original type and function.

Pure breeding and purebreds are vital in all species of domesticated animals, so the issue of upgrading does need to be evaluated for its place in breed maintenance, management, and conservation. If carefully managed and operated, upgrading does not threaten the status of any breed as a genetic resource. This is counter to the politics of many breed associations, so upgrading is likely to remain relatively rare. For international breeds, associations must fit their policies and procedures into those accepted in other countries, and generally the most restrictive country sets the policy on this issue. All breed associations will eventually need to address the issue of upgrading versus absolute breed closure.

The downside of completely closed populations is gradually making its power felt as evidenced by a slow erosion of vigor in breeds such as the Thoroughbred horse, Holstein cattle, and several dog breeds. Such declines, if they become widespread, may give breeders cause to evaluate what a breed is, why it is valuable, and how best to manage its genetic status.

Due to the complicated character of breed identity, it is nearly impossible to make general recommendations on upgrading programs. Each breed has a unique background, history, and present status, both genetically and culturally. At one extreme are breeds such as the Thoroughbred horse, with centuries of pure breeding and a great deal of mystique surrounding its identity and breeding. As a result, any inclusion of outside breeding must be done carefully and in light of the rich history of the breed. One option might be to reinvigorate the breed by a few allowed outcrosses to the Akhal-Teke or other Turcoman horses, which is historically appropriate due to the role of Turk horses in the original foundation of the Thoroughbred (Figure 3.19). It likely makes more biological sense to upgrade some animals to Thoroughbred from a Thoroughbred x Akhal-Teke base in an upgrading plan, rather than to include early outcrosses as purebreds and thereby run the risk of a sudden change in the genetic makeup of the breed. By this strategy, the breed package remains intact and loses no predictability. In contrast, a widely divergent cross such as to a Brabant Belgian has little to offer the breed genetically or culturally, even if a long series of upgraded generations could theoretically replace the genetic material with Thoroughbred influence.

On the other hand, relatively recently defined landraces, such as the Pineywoods cattle or Navajo-Churro sheep, have to consider upgrading very carefully. These breeds, though centuries old, retain a great deal of genetic diversity and face the challenge of restrictive breed definition even more than they face any challenge of viability. For these breeds, upgrading offers little, if anything, at this point in time.

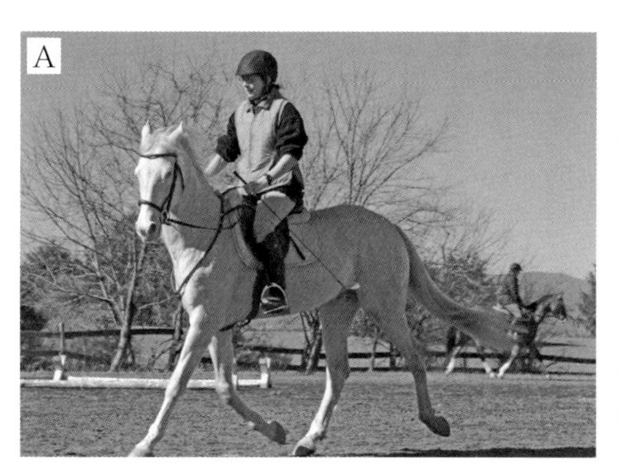

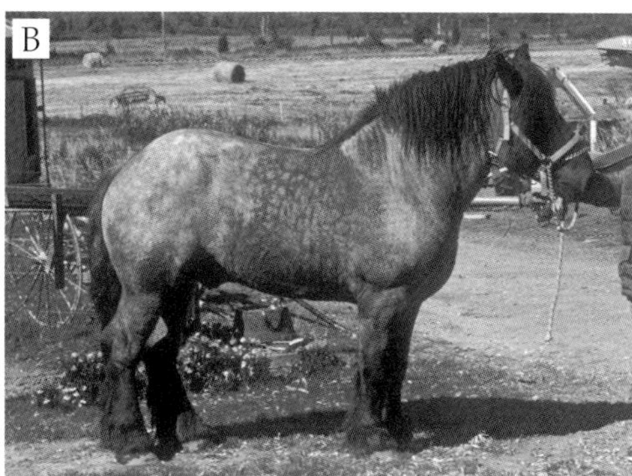

Figure 3.19 The Akhal-Teke (A), one breed of Turcoman horse, figured in the foundation of the Thoroughbred horse breed and is a logical and related source of influence if upgrading is ever to be allowed. In contrast, the Brabant (B) would be a very poor choice for an upgrading base for Thoroughbreds. Photo A by JB, B by DPS.

Upgrading, if carefully managed and monitored, can help pure breeds remain viable and vital. Upgrading can also assure that breeds retain their status as genetic resources. Any upgrading program must be carefully monitored to achieve appropriate levels of grade before inclusion of animals into the purebred breed. One strategy that assures this is the registration or recording of all the generations of grade so that the association is confident of the genetic status of each animal. A final criterion might be to inspect those animals before inclusion in the main purebred herd book, either by photograph or physical inspection, to confirm congruence with breed type.

At the same time that breeders protect breeds from too radical an inclusion of grades and outside influences, it is also important for breeders to recognize the value of grades to the viability and production of the breed. The value of grades can be quickly negated by the political view in many breed associations where upgraded animals are considered second-class citizens. For a breed to fully reap the biological benefits of upgrading (numerical expansion, increased market for breeding males, some gain in genetic vigor), the upgraded animals must at some level of grade indeed be considered as full members of the breed. That is where breed politics get into the picture, and breed politics frequently do not have an answer in biology.

The controversies of whether or not to allow upgrading can often generate huge amounts of passion and friction. Some breeds have little to gain from upgrading, but few have much, if anything, to lose. The final determination of the appropriateness of upgrading for any breed will be decided by tricky issues such as breed politics and reciprocity between national herd books, which is absolutely essential for international breeds. Upgrading in some form does, however, make good genetic sense for many breeds, but only if upgraded animals can be eventually included as full members of the breed.

3.4.2 *Upgrading and Bloodlines*

Bloodlines are important as reservoirs of genetic diversity within a breed. Maintaining bloodlines as genetically healthy resources for the breed is necessary. Having distinct bloodlines within a breed helps breeders to manage the genetic material of the breed so that relatively isolated pockets within the breed maintain some genetic distinctiveness. This is useful for sustaining viability in the breed, but only if these bloodlines remain functional and robust. Similar to the situation of a breed as a whole, bloodlines within a breed also gain important and necessary benefits by upgrading using other lines within the same breed. The issues of upgrading to a pure breed from crossbreds are slightly different than those concerned with upgrading of a bloodline from within a single pure breed.

The level of genetic distinction between bloodlines is much lower than is present between breeds. This is because bloodlines within a breed are indeed all members of that breed's gene pool. The level of breeding of a candidate animal to be considered as of a strain or bloodline is therefore not as stringent as that required for inclusion of a true upgrade into a breed. This is, of course, only true if the grading animals are of the same parent breed. A purebred animal that is only 87.5% of a specific bloodline is for most purposes essentially of the bloodline in question. The inclusion of 87.5% or 94% animals into old established foundation bloodlines can meet some political resistance, but is essential if the older bloodlines are to remain viable and contributing members of the breed. To lock them down genetically is to assure their eventual demise, and they offer too much benefit to breeds to allow that to happen.

One very useful application of upgrading is the rescue of bloodlines that have become endangered. The details of this are explained in Chapters 15 and 16. This is an especially appropriate tactic for recovering old family strains that have been reduced to a handful of older females and no males. In this situation, it is all too common for breeders to then use a sequence of outside males, the result being a steady dilution of the original genetic material of the strain. The first crop of offspring is 50% the original strain, the next generation is only 25%, then 12.5%, until finally very little of the old strain genetic material remains. An alternative approach is to use the females to produce sons that can be taken back to the original group of females. This is somewhat the reverse of more usual approaches to upgrading, which depend on using males from the target line or breed that is desired (Figure 3.20).

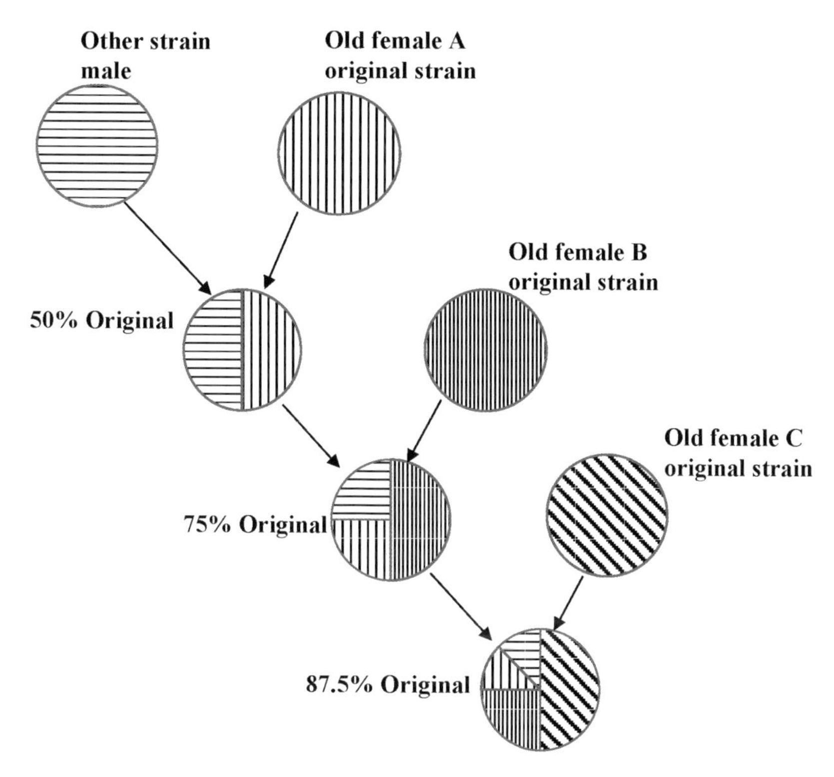

Figure 3.20 Upgrading to a bloodline, rather than a breed, usually relies on sequential mating back to the original females. Figure by DPS.

CHAPTER 4

Defining an Individual Breed

Accurately defining the characteristics of an individual breed is an important step in conservation. This step has obviously been accomplished long ago for most recognized, standardized breeds, but even in those situations a good understanding of the process of breed definition can help to guide effective breeding and conservation decisions. Definitions for specific breeds vary, but should ideally focus on aspects of foundation, isolation, and selection pressures that first formed the breed. It is also important to recognize the cultural and management environment that typifies the breed so that this important aspect of a breed's function is not lost when defining the breed.

It is important to reflect on the essential character of the breed concept. Breeds, as biological entities, exist somewhat independently from any cultural trappings that their human caretakers impose upon them, despite those interactions having important consequences. Basically, breeds pre-exist their official recognition. Consequently any definition or recognition of an animal population as a breed should take every effort to discover and describe what is actually present rather than what the observer might hope should be out there. Those two approaches can lead to very different results.

As an example, hair sheep on the island of St. Croix in the Caribbean are variable for color and horns. A white, smooth, polled subsample of this population was brought to the mainland of the USA in the 1970s, and was defined as the white, polled "St. Croix sheep." The question then becomes which version is indeed the St. Croix sheep breed? The variable island population, or the more uniform mainland population? The answer depends on the specific viewpoint adopted by the observer, and each answer has different consequences for maintaining the genetic resource (Figure 4.1).

4.1 *Which Animals to Include*

The question of which specific animals to include within a breed population is an interesting and thorny problem, especially at the outset of breed definition. This problem plagues rare breeds that are of conservation interest much more than it does common breeds, and occurs most frequently with landrace breeds. The goal of breed conservation should always

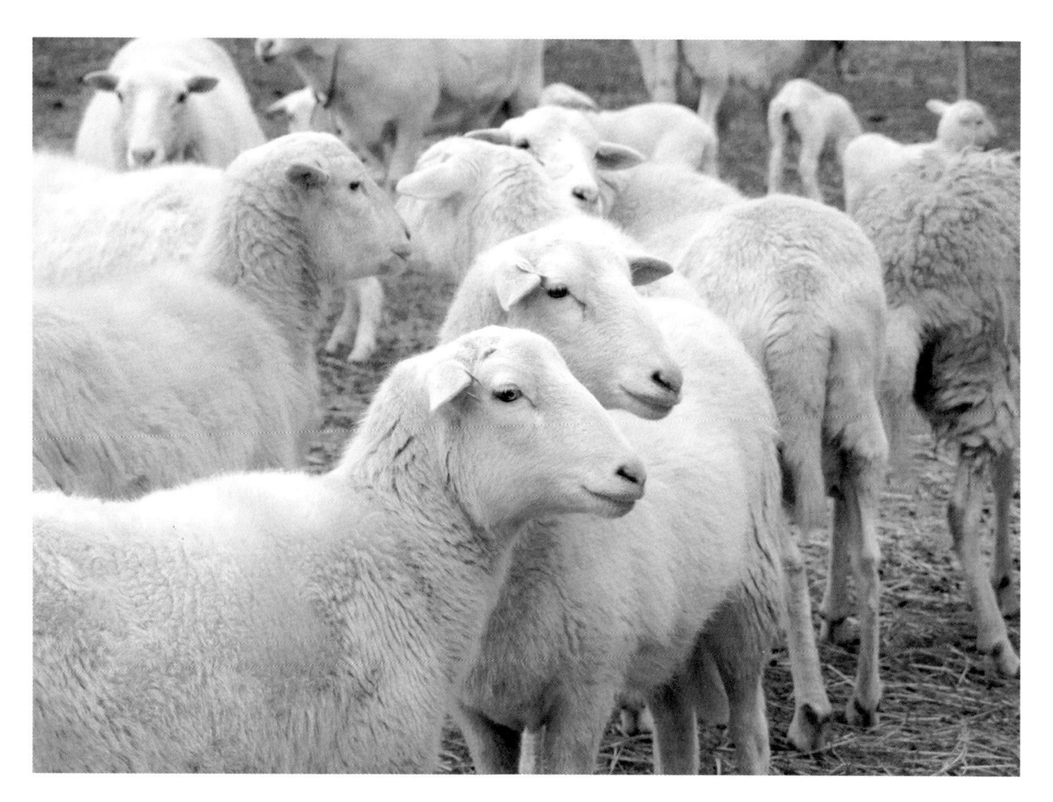

Figure 4.1 St. Croix sheep on the mainland are much less variable than those on the island. Photo by JB.

be to try to exclude all animals that are not of the breed, and to include all of those that are. Rarity of a breed imposes the need to include every individual that is truly of the breed. Decisions are thereby pulled in opposing directions to avoid leaving anything out that should qualify for inclusion, while also avoiding inclusion of extraneous and nontypical animals. Achieving the right balance can be difficult. It is easy to state the goal to be "include all the purebreds" and "exclude all the partbreds," but this is difficult to actually achieve.

Determining the boundaries of a breed, especially a landrace, is a challenging and complicated task. Reflecting on the identity and character of breeds can greatly aid this process.

- Breeds result from foundation, isolation, and selection.
- Breeds are repeatable genetic packages.
- Breeds develop and function within specific human culture and use.

Good breed definitions reflect all three of these components and direct the decisions about which specific animals should be included in a breed population.

The three most useful means to evaluate animals for inclusion as members of a breed include phenotype (external appearance), history, and genetic analysis. Any of the three, if used alone, can lead to a wrong conclusion. In contrast, when all three are used in concert it is rare to misclassify animals.

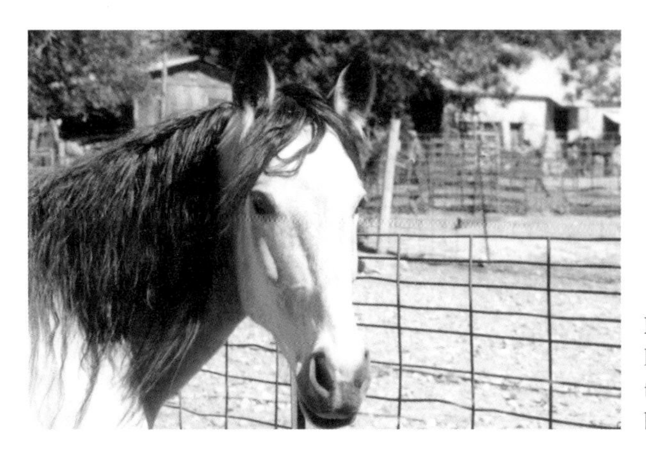

Figure 4.2 Colonial Spanish horses have a typical appearance that distinguishes them from other breeds. Photo by DPS.

Phenotype is important because all members of a breed should consistently reflect breed type and conformation, despite any variation in superficial cosmetic characteristics. The external indicators of breed membership are not trivial, for they mirror the underlying genetic package. External clues are therefore very good and easily observed indicators of relative congruence with what is expected of members of the breed. Phenotype can be misleading in the case of individual animals, but is much less likely to be so when considering entire populations. An individual horse presented as a Colonial Spanish horse is much more difficult to assess than a herd of 100 individuals (Figure 4.2). This is true because the 100 individuals are much more likely to betray any deviation from the breed package than a single selected individual is. Because the investigation of the phenotype of candidate animals and populations is relatively easy and economical, it is often used as a first step when deciding whether or not a population qualifies as a breed, or making decisions about inclusion of a group or an individual animal into a breed.

A useful strategy for evaluating animals for potential inclusion into a conservation program is to use a phenotypic matrix. This should emphasize breed-specific points of conformation and breed type, and should be individually tailored for each specific situation involving a single breed. The matrix emphasizes the pure type, and also pays attention to the phenotypes that result from introgression from the most common other breeds used in the area. Multiple traits can be scored, with "1" being most typical of the breed and "5" being obviously crossbred. While it is tempting to compute the final score from an average of the scores of each individual trait, this can often lead to poor conclusions. A more accurate outcome is achieved when the matrix is used to detect specific off-type traits, and then to explore the significance of these for purebred status. Some traits are likely to be more important than others. The important few can veto the inclusion of a candidate animal, so that a poor score in one important trait might automatically eliminate the animal despite good scores for other traits. The components of a matrix vary from breed to breed. Chuck Reed of the Bureau of Land Management (BLM) first developed this idea for Colonial Spanish horses (New World Iberian horses). This matrix is long and complicated, and is presented in Appendix 1. Breed-specific influences in this situation are included from nearly all body regions of the horses, and so a good whole-animal inspection is required.

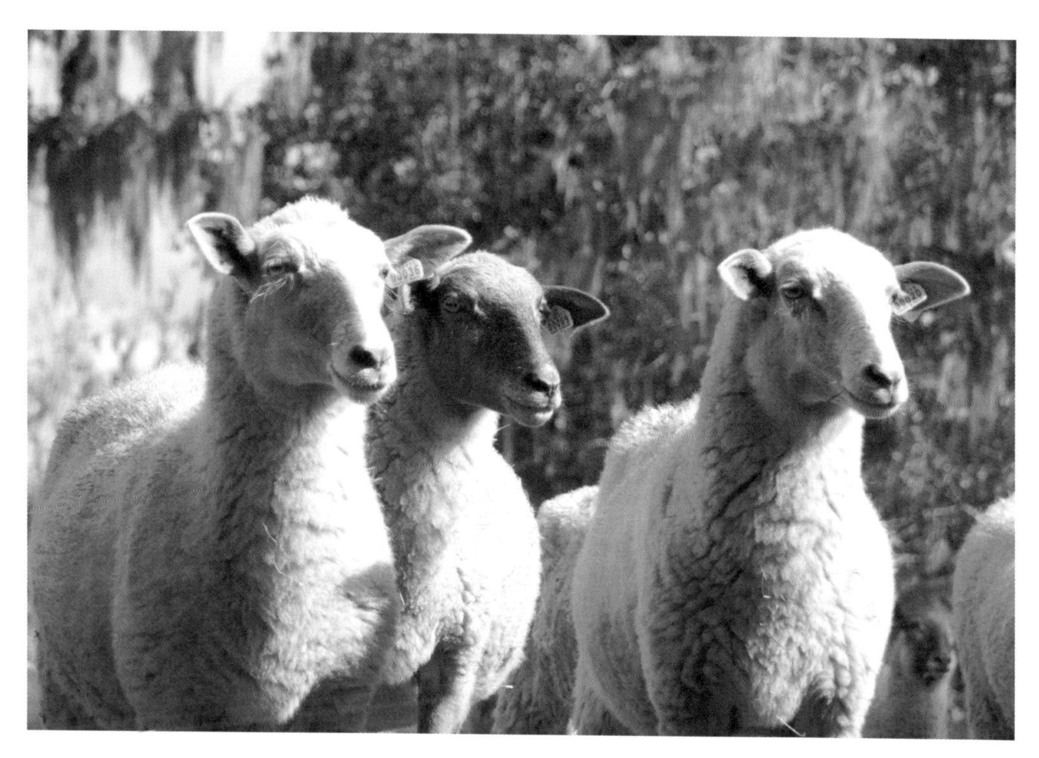

Figure 4.3 Florida Cracker ewes all have similar head shapes, betraying their breed origin despite variation in color. Photo by JB.

The development of a phenotypic matrix varies from species to species, and from breed to breed. The important concept is that the matrix should focus on breed-specific traits, and not on traits of general productive quality. Horses tend to have important clues in most body regions. Sheep and goats have little breed-to-breed variation in most body regions, so most breed-specific traits center on the heads, horns, ears, tails, and fleece character (Figure 4.3). Cattle and hogs are somewhere between these two extremes. Poultry tend to have telltale clues throughout body regions.

People familiar with the candidate population and its breed type can evaluate phenotype, even if somewhat subjectively. This process may not satisfy all challenges to scientific accuracy, but is frequently all that can be accomplished for large, extensively raised populations such as feral horses or range cattle. This rather simple approach has cost advantages, and whenever the results have been compared with lengthier, costlier, and more intrusive DNA-based methods the conclusions have been in consistent agreement. This means that the rather low-tech approach of "just looking at them" does indeed have merit.

An alternative to the somewhat subjective analysis involved with using a matrix is to assess linear measurement. In this type of assessment very specific measures are made on a number of animals in the population. These measurements, when analyzed in their totality, are remarkably accurate in pinpointing membership in the breed, and are likewise good at eliminating nonconforming animals. The sorts of measurements vary with the different species, but usually include height at withers, height at top of croup, height in middle of back, distance halfway from topline to belly, width of croup, anterior width of croup, posterior width of croup, heart girth, width of head, length of head, length of face, distance between eyes, circumference of muzzle, width shoulder to shoulder, length of body, depth of body, and topline from poll to rump. The disadvantage of this approach, in many situations, is that the animals are not tame enough to accomplish the measurements without considerable risk to the evaluator.

Investigation into the history of candidate animals or populations is either accomplished after the phenotypic investigation or concurrently with it. History is important because most breeds spring from a limited area or have a limited influence of founders that can be traced historically. Colonial Spanish horses (Spanish Mustangs and Barbs) provide a good example. Feral horse herds with appropriate phenotypes continue to come to light, even if increasingly rarely as time goes on. The history of these newly discovered herds must be evaluated to identify known or suspected introductions of outside horses. Historical investigation can be quite difficult because many of the people involved have a vested interest in the outcome of the process. Those who favor inclusion of the population into the breed will often indicate a pristine history of absolute purity with no outside influences. Those who would detract from it will point to long and consistent inclusion of outside influences. Sorting through these different threads can be quite difficult, although weighing the history against the external phenotype can greatly aid in coming to an accurate conclusion. A history of constant introduction of outside animals is simply not consistent with a uniform population, and neither is a long history of isolation with a highly variable population.

Wherever possible, animals and populations that pass muster from the phenotypic and historical aspect should be investigated genetically. In decades long past, most cattle and horse populations were blood typed as a final step to assess candidate animals and decide on breed membership. Recent advances have allowed DNA analysis techniques to largely supplant blood typing as an investigative tool. Unfortunately, blood typing and DNA analysis provide different information, and these are not interchangeable. The main commercial use of the DNA technique is parentage evaluation of animals presented for registration into existing herd books. Exploration of breed origins is a secondary endeavor that can be tacked on with varying degrees of success.

The strength of blood typing was the huge repository of information acquired over a long period of time that allowed breed-to-breed comparisons to be made. In addition, many breeds had "private" variants limited to that one breed. The presence of these private alleles was extremely helpful because they helped to validate breed membership, but also helped to detect introgression from other breeds when they popped up where they should not be present. This once provided a strong advantage over some of the DNA techniques, although for most species blood typing is no longer widely available, so this is a moot point. As a greater volume of DNA results are amassed, it will likely prove equal to the task of evaluating the purity of candidate populations, although that capability is currently not uniformly present across all species or breeds.

DNA analysis for parentage validation is most routinely used for horses, cattle, and alpacas. It can present a challenge when investigating other species because the relatively low value of individual animals usually does not warrant the expense of DNA validation

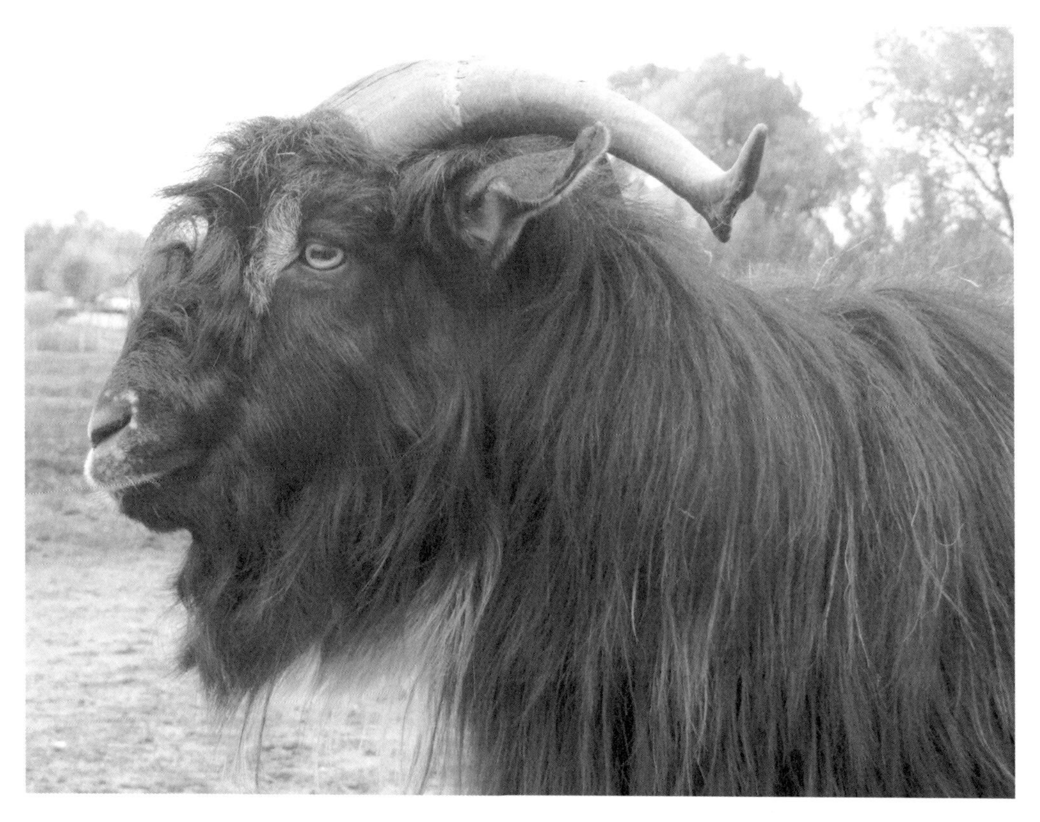

Figure 4.4 Arapawa goats are typical feral goats from an island. The small founder population and subsequent long isolation have led to very low genetic variability, which makes identification of purebreds by DNA analysis quite easy. Photo by JB.

of parentage for routine use in registrations of animals into herd books. As a consequence, the smaller species lack the deep backlog of information that routine validation provides for horses and cattle. For several species, the decisions on the accuracy of breed identity therefore rest more on phenotypic and historical investigations simply because the extensive information needed to accomplish across-breed DNA evaluation do not currently exist.

DNA analysis techniques need to be considered in light of the type of population that is being considered. Some populations are inherently more variable than others. These include landraces, especially those that have several relatively isolated founder subpopulations. At the other extreme are populations with minimal variation. These are usually long-isolated populations that had relatively small numbers of founders. Many island populations of feral animals, such as Arapawa and San Clemente Island goats, fit into this group (Figure 4.4). Other breeds, such as Randall Lineback cattle, also fit in here. At the more variable extreme are landraces such as Gulf Coast sheep or Spanish goats with numerous foundation herds that each have long periods of isolation from one another. The evaluation of DNA variants must take this history into account.

A good example of a potential pitfall with DNA analysis comes from the Dexter cattle breed in the UK. A recent DNA study revealed that the Woodmagic herd has genetic differences from the balance of the breed. The tempting interpretation is that this is due to introgression from other breeds. In this case, though, the Woodmagic herd has a long history of isolation from the rest of the breed, and in those years the animals were under the selection protocol of a single devoted owner. This is the sort of situation that easily leads to consolidation of differences, even within a single breed. A conclusion of introgression versus purity must go beyond simply noting genetic differences in subpopulations, and must compare these unusual DNA variants with those of breeds that could have provided for any introgression. The existence of the variation, by itself, is not adequate proof that the herd should be removed from consideration as purebred, especially when no information exists on the suspect variants and their occurrence in other breeds. The conclusion as to whether to exclude such animals must rest on a complete evaluation of all the evidence.

Examples of the value of employing all three approaches (phenotype, history, DNA studies) occur in many breeds of many species. Colonial Spanish horses stand out as one breed for which the three approaches have been successfully used for several decades. A few populations can demonstrate how these have helped to either include or exclude candidate populations.

The Nokota horses have a history of descent from Chief Sitting Bull's herds. From there they went to the Teddy Roosevelt National Park, and the story becomes clouded with the possibility of crossbreeding on at least some parts of the range. The horses have variable external types, but the most typical individuals are very good representations of the Colonial Spanish horse type (Figure 4.5). In this situation it is important to decide whether the few typical horses are remnants of a historically important population, or are simply a phenotype that occasionally resegregates from a crossbred population. Unfortunately, the DNA results clearly point to recent crossbreeding across all of the types within the population. Importantly, as the more traditional type is segregated and mated within its own group, the long-term trend will be consolidation of this type to make it more uniform throughout that sub herd. This uniformity, derived from recent selection, will mislead future observers as it will have come from recent selection rather than the longer-term factors of foundation and isolation that are associated with genetically based breeds.

Other populations yield yet further illustrations of the importance of all three evaluations. Wild horses on Jarita Mesa in New Mexico are from an isolated region. A phenotypic evaluation showed the horses to be very uniform, but also very slightly "off type" for the usual Colonial Spanish horse herd. The deviations from usual type included the horses being somewhat shorter and having shorter heads with consistently plain and rounded muzzles. A close evaluation of the history of the herd pointed to the release of a herd of Welsh ponies into the area during the drought of the 1930s. DNA evidence pointed to the same conclusion of a relatively recent composite foundation. The intervening years of maintenance as a closed population resulted in a very uniform population of handsome horses, although with nothing to offer to the conservation of the Colonial Spanish horse.

A more reassuring study involved the feral horses on Fort Polk in Louisiana. These have a long history of isolation, with a few hints of introgression from Tennessee Walking horses. The history is therefore somewhat problematic, but that is common among feral horse herds. The external type of many of the horses is an Iberian type, making the herd a candidate herd as Colonial Spanish horses. This, however, would be unusual given the location of

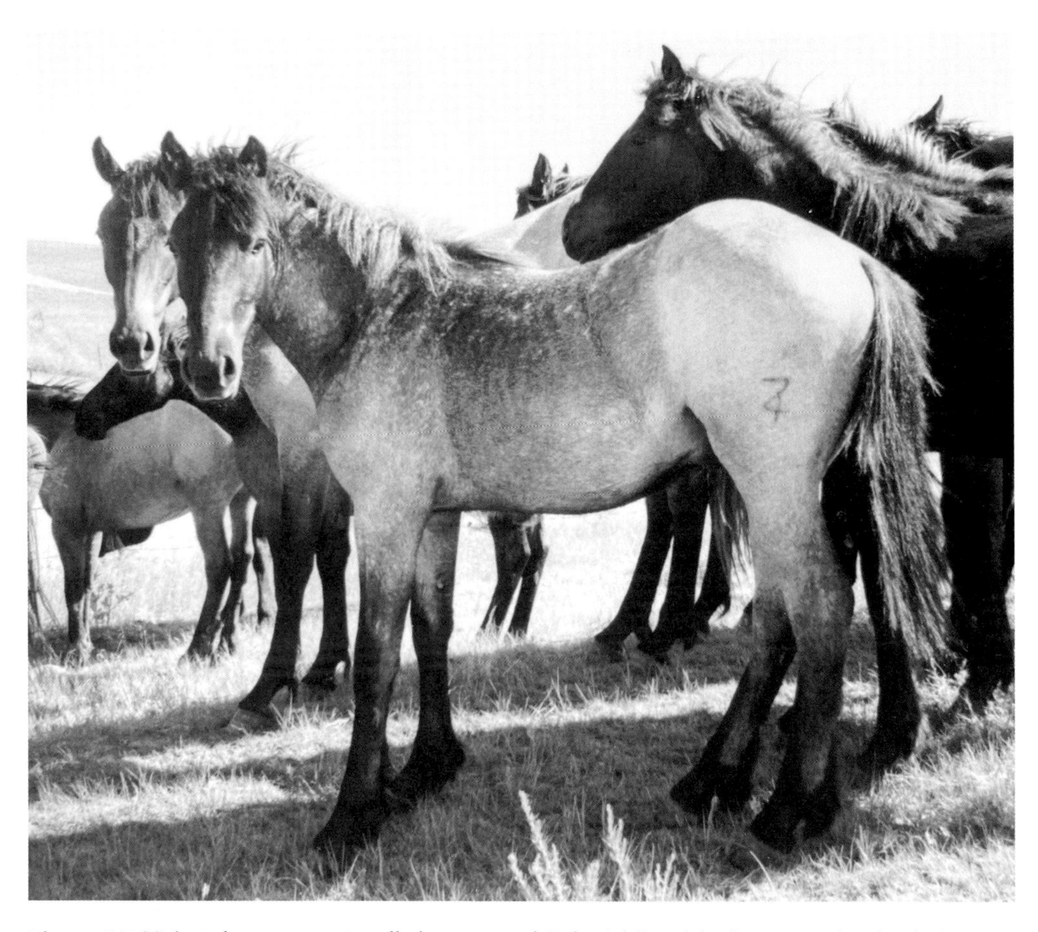

Figure 4.5 Nokota horses occasionally have a good Colonial Spanish phenotype despite their mixed foundation. Photo by DPS.

the horses and the long period since the 1830s in which the Spanish and Native American human influences in the region were minimized. However, DNA studies grouped the horses very cleanly and strongly in the Colonial Spanish group, with a somewhat surprising close connection to Caribbean horses that tend to betray very strong links to Iberia. These Fort Polk horses therefore emerge as a high priority candidate for conservation.

In contrast to horses and sheep, the phenotypic traits of interest in goats are nearly all on the head (Figure 4.6). The matrix approach to phenotypic evaluation still proves useful, though. Goats that score as typically Spanish in the USA have had their DNA compared to others of similar type in Mexico, Central America, and South America. These phenotypically similar goats are all indeed genetically similar, and are a high priority for conservation.

While less formal than a matrix, the evaluation of Texas Longhorns by the Cattlemen's Texas Longhorn Registry (CTLR) also yielded a highly accurate result that has been validated by genetic results. The CTLR characterizes the pursuit of breed purity as "Longhorn versus Wronghorn." A number of characteristics help to identify authentic Texas Longhorns that have an Iberian origin, and to distinguish them from cattle that are more recently crossbred

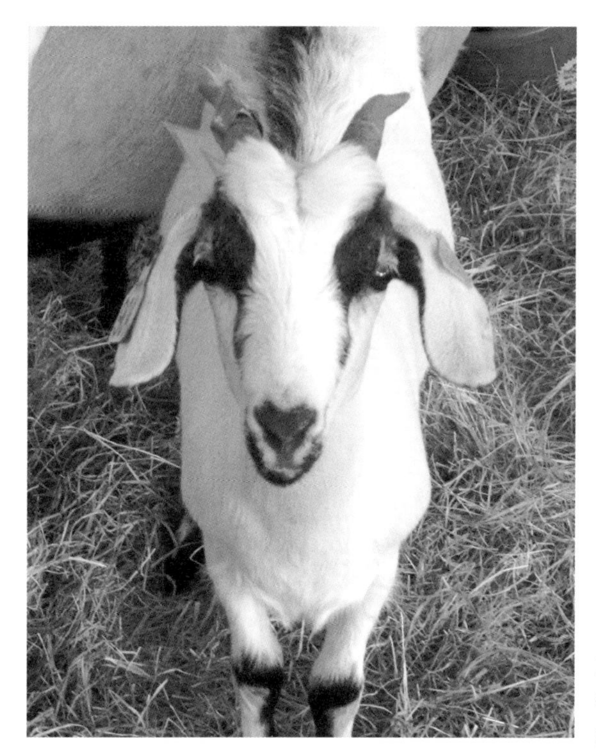

Figure 4.6 Head and ear conformation is especially useful when evaluating Spanish goats. Photo by DPS.

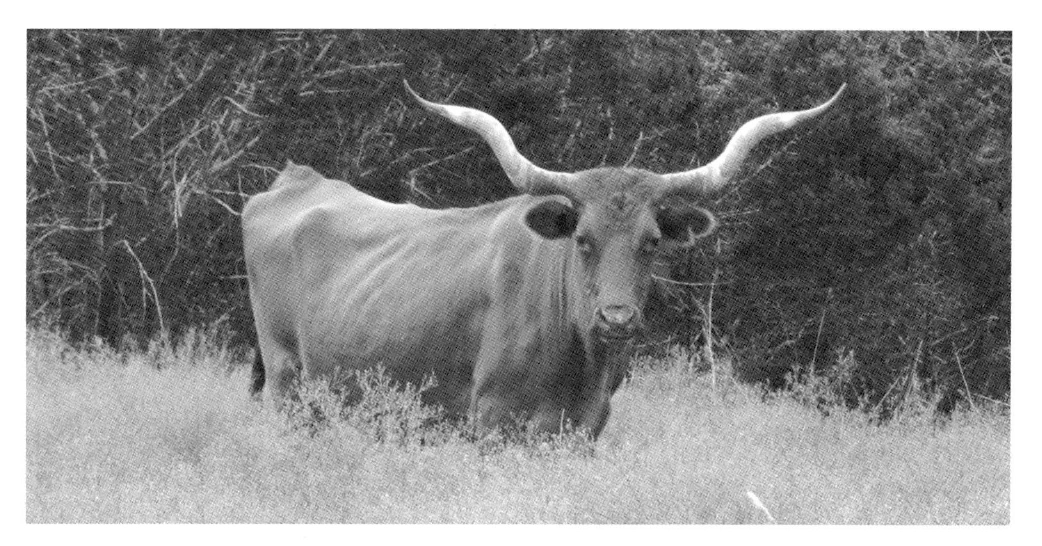

Figure 4.7 The distinctively Iberian character of Texas Longhorns is expressed throughout the body, but especially in the head. Photo by JB.

(Figure 4.7). One striking difference is the horns, but heads, legs, tails, and ears also have contributions to make in the final analysis. The "Wronghorns" have a foundation in the Texas Longhorn, but have also included influences from breeds such as Ankole, Africander, English Longhorn, and Hereford to create specimens with enormous horns. Wronghorns are very popular because of their impressive heads, but they are no longer genetically typical historic Texas Longhorns. One especially consistent finding is that Longhorn cows and steers have relatively narrow skulls, and usually have a typical twist to their horns as they mature.

It is wise to decide about the inclusion or exclusion of rare variants such as color or horn status early in the process of breed definition, and it is important to remember that the single genetic alleles that cause these variants occurred long before breeds were developed. It is especially common to have variation in these characteristics in landraces. These variants pre-date breeds, and can easily be shared among several breeds. Put another way, the presence of these variants in some animals of a breed does not necessarily indicate that there has been crossbreeding in the past. Instead they are a reminder that almost all of today's breeds descend from groups of animals with more variation than is typical of today's standardized breeds. One example is the presence of a small number of polled cattle in older, pre-registry herds of Texas Longhorns. Due to the exclusion of polled cattle from registered populations, this variant is now extinct in the breed. In contrast, the Shorthorn breed has always included polled animals, despite the breed name. They have persisted, and today have become the most common phenotype in the breed.

Many breeders jump to the conclusion that recessive phenotypes that pop out as surprises are always the result of fraudulent introgression from crossbreeding. Introgression can and does happen, and always detracts from breeds as genetic resources. It is also true that nearly all breeds, all the way from landraces to industrial strains, harbor recessive genes that can dramatically change color or horn type without fundamentally changing the underlying functional breed package. In suspect cases, DNA analysis should quickly put to rest any question of crossbreeding. For rare breeds especially, it is important not to jump to the conclusion that recessive variants are the result of crossbreeding, because eliminating these animals can also eliminate the genetic variation needed for future breed viability. Nearly all breeds have recessive traits that crop up as surprises from time to time. The question facing conservation breeders is just what to do with these when they do occur.

Randall Lineback cattle provide a good example of variation popping up as a surprise. All of the founders of the current breed were black and white. After several years of breed rescue and conservation breeding, red and white calves began to appear. Rather than reflecting any crossbreeding, these were in fact consistent with the longer-term history of the breed, which always included red and white in addition to the more common black and white cattle. In this case, the genetic code for red is recessive, and can be carried along for several generations while hiding under the black-based color of most of the cattle.

DNA analysis is useful in laying to rest some of the doubt that rare variants can incite, but in rare breeds DNA analysis can occasionally be misleading. A specific situation arises in several rare breeds when DNA is used for inclusion or exclusion of candidate animals or herds. If a candidate herd has been isolated for several decades from the rest of the breed, founder effects as well as genetic drift can lead to genetic differences. If the DNA profile of the breed has been defined from only a portion of the breed, then isolated groups may have been excluded from that documentation. These groups can be different enough to lead to their exclusion, despite their being truly of the breed by foundation and isolation. As a result, the best analysis includes history, physical evaluation of phenotype, and DNA investigations. All three must be used in concert, and must be used wisely, because each is subject to error if used in isolation.

Inclusion of foundation stock for breeds should ideally be as free from political agenda as is possible. It is all too common for landrace herd books to be closed prematurely, before all representative individual animals have been included. This is greatly to the detriment of the breed over the long term, and is an approach to avoid. The most common situation is for politically powerful individuals to favor inclusion of only their own animals, and to exclude influences from other herds that can often be essential for long-term breed survival.

It is important to keep in mind that breeds exist independently of social constructs like registries and associations. Breeds reflect their unique combination of foundation, isolation, and selection. The process of recognition and definition is ideally one of describing what is actually present, rather than imposing any sort of constraint from the outside. Breeds are breeds, regardless of whether or not they are recognized as such. The main goal of defining and officially recognizing them is to assure their survival.

4.2 *One Breed or Two*

Splitting and branching from a root of domestication have produced the breeds of today. That process continues within breeds, and if the relationships are taken below the breed level the branches are usually referred to as bloodlines, strains, or varieties. These are all generally considered to be subunits within the single breed, but are distinct enough by history, genetics, or phenotype to warrant some additional identification.

The mental picture of a tree of breed groups, breeds, varieties, and strains is useful in pointing out a very real and confusing issue in breed definition. At what point along a branch should populations be considered distinct enough for independent maintenance and conservation? This question has no easy answer, because the answer is rooted not only in biology but also in the political and cultural environment surrounding breeds. One useful strategy is to link together into one breed those populations that are more like one another than they are like any other breed. This strategy includes in a breed some close cousin populations that have been separated for only a short while. Decisions to group together or split apart should be based mostly on the similarity of the animals to one another, their distinctiveness from other breed resources, and the likelihood of successful persistence and viability of the population. Politics or personal preferences should have minimal influence in these decisions.

Pineywoods cattle can serve as an example of the difficulties encountered in deciding to group or to split (Figure 4.8). Pineywoods cattle persisted in the hands of a very few dedicated breeders whose numbers dwindled in the last half of the 1900s. As a result of fewer and fewer breeders, the herds became increasingly isolated from one another, both geographically and genetically. By the late 1900s the few remaining herds had histories of complete isolation for several decades, and in most instances over a century or more. In one sense, each could have been considered to be a separate breed and each could have then been managed separately in order to maintain the historic genetic isolation. However, the resulting lines would have been critically endangered. All of them would be in peril of extinction due to low numbers and unavoidable inbreeding depression.

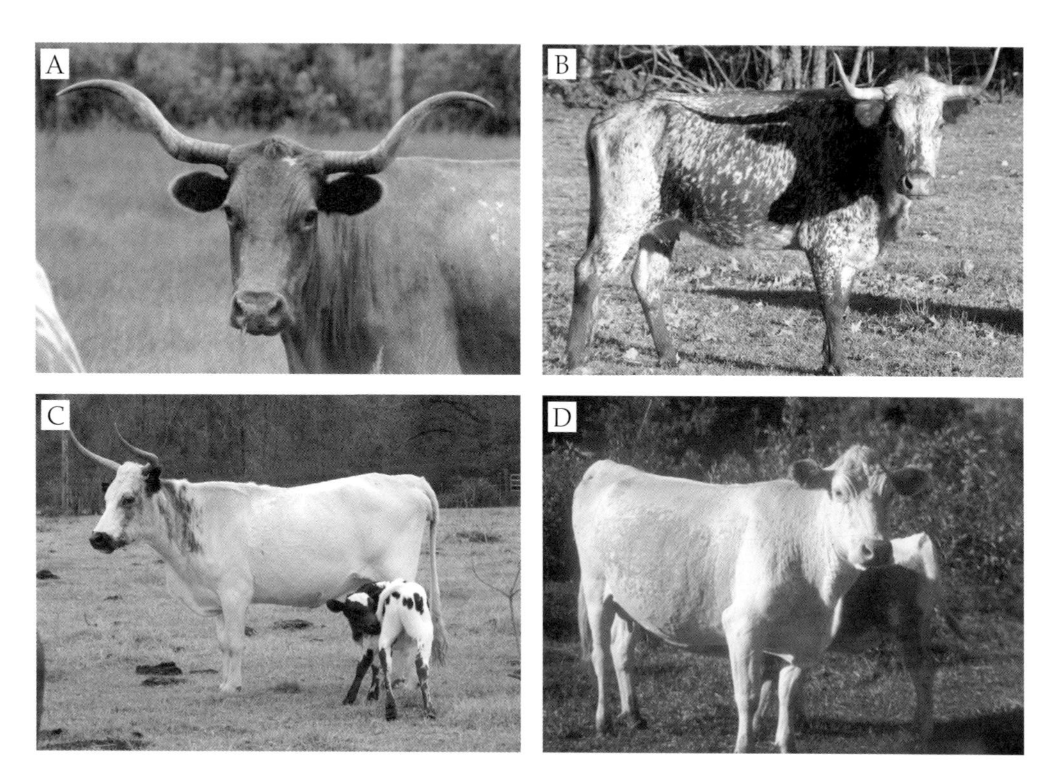

Figure 4.8 While differences exist among the strains of Pineywoods cattle, they are all much more like one another than they are like any other breeds in the region. These cattle come from Griffin (A), Conway (B), Hickman (C), and Barnes (D) stock, isolated from one another for a century, but still similar due to a common foundation. Photo A by Jess Brown, Cowpen Creek, B and D by DPS, C by JB.

All of the different strains of Pineywoods cattle have historic links to a single earlier population of humpless cattle in the Southeastern USA. That origin led to a similar phenotype across all the strains, and a phenotype that was unlikely to be confused with later introductions of zebu (humped) or northern European (nonhumped) cattle. Grouping the strains together in a single breed makes it easier to manage the population for viability into the distant future, while at the same time not endangering the distinctive characteristics of the cattle.

The answer to the question, "At what level to group?" is never simple. In some situations closely related breeds are kept separate by registration in separate herd books due to the history and politics of the breeds involved. Examples are the Dales and Fell ponies from England. In other situations, history and phenotype consolidate considerable variation into a single landrace breed group, such as the Colonial Spanish horse group, which has strains as geographically diverse as Marsh Tacky, Florida Cracker, Choctaw, Wilbur-Cruce, and Baca horses.

Dog breeds within a single breed group are also perplexing examples of just exactly where to lump and where to split. Small terriers tend to share relationships, some of them quite recently. Likewise, most of the retrievers are fairly alike if subtle differences of coat and color are disregarded. Large hounds, especially coonhounds, represent a similar

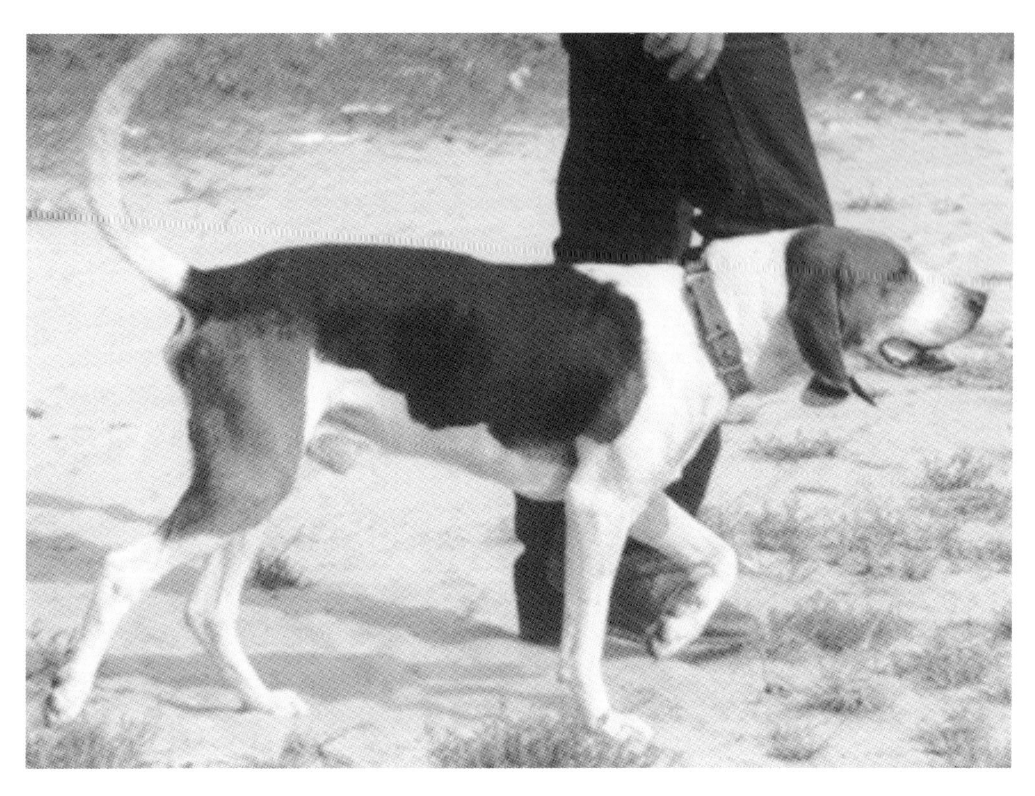

Figure 4.9 Coonhounds in the USA nearly all descend from a single genetic pool, with later differentiation into breeds based on color. Photo by DPS.

phenomenon. Coonhounds, other than the Blue Tick, all originate from a single early gene pool from which the various colors were subsequently standardized into separate breeds. The recent common origin of these has resulted in a fairly similar size, type, and function for all of them (Figure 4.9). The Belgian group of herding dogs is another good example. All of the different coat types and colors are considered one breed in Europe, while each is viewed as a different breed in the USA. Exactly where to establish firm breed boundaries can be tricky and somewhat subjective. Drawing these boundaries needs to be done with appreciation for not only distinctions, but also commonalities. Breed boundaries also need to account for the likelihood of long-term breed survival, especially when population sizes are small.

Poultry present yet more challenges in breed definition. Poultry breeds are placed into large groups by their geographic origins, but are then split into breeds by overall body type. Many breeds are further split into varieties that vary from one another in details such as comb type or color. At a superficial glance, this leads to the assumption that the varieties within a breed are different from one another by traits caused by single, or a few, genes. In many breeds this is not the case. While some varieties within a single breed are indeed closely related, others share very little by way of foundation.

Wyandotte chickens are in the American breed group. The Silver Laced Wyandotte variety was derived from crosses of local birds with influences from Silver Hamburgs, Dark

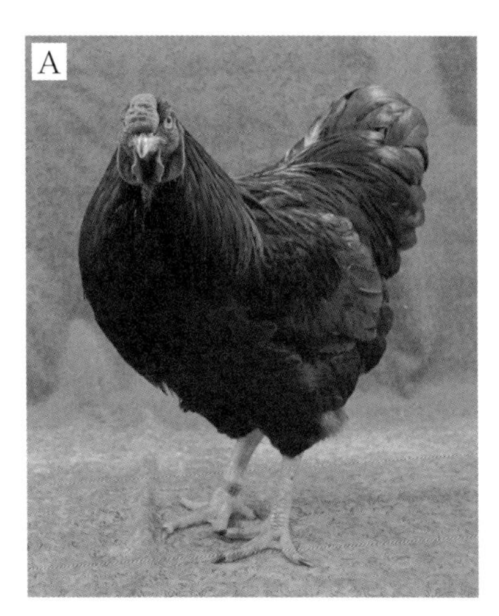

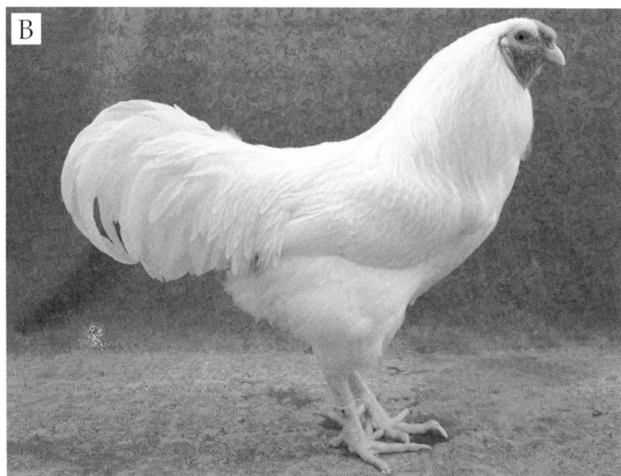

Figure 4.10 The different color varieties of Chantecler chickens, including Partridge (A) and White (B), share very little common genetic background, despite their superficial resemblance one to another. Photos by JB.

Brahmas, and a few others. White and Black Wyandottes descend from the Silver Laced as sports (mutants), so these are three closely related varieties that share a common foundation. The Golden Laced Wyandotte, in contrast, hails from crosses of Partridge Cochin, Brown Leghorn, Buff Cochin, and Golden Sebright, a different foundation from the previous three varieties. The Partridge Wyandotte comes from crosses of Cochin and Cornish stock. Buff, Silver Penciled, Columbian, and Blue varieties also have different origins. Each of these varieties, aside from color, resembles the others closely in size and type, despite the underlying genetic differences due to the vastly different foundations. The result is that within this one breed, some varieties are close kin while others are only distantly related.

The three varieties of Chantecler (White, Partridge, and Buff) share minimal common genetic ancestry with one another despite their similar size, comb type, and production characteristics (Figure 4.10). Their similarities are nearly all from selection, and not from a common foundation. For poultry especially, it is necessary for conservation breeders to be very familiar with their breed of choice and the relationships between the varieties. In many breeds, some varieties are as distinct from one another as whole breeds would be in other species.

4.3 *Breed Histories*

Understanding breed history is essential if breeders are to adequately steward breeds as genetic resources. Each breed has been shaped into its current form by a unique history. Breed histories must be as clear and accurate as possible. Clarity is essential because most breed origins are at least somewhat obscure and shrouded in mystery. Nearly all breeds claim to have originated long ago in the mists of time and are consequently "one of the oldest pure breeds in existence." This is clearly not true of most breeds. Understanding the relationships of the breed, the influences of its foundation, its early and present environment, and the history of selection pressures can help to guide successful management and conservation of breeds as genetic resources.

Breed history should accurately reflect the source of founders and the way in which they contribute to the current breed. What founders were involved? Were outside influences common or rare? How did selection produce the animals that survive today? In what environment did the breed take form? For what purpose was the breed developed? Each of these is a key aspect in forging a breed as a genetic resource, and each should influence decisions for breed maintenance and conservation.

Breed histories can be complicated. Most of them involve a reasonably well-documented early foundation. Then, in the case of many rare breeds, a period ensues in which very little is documented or known. If the breed had remained popular, then it is obvious that people would have taken more interest in documenting what was happening. A breed often slips into rarity because people quit caring about its fate, with the result that many unique and useful rare breeds have lapses in their history.

Examples of breed histories with gaps in the middle include the Colonial Spanish horses and Florida Cracker cattle. In both cases an exciting amount of detail is known about the founding events, even though these occurred centuries ago. Details also tend to be known about the expansion of these breeds as they became numerous into the 1800s. Then silence falls on documentation for a century until recent conservation efforts began. Today's conservationists are only able to focus on the few traditional family lines that have survived from those earlier large populations. It is from these alone that the present-day breeds descend. Breeds such as the Texas Longhorn do indeed go back to the millions of such cattle on the plains of Texas in 1850, but only do so through a limited number of family lines, each of which has become a bottleneck and a small sample of those original huge populations. Understanding history can help breeders to manage and conserve these breeds more effectively. The histories of these breeds are very different from one in which a wider sample of numerous ancestral lines persists to the present.

4.4 Geography and Source Herds

Geography can play a large role in discovering and identifying source herds for many breeds. This is especially true for landrace breeds, which present complicated conservation challenges. The original geographic region of a landrace is likely to provide newly discovered herds, while regions outside of the geographic region are very unlikely discovery sites. The Tennessee Myotonic goat can serve as a useful example. Herds of traditionally managed goats survive in Middle Tennessee. Their owners persist outside of the formal structure of breed associations and registries. A typical Tennessee Myotonic goat is much more likely to pop up unannounced from this region than it is from northern Idaho, especially when considering historic documentation of the herd's foundation and other details of its lineage.

The link of geography and landraces is essential to their status as genetic resources because they were forged for adaptation in specific environments. Taking geography into account when considering "found" or newly discovered herds or individual animals is therefore appropriate and helpful in bringing these animals into conservation programs. The link between geography and genetic resources can also point to regions where active

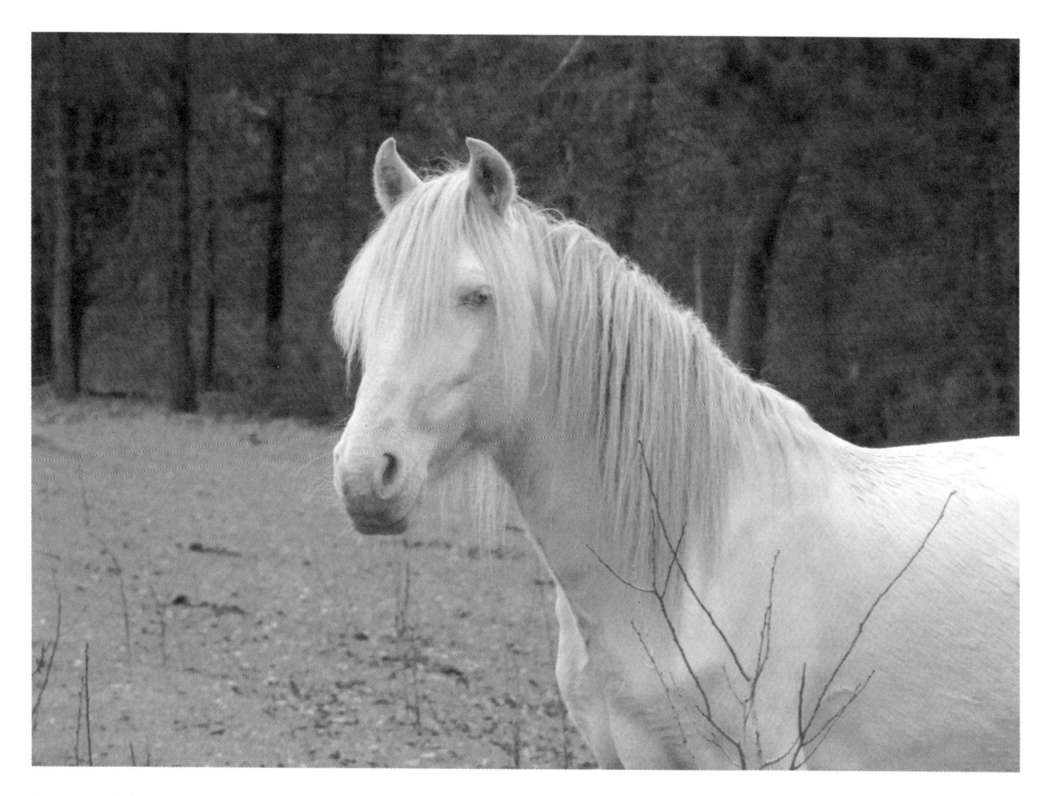

Figure 4.11 Pine Tacky horses, from Mississippi, hail from the same origin as Choctaw horses in Oklahoma. Photo by JB.

searches are needed to identify any remaining isolated and overlooked herds of landraces so that they can be brought into effective conservation programs. An example demonstrating success using a geographic approach to conservation work is the rediscovery of the Baca and Mount Taylor strains of Colonial Spanish horses in New Mexico, right where the hub of the diffusion of this important North American breed occurred.

A second equine example is the discovery of Pine Tacky horses in Mississippi, Fort Polk horses in Louisiana, and their relationship to Choctaw horses in Oklahoma (Figure 4.11). Mississippi was the original homeland of the Choctaw nation before forced removal to Oklahoma in the 1830s, and so it is logical that a few isolated pockets of the horses might have survived in this area. The discovery of a few horses of appropriate type was followed by DNA validation, allowing them to be used in conservation programs.

History, geography, and genetics usually all go hand-in-hand for effective breed definition and breed conservation. All avenues should be thoroughly explored in order to ferret out what is most likely to be true, and most likely to result in meaningful conservation of legitimate genetic resources.

4.5 Recovery of Purebred Animals into Registries

While inclusion of "recovery" or "rescue" animals into breeds can be controversial, the goal of breed associations should be the inclusion of all purebred representatives of the breed on equal footing. From time to time situations occur in which registrations have lapsed, but the pure breeding of a group has been maintained. Often this is due to owner laxity or outright laziness, and in these situations, it can be annoying to reward such behavior by including these animals back into purebred populations. Recovering animals can be controversial, and one way to view this is to reflect on the relationship of a breed, its association, and its registry. The breed has an independent existence outside of the human constructs of association and registry. The association and registry should have the goal of stewarding this independent entity, and not serving as a restrictive point such that the breed's existence becomes secondary to the association instead of primary to it.

Advocates of rescuing any lapsed herds do need to assure the purebred status of the candidate populations. This can be done using their history. The ideal history is one in which a purebred foundation has simply lapsed in registration, but has been maintained in isolation since its origin in purebred animals. Each recovery is different, and general rules can fail to achieve a wise outcome in some specific situations. Each case must be considered individually, with the goal of assuring a good outcome for breed conservation. A few examples of situations requiring different approaches can be given.

One example involves a flock of 3000 Leicester Longwool sheep that are kept in New Zealand under commercial management practices. The flock ceased registration, but continued purebred breeding. In this situation the potential benefit to a rare breed is significant because no other flocks of this size still exist within the registered populations of this breed. Additionally, at least in New Zealand, no other breeds could easily be confused with Leicester Longwools. This assures that mistaken inclusion of crossbred animals is highly unlikely. For this case, it makes sense to inspect the entire flock to validate that the appearance of the sheep is consistent with the history of being purebred Leicester Longwools. If the flock consists of sheep that consistently look like Leicester Longwools, then they no doubt are. The flock could then be recovered into the flock book. This could be done for all sheep in the flock, or for a select representative sample. In either case the breed would benefit from the inclusion of Leicester Longwool sheep that had several generations of selection for commercial production.

A second case involves a herd of Dexter cattle in the USA that descends from early Irish and English imports. The herd was founded on five cows and two bulls, and has been closed since the 1970s. The herd now has about 40 animals. In this situation, an accurate assessment has been possible with DNA technology. A population with this history should have a high degree of genetic consistency, and should only have variants typical of Dexter cattle (barring any role of genetic drift and founder effect). At the very least, any crossbreeding should be easily detected. Herds such as this that pass both a visual and genetic inspection offer a great benefit to what is otherwise a very small population of Dexter cattle that go back to this unique foundation.

Other recoveries are more difficult. Several years ago a breeder of Milking Devon cattle died suddenly from a heart attack. Unfortunately, the last few calf crops had not been ear

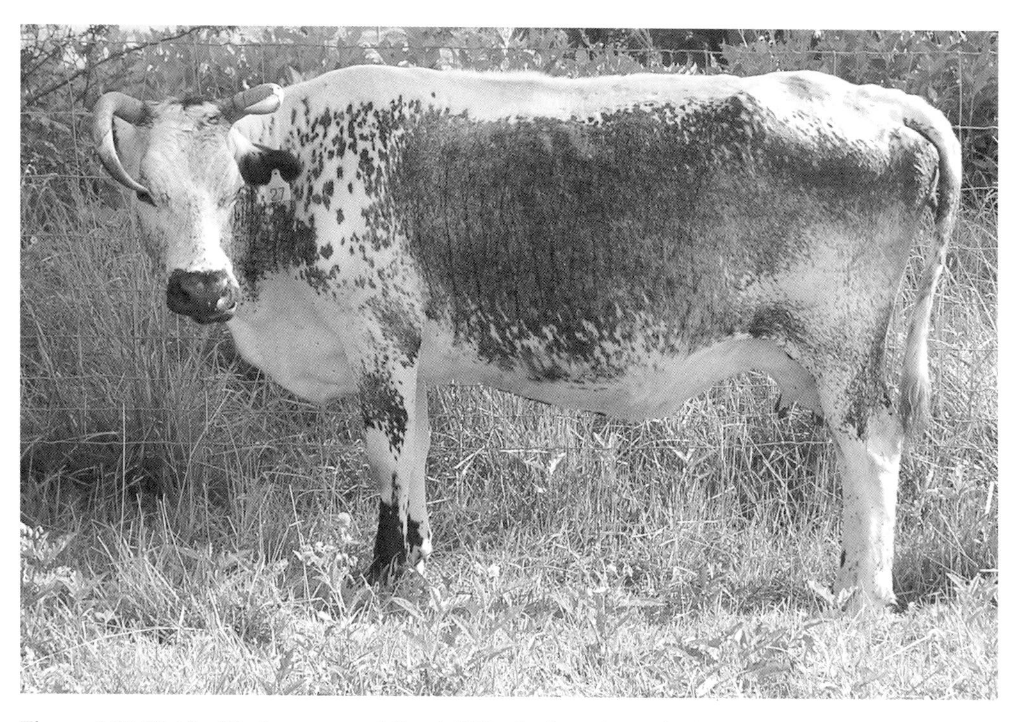

Figure 4.12 Unidentified or untraced Randall Lineback cattle, and other breeds with low levels of genetic variation, can easily be recovered as purebreds by DNA validation. Photo by DPS.

tagged, and so could not be connected back to registration certificates. While the full impact of this was only revealed years later, had other breeders been alerted sooner it would have been possible to sort out pedigrees and individual identities from DNA investigations of calves and cows. After the passage of time, and more generations of undocumented breeding, this becomes less and less likely to succeed. In this situation the cattle were lost to the breed.

In another example, the owners of a flock of elite Lincoln sheep faced various challenges, such that the flock was essentially feral for six years. In this situation the genetics were known and had definitely been isolated. Even though pedigree information was sketchy at best, the type and background of the animals argued strongly for renewed inclusion into the registered population.

The Postell bloodline of Marsh Tacky horses was recovered back into the breed following detective work using breeding calendars and memories of family members and friends that were able to piece together pedigrees on the horses. This established the purity of the horses, and enabled their inclusion in conservation breeding programs.

Recovery efforts for some breeds, such as the Randall Lineback, benefit from the fact that the cattle are distinctive and have very limited genetic variation (Figure 4.12). In this case, evaluating DNA can quickly validate cattle as purebred or not, even if specific pedigrees are difficult or impossible to reconstruct.

Recovery efforts such as these are important because the animals involved can have genetics that are distinct from the remainder of the breed. This means that they can play a constructive role in breed conservation and maintenance, but their inclusion must only occur after assurances that the animals are indeed purebred. It is also important to avoid a few traps that can seem logical at the outset but that have negative consequences. Some breed associations have recovery programs where the qualifying animals are required to be mated to registered stock for multiple generations before being fully accepted into the herd book. This essentially imposes a system of upgrading these recovered animals, and ends up replacing their unique genetics with the genetics of what is already registered within the breed. The important issue here is that the recovered animals are either purebred or not. If they are purebred, then they need to be fully accepted into the breed, and not relegated to some sort of second-class status that precludes their making the maximum contribution possible for breed vitality and viability.

4.5.1 *Native on Appearance*

A few breed associations have adopted a procedure known as "native on appearance," which allows animals with the breed phenotype to be included in the registry. Often this is not accompanied by any sort of investigation of history or genetics, and the procedure stands on its own.

In many associations the acceptance of an animal that is native on appearance comes along with further stipulations on how that animal and its descendants must be bred for at least a generation and sometimes for several generations. If an animal is accepted but then, along with its descendants, must be mated to purebred animals for several generations, this is essentially an upgrading program. This does work to protect the breed's integrity, but also diminishes any potential benefit from including a truly purebred animal that is native on appearance. The opposite situation, of simply accepting such an animal on equal footing with those previously registered, has the exact opposite weaknesses and strengths: the risk of inclusion of an animal that is not truly purebred, or the potential and beneficial wide use of one that is indeed purebred.

The wisdom of accepting animals with a breed phenotype varies considerably from breed to breed and depends on a host of factors. Breeds that are numerous and variable have little to gain from this strategy, although equally, little to lose. Breeds with small numbers have a great deal to gain from any purebreds that are located and accepted, and a great deal to lose if animals that are not purebred simply "look right."

At the core of deciding whether or not this is an appropriate approach are the various details of the breed in question. A major issue is the phenotypic uniqueness of the breed, and the ease with which it could be confused with other breeds. Extreme phenotypes generally cannot be achieved by anything short of pure breeding, and there are examples in most species, including Mammoth Jackstock donkeys (Figure 4.13), Ankole cattle, African geese, Chinese geese, Brahma chickens, Myotonic goats, and Flemish Giant rabbits. Candidate animals from breeds with less distinctive phenotypes should likely be investigated a bit more thoroughly than a simple external evaluation.

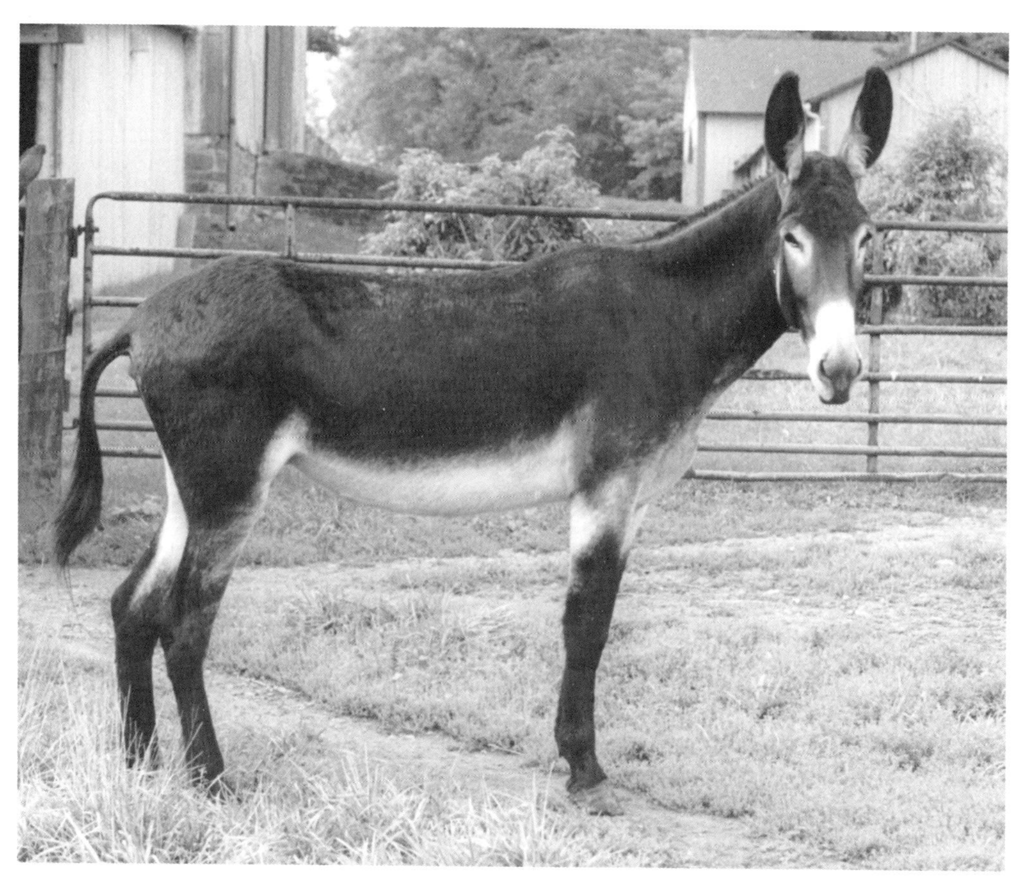

Figure 4.13 The extreme phenotype of a Mammoth Jackstock donkey cannot be duplicated by other breeds. Photo by Mary Ellen Nicholas.

CHAPTER 5

Breed Standards

A breed standard is a formal description of the ideal animal in a specific breed, and is therefore an important tool in breed management and conservation. Breed standards straddle a delicate line between reflecting the actual animals within the breed, while also being a target to aim for as breeders strive for excellence. Balancing these aims depends on the general sort of breed being described.

5.1 Breed Type

"Breed type" is difficult to define but includes all aspects that make each breed unique. "Type traits" are those characteristics that set one breed apart from others in the same species. The individual animals of any breed vary in "typiness," which is the relative degree to which individuals express their breed's type traits, and therefore represent the breed and accurately reflect the breed's uniqueness within the species. Animals that strongly express their breed type are generally referred to as "typey" and are difficult to misclassify into a breed other than their own due to their strong expression of breed-specific characteristics (Figure 5.1). Most breeds also have animals with a somewhat weaker expression of breed type, and although these must be managed carefully, they should not necessarily be eliminated from breeding.

Each breed has a unique combination of appearance, performance, and behavior. Superficial elements, such as color, size, general shape, and conformational peculiarities, are the easiest to quantify and describe. A breed is much more than these, however, and behavioral, production, and adaptation traits are all important, even though they are difficult to describe. All of the repeatable traits of a breed go together to yield a "breed type" that reflects the overall appearance and ability of the breed.

Typey animals have a subtle but important overall appearance that stamps them as not simply random-bred. This is well illustrated in cats. A purebred American Domestic Shorthair cat has a harmonious smooth conformation that sets it apart from the more random-bred shorthaired cats that are commonly produced by unselected feral parents throughout the USA. The two are often confused in people's minds, but they are quite

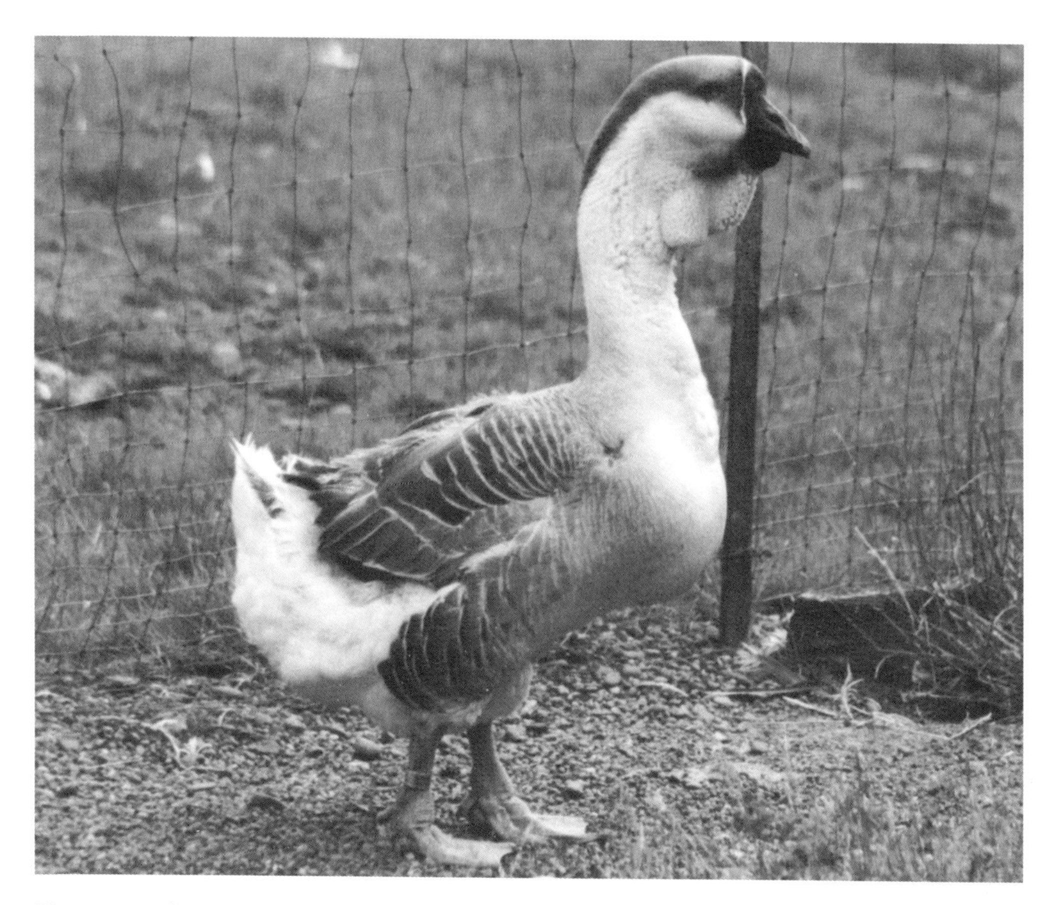

Figure 5.1 African geese have distinctive breed type traits and cannot be confused with any other goose breed. Photo by DPS.

different. One is a defined purebred betraying its status through an overall conformation and type that reflects its selected gene pool background. The other is a random-bred feral that is the product of whatever genetic influences happened to be combined. The type of the purebred American Domestic Shorthair reflects the conscious selection decisions made by cat owners over multiple generations.

Breed type is critically important to the conservation of a breed, and is a concept that is increasingly ignored in modern animal breeding and evaluation. The trend in most classes of production livestock is to encourage most or all breeds to converge onto a single generalized type. This trend is largely being driven by the industrialization of livestock and poultry breeding, and is a response to market pressures for large quantities of a narrowly consistent product. Warmblood horses, beef cattle, swine, and dairy goats are all good examples of classes of livestock where once unique breed types have tended to converge. The result has been that many animals of several breeds are now nearly identical for type, and the underlying uniqueness of the various breeds has been compromised. Most of this has been accomplished by selection, rather than by crossbreeding, but crossbreeding has certainly been used in some instances to erase breed type.

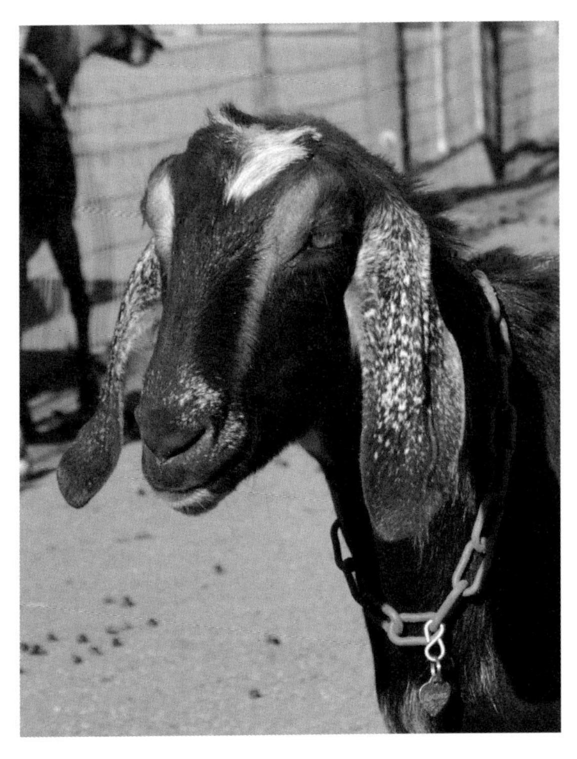

Figure 5.2 Nubian goats have not only distinctive type traits, but also production and behavioral characteristics that go along with these. Photo by JB.

An odd quirk of breed type for many species of livestock is that type centers on the head, which is generally the only part of the animal that is not directly consumed or shorn. Heads do, obviously, have importance in being the major thinking and food-gathering organs of the body, but have even further importance in revealing overall breed type. Head character, shape, and carriage are important signals of breed type in most species and are often the most breed-specific components of an animal. Horns and ears can be especially important in contributing to breed type, and while they are not directly involved in production, they are important clues to the genetic background and breed affiliation of animals. This is especially true when specific features of type are extreme, such as the short ears of LaMancha goats, the long ears of Nubian goats, the domed head of Gyr cattle, or the four horns of Jacob sheep.

Type traits set one breed as distinct from all others. Breed standards should emphasize these traits because they most accurately reflect the breed as a distinct genetic resource. Evaluation of type traits presents many observers with a philosophic problem because type traits are usually not production traits. However, the presence of type traits indicates breed identity quite clearly, and serves to indirectly predict production, behavioral, and adaptive characteristics associated with that breed.

Nubian goats betray their breed identity by their conformation and type traits, including a Roman nose, long ears, and dairy conformation (Figure 5.2). A buyer can expect a goat that has good fecundity, nonseasonal breeding, ample quantities of rich, sweet-tasting milk, that is minimally aggressive to other goats, and that vocalizes a lot. All of these characteristics form part of their breed identity. The external breed type has betrayed these characteristics to the observer, even though most of the traits of production interest have been delivered by the underlying genetic package that cannot be observed directly. A Texas Longhorn cow, in contrast, betrays her breed identity by horns, ears, body, and head conformation. That package of characteristics should ideally go with a cow likely to rebreed quickly after calving, raise calves well, forage well, and resist droughts well, and to do all of this over a very long life.

General traits of conformation, production, and soundness are more likely to be shared across breeds than type traits are. The more broadly shared traits are essential to animal function and well-being, and as a result these tend to receive considerable attention in breed standards even though they are not breed-specific. The boundary between general traits and type traits can be blurry, but they do overlap. Realizing the difference between type traits, soundness, and production traits as they relate to breed character can be essential in understanding how the breed standard relates to the maintenance of a breed. Soundness and production traits usually answer the question of "how good is this animal?" while type traits answer the question of "how typically does this animal represent this breed?" Those two questions are different, and confusing the two muddles breed distinctiveness and management. Both questions are essential when evaluating animals, but each question targets different information.

Although type traits are the most essential for breed character, it is also true that conformational and soundness traits are equally if not more important for production and longevity. With both sorts of traits it is important to allow some leeway for variation. It is important to put type traits in an appropriate context, and a very typey but poor-performing animal is of less value to a breed than a less typey animal with excellent performance. In either case, animals deviating greatly from the norm have little or no role in breed conservation or breed maintenance.

5.2 *Different Sorts of Breed Standards*

A good breed standard is an essential tool that greatly helps breeders to maintain and manage their animals as a genetic resource. The standard should be the mental picture that drives selection decisions by all breeders. The concept of standard can be a tricky one, and has important and distinct interactions with the various major classes of breeds. Standardized breeds, landraces, and island-based feral breeds need different sorts of standards.

Standardized breeds, logically, have a standard. The standard is indeed integral to the overall culture of breeding, and is nearly always an assumed underpinning of much of the breed community. Breeders of standardized breeds use breed standards alongside other major defining concepts to establish breed identity. The standard works alongside restrictions on registration requirements to shape the breed. Standards for most breeds are "prescriptive" and prescribe what the ideal animal should be. This ideal may or may not actually exist, but it is a target for all breeders to aim for. An example is the standard for Lincoln Longwool sheep (Figure 5.3), which prescribes a very specific combination of head shape, head carriage, color, leg conformation and placement, body size and style, and fleece characteristics. By the standard, the ideal Lincoln sheep can be seen as a single sheep, and this is the guide for breeders' selection decisions as they aim to produce that ideal Lincoln sheep.

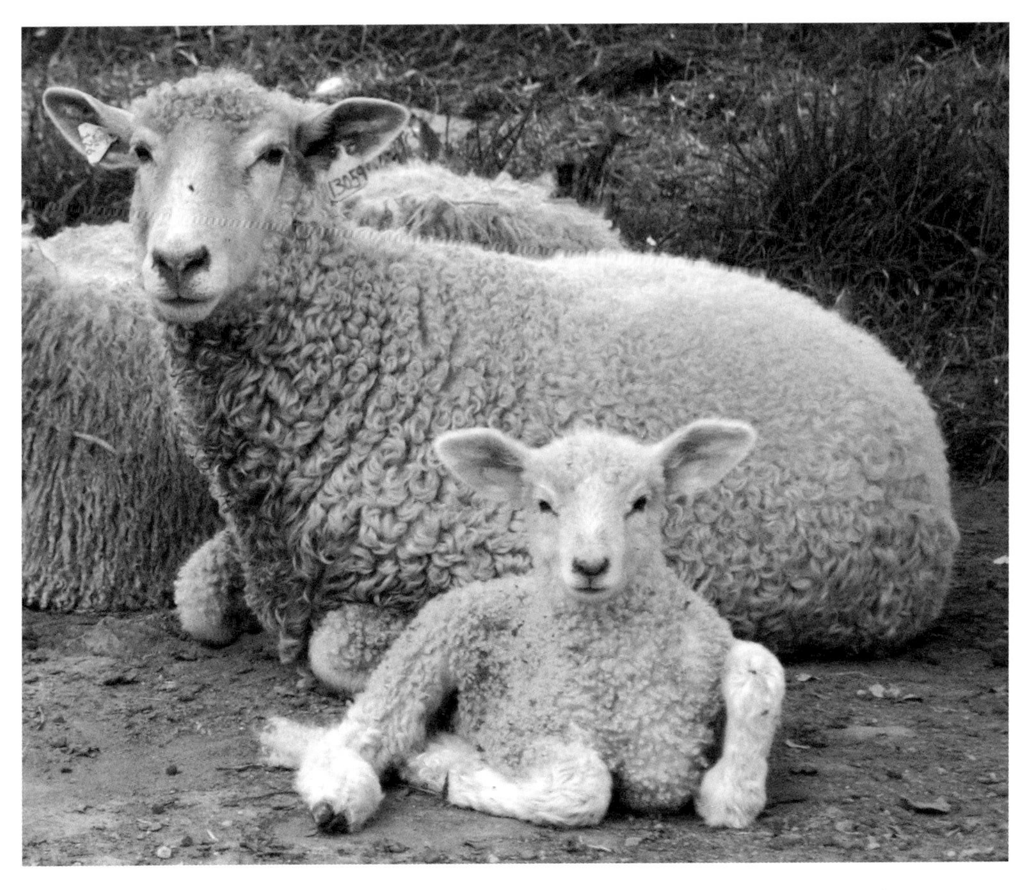

Figure 5.3 Lincoln Longwool sheep have a prescriptive breed standard that gives breeders a target to aim for in breeding programs. Photo by JB.

Nearly all dog breeds have a prescriptive standard that allows for minimal variation. This is a logical consequence of so few dog breeds being landraces or local breeds. However, in numerous cases the standardization has occurred through the process of gentrification. This process occurs distant from a breed's place of origin and is often used for purposes other than those for which the breed was originally developed. Afghan hounds, for example, are unlikely to be used for hunting in the USA, although that was their original purpose in Afghanistan. Often the dogs of the homeland encompass more variation than those that have been taken out of it. Color, coat type, and eye color are especially susceptible to standard definitions that are narrower than the actual range of variation present in dog breeds in their homelands.

The challenges of a prescriptive breed standard are well illustrated by the historic standards for some chicken breeds. Some poultry breeds have long had standards in which the color prescriptions for males and females could not be met by a single interbreeding population. In those cases breeders resorted to a strategy called "double mating." Show ring breeders have "male lines" ("cockerel breeders") to produce show males, and "female lines" ("pullet breeders") to produce show females. Males from one line and females from

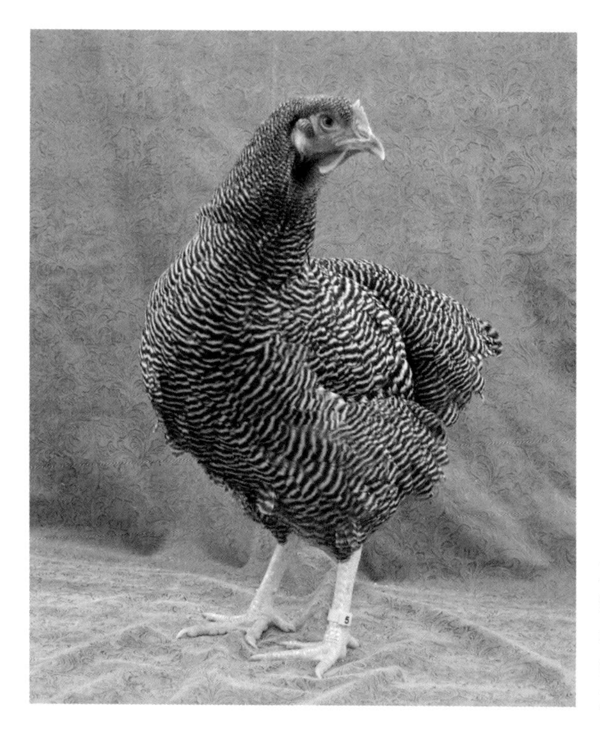

Figure 5.4 Barred Plymouth Rock color is ideally the same very uniform bars on males and females, yet this is impossible to attain in a single breeding population. Photo by JB.

the other were put together in show pens in order to assure winning groups at shows (Figure 5.4). The two lines were never crossed, because the females of the male line and the males of the female line failed to meet breed standards. These off-standard birds were essential to produce the show winners of the opposite sex. Experienced breeders realized that this prescriptive approach did not reflect the reality of the breeding yard, because single populations could not meet the standard. A more descriptive standard would have allowed for the males to be appropriate for females of the same breeding line. Some clubs of specific breeds have now changed their standards to reflect the reality of the type within a single true breeding population.

In many cases, poultry breed standards have also confused the definition of the breed with the external appearance only and with no consideration of the underlying foundation, isolation, and selection essential to the character of any breed. Creative breeders have, in some rare cases, been able to win at the shows by blending a range of parental birds of different breeds that produces the package described by the standard. They show these birds as representatives of a breed with which they have no or little connection. This practice does little to promote effective breed conservation, but it is important to note that it would not be considered fraudulent given the widespread ideas that surround the definition and standardization of poultry breeds. This occurs for rabbit breeds as well.

In contrast to prescriptive standards, the best breed standards for landraces are "descriptive." This sort of standard describes what the animals actually are rather than prescribing what they should be. This is subtly different from a prescriptive standard, but understanding this difference is essential if the genetic variability within landraces is to be successfully conserved. While standards for standardized breeds select a target to aim

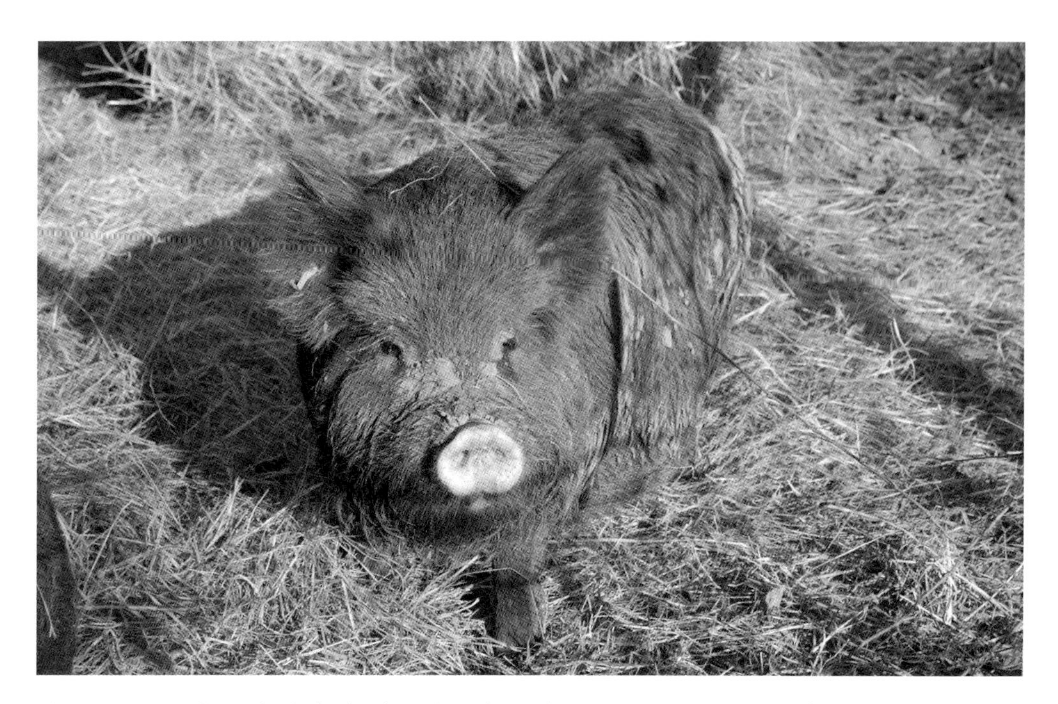

Figure 5.5 Breed standards for landrace breeds, such as Guinea Hogs, walk a fine line between describing allowable variation while also assuring enough consistency to reflect traditional heritage. Blue Guinea Hogs are a rare variant historically present in the breed. Photo by JB.

for, standards (or descriptions) of landraces are often used to either include or eliminate animals from participation in the breed.

Making a descriptive standard is more difficult than making a prescriptive one because most breeders are interested in some degree of uniformity and superiority for their animals. These goals can tug against the variability inherent in landraces. An example of descriptive standards is used by breeders of Colonial Spanish horses within the Spanish Mustang Registry, Horse of the Americas, and Southwest Spanish Mustang Association. These standards give a range of types varying from a heavier, generally northern, type and a lighter, generally southern, type, with a range of variation between these extremes. The Colonial Spanish horse matrix score sheet for type includes acceptable variation in such details as head shape (see Appendix 1). A range, rather than a specific single type, is appropriate for this landrace breed. The ideal Colonial Spanish horse is not a single horse but instead fits within a range of acceptable types that accurately reflects the genetic origin of the breed.

One problem with descriptive standards is that they do allow variation. Many local and landrace breeds have had situations where rare variants within the acceptable range became the target of fads among breeders and thereby increased in popularity and frequency. This changes the original and traditional form of the breed as the rare variant becomes more common at the expense of those that were frequent in the original breed. This is especially likely with color traits, such as moon spots or blue eyes in Myotonic goats, or red or blue coat color in Guinea Hogs (Figure 5.5). Color traits in historically white breeds of sheep also fit in here, as does the polled variant of Criollo Argentino cattle. Each of these traits occurred at low frequencies in the original traditional breeds. Selection can change the frequency, and thereby subtly or even radically change the character of the breed. The challenge is to allow these variants to persist without having them overwhelm the rest of the breed when some breeders focus on them as desirable only because they are unusual.

A potential problem with landrace standards is that including the more divergent foundation strains under a single breed umbrella does not always sit well with the very folks that saved the divergent strains in the first place. This can seem something of a paradox, as these are the very people who should be most interested in the conservation of the breed. Breeders of the various strains are likely to consider their own strain as the only strain that is a true representation of the breed. These important breeders often feel that including strains other than their own diminishes, rather than enhances, conservation, to the extent that some traditional breeders refuse to participate in any effort that includes more than their specific strain. To succeed as effective conservation tools, the standards for landraces must address these concerns and must be clear to define acceptable ranges of variation. The standard must be specific in describing allowable variation so that it does not become so vague as to be overly inclusive. At that point, the standard is not useful for weeding out variation that is outside the limits of the landrace. Standards can specifically address strain-to-strain variation if that helps to communicate the essence of the breed.

It is important to realize that most landraces and other local breeds existed before a breed standard was created for them. This is an essential detail if important variants are not to be lost for future generations. Standards for landraces must allow more variation than those for standardized breeds, even though most landraces eventually move toward standardization. They can lose much in this transition. People that design a standard for a landrace breed need to be specific enough to safeguard the status of the landrace as a genetic resource while not being overly strict and thereby excluding legitimate variation. Breed standards (or descriptions) for landraces are useful in accepting or eliminating candidate animals for inclusion into the breed. This is an important function, and the best standards for landraces address this specifically. The standard can serve to protect the breed from introgression while at the same time allowing newly discovered sources of the landrace to be fully included.

The standard for St. Croix sheep from one of the breed associations is an example of a breed standard that recognizes only a portion of the variation in the original breed (Figure 5.6). The standard calls for white, polled sheep. However, on the island of St. Croix the local hair sheep vary considerably in color. They also occasionally have horns. When the sheep were first brought to the mainland USA, only white, polled sheep were included, and the breed standard reflects that uniformity. The other variants still do appear from time to time, but have historically been barred from registration because they do not meet that breed association's standard. The standard is prescriptive rather than descriptive despite these sheep coming from a variable landrace on the island. Another breed association has modified its standard and registration definitions to include more of the island variation. Each strategy has consequences for the breed.

A few breeds stand apart from most standardized breeds and most landraces. These few have very isolated foundations with very little question as to which animals descend from

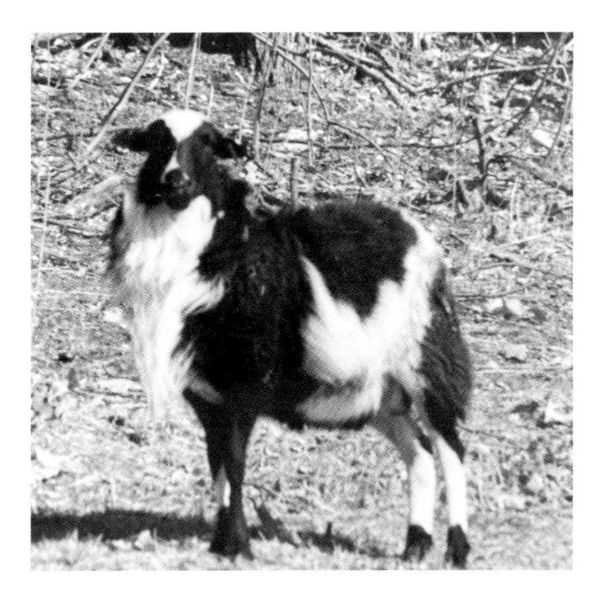

Figure 5.6 Tight definition of St. Croix sheep as polled white sheep ignores some of the variation in hair sheep on their home island. Photo by DPS.

that foundation. Standards for these breeds can become a complicated issue because the main definer of these breeds is the isolated foundation rather than the appearance of the animals. Many of these breeds are from feral island sources, including San Clemente Island goats, Santa Cruz sheep, Arapawa Island goats, and others. Randall Lineback cattle, while never feral, also descend from a known and specific source. For these breeds it is important that a standard or description is not used to eliminate animals, because the breed definition is entirely related to the line of descent from the original defined foundation. Standards for these breeds, especially if used in a manner typical of standardized breeds or landraces, run a very high risk of eliminating variation that truly belongs in the breed. This difference in philosophy of breeding is easily ignored by breeders, to the potential detriment of these breeds.

5.3 *Breed Type Reproduces Breed Type*

For breeds to be useful genetic packages, they must be genetically consistent enough to predictably reproduce themselves. Breeds breed true. The standard, and the rules and regulations of the association, should be targeted toward the goal of assuring that the breed maintains its status as a consistent and predictable genetic package. Standards serve their breeds very poorly if they fail to adequately define breed type, overall performance, or conformation. Such loose standards result in the breed becoming too loosely defined to serve as a genetic resource.

Breeds must be subjected to ongoing selection that reflects and emphasizes breed type. For any breed to maintain a useful status as a genetic resource it must maintain its genetic integrity. While genetic integrity can be lost in several ways, selection away from breed type is one common avenue to lose breed integrity.

Breed type has a powerful role in the conservation of breeds, and breeders need to pay close attention to it. For example, the Guinea Hog is a genetically unique breed found only in America. It is a small hog with a very specific body and ear type that cannot be confused with other breeds. When crossed with other smallish hogs, the resulting offspring diverge from the classic body and color of the original breed. These changes in type reveal a great deal of the underlying loss of genetic consistency, and a good breed standard can help breeders to reject these off-type animals as breeding stock.

5.4 Developing a Breed Standard

Breed standards range from very narrowly defined to more broadly defined. It is common for standards to be so broad and vague that they could describe just about any well-conformed animal. In order to be truly useful, breed standards should be specific and should include a description of the breed that could not be confused with descriptions of other breeds. Breed standards that indicate only how animals should be conformed usually relate to overall soundness, with descriptors such as "level," "broad," "well made," and "strong." These terms do little to convey the uniqueness or character of any animal or breed. The more precise and breed-specific the standard is, the better it serves to guide breeders in maintaining the breed.

It is common for breed standards to emphasize external and easily observed characteristics, such as color, and to skirt discussion and description of breed-specific traits. The breed-specific traits are generally difficult to describe because they are complicated, and it is difficult to marshal the vocabulary that can convey the subtleties of breed type. A good example is that the shape of the head is often difficult to describe. However, it is in the arena of type traits that a breed standard is most useful, but only if it can be written to truly convey the uniqueness of the breed type. A possible description of a sheep head is:

> Broad muzzle with a straight profile, with lower teeth meeting the upper dental pad evenly. Ears are fine and moderately large, and carried horizontally from the head. The jaw is deep, wide, and full. Skin is dark with hair usually white, producing a blue appearance. Long, lustrous wool grows from the topknot, but cheeks lack wool with no tendency toward wool blindness. No presence of horns or scurs.

This head description fits Leicester Longwool sheep and very few others. Those others could easily be eliminated by description of the breed standard for other body regions. The overall result of descriptions like this is a breed-specific document that can help to guide breeders.

A more mathematical approach to breed documentation is that of linear assessment, which compiles several specific distances (eye to eye, shoulder to hip, and many, many others). In most situations, these differences are assessed on several animals and then are given as an average and a range of values. These measures, when combined, fairly accurately reveal breed-specific conformation, although they lack the ability to instill a mental picture that the more traditional written breed standard allows.

Functional traits are as important as physical traits for breed function and integrity. For these, breed standards can include mothering ability, foraging ability, parasite resistance, ease of parturition, fertility, breeding season, and longevity. In some horse breeds gait is an essential component of the breed standard. These functional traits are difficult or impossible to assess by visual inspection, so most breed standards do not include them.

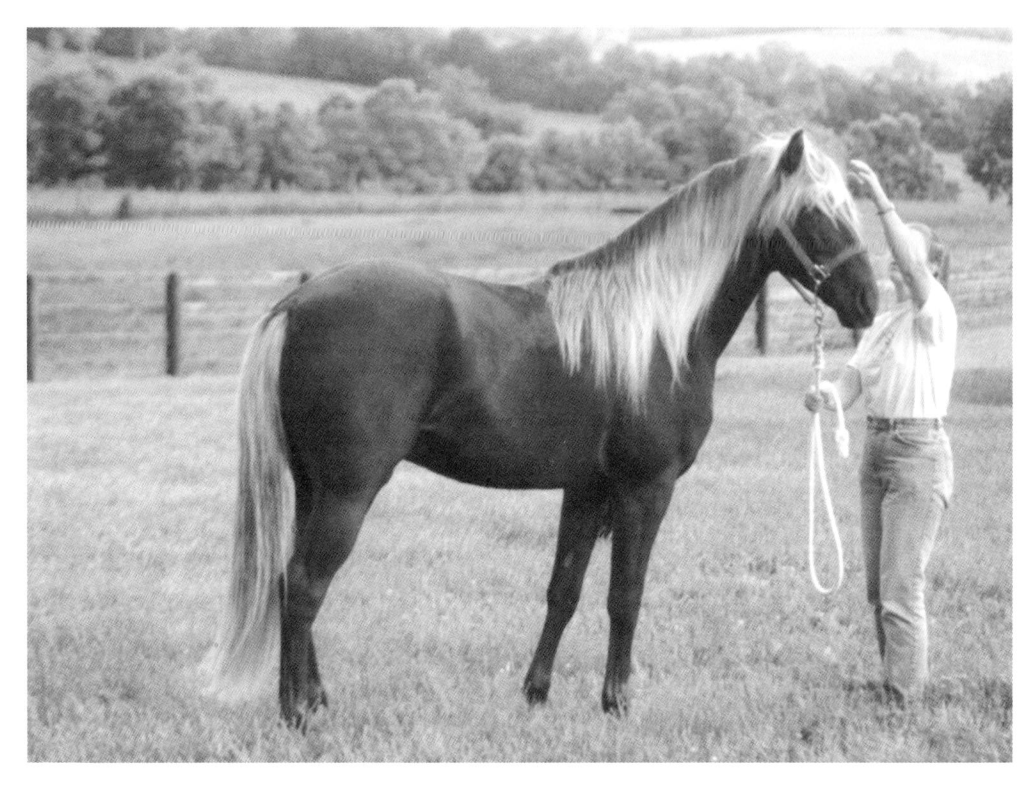

Figure 5.7 The distinctive gait of a Rocky Mountain horse is essential to the breed's character. It is important to include such traits in breed standards. Photo by DPS.

This is unfortunate because the non-visible traits are often key to a breed's success (Figure 5.7). This is especially true of dog breeds, for which temperament and ability are key components to success.

Some of the best breed standards are annotated to indicate the reason why certain traits are important. For example, it is fairly easy to describe a goat's pasterns as upright and strong. Explaining that such conformation leads to a long, sound lifetime can help breeders, especially inexperienced breeders. Breeders need to realize that these descriptions actually relate to function. Including reasons helps to educate breeders as to the reasoning behind the fine points of the breed standard, which provides breeders with powerful tools for evaluating their animals.

5.5 Breed Standards and Genetic Diversity

The goal of any breed standard is to help breeders recognize characters and traits that are typical for their breed. The standard guides observers (especially breeders and judges) as to what should be ideal, what is marginal, and what is outside of breed parameters.

The level of specificity of a breed standard can vary from breed to breed. For standardized breeds, it is common to have a fairly narrow standard that is based on an ideal that may or may not ever have been achieved, or may not even be achievable! In many standardized

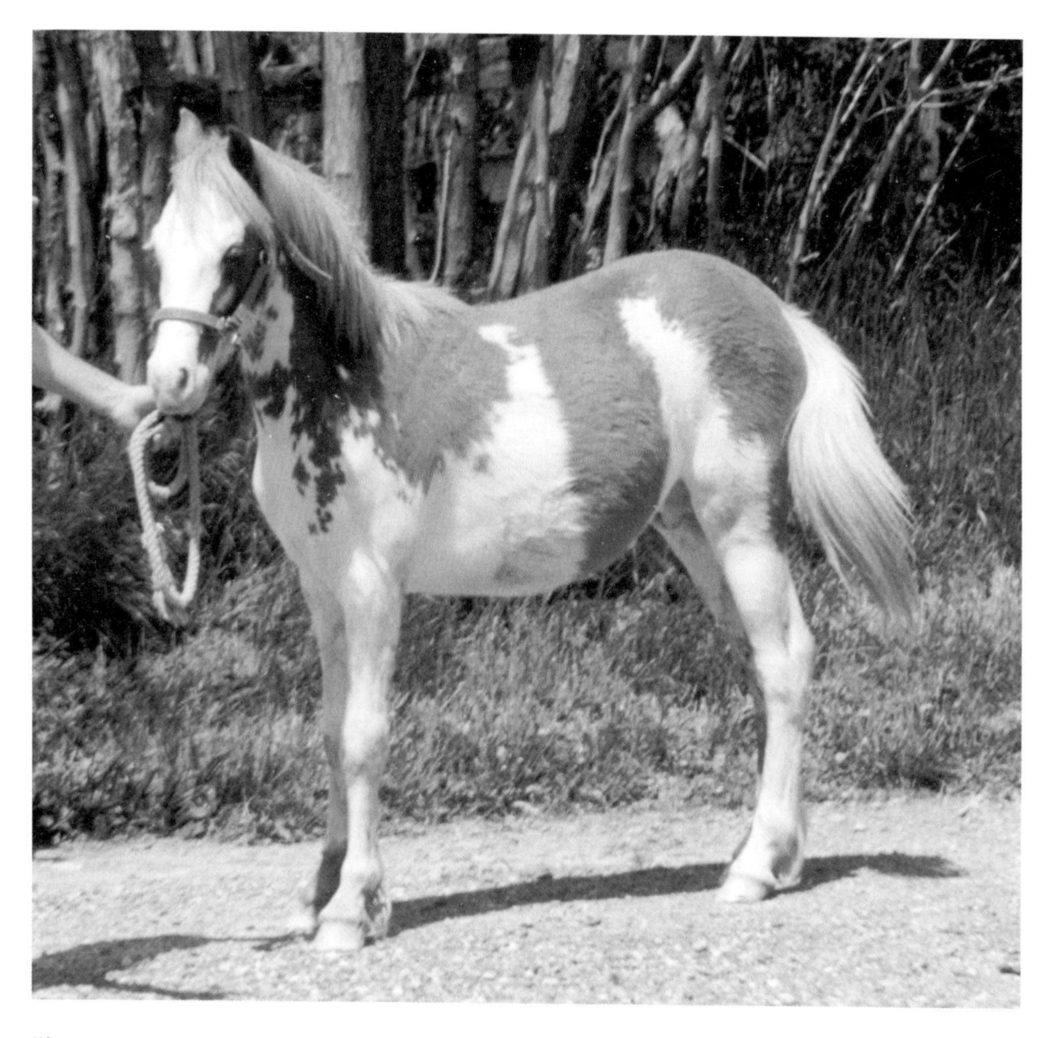

Figure 5.8 In many breeds, ponies with body spots are denied registration, even when such ponies (such as this Welsh pony) come from registered parents. Photo by DPS.

breeds, it is common for the standard to specifically penalize certain variants that appear in the breed from time to time. This is especially true of color traits, such as red in Angus cattle, or body spots in many horse breeds (Figure 5.8). Such exclusion can also be given for physical traits such as a split scrotum in many goat and sheep breeds, or polledness or horns in several species. Some breed standards specifically fault traits that are considered to be defects by the breed association, such as supernumerary teats in goats or an overshot or undershot jaw in several species. These traits are deemed objectionable, even though they do indeed occur from time to time in the breed. Standards can help to eliminate these traits from breeds. Such targets vary in their importance to animal function, and must therefore be chosen carefully.

Restrictive breed standards can have the unintended, and potentially dangerous, side effect of narrowing genetic variation because certain variants are excluded. For breeds with

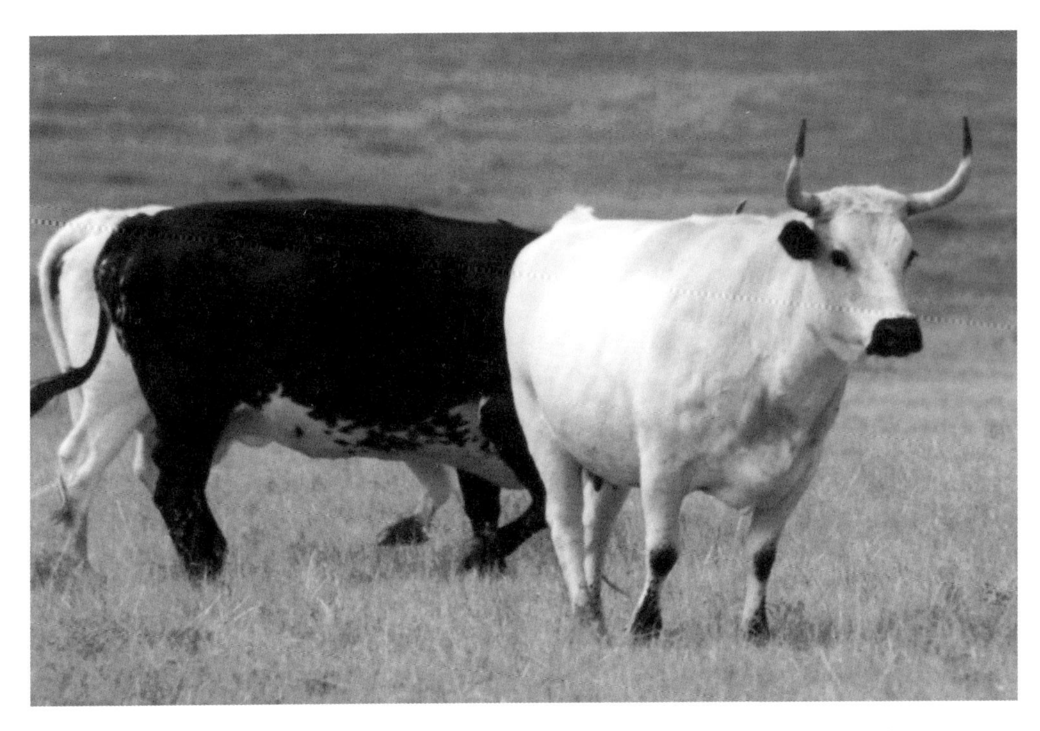

Figure 5.9 Black calves are common in herds of White Park cattle, with roan or spotted variants appearing more rarely. Many breeders discriminate against these "non-white" White Park individuals, while others retain them in the breeding population. Photo by DPS.

high census numbers and great genetic breadth this narrowing is probably of little or no significance. For rare breeds whose population sizes are barely viable, the standard must be a part of the breed's conservation strategy. Standards for rare breeds must focus on the larger issue of breed survival and less on the presence of trivial variation. This does not hold true for fitness traits that are lethal or debilitating, but certainly does hold true for more cosmetic traits such as color. The philosophy behind determining which traits to penalize varies breed to breed. If standards and practices are too lax, the result can be unsound or poorly conformed animals. If too strict, the level of variation in the population can be too restrictive to allow for effective breeding strategies focused on long-term survival of the breed. The goal is an effective balance between these extremes.

Color is an especially easy target for breed standards, and a few examples can flesh out its effects on different breeds. Welsh Black cattle descend from a local landrace. The breed lost many color variants as it was standardized for the black color that was most common in the landrace. Fortunately, black cattle were numerous enough to provide for breed viability, and this breed still occurs in numbers sufficient to form a genetically viable population. The few breeders of non-black cattle of the original landrace have recently organized in order to assure the conservation of the colors that were nearly lost through standardization. For other breeds, color bias can have more deleterious effects. Ancient White Park cattle, already in very low numbers, could easily slip further as a result of draconian measures against solid-colored animals (Figure 5.9). A few rare breeds, such as Randall Lineback cattle, have a common color (black lineback in this case), but have fortunately embraced and encouraged the use of the few red individuals in the breed. This acts to save the genomes of these cattle with unusual colors.

A few breeds, such as the Navajo-Churro sheep breed, have very active procedures to embrace and celebrate the variation present in the breed as a positive and desirable part of breed identity. These include a wide range of characteristics such as colors and horn status (polled, horned, or multiple horns). Navajo-Churro breeders track the many variants of color and horns, and when one variant becomes rare the breeders act to recruit sheep carrying the trait as future breeding stock. This succeeds in maintaining the diversity long present in the breed.

Eye color in many dog breeds can serve as an example of a trait that had little practical importance but can have a huge influence on breeding practices. Some standards call for dark brown eyes, when certain coat colors more typically have amber or yellow eyes. This raises a very real issue in that some prescriptive standards actually require traits that are difficult or impossible to achieve. Standards should always be based on what is actually possible, especially for the more cosmetic traits.

5.6 Breed Standards and Breed Loss

Breeds can be lost in various ways, and breed standards affect a few of these. One way is the insidious loss that can occur through large changes in type. This usually occurs when breeders ignore or modify the breed standard to the extent that the original genetic package is gone even though the name remains. Modern lean swine breeds are dramatically different from their exceedingly fat, lard-producing ancestors. Even though the modern hogs are known by the same breed name, the genetic package beneath that name is drastically changed from the original. While the practicality of the change can be debated, the fact remains that changing standards, and the resulting selection pressures, do indeed change breeds.

Changes in breed type change the underlying breed. The Marsh Tacky is a horse breed developed in the wet coastal low country of South Carolina as a superb hunting horse that could navigate in remote and swampy areas. They are smallish horses which average 14 hands high, and perform better than much larger horses because of the challenging terrain in which they are expected to work and live. Some breeders have tried to change the traditional type by increasing size. The result inadvertently reduced the athletic ability of the Marsh Tacky as a hunting horse. As one hunter put it, "Once they get up near 15 hands, they can't get out of their own way."

Another way in which breeds can be lost occurs when small populations are managed so stringently and strictly that eventually the genetic variation needed for viability is no longer available to the breed. It then succumbs slowly and inexorably to extinction through loss of usefulness, vigor, and viability. Examples of this are hard to cite because the loss is insidious and slow.

Standards should be carefully constructed because they greatly affect the breeding selection of breeds. Making decisions on what traits are desirable and what are undesirable can be controversial. It is important for breeders to be clear-headed in defining the most important traits central to a breed's identity and function. Traits that are minimally important to true breed character are best left out of standards.

5.7 Standard Traits That Can Be Detrimental

Some breed standards include specific traits that are desired in the breed but that have detrimental effects. Many of these occur due to specific genes that are favorable and create the breed type when present in one copy (heterozygous), but detrimental when present in two copies (homozygous). These traits and their mode of inheritance present real challenges to breeders. In the case of rare breeds, it is often wise to allow great laxity in the expression of some of these traits in order to be able to recruit a broader sample of the breed into the reproducing population.

An example of one such trait is the rose comb of many chicken breeds. Roosters that are homozygous for one type of rose comb have defective sperm motility. While some fertility is present, the sperm from homozygous rose-comb roosters have lower motility and longevity than those from heterozygous rose-comb or single-comb birds. This is the reason that most rose-comb chicken breeds also produce single-combed chicks. The very genetic mechanism that causes rose combs also favors heterozygotes and assures the occasional production of single-combed birds (Figure 5.10).

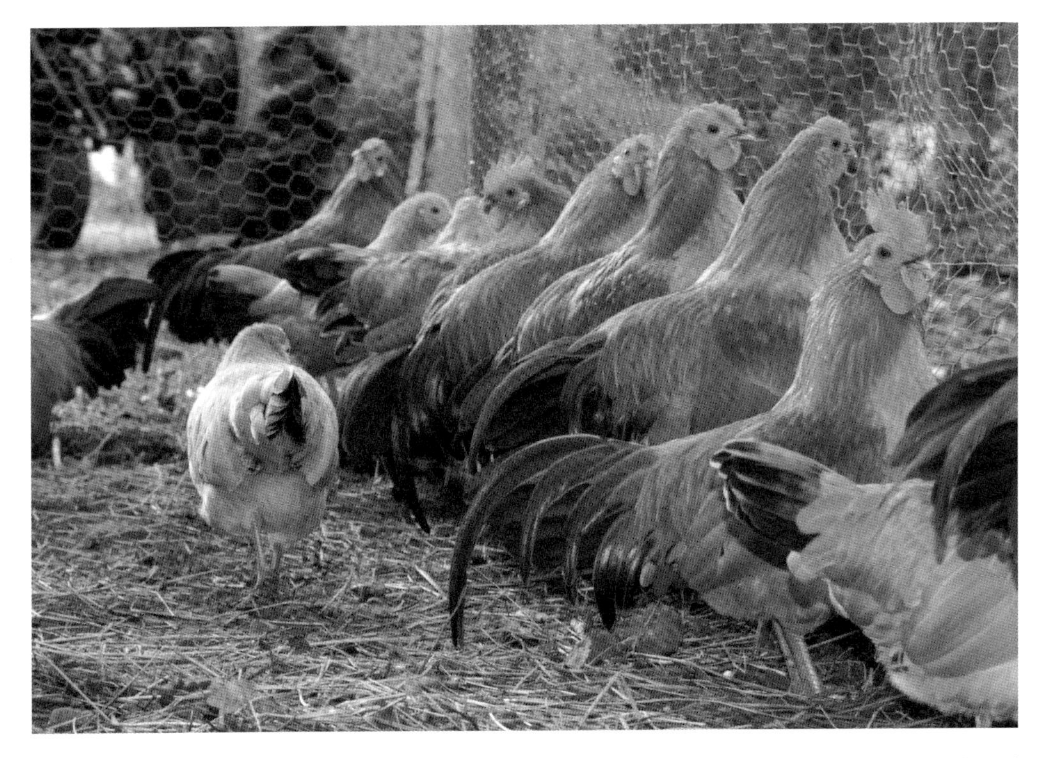

Figure 5.10 The Nankin bantam chicken breed is a good example of a generally rose-combed breed that often produces individuals with single combs. This is due to the inherent genetics of rose-comb birds. Photo by JB.

The "creeper" short-legged dwarfism in chickens is similarly deleterious to homozygotes, but in this case, it is lethal to the developing embryos. As a result, all Scots Dumpy chickens are heterozygous, and will produce normal-legged chicks in addition to the desired short-legged ones even if both parents are short-legged. When mated together the Scots Dumpy produces many eggs that simply fail to hatch. Similar dwarfism is common in Dexter cattle, and breeders are careful to manage the gene to avoid the production of defective calves, while also producing the historic dwarf cattle that are so integral to the breed identity.

Several prescribed color traits are heterozygous. Palomino horses, mated together, produce the desired palomino foals, but also chestnut and blue-eyed cream-colored foals. This phenomenon has made some blue-eyed cream horses highly desirable as breeding stock, because when mated to chestnuts they produce 100% palomino foals. In many breeds, though, the homozygous blue-eyed cream horses are denied registration even though the genetic machinery for producing them is present in the breed. Breeders may be biased against these horses because of their appearance and an assumption that they are weaker than other horses, even though this does not appear to be true.

Blue chickens are heterozygous, with one homozygote being black and the other a "splash" color that is white with occasional splashes of blue or black. In this case the selection process is very complicated because the final shade and character of the blue is highly modified at other loci. As a result, the mating of splash to black birds can produce chicks that are either too light or too dark for the standard. Most breeders use the blue-to-blue matings because the shade of blue can be more easily controlled, despite the production of unwanted black and splash birds.

5.8 *Qualitative and Quantitative Traits*

Breed standards usually dictate both the qualitative and quantitative elements of breed character and type. Qualitative elements are "either/or" traits such as coat color and length, class of wool, presence or absence of horns, and similar characteristics that are usually easy to classify as to their presence or absence in an animal. Most standardized breeds have a limited array of choices in any of several qualitative traits. Included among these are a tendency in most standardized breeds to limit the color array (frequently to a single color or pattern), and a single choice for horn presence or absence. Variation in qualitative traits is usually greater for landrace populations than for standardized breeds. This subtlety often results in the uninformed observer failing to recognize landraces as legitimate breeds, as it is difficult to see past the superficial variation in color and horns to detect the underlying conformational and performance similarity.

The Beechkeld herd of Myotonic goats deliberately fosters a good degree of variation in color and coat length, and always has both horned and polled individuals. One astute guest observer paused after looking at the herd, and commented, "It's them heads and ears, ain't it?" He had quickly picked out the essence of the type traits in the herd, despite some superficial variation in other traits.

Quantitative traits are those that vary along a continuum, such as height, weight, quantity of milk, linear measurement traits, and other similar "how much" traits. Quantitative traits are as important to a breed as qualitative traits, but are much more difficult to capture in a

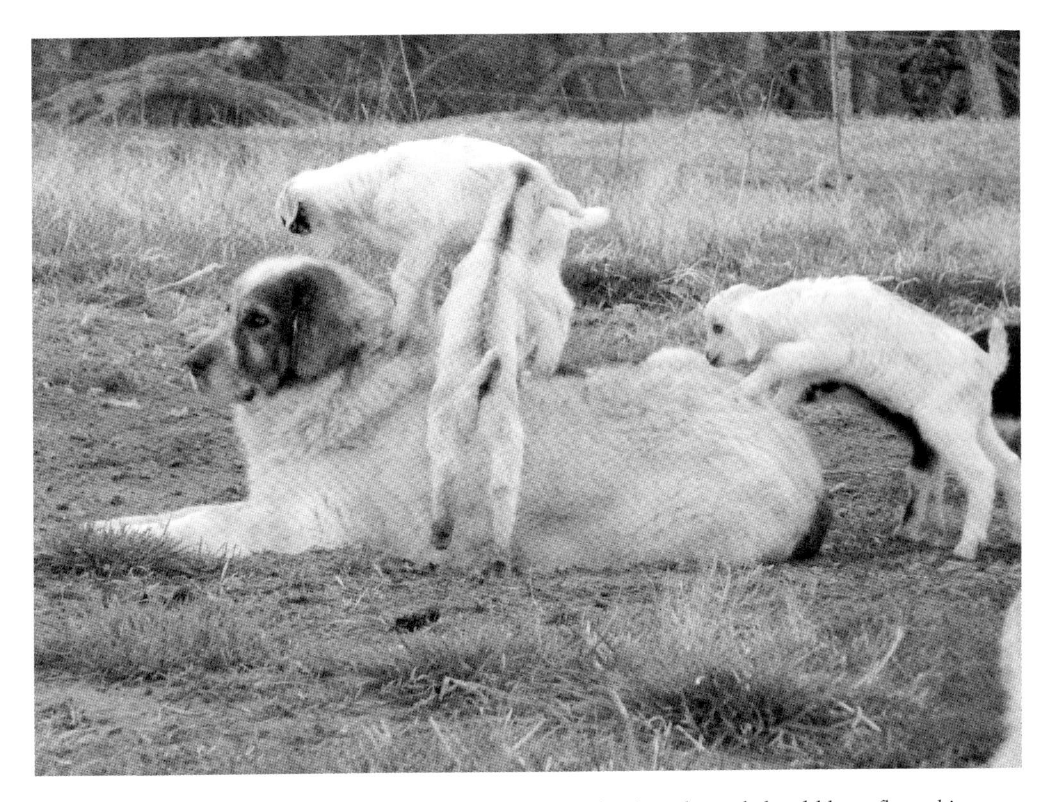

Figure 5.11 Behavioral traits are especially important in dog breeds, and should be reflected in their breed standards. Effective livestock guardian dogs have a host of traits that all combine for a successful final package. Photo by DPS.

breed standard. Certainly, size parameters can be described, but traits such as growth rate, milk production, fecundity, and egg size are equally critical to defining a breed and yet are much more difficult to detect by a casual one-time observation such as occurs in a show ring.

Traits such as hardiness, parasite resistance, fertility, and other complex characteristics are even more difficult to classify as either quantitative or qualitative. These traits frequently have contributions from a wide variety of genetic mechanisms, some of which are simple and some more complex. These are among the hardest of all traits to describe or evaluate, but are also among the most important for many breeds of livestock. Traits of adaptation and function can be especially important in landraces. Behavior traits, such as guarding or herding ability, are especially important in dog breeds, but notoriously difficult to capture in a breed standard that focuses mostly on visual appearance (Figure 5.11).

5.9 Changes to the Breed Standard

Breed standards should be thoughtfully and carefully constructed from the outset. Changes should be rarely needed or advised. For some breeds, though, experience and improved information might well indicate that some changes are needed. Changes should be agreed

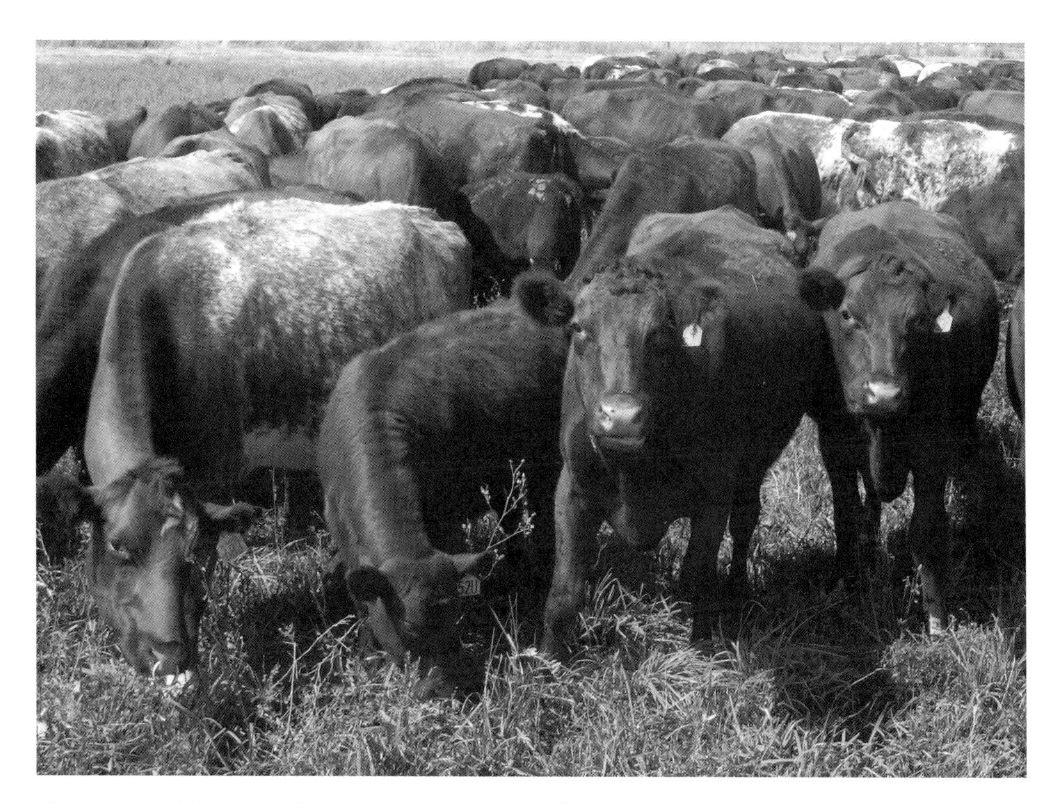

Figure 5.12 Today's Shorthorn cattle breed benefits from centuries of careful breeding toward a standard. Photo by JB.

upon by the general membership in an association, and are best accomplished following an extensive educational campaign concerning the breed, its history, its type, and the potential effects of the changes on the breed as a genetic resource.

It is especially necessary for breed standards to reflect the biological realities of the breed. Breed standards should be realistic portrayals of the breed's appearance and optimal biological function. The ideal, or standard, should reflect the reality of the breed so that pure-breeding populations that meet the standard can be achieved. This is especially true of poultry standards, which should be achievable using a single pure-breeding population rather than having separate cockerel breeding and pullet breeding groups for the production of exhibition birds.

Changes in breed standard are always politically highly charged because these changes necessarily indicate a change in the direction that the breed is being taken. This also means that some breeders come out ahead because they own animals that are more in keeping with the revised standard, while others are disadvantaged by the change because they own animals less in keeping with the revised standard. The political and economic aspects of such changes can become very highly contentious and need to be handled openly and fairly in order for the breed and its breeders not to suffer. Most breeds benefit from a breed standard that is thoughtfully constructed and therefore needs to be changed rarely, if ever (Figure 5.12).

CHAPTER 6

Principles of Genetic Management

Maintaining breeds as healthy and viable genetic resources should be the goal of each breeder and every breed association. This effort ideally involves different breeding strategies both within breeds and across breeds (Figure 6.1). Each breeding strategy has different consequences for the individual herd as well as for the breed. Each breeder must tailor a

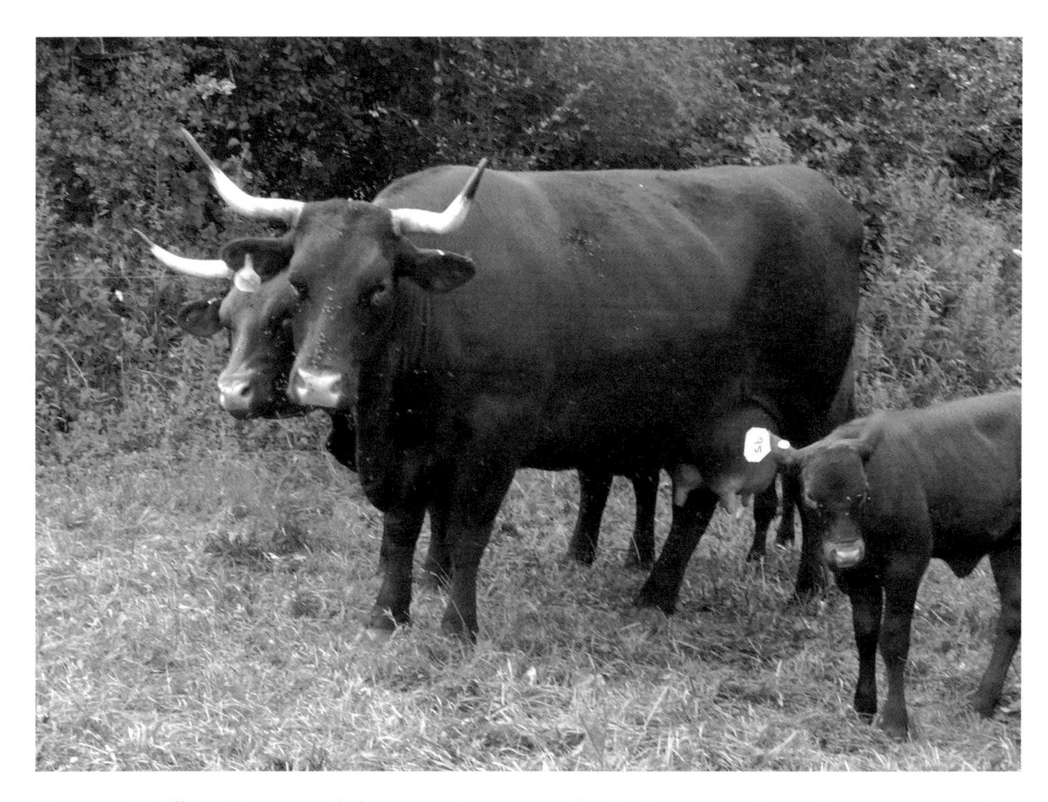

Figure 6.1 Milking Devon cattle have a unique array of traits, history, and population structure that benefit from breeding practices tailored specifically for this breed. Photo by DPS.

strategy for the specific mix of philosophies, situations, and goals that are unique to the herd being stewarded. The overarching goal is to assure a viable genetic structure for individual herds and also for the entire breed in order to assure the best chance for the breed's long-term survival and productivity.

The mating strategies most commonly used include inbreeding, linebreeding, linecrossing, outcrossing, and crossbreeding. Understanding how each of these strategies is used is important for breeders whether they emphasize conservation, production, or performance. These terms are all defined differently by different groups of breeders, but the key fact is that the pairing of animals for reproduction has varying outcomes depending on the degree of relationship between the animals that are mated. The results of each of the different breeding strategies are subjective points along a single line that vary from completely inbred and uniform at one end, to completely crossbred and variable at the other end. The exact point along this line that the boundaries are drawn between inbreeding, linebreeding, linecrossing, and crossbreeding is subjective. Despite that lack of tight definition, the effects of these strategies on populations are very real and need to be understood by conscientious breeders. Each strategy has an important role in shaping animal populations, and for most breeds a combination of them is advisable for managing long-term success.

At the outset, it is important to note that selection is the factor that can change allele frequencies in a population, in contrast to the effects of the different breeding strategies. Selection changes allelic frequencies, which in turn changes the genetic package of a breed. The various breeding strategies do not change allele frequencies. The strategies can, and do, change the relative number of heterozygotes and homozygotes, which exposes the genes to different levels of selection pressure. The final makeup of the population looks somewhat different depending on the breeding strategy, but the only way to deliberately change allele frequencies is through selection.

6.1 Linebreeding and Inbreeding

Linebreeding and inbreeding are only different from one another in degree. Both of these involve the mating of related animals. One definition that separates these is "it is linebreeding if it works, and inbreeding if it doesn't work." This definition has some merit, but does not serve as a very good guide for breeders as to the specifics of the two techniques.

Any mating of related animals is technically inbreeding. Related animals vary in their degree of relationship, and can be either distantly related or closely related. A practical definition that can help guide breeding practices is that the cutoff point for inbreeding is arbitrarily set as the mating of first-degree relatives. First-degree relatives include offspring, parents, and siblings. Although this is only one possible definition among many, it usefully separates inbreeding from linebreeding at a defined point. This definition works fairly well as a boundary between lower levels of related breeding that are generally tolerated quite well in all populations, and higher levels of related breeding that can hit barriers in some populations if not carefully monitored. Linebreeding can then be considered as the mating of related animals that have more distant relationships than first degree. Matings of aunt to nephew and grandparent to grand offspring could all be included here, as well as more distant matings such as between cousins.

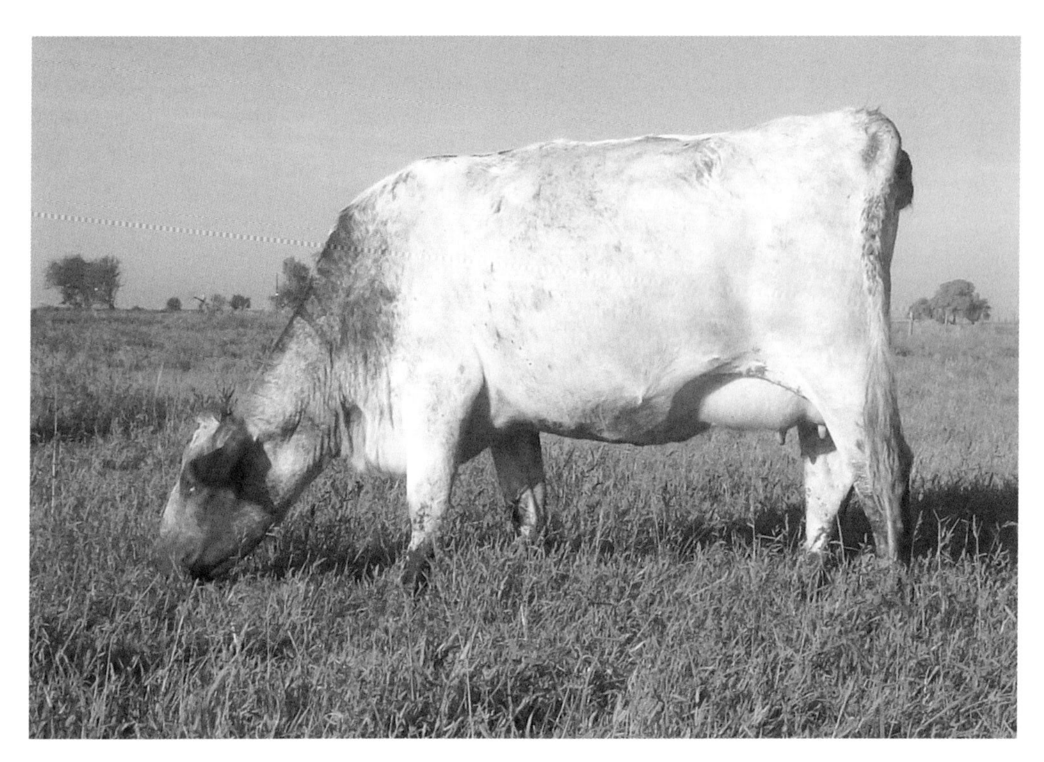

Figure 6.2 The development of the Shorthorn cattle breed involved varying levels of linebreeding and inbreeding and resulted in the productive breed that survives to this day.
Photo by Winifred Hoffman.

Linebreeding and inbreeding both result in increased genetic uniformity of offspring. This occurs through an increase in homozygosity. The genetic uniformity can be especially noticeable if these strategies are accompanied by appropriate selection. Linebreeding increases genetic uniformity because parents are related and therefore descend from a common and limited gene pool, which means that they have limited genetic variation to pass along to their offspring. Uniformity of appearance and performance of linebred animals springs directly from this fact. The uniformity can apply to very good looks and performance, or to very bad looks and performance. The initial animals that are mated, as well as selection practices, determine the relative quality of the end product. In addition, the degree of relationship of the parents helps to influence the degree of uniformity in the offspring. The closer the relationship, the more uniform the offspring. And, if inbreeding is practiced over several sequential generations, the relationships become ever closer, and uniformity also increases.

A very important historic note is that linebreeding and inbreeding were the usual strategies for the establishment of breeds (Figure 6.2). These two breeding strategies can be coupled with selection to increase uniformity, and therefore predictability. The very essence of a breed is sufficient uniformity for predictability. In that regard, both inbreeding and linebreeding can be effective in achieving the status of animal populations as true genetic breeds.

When linebreeding is coupled with selection, which it usually is, the result is a productive, predictable gene pool. The key importance of a purebred animal is the predictability of production. Despite the very real advantage of this strategy, potential problems can occur in linebred populations, and these are even more common in inbred groups. Common problems include loss of general vigor and especially loss of reproductive performance. In addition, inbred groups can have a concentration and expression of undesirable recessive traits. Skilled selection can help offset these so that several linebred and inbred resources (including entire breeds or strains within breeds) are indeed productive, vigorous, and reproductively sound. These exceptions in no way eliminate the need for caution when breeders embark upon a strategy of inbreeding or linebreeding.

It is vitally important to manage all inbreeding within limits due to its potential negative aspects. It is also wise to assure that outcrosses to other lines are available within the breed or herd in the event that production and reproduction begin to suffer in any linebred group. Every animal in every breed should have a potential outcross mating available, otherwise the breed will find itself perched on a dangerously narrow genetic foundation. This usually happens in breeds when all breeders chase after a few specific bloodlines. For example, all matings of current Lusitano horses are assured to be linebred or minimally inbred because all pedigrees go back to a single popular stallion from the early 1900s. At this point there is no way to get around inbreeding, because no completely unrelated animals are available. This is unlikely to play out to the detriment of the breed due to its large numbers, but is an example of a situation that could have been avoided with better long-term planning to assure that unrelated animals were always available to the breeders. Similarly most, if not all, Ayrshire cattle in the USA include a single popular bull from the 1950s, so this breed is also now limited to linebred matings (Figure 6.3).

An extreme example of inbreeding involves a Texas Longhorn cow from a line that was resistant to inbreeding depression (Figure 6.4). This cow had the same bull as sire, grandsire, and great grandsire. As a result she was 87.5% the genetic influence of that one animal. She continued producing calves at intervals of little over ten months during her long and useful life. But she is the exception to the general rule that close inbreeding results in depression. Usually, this sort of animal results from breeders not planning for future generations (as was the case in this instance), and only rarely is such a highly inbred animal productive and well adapted.

A few breeds have shown great resistance to inbreeding, and these exceptions to the general rule are important. Unfortunately, they also can lull breeders into a false sense of security in believing that inbreeding does not pose a threat to any line. Ancient White Park cattle come down to the present after centuries of isolation and inbreeding. They remain viable and productive. Exceptions are interesting, but they are the successes that just happen to survive and therefore are noticed while the failures are not around to gain that same notice. If 20 or so lines are started with intense inbreeding, only about two are likely to survive for several generations. The remainder will succumb to inbreeding depression and to eventual extinction if outcrosses are not used to reverse the effects. Unfortunately, it is impossible to predict which strains will survive and which will succumb, so they should all be managed as if inbreeding depression is a real threat.

Inbreeding is not without risk, and this risk needs to be acknowledged and planned for

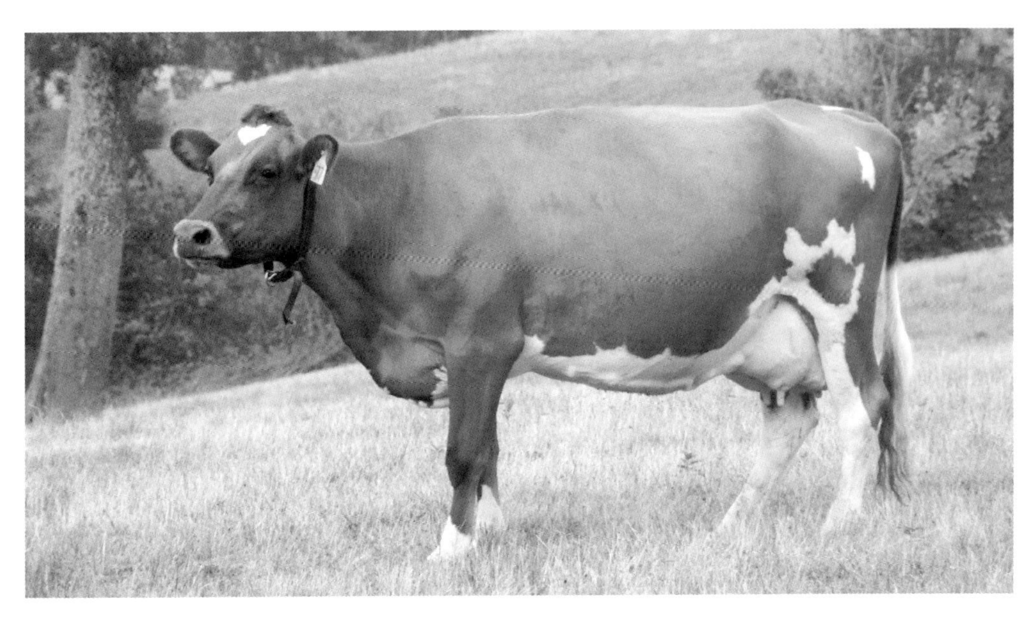

Figure 6.3 Ayrshire cattle in the USA all go back to a single popular bull used in the 1950s, although some breeders are now avoiding or minimizing this by using frozen semen from early unrelated bulls. Photo by JB.

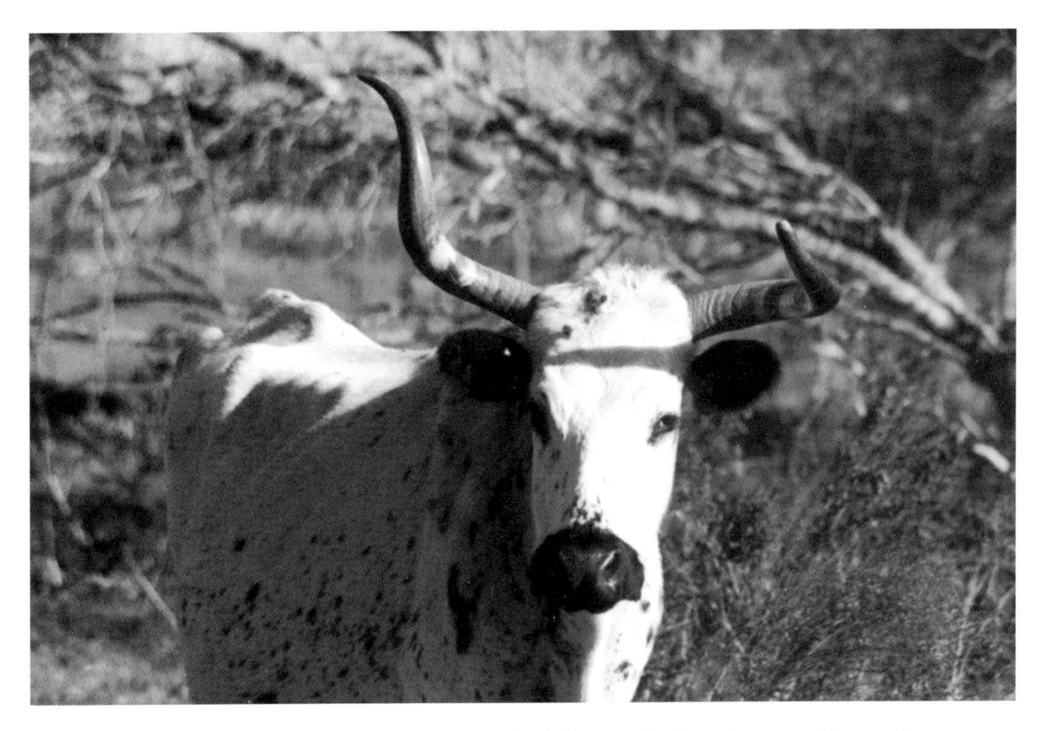

Figure 6.4 This productive Texas Longhorn cow had the same bull as sire, grandsire, and great grandsire. She is the exception that proves the rule that inbreeding usually causes declining vigor and vitality! Photo by DPS.

in any long-term breed maintenance program. Both linebreeding and inbreeding expose recessive traits in a homozygous state, whether these are positive or negative. These two strategies must only be employed with a firm and resolute commitment that deleterious traits be rigorously culled out of the breeding population.

Some herds have long practiced linebreeding or inbreeding as a successful strategy over several generations. In these situations the breeders tend to ignore the very real risks of long-term inbreeding strategies because their own personal experience varies from the general rule. In multiple cases, the inbreeding that continues successfully for several generations suddenly hits a generation where vitality and reproduction fail precipitously. This provides an important warning. Many populations reveal very little sign that inbreeding is reaching unacceptable levels until it is too late! Many breeders firmly believe that their own breed is completely resistant to inbreeding, only to find out that the next generation proves them wrong.

While several cautions have been raised against inbreeding and linebreeding, it is very important to remember that these are extremely useful breeding strategies in some situations and for some specific goals. The deleterious effects usually surface after several sequential generations of linebred or inbred matings. Over shorter periods they can each serve very positive roles in the management of gene pools. Inbreeding and linebreeding are power tools. They are effective when used appropriately, and dangerous when used carelessly.

6.2 Outcrossing: Crossbreeding and Linecrossing

Outcrossing involves the mating of animals that are not related and is the philosophical and biological opposite of linebreeding. Outcrossing and outbreeding are synonyms, and the results are commonly characterized as outbred (as contrasted to inbred). Outcrossing can be divided into two subgroups: crossbreeding and linecrossing. Crossbreeding is the mating of animals from two different breeds. Linecrossing is the mating of unrelated animals from within the same breed. Usually these matings occur between animals from two different bloodlines within the breed, which leads to the term "linecrossing" (Figure 6.5).

Crossbreeding is a fascinating phenomenon, partly because different results occur depending upon which generation is considered. The first stage is the initial cross. A useful example comes from cattle. When Angus (black, polled) and Hereford (red, white-faced, horned) cattle are crossed, the initial result is a uniform crop of "black baldy" calves. The calves exhibit the dominant traits of both breeds: black and polled from Angus, and white

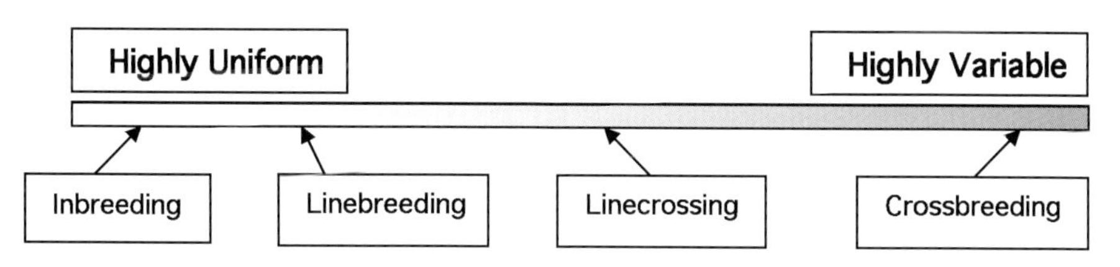

Figure 6.5 Relative degrees of genetic relatedness resulting from different breeding strategies. Figure by DPS.

Table 6.1 Variations in calves produced from black baldy to black baldy matings. Despite the superficial uniformity of the parents their hidden genetic variability is expressed in the next generation.

Body color	Head color	Horns
black	white	polled
black	white	horned
black	black	polled
black	black	horned
red	white	polled
red	white	horned
red	red	polled
red	red	horned

face from Hereford. These offspring have benefitted from the specific combination of the genetic array of the parental breeds. This generation is called the F1 (first filial) generation. Each parental breed is uniform, each calf gets half of its genetic makeup from each parental breed. The result is great uniformity. This first calf crop is reaping the benefits of the two homogeneous parental breeds, as well as hybrid vigor that results from the two breeds being unrelated.

When these crossbred calves are mated to each other the result is the F2 or second filial generation. Variability increases because the calves of the F2 generation are varying mixes of their parents. Those parents are half one thing, half another thing, and their combination yields a variety of different phenotypes among their offspring. The color and horns, let alone other characteristics, can serve to illustrate what happens when a crossbred animal is used for reproduction. Breeding black baldies among themselves produces black, black baldy, red, and white-faced red calves, some having horns, and some being polled. The initial consistency present in the F1 generation is gone, and the result is a variable group of calves (Table 6.1 and Figure 6.6).

This variability is not all bad. When combined with selection the excellent individuals can be skimmed off the herd and used to good advantage in the show ring and other situations. They may indeed have excellent type and performance. What they lack is the ability to consistently pass along this excellence to the generations following that initial F1 generation. They are something of a dead end for a breeder, even though as individuals they may be wonderfully productive animals. The phenotypic excellence of the F1 animals from many different species has repeatedly lulled animal breeders into thinking that this strategy works over the long term. It is a wonderfully productive strategy, but only works in the short term and requires a constant supply of purebreds to put into the initial cross that the system depends on.

Many of the advantages arising from a crossbreeding strategy (increased vigor and reproductive efficiency) are diminished under a linebreeding strategy. Conversely, the advantages of using a linebreeding strategy (consistency and predictability) are diminished under a crossbreeding strategy. Each therefore has a place in wise animal breeding systems.

Linecrossing is less extreme than crossbreeding because it occurs within a single breed. It has some of the same biological consequences as crossbreeding even though the crossing

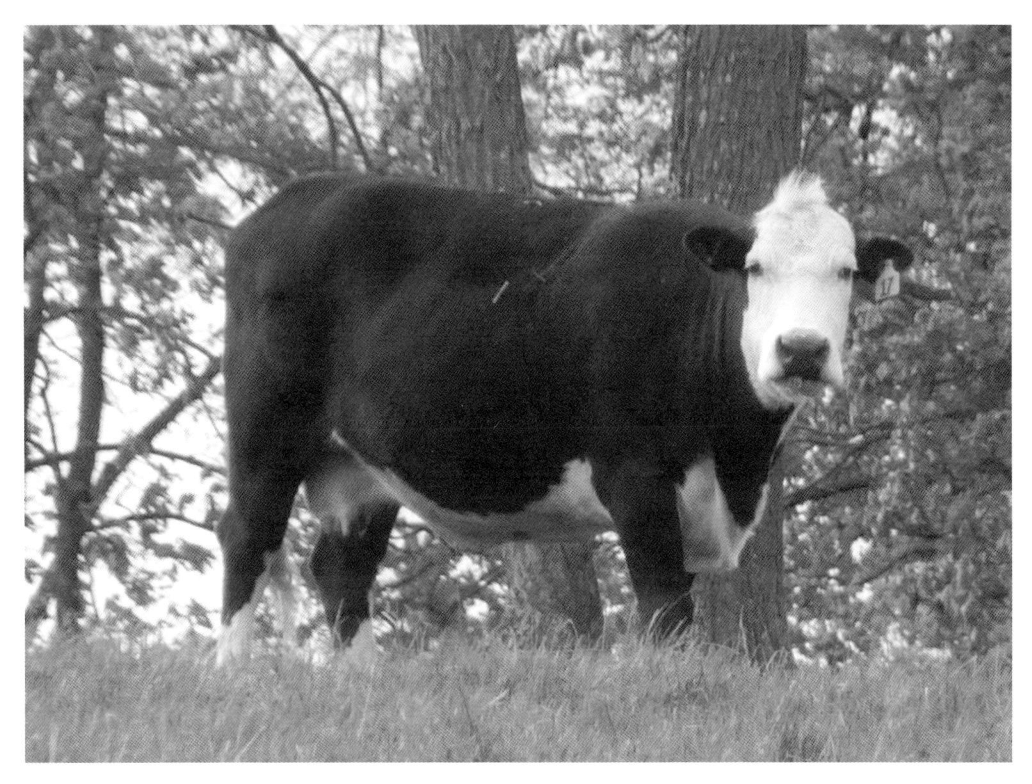

Figure 6.6 The "black baldy" is the first-generation cross of Hereford and Angus cattle and is visually uniform. Their underlying genetic variability is easily expressed when they are mated to one another. Photo by DPS.

is contained within a single breed. This can provide the benefits of crossbreeding without the loss of breed character and type. As a result, the variability is not as great as that produced by a cross between breeds, so the boost from hybrid vigor is not as great. This technique can be used to good advantage in certain breeds, such as the Angora goat, where interbreed crossing would make no sense at all because no other breed could be crossed without causing the loss of the Angora's distinctive and valuable fleece characteristics. Linecrossing can contribute to the vigor associated with high production, but it lowers the predictability of production in following generations by virtue of creating animals that are more genetically mixed than linebred animals. Only a careful analysis of each individual situation will indicate whether or not this is a good tradeoff.

6.3 Defining Matings as "Related" or "Unrelated"

The exact point at which matings are classified as "related" (contributing to inbreeding) versus "unrelated" (not contributing to inbreeding) is impossible to define in absolute terms. Nearly all purebred matings are more closely related than matings to another breed are. This, after all, gets back to the whole point of breeds being genetic resources that spring from a single foundation with enough genetic uniformity to be predictable.

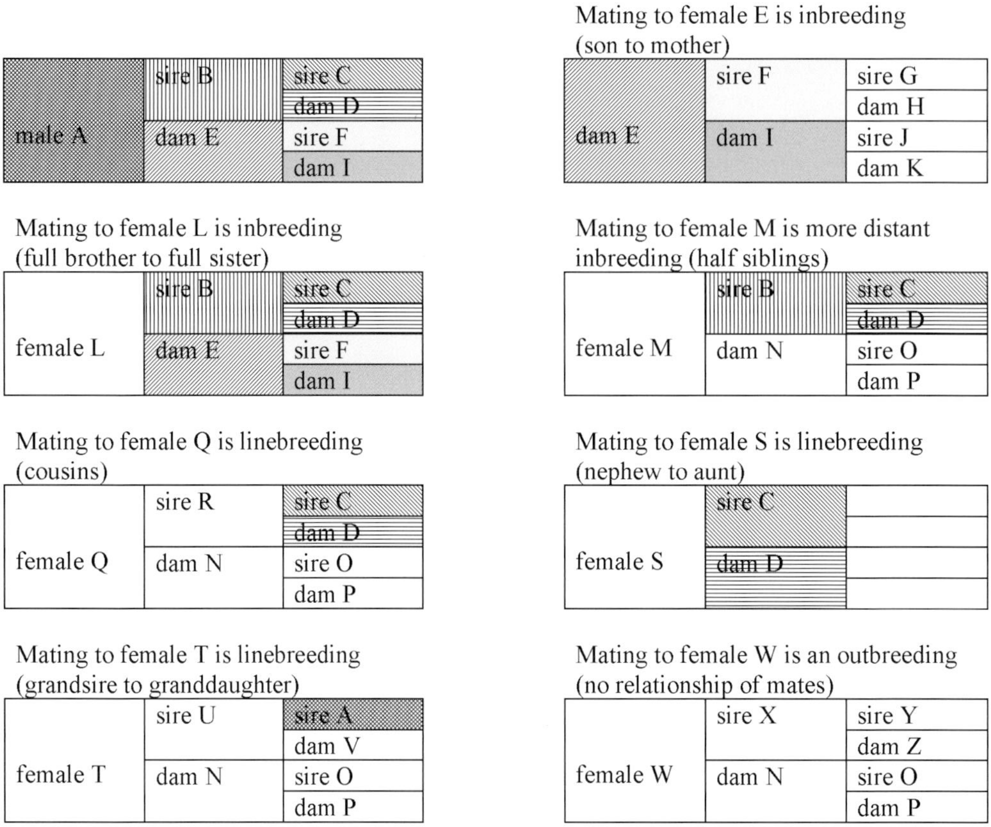

male A	sire B	sire C
		dam D
	dam E	sire F
		dam I

Mating to female E is inbreeding (son to mother)

dam E	sire F	sire G
		dam H
	dam I	sire J
		dam K

Mating to female L is inbreeding (full brother to full sister)

female L	sire B	sire C
		dam D
	dam E	sire F
		dam I

Mating to female M is more distant inbreeding (half siblings)

female M	sire B	sire C
		dam D
	dam N	sire O
		dam P

Mating to female Q is linebreeding (cousins)

female Q	sire R	sire C
		dam D
	dam N	sire O
		dam P

Mating to female S is linebreeding (nephew to aunt)

female S	sire C	
	dam D	

Mating to female T is linebreeding (grandsire to granddaughter)

female T	sire U	sire A
		dam V
	dam N	sire O
		dam P

Mating to female W is an outbreeding (no relationship of mates)

female W	sire X	sire Y
		dam Z
	dam N	sire O
		dam P

Figure 6.7 Pedigrees of a male and several potential female mates demonstrating varying levels of inbreeding and linebreeding. Male A could be mated to each of these females. The common ancestors are coded to indicate the ancestors that are identical. Figure by DPS.

Animals are unrelated if none of the ancestors on the sire's side also occur on the dam's side. As a useful general rule, the mating of any two animals that have no ancestors in common back to grandparents can be considered as outbreeding. The offspring will have no ancestors in common on the sire's side and dam's side back to the great-grandparents. Any relationship beyond this level is generally trivial and contributes so little to an inbreeding coefficient that it is generally safe to ignore. At the other extreme, the mating of first-degree relatives (parent to offspring, full and half-siblings) can be considered inbreeding because these animals are very closely related. Between these two extremes lies linebreeding, which varies in degree but still lies at a level below severe inbreeding and above outbreeding (Figure 6.7).

A minor warning is warranted. Some populations are linebred in consistent ways to a few founders that were used to expand a population. As the generations continue to develop, these relationships can exist so far back in the pedigree that breeders are unaware that animals are indeed fairly highly inbred. The Farceur line of Belgian horses went back to a single founder stallion imported in 1912. Many generations (and decades) after the

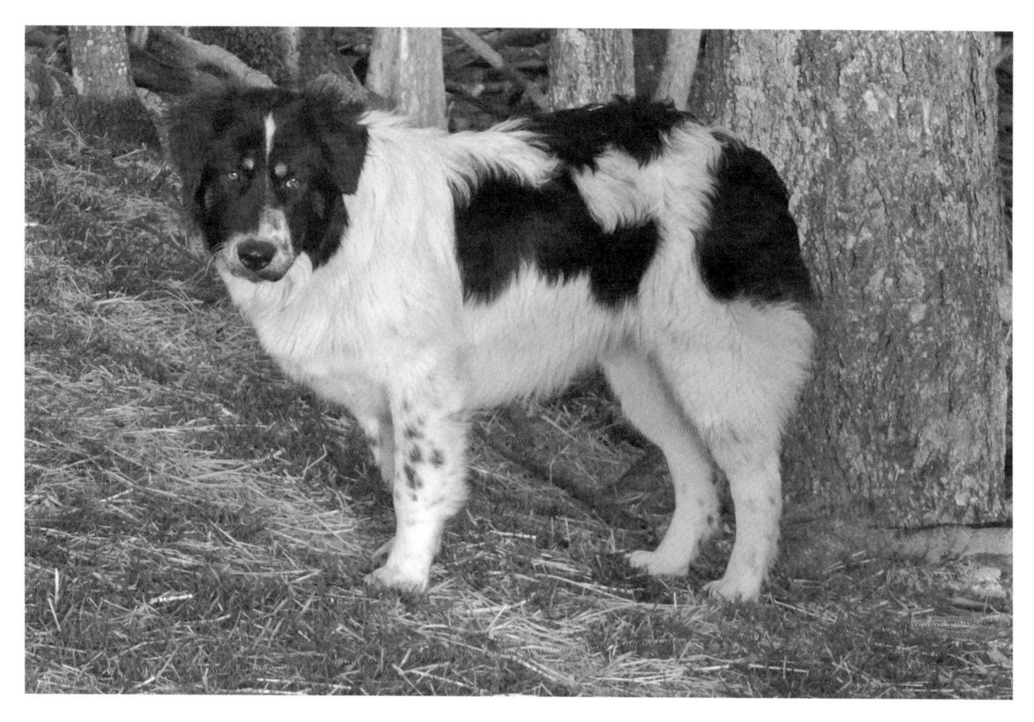

Figure 6.8 KaraKitan kennel used linebreeding very effectively to produce their reliable Karakachan livestock guardian dogs. Relationships between animals can only be determined by examining extended pedigrees. Photo by DPS.

importation of this horse it was still easy to find horses that were 50% his influence due to the initial production of many sons and daughters that were used in breeding programs. Similarly, the KaraKitan line of Karakachan dogs is largely based on two founders, but this relationship might not be obvious unless extended pedigrees are examined. In some cases dogs that are four or five generations removed from these founders are still up to 40% their influence. A mating between two such dogs is indeed an example of inbreeding despite them having no ancestors in common back to grandparents (Figure 6.8).

The consequences of inbreeding that occurred in recent generations may be different from those that occurred in more distant generations. The devil is in the details. Parental genetic material is blended by a few different processes at each generational step, and these compound over several generations.

One mechanism derives from the fact that the genetic material of an individual is housed in different chromosomes, a different number for each species. Chromosomes occur in pairs, and one from each pair sorts out randomly into the next generation. This is one mechanism for blending genetic material, because each offspring gets a different mix of the maternal and paternal chromosomes.

A second powerful mechanism is that at each generational step the two pairs of chromosomes "cross over" which means that they swap portions of the genetic material with their partner. This occurs at a rate of a little over one crossover event per chromosome per generation. The consequence of this is that after many generations the genetic material from a single ancestor is no longer as intact as it was after only a few generations. The practical implication of this is that inbreeding that occurs to ancestors that are back several generations is unlikely to be as risky as inbreeding that occurs from ancestors that are more recent. This is due to the original genetic sequences no longer being intact as long stretches of DNA, and therefore being less likely to be identical in the linebred descendant.

6.4 Linebreeding or Outcrossing: Which Is Best?

The phenomena associated with crossbreeding and linebreeding have different consequences for different breeders. These strategies each work well for specific philosophies and goals. Different breeders have different philosophies and goals, and this is healthy for breeds. Philosophies might include strict conservation principles, strict commercial utility, or high-profile programs with name recognition, among others. Goals might include excellent temperament, maximum weight gains, production on minimal inputs, easy births, prolificacy, and many others. These different philosophies and goals are all legitimate underpinnings for a breeding program. The specific goals and philosophies are important in driving decisions as to which strategy to use, and when to use it. Underlying philosophic questions (why is the breeder breeding livestock in the first place?) are essential for all breeders but are frequently not asked. In the absence of a guiding philosophy and set goals, breeding programs generally fail to make much progress toward any goal. All breeders should develop a guiding philosophy, for this assures better progress and a more focused breeding program. Only then can the breeding strategies be used for maximum benefit.

Inbreeding tends to firmly establish traits in the offspring. Inbred offspring, ideally, are more consistent in reproducing their own type than are outbred individuals. Breeders can use this to good advantage. However, breeders must keep in mind that prolonged multigenerational inbreeding will likely bring a decline in vitality and reproductive fitness. The real risks of long-term inbreeding in no way limit the usefulness of short-term inbreeding that is targeted to accomplish specific goals within a herd or breed. Specific strengths and uses for inbred animals include using them for outcrossing to other lines to balance genetic founders within a breed or herd, to increase vigor and vitality, or to reap the benefits by adding in some specific trait in a given line. Another wise use of inbreeding is to concentrate the genetic material of a superior animal so that the offspring can be used more broadly than is possible with a single animal.

For example, the Randall cattle breed traces back to only three founder bulls and nine founder cows, all of which were related to one another (Figure 6.9). Using bulls that are linebred to only one of these founders makes it possible to assure the production of calves that are relatively high percentage breeding of that founder so that the founder's influence is not lost to the breed. In contrast, by using non-linebred matings it is impossible to avoid diluting the founder contribution to the point that no individual cattle of the breed have any high percentage of any individual founder, and all cattle become fairly equally related to one another. Only by resorting to the occasional inbred mating is it possible to assure some genetic distance between members of this breed, although it must be done strategically and with a view to the population structure of the entire breed.

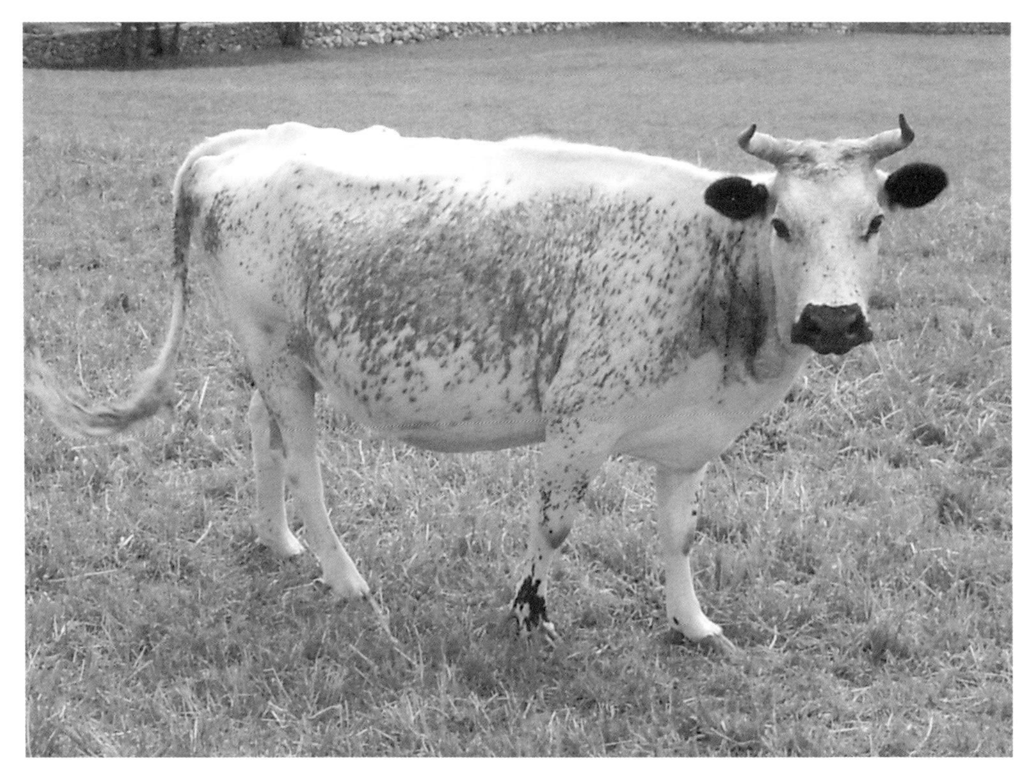

Figure 6.9 Randall cattle trace back to very few founders, but breeding strategies can manage their influence to assure productive individuals on into the future. Photo by JB.

Uniformity of progeny is important for breeding operations that are oriented toward commercial production. Linebreeding is one strategy used to achieve this end in a purebred setting. Reasonably uniform animals that perform predictably are of great value to farmers, enabling them to target management for the expected level of production that the animals are going to achieve. Obviously, the animals are never going to be entirely uniform, and the better producing animals will always be retained in favor of the lower producing ones. However, as the variation diminishes, the top and the bottom performers of the population approach one another (hopefully by the bottom coming up toward the top), so that the casual viewer is struck by how much the animals resemble one another and make a uniform group. This is indeed the impression received by viewing animals from many long-term and successful purebred operations.

Linebreeding takes time and commitment, while linecrossing and crossbreeding can be quick fixes and are tempting strategies for a variety of reasons. One outcome of crossbreeding is initial phenomenal results, especially if the parents that are recruited for the crossbreeding are thoughtfully selected for complementary strengths. The boost of crossbreeding comes from hybrid vigor and can easily be seen in several breeds of many species, especially those used for meat production. The boost in overall vigor is of very good benefit in several production systems, and some examples illustrating this are discussed below.

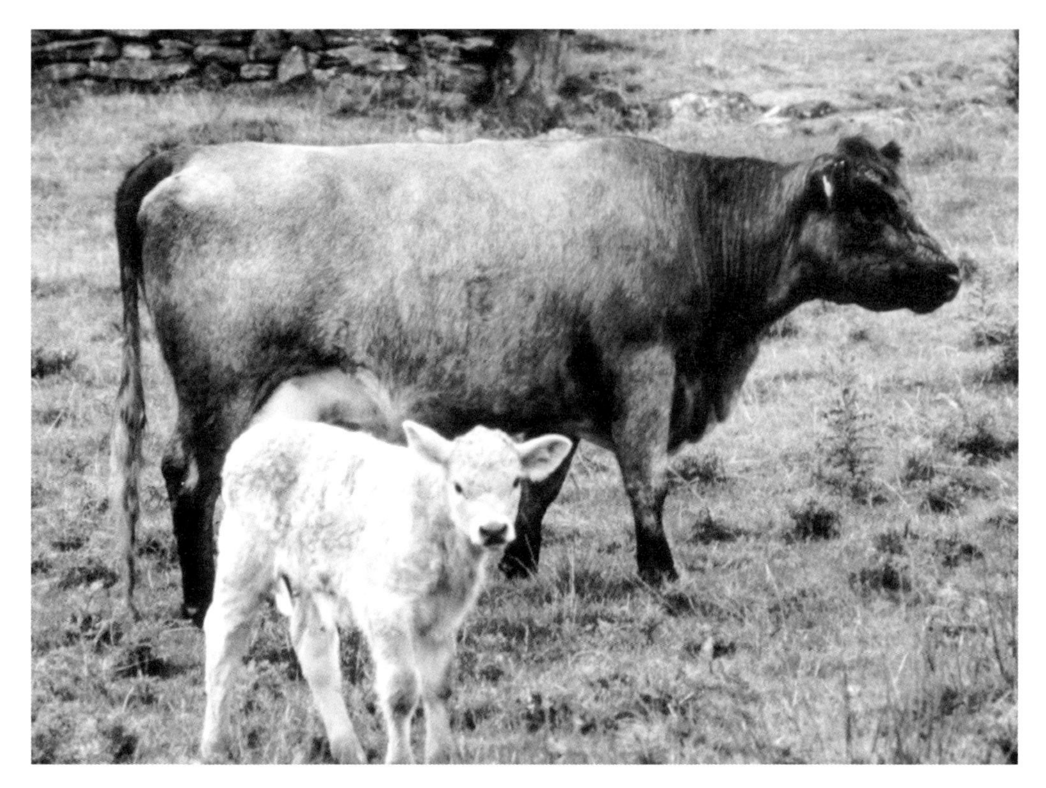

Figure 6.10 White Shorthorn to Galloway crosses have long been used to generate productive commercial brood cows in the United Kingdom. Photo by DPS.

Crossbreeding makes less sense if the goal is consistent production generation to generation. Crossbreeding does indeed make sense in many other circumstances. One of these is the production of a terminal production animal. Show ring animals and meat-producing animals provide useful examples of situations in which the boost from hybrid vigor can be put to very good use. One very well-established system is the British system of mating hill-breed ewes (small, adapted, with less growth rate) to longwool rams (large bodied, heavy fleeces, good maternal characteristics, prolific) to produce vigorous crossbred ewes for production in more favorable environments. These crossbred ewes are medium to large, fertile, prolific, and shear adequate amounts of good wool, having inherited a combination of production and adaptation traits from their divergent parent breeds. The crossbred ewes are mated to large, fast-growing meat breeds to produce large numbers of fast-growing lambs for the market. The lambs of this last stage are not retained for breeding because at the end of this three-breed cross, the genetic variability is such that they would not reproduce consistently enough to be useful. A similar system is used with Galloway cows and White Shorthorn bulls to produce blue roan crossbred brood cows that cross well with terminal beef sires (Figure 6.10).

Crossbreeding has also been used to good effect in dogs. "Lurchers" are used for vermin control, and usually are sighthound to terrier crosses or herding dog to terrier crosses. The goal is to combine the traits of both of the parental breed groups in the final effective dog.

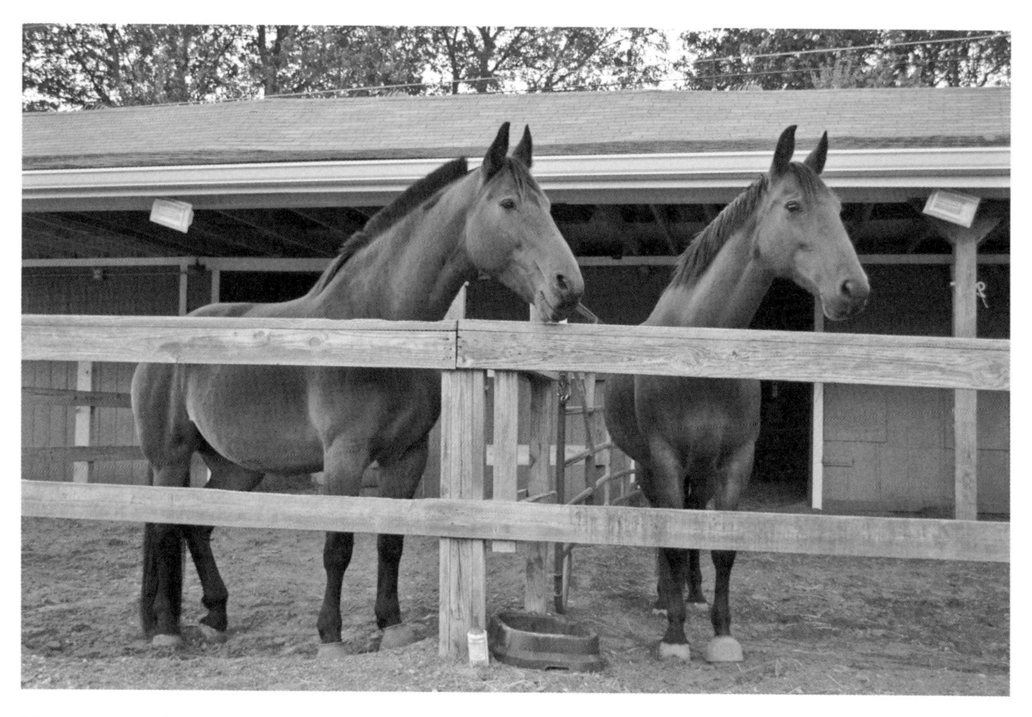

Figure 6.11 The Cleveland Bay breed is a victim of its own crossbreeding success, as purebred foals are produced less frequently than crossbreds that are used as sport horses. Photo by JB.

Similarly, a century ago dogs used for coursing coyotes were often crosses of Greyhounds (for speed) with Borzois or Scottish Deerhounds (hunting prowess). The Texas prison system originally used purebred Bloodhounds for tracking escaped prisoners but was disappointed that the dogs tried to befriend the escaped felons upon finding them. An outcross to Foxhounds assured that friendship would not be the ultimate goal. The current trend in "designer dogs" such as the Labradoodle is to cross pure breeds that are chosen with specific goals for the predictable first hybrid generation. Designer dogs also illustrate the main weaknesses of crossbreeding, because succeeding generations after that first one result in highly variable dogs.

Note well that crossbreeding systems depend on a reliable, long-term continuous source of the female line as well as the male line that goes into the cross. Crossbreeding requires different and divergent pure breeds for its success. Without pure breeds, crossbreeding quickly fails. The Cleveland Bay horse is falling victim to the success of its crossbred offspring (Figure 6.11). Cleveland Bay mares are frequently crossed with Thoroughbred stallions to produce valuable sport horses. The purebred Cleveland Bay foals often have lower market value than the crossbreds, so that purebred recruitment is diminishing and could eventually lead to the point where the cross is no longer possible due to loss of the purebred Cleveland Bay mares.

Industrial egg-laying chickens are produced in a very clever scheme that manages genetic material for maximum production as well as maximum corporate security over the genetic resources. The primary breeding lines are very highly selected and very closely guarded.

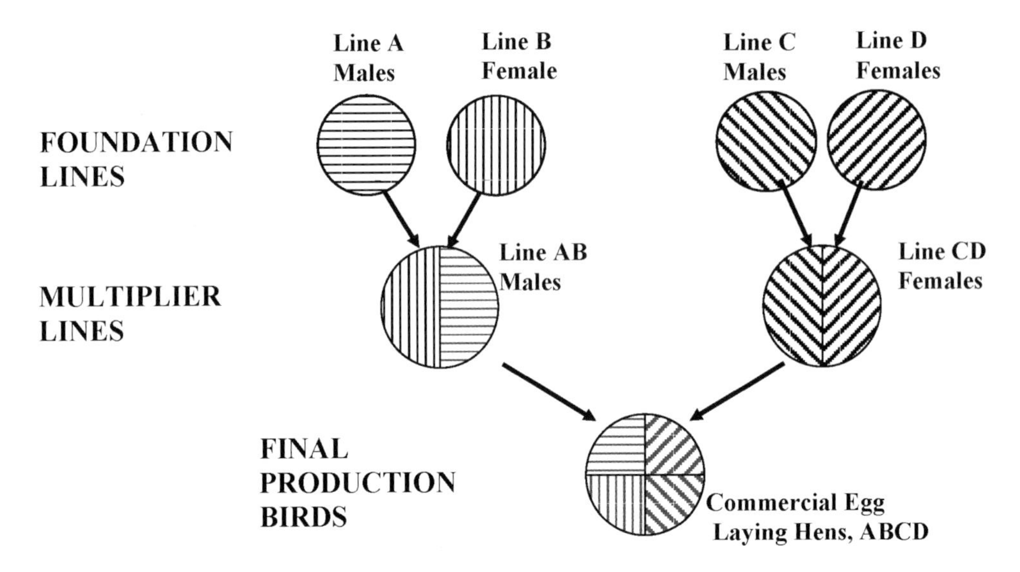

Figure 6.12 Genetic production of industrial egg-producing hens relies on the hybrid vigor assured by the crossing of unrelated foundation lines. Figure by DPS.

These include two lines that are crossed to make up the male side of multiplier flocks, and two lines that are crossed to produce the female side of multiplier flocks. The multiplier flocks are much less closely guarded than the primary breeders because they are each the hybrid result of two lines and therefore cannot be used effectively to regenerate the original resource. The resulting two hybrids (one the source of males, the other the source of females) cross well with one another to produce the final egg-laying hens. These hens benefit from great vigor and productivity provided by their four-way hybrid, outcrossed genetic makeup. They are superb layers of eggs of consistently high quality, but would be very substandard as breeding animals because their offspring would be too variable to be at all predictable. As a consequence, the industrial breeders need to have no control over where the production birds go. The corporate resource is safely back at home in the grandparental lines. Pure breeds of livestock are a similar resource, to be guarded and not squandered on crossbreeding without replacing the purebred resource (Figure 6.12).

Crossbreeding basically "uses up" genetic material without contributing to its maintenance within predictable and useful breed packages. It therefore has little role in breed conservation despite its very useful role in animal production systems. The production value derived from crossbreeding ultimately depends upon those segments of agriculture that are committed to purebreds, more specifically purebreds of different breeds for different production and market niches. The importance of this cannot be overstated, and all of production agriculture owes a huge debt to dedicated purebred breeders who maintain pure breeds as genetically distinct and useful entities.

Is crossbreeding bad? Absolutely not, although if breeders go for the fad of the moment, they can use up adapted breeds by crossbreeding without purebred replacement. Uncontrolled crossbreeding leads to diminished choices for future breeders. An example of this is the feral goats of Britain that have been incorporated into cashmere producing

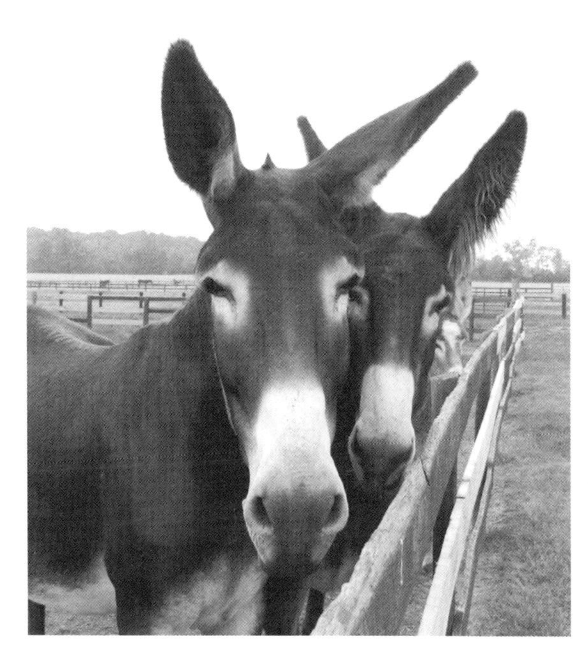

Figure 6.13 American Mammoth Jackstock breeders have long destined the most excellent jacks for pure breeding to produce replacement breeding. This strategy assures the long-term production of excellent sires for crossbreeding to mares for mule production. Photo by JB.

systems. Some of these ferals were likely to have been the remnants of the old type of North Atlantic goats. These had exquisite environmental adaptation. It is too early to say if something potentially useful has been lost, but it is not too early to say that we have indeed lost something.

In contrast, crossbreeding only some portions of a population while assuring purebred breeding of other portions can be an excellent strategy for breed conservation. This is especially true if the pure-breeding population is the portion of the breed tested as having superior performance. This was long the practice of American Mammoth Jackstock breeders, who destined the top-end jacks as "jenny jacks" to produce donkey foals, and the second tier as "mule jacks" to be mated to mares for mule production (Figure 6.13). This breed also illustrates a second subtle phenomenon associated with breeds destined for crossbreeding. Many of these breeds, especially those used on the male side of the pairing, have very low census numbers because this is sufficient to produce the males used for crossbreeding. These breeds, especially, need to have wise and careful genetic management due to their inherently small population sizes.

Similarly, throughout most of the Americas, many of the adapted and productive Spanish-based Criollo cattle have disappeared as a result of being crossbred out of existence. Included in this loss were several strains of Pineywoods and Florida Cracker cattle from the Southeastern USA. The crosses were generally to zebu-type cattle. The first crossbred generation had phenomenally good production and vigor. Subsequent generations began to lag in production until eventually they were below the level of the original Criollo base from which the crossbreeding began. At that point, the Criollo genetic resource was gone because it was used up in crossbreeding. It is now impossible to recover that original resource. Crossbreeding is a very real threat to local, purebred, long-adapted landrace animal populations.

In contrast to crossbreeding and linecrossing, many older, high-reputation breeders of most breeds have used a linebreeding strategy (coupled with selection) to produce the animals and breeds that breeders today highly desire. For most breeds, too few breeders have long-term commitments to linebreeding and the development of consistent, productive lines that are predictable for performance. A new generation of committed knowledgeable breeders is desperately needed.

The benefits of linebreeding and linecrossing can both be exploited by alternating these strategies from generation to generation within a single herd. This is accomplished by assuring that linecross animals, rather than being further linecrossed, are preferentially linebred back to one of the specific lines that is in their own ancestry. Mating linecrossed animals back to one of their parental lines accomplishes this. That sort of mating then produces linebred animals once again, which can then be used in linecrossing. This strategy avoids multigeneration linebreeding with its attendant risks. While the resulting population will not be intensely linebred, some portions of the overall population will indeed be moderately linebred. This portion will have the benefits of linebreeding, but without much risk of the drawbacks that can possibly plague more long-term, multigenerational linebreeding programs. A breeding program that accomplishes the alternation of these strategies needs to be carefully planned and executed, and the results will usually reap great benefits for both the breeder and the breed. Such a protocol (Figure 6.14) is explored further in Chapter 13.

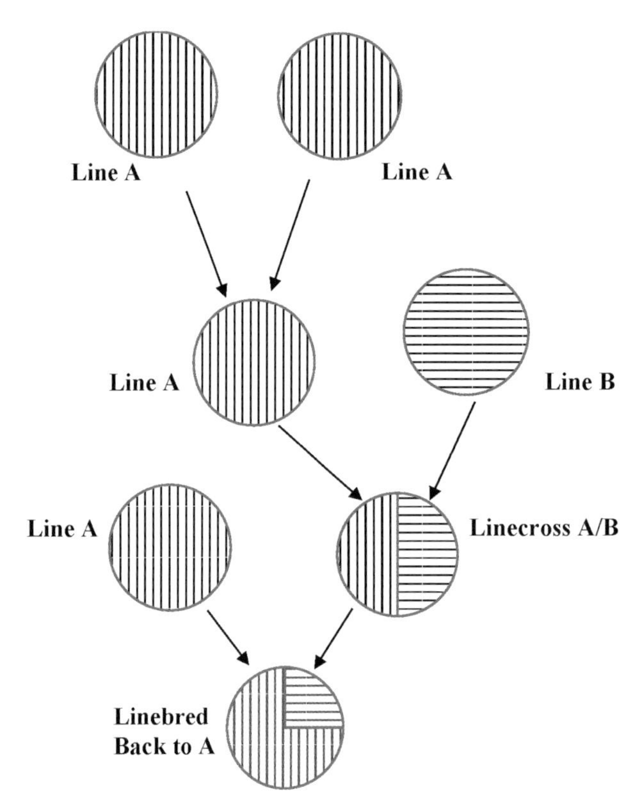

Figure 6.14 The effects of alternating linecrossing with linebreeding generation to generation. The proportion of genetic material from the different lines in each generation is indicated by the different proportions of each pattern. Figure by DPS.

A breed population is best served if several breeders are using slightly different breeding strategies, philosophies, and methods. The genetic health of a breed benefits if some breeders are linebreeding and others are linecrossing. This allows for successful genetic combinations to be developed in a variety of locations and conditions. This is good for both breeds and breeders. A single program and philosophy will not fit all situations, and breeders need to encourage diverse approaches and techniques. This requires coordination and cooperation among purebred breeders, and overseeing and facilitating this is an important role for breed associations.

6.5 Rational Crossbreeding

Crossbreeding poses a very real threat to purebred breeding if it is done so extensively that there is limited replacement of the purebred resource. Managing for adequate purebred replacement is difficult in situations where crossbred offspring bring higher economic return than purebred offspring. This can occur despite a relatively high economic value of individual purebreds in crossbreeding situations. Combining commercial production with conservation breeding is possible by carefully constructing crossbreeding plans that can provide for commercial animals as well as purebred animals. Ideal candidate breeds for such a program are those that are well adapted to difficult environments and that have good maternal qualities. Texas Longhorn cattle, Gulf Coast sheep, and Spanish goats are good candidates, as are several other breeds. Criollo cattle breeds throughout the Americas have been used in this way and unfortunately several have been lost by being completely absorbed by crossbreeding. Loss of well-adapted breeds that are rugged, long-lived, and reproductively sound is a danger in such programs of breeding as these are the very characteristics avidly sought in commercial crossbreeding endeavors (Figure 6.15).

In this situation, it is possible to organize breeding programs so that purebred females have opportunities in both crossbreeding and pure breeding. This works especially well for adapted breeds, most of which have somewhat smaller stature than animals of the usual commercial breeds. Females can be taken to a male of the same adapted breed for the first offspring. This assures an easy birth and sets the female up for a long, sound, and productive life. This first offspring is usually not "top end" due to the inexperience and immaturity of the dam, and may not be a good candidate for retaining in the breeding herd. Following this first purebred offspring, the female is then mated to a sire of a different breed, providing crossbred offspring with high economic return. After several years of commercial crossbreeding, the purebred female is then returned to a pure-breeding situation. This is the essential step for conserving the adapted resource. The female is mated to purebred mates from the adapted breed late in life. This can continue until they play out from old age or other loss. This provides the chance for the last several offspring to be purebred, and therefore potential replacements for the purebred herd (Figure 6.16).

This type of system does require enough infrastructure to provide for both commercial and purebred herds, usually in separate pastures. The main advantage of this system is that the purebred replacements are coming from the females with proven success in production. Females that are culled or lost along the way are simply unavailable. Consequently, the older dams that are being used for pure breeding have been well proven as successful in the

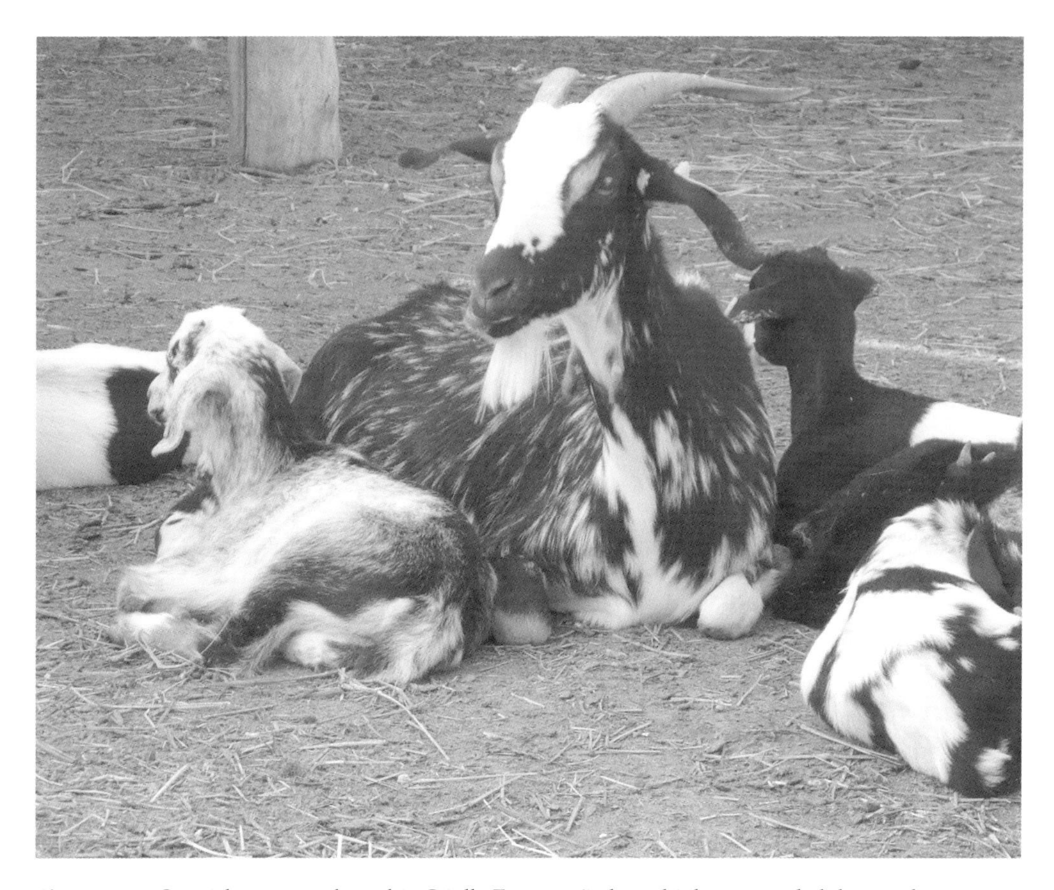

Figure 6.15 Spanish goats such as this Criolla Formoseña have high maternal ability, and are sought after in crossbreeding systems. Photo by DPS.

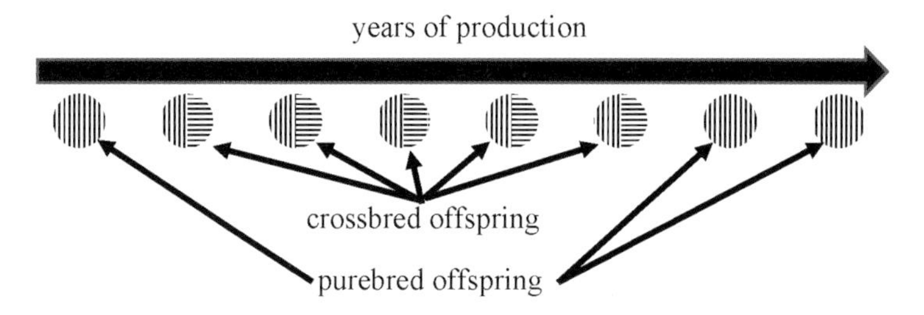

Figure 6.16 Rational crossbreeding devotes a female to sequential years of either pure breeding or crossbreeding. Figure by DPS.

very system in which they live. It is important, though, to not delay the pure-breeding stage too long, because the last few offspring of a very elderly female are likely to be somewhat compromised when compared to the ones produced a few years earlier. There is no single cutoff age for females to be transferred from crossbreeding to pure breeding. This is due to the variability in productive life from species to species and breed to breed. It is best to be sure that the last three or four offspring are purebred. In well-adapted cattle breeds such as

Texas Longhorns, it can be safe to resume pure breeding at about 12 or 13 years old. This provides for a first purebred calf at about two years old, later about ten crossbred calves, then several purebred calves at the end of her career.

This strategy has several advantages. It provides conservation breeders with a ready source of commercially acceptable offspring. In addition, it provides for purebred recruitment from a portion of the gene pool that has been tested and proven to be effective. These are the very sorts of animals that should contribute most to pure breeds. This strategy selects for productivity, longevity, and fertility, as well as adaptation. It is a good fit for many of the goals of maintaining adapted breeds.

In a few situations, it is the male rather than the female that is the desired component of a crossbreeding system. This is a more difficult situation to manage because the purebred females are viewed as less economically valuable, and this imposes a real cost to their maintenance for the production of the desired purebred males. The Criollo Saavedreño cattle of Bolivia are a good example of this. Dairy producers want about a quarter of this breeding in their commercial dairy cows. They manage to get this by using purebred bulls for half-bred daughters who are then taken to bulls of other dairy breeds (usually Holstein or Gyr). The government maintains the purebred herd of about 200 Criollo Saavedreño cows and sells the bull calves to dairy producers. This system does succeed but is at least moderately precarious because it depends on the whims and resources of the government (Figure 6.17).

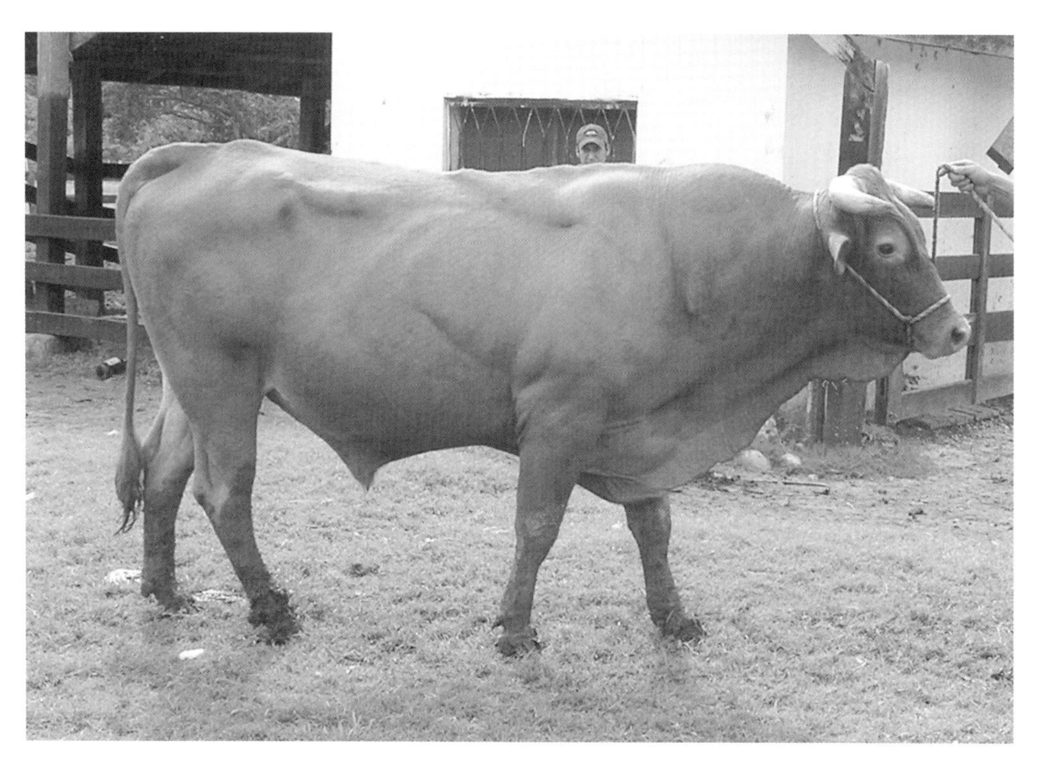

Figure 6.17 Criollo Saavedreño cattle in Bolivia are highly regarded for their inputs into adapted crossbred dairy cattle. Rational crossbreeding plans can maximize their production while also safeguarding the pure breed resource. Photo by DPS.

CHAPTER 7

Selection as a Genetic Management Tool

Selection and culling are the two sides of a single coin. "Selection" is usually used in a positive sense for the act of saving an animal for reproduction. "Culling" is the act of removing an animal from reproduction. Some breeders find references to culling distasteful due to the negative aspects of denying an animal the chance to reproduce. Selection and culling are both essential components of the maintenance of all breeds.

Selection is a power tool, and as with most power tools it can either accomplish good work at a rapid rate or it can be incredibly dangerous and can end up causing great damage. Selection tends to reduce genetic variation, and if not managed carefully it can do this precipitously. Selection can be imposed by breeders, and is also always imposed by the environment (Figure 7.1). The consequences of selection are obvious. Selection works by assuring that some animals reproduce, and others do not. This directs the flow of genetic variation from generation to generation. A breeder's role in directing that flow is all important in shaping the final product.

Selection assures that the more desirable animals produce more offspring than the less desirable animals do. The definition of "more desirable" and "less desirable" varies with situation and philosophy, and from one breeder to the next. The assignment of relative desirability of an animal is usually determined by performance testing in its various guises, which is discussed further in Chapter 8. Selection practices have profound repercussions on

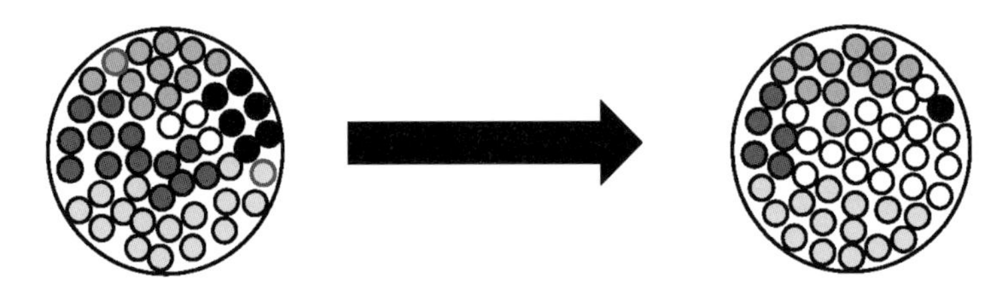

Figure 7.1 Selection reduces genetic diversity by deliberately removing some characteristics, while favoring others. In this example, breeders have selectively retained white circles at the expense of black and dark grey circles. This changes the frequencies of these in the descendant population. Figure by DPS.

the breed and its future and must therefore be chosen carefully. Selection is an important aspect of breed improvement and breed maintenance because it can either strengthen or weaken the status of a breed as a genetic resource.

Selection has a role in maintaining pure breeds, regardless of the mating system and breeding strategy used by breeds and breeders. Even among those animals that do reproduce, each individual animal's relative contribution to the next generation can (and usually should) vary considerably. Choosing which specific animals should reproduce, and the relative contribution of each, is determined by different goals that not only guide individual breeders, but that also vary breed to breed.

Selection has a role in changing or maintaining an animal population and is a critically important aspect of breed maintenance. Selection is the most common way that gene frequencies are changed and is an important source of uniformity within breeds and herds. Any individual breeder tends to favor a certain look and function over others. Over time a herd under a single breeder's care and selection will tend to express that look more and more strongly. Selection and linebreeding frequently act together as potent forces for this uniformity. The selection piece of the puzzle is an essential one.

The two major factors to consider in selection decisions include production traits on one side and aspects of population structure on the other. Especially for rare breeds, selection should emphasize the genetic structure of the breed while never ignoring the performance characteristics of the animals (Figure 7.2). Breeds that are the "rarest of the rare" will have this balance tilted more toward management of the breed's genetic structure in order to first assure breed survival. Breeds with a larger population can more safely emphasize the production performance end of the spectrum with minimal long-term threat to breed survival. Focusing narrowly on only one of these two aspects while ignoring the other is a mistake for any breed. In breeds with large numbers of animals it is usual for production performance to drive most selection decisions, and breeders can easily overlook the importance of maintaining a healthy genetic structure for the breed. Population structure is important to overall breed health and long-term productive potential even in the most populous breeds.

Some breeds unfortunately have moved from being common in the past to being rarer currently. Breeders of such breeds usually fail to make the important shift in philosophy that accompanies this change. Their selection decisions are often still driven by fine points of breed standard or by performance criteria, while ignoring the genetic structure of the breed. This situation can find the breed structure collapsing precipitously as breeders disregard the importance of maintaining rare bloodlines for the genetic diversity that is essential for breed survival.

The consequences of selection work out differently in populations with different histories of past selection. Breeders are often amazed at the rapid changes that can happen in the first few generations of targeted selection in landraces that previously have not undergone much human selection. This is a direct consequence of the fact that selection changes gene frequencies, and that landraces have variable genetics upon which selection can act. In contrast, selection in a long-standardized breed that has had multiple generations of selection for performance is unlikely to yield such dramatic results because the genetic variability so necessary for marked change is simply not present. The lower end of

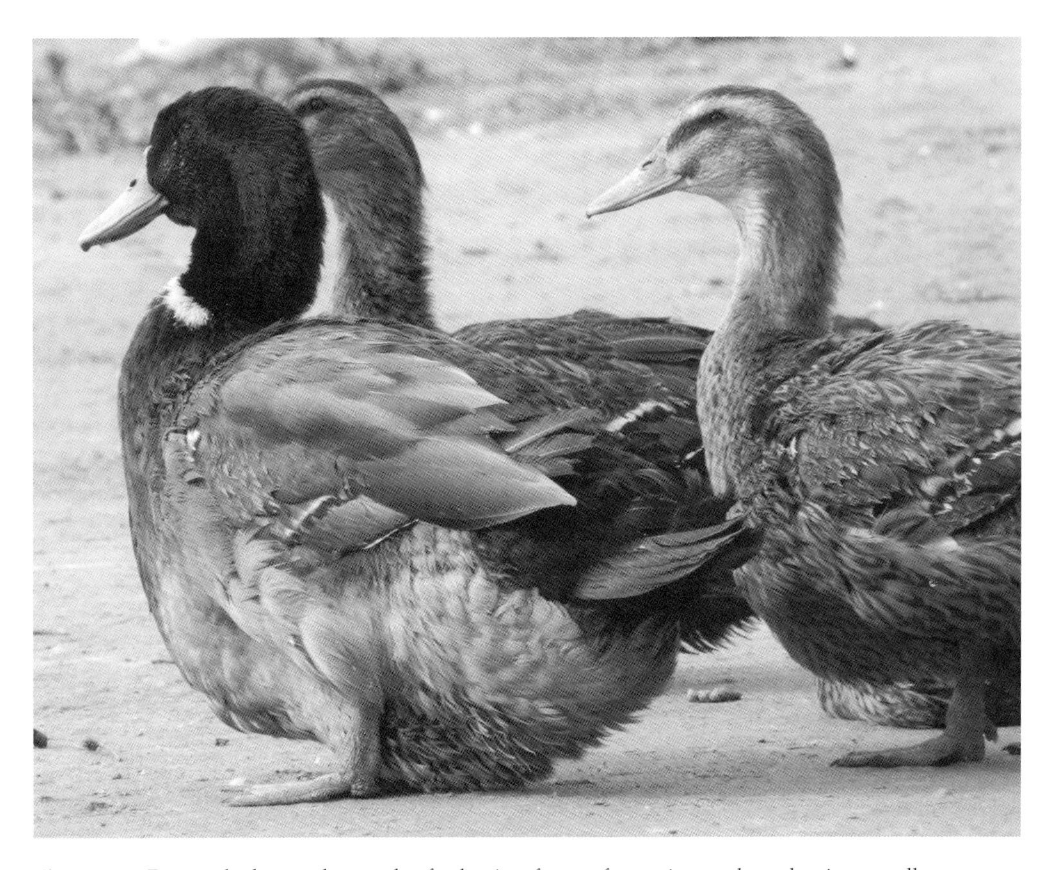

Figure 7.2 Rouen ducks are the result of selection for conformation and production excellence over many generations while not ignoring aspects of population structure. Photo by JB.

potential for performance is long gone. Selection requires genetic variability in order for it to work.

Varying selection goals have caused differences in the style of animals produced by different breeding programs. The Pineywoods breed illustrates this tendency. More traditional breeders hark back to the use of oxen in the breed, and insist on horned cattle. Some breeders more interested in beef production have favored polled animals. Conway strain cattle, as a result of selection, are nearly all red and white in some combination. Hickman cattle have no such color theme, and selection favored color variation instead of uniformity, while also favoring lyre-shaped horns. Some breeders liked and kept a few guinea dwarf cattle in their herds, others avoided these, and the result is the absence of guineas in some strains but the persistence of them in others. No single approach is inherently "right" or "wrong," but each does take the herd, and the breed, to a different destination by shaping the genetic material differently.

Animals not chosen to reproduce in a selection strategy can still have important roles, whether that be fiber production, food production, draft power, other performance, or life as a pet. Each of these roles can be important for breed promotion, despite the fact that the animals are not reproductive.

7.1 Degree of Selection

The degree of selection that occurs in a population depends on the relative number of animals used for reproduction. The degree of selection for some populations of rare breeds is fairly low. This is especially true for females. That is, nearly every female is used for reproduction and therefore gets a chance to pass along her genes for good or ill. In essence this means that little selection is occurring on the female side of the equation. This situation is typical of breeds or species that are involved in the novelty market or that are newly present in the marketplace. Recently imported breeds often go through a phase of minimal selection pressure on the female side.

For most breeds, the degree of selection for males is higher than that for females. How much higher varies with individual breeds as well as with individual breeding programs. In some herds nearly every male that is born is used for reproduction, while for other herds, only a small percentage has the opportunity to reproduce. The overall result is that the degree of selection for males is higher than for females and varies from moderate to extreme. This can be good or bad depending on how selection is used.

Dairy cattle illustrate the extreme to which the degree of selection can go. The degree of selection for dairy bulls (especially Holsteins) is probably the highest of the common domesticated species. Artificial insemination allows the use of only one bull in thousands, and that one is likely to produce tens of thousands of calves. Over several generations this strategy has profound consequences for the genetic composition of the breed. In each new generation, the bulls selected for semen production are nearly invariably the offspring of a previously selected semen sire. The result is that the new sire is related to many of the females of the breed (his half-sisters). A trend to save bulls out of certain cow families (half-sisters from specific sires) also contributes to an increasing concentration of the genetics as each new generation is produced by only a very few individuals. Over several generations this breeding strategy compounds the narrowing of the genetic base. The intense degree of selection and the resulting narrowed genetic base have long-term consequences for the overall genetic health of the breed because this strategy assures an increase in the level of inbreeding across the entire breed.

In contrast, many alpaca herds have a relatively low degree of selection because many males see at least some use, and very few males are used all that widely. In this situation, more genetic change is easily possible than is currently being realized. This can be accomplished simply by increasing the degree of selection used among the males, by using fewer males, each of them with a higher number of females (Figure 7.3).

To effectively manage the genetic structure of breeds, and especially those with small populations, it is generally wise to not have a degree of selection as high as is typical of mainstream industrial dairy cattle. Progress for genetic potential for production can be rapid under high degrees of selection, but the disadvantage of this tactic is that a great deal of genetic material is discarded in unused males. The result can easily be very restricted genetic variation that approaches nonviability, especially if such high degrees of selection are used for several generations in a row in a breed with a small population. The other extreme uses each and every animal for reproduction and assures that no improvement in performance is achieved in the population, along with no penalty for nonperformance.

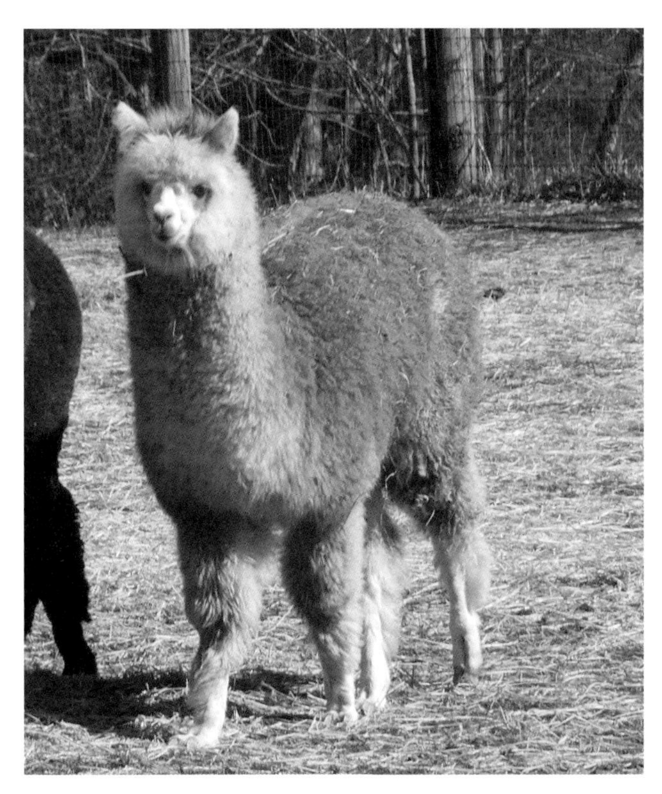

Figure 7.3 Most alpaca herds in North America have a fairly low degree of selection, with many males seeing at least some use as sires. Photo by DPS.

While this strategy maintains high levels of genetic variation, it does this to an extreme that can easily detract from the predictability of the animals that is at the core of the utility of breeds. Lack of selection also leads to lack of a performance potential such that the breed is rejected by commercial producers for that very reason. Both extremes of selection work to the detriment of a breed, and the best strategy usually lies somewhere in between. A balance of selection for performance and for maintenance of good population structure is wisest for all breeds.

Turkeys provide examples of both extremes of degrees of selection. At the industrial end, turkeys are the result of an extraordinarily high degree of selection and are very genetically uniform. They are exquisitely productive, but only in the narrow industrial environment because they lack the ability to adapt well to other environments. In contrast, many backyard flocks have very limited selection and may use a tom on only one or two hens. Consequently, many backyard flocks have relatively low potential for production. However, heritage turkeys of the standardized varieties were once commercially important. The historic system, never abandoned by some and increasingly adopted by others, included mating individual toms to groups of about 12 hens each. This provides for a degree of selection that is adequate to assure constant progress in the commercial utility of this important type of turkey, without losing important performance in traits of adaptation to the environment (Figure 7.4). Fortunately, more and more breeders are learning the techniques of selection that can be applied to this type of bird, and their important historic role is increasingly being recaptured. Turkeys therefore illustrate all levels of selection,

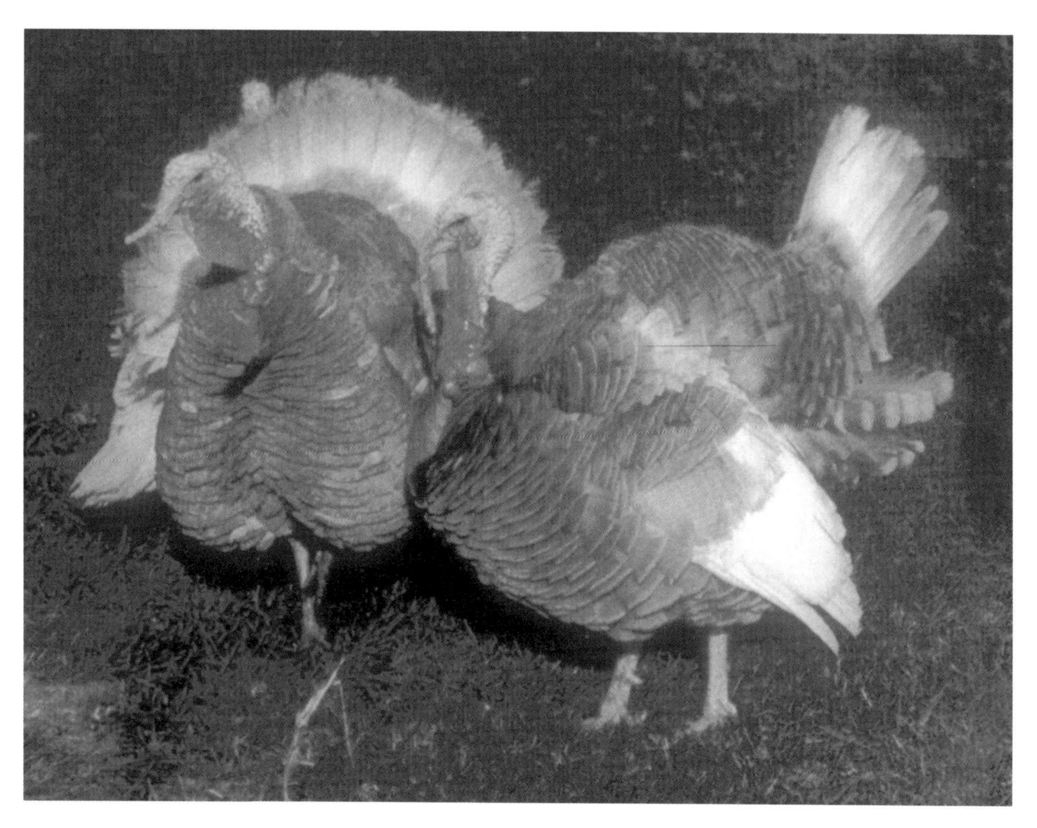

Figure 7.4 Heritage turkeys, because they reproduce naturally, have a lower degree of selection than the industrial varieties that depend on artificial insemination from a relatively few breeding toms. Photo by DPS.

including that balance point between the extremes where production levels increase while a good population structure is maintained.

7.2 Selection and Breed-Specific Traits

Selection is a sword with two edges. Selection is a powerful tool for change, but not all change is good. The loss of a breed's genetic heritage is obvious when it occurs through the outright extinction of the breed, but a more insidious loss involves deviation from the original type of the breed such that it no longer represents the original gene pool. This second kind of loss can occur rapidly and completely if crossbreeding is occurring. A similar loss occurs, if more slowly, by selection within the breed but away from the traditional form of the breed that includes breed-specific traits that are not shared widely across breeds. As a result of recent selection pressures, many mainstream beef cattle breeds are all remarkably similar in overall conformation. A can of spray paint could render them impossible to distinguish by breed. One underlying philosophy of breed conservation is that the original forms of breeds are important to keep so that real choices remain available to future agriculturalists.

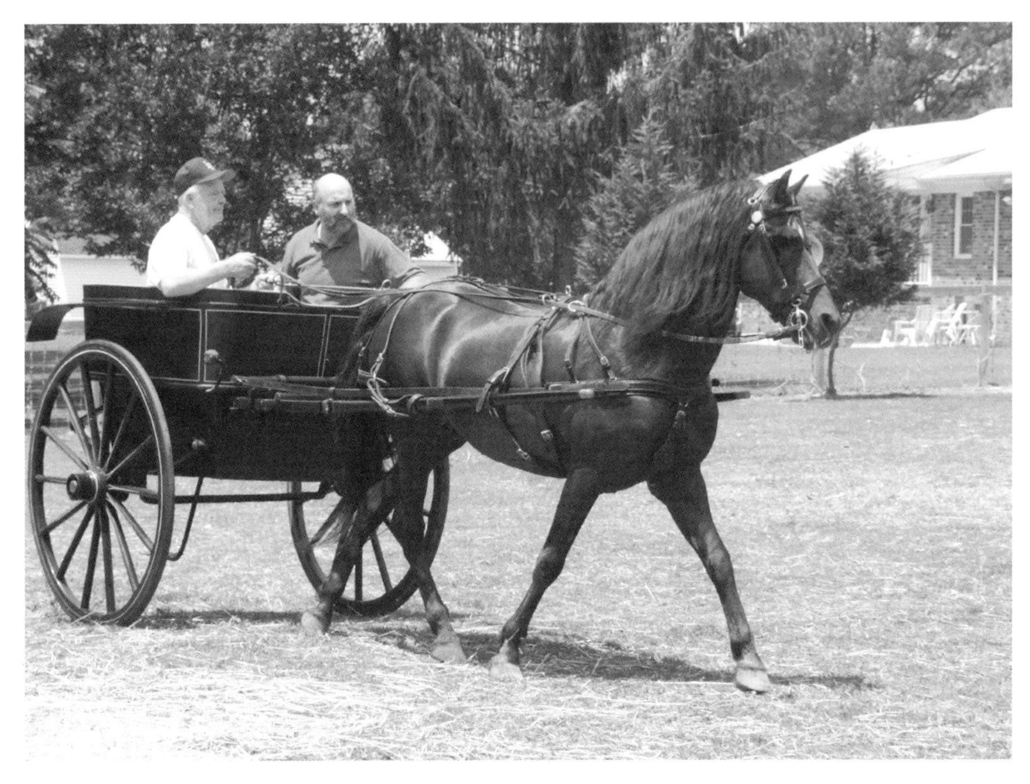

Figure 7.5 Morgan horse breeders have diverged widely in their selection goals, but fortunately a dedicated group works together to keep the original horse available for future generations. Photo by JB.

To preserve breed uniqueness, it is important for breeders to constantly select animals that reflect the original breed-specific traits and to reject those that deviate from it. Some of the experiences of South American breeders of Criollo horses are instructive in this regard. In the mid-1900s, selection began to produce animals that were taller than their traditional height of 14.2 hands. With that increase in height came a perception of great beauty and eye appeal, but much less athletic prowess. Breeders wisely abandoned the quest for height in the breed and returned the breed to its original form before irreparable loss had occurred.

Other examples of changes in breed-specific traits are numerous. Today's Morgan horses vary in type all the way from the original multipurpose farm horse to a very specialized park-type show horse (Figure 7.5). Many hog breeds have varied over time as they abandoned very obese lard types that lapsed in demand. Hog type in many breeds then changed to very lean hogs. This change occurred all within individual breeds as they responded to the pressure of selection over decades for a new and different ideal type. Angus cattle have changed from low, wide, fat cattle to much taller, rangier, muscular cattle over the last 60 years.

Controversies over breed type that comes from breed-specific traits have no easy answers, but maintaining a breed's type is fundamental if conservation is to truly save the unique genetic packages that breeds are. Breed-specific traits, or combinations of traits, are essential to breeds and must be closely safeguarded rather than allowed to drift too far. Breeders must be able to understand and appreciate type in order to conserve it. Guarding these traits can become an extremely difficult issue in some breeds where historic types (lard hogs, dual-purpose cattle, farm horses) meet with little current demand. For those breeds, changes in breed type can help them to compete in the modern marketplace more successfully. These are complex issues with no easy remedies because guarding historic types that are undesired in the contemporary marketplace nearly assures relegating some specific breeds to rarity. Losing these breeds and their breed-specific traits, though, can easily erase them from the range of options available for future animal breeders.

While breed-specific traits are important, they need to be put into the context of the entire package that an animal represents. Culling an exceptionally productive animal makes little sense if that decision is based on minor deviation in a trait related only to breed type. A better strategy is to selectively mate such an animal to one that excels in that specific trait. For example, many breeders of Leicester Longwool sheep are diligent to fault animals with weak skin pigmentation. While dark skin pigment is a specific trait for that breed, it is much less important than overall body length, size, wool character, and fecundity. While an animal that is generally weak over all should be culled for having little pigment, it makes no sense to follow that course of action with an exceptional animal that is otherwise outstanding for the breed. The minor weakness in a breed-specific trait can be corrected in the next generation by mating to an animal with stronger expression of that trait. Traits that are breed-specific should not be ignored, but neither should they have complete veto over the rest of the animal's attributes or contributions to purebred breeding.

7.3 Genetic Drift

Genetic drift is a second way that a population's genetics change. Genetic drift is more subtle than selection. It is the loss of gene variants by random effects related to the chance events of genes passing along at each generational step (Figure 7.6). Drift is not a response to directed selection. Chance, as opposed to conscious selection, is especially likely to eliminate relatively rare genetic variants from small populations because they can simply fail to make it to the next generation. Subdividing a population reduces the risk of genetic drift contributing to loss of variation in a breed because it is unlikely that each subpopulation will be affected in the same way by the random events that cause it. Subdivision also tends

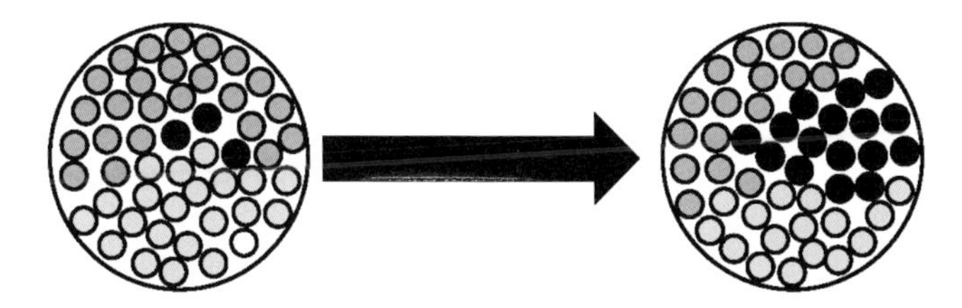

Figure 7.6 Genetic drift changes allele frequencies through random effects. Rare variants are especially likely to be lost. In this example, the one individual (white circle) failed to make it to the next generation, while another contribution (black circles) was boosted, all by chance events. Figure by DPS.

to reduce the effects of selection if the subpopulations are under different managers. It works well in most situations to maximize the opportunity for survival of genetic variation within breeds.

The consequences of genetic drift can be imagined as a jar of mixed dried beans. A large jar has 500 pinto beans, 500 red kidney beans, 100 black beans, 50 cranberry beans, and only 10 Mayflower beans. If a random sample of 50 beans is taken out, it is very likely that Mayflower beans simply do not make the cut. It is also more likely to lose cranberry beans than it is pintos or kidney beans. Genetic drift is a real threat to rare variants, even if it does sometimes work out in the other direction.

An example of the interaction of genetic drift and subdivision comes from a recent study of the microsatellite DNA analysis of Randall Lineback cattle. Microsatellites are discussed in detail in Chapter 12. The important detail here is that certain microsatellite variants are relatively rare in the breed. These are present in some herds, and completely missing in others. Subdivision therefore changed the frequency of the alleles among the various herds, just by the chance of which cattle ended up in which herd.

7.4 Single Gene Traits

Many traits are controlled by single genes. Some of these lead to weakness; others are related to traits that are more cosmetic. Color comes to mind as one obvious trait that is important in many breeds and is controlled by only a few genes. The advantage of working with single genes is that they are relatively easy to track, identify, and manage. This is especially true currently because the technology to probe and track many of these genes has become routine. This has the very important practical consequence that in rescue situations it is possible to relax selection for these single genes while animal numbers are expanding, because those single genes can then be tackled later when the population is more secure.

A few examples of single genes that are important to rare breeds include the *champagne* allele that gives rise to the color of the American Cream Draft Horse (Figure 7.7). Horses of the breed that lack this allele are usually sorrel, a color that is not favored in the breed. But selectively removing all of the sorrel horses imposes a shrinking gene pool on a breed already perched on the verge of extinction. Including those sorrel horses in the breeding population can be important to the future of the breed. An even more drastic action, made possible by the advent of genetic testing, would be to insist on all horses being homozygous (two copies) for the *champagne* allele. While this would assure uniformity for the desired color, it would remove so many horses from reproduction that an already rare breed would rapidly approach the threshold of nonviability. Similar principles are at work in other breeds such as Cleveland Bay horses and Friesian horses. Removing the occasional chestnut horses of these breeds, or carriers of the genes for chestnut, ripples through the population and makes breed survival all the more tenuous.

Single genes related to disease traits have slightly different consequences when compared to those for color, but these can still be managed creatively and successfully in small populations. Most breeds have a few such genes, and the underlying principles work equally well for all of them. The gene for *junctional epidermolysis bullosa* (JEB) trait is a recessive gene that occurs in some American Cream Draft Horses, as well as in other breeds. In this

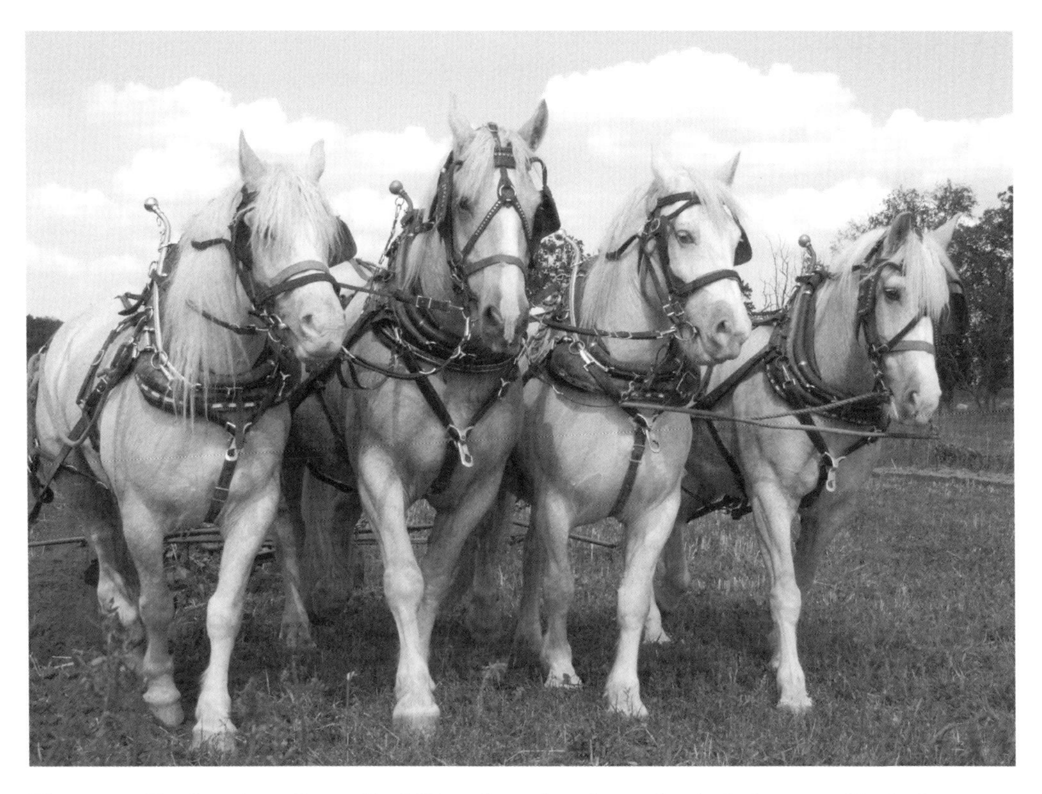

Figure 7.7 The American Cream Draft Horse has a breed type that includes a specific single gene related to the typical color of the breed. Photo by JB.

case, the animals with two copies of the gene fail to survive, so obviously "doing nothing" is not an option as was the case with the color genes. However, removing all of the carriers of this gene is likely to have drastic consequences for the population structure because entire families are likely to be removed. The breed cannot withstand that loss and still maintain genetic viability for other traits. In this case, as with many single genes, the animals with only one copy are perfectly normal. In such situations it is wisest to test horses, and not mate one carrier to another. This strategy instantly assures that no affected foals will be born despite the presence of the gene in the breed. A slight modification of this strategy is to test all stallions, and require that carrier stallions only be mated to tested mares that are non-carriers. The non-carrier stallions can be safely mated to any mare, including mares that have not undergone the genetic test, because non-carrier stallions have no risk of ever producing affected foals.

The demand for breeding animals is going to be an issue for any single-gene disease trait. Animals that are carriers, even though they are normal, are going to be less economically desirable than animals free of the trait. Some level of this preference is going to be nearly impossible to avoid. It is essential, though, to be sure that carriers of rare bloodlines are used for breeding. This assures that the breed does not lose the remaining balance of their genes that offer so much to breed viability. Carriers can be safely used, with the single stipulation that they are not mated to other carriers. In the next generation the non-carrier

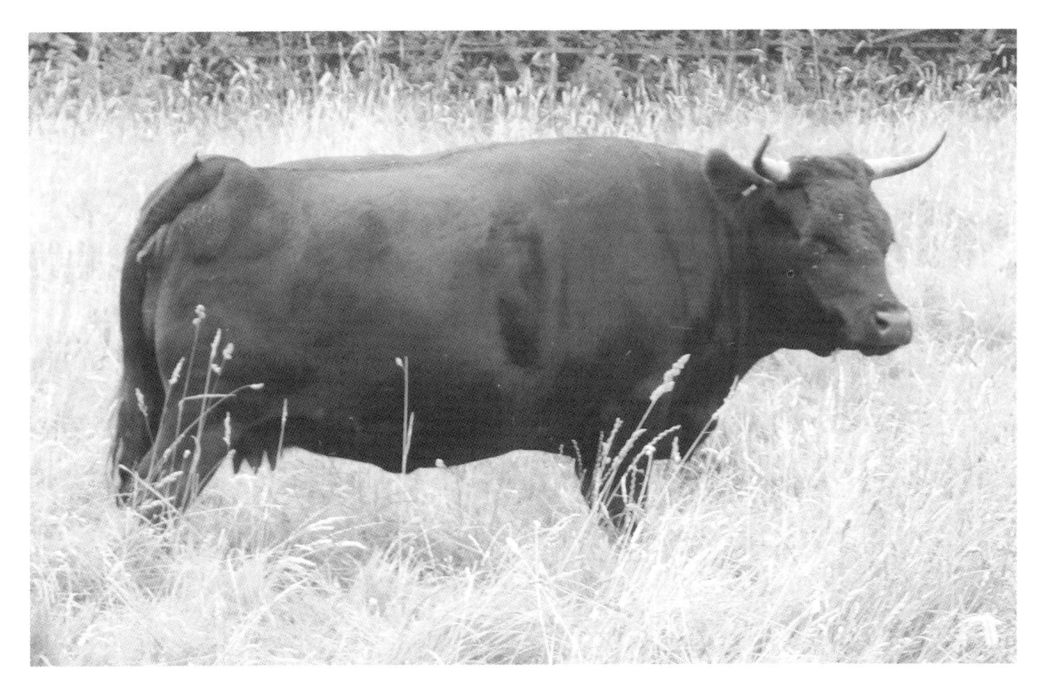

Figure 7.8 Dexter cattle are a breed that needs careful attention to underlying genetics in order to assure viable, productive cattle that are typical for the breed and have the full potential for adaptation and productivity unique to the breed. Photo by DPS.

offspring can be selectively retained. This is an effective strategy that allows carriers to contribute to the genetic future of the breed without passing along the disease coded for by their deleterious gene. It is vitally important to realize that carrier animals have many more genes than this single one, and to balance the potential negatives (which can usually be fairly easily managed) against the positive contributions that the rest of their genome can make.

A few genes are a bit more complicated because they are related to phenotypes that are desired when the gene is present in one dose, but that are deleterious when present in two doses. The dwarfism of Dexter cattle is one such gene (Figure 7.8). Homozygous calves are aborted rather than born viably, and this greatly diminishes the productivity of the cow producing such a calf. Heterozygous cattle, though, are the short-legged type of dwarf form long associated with the breed. The experience of some breeders is that these animals have other advantages in production and adaptation in addition to their desired short stature. This is a situation where mating of carriers can be avoided, as long as both non-carrier bulls and cows are available to mate to carriers. This strategy provides for uniformly viable calves, including those that have the short-legged dwarf type long associated with the breed. The availability of a test for this gene has had the consequence that bulls carrying the gene face considerable negative discrimination. However, these carrier bulls do indeed have a very clear and constructive role to play in maintaining a traditional type within the breed, and hopefully will see wise use by being mated to non-carrier cows. Failing to be wise in decisions for managing single genes like this one brings a very real risk of forever changing

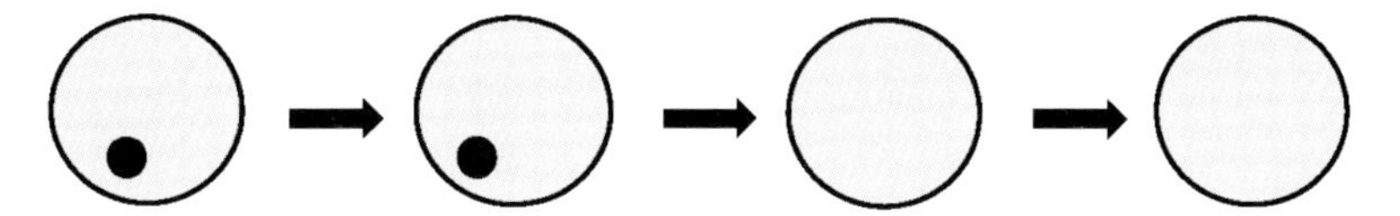

Figure 7.9 This single allele (the black dot) is passed along through the first generation to the second, but then fails to make it to the third generation. That makes it unavailable for the fourth and all succeeding generations. Figure by DPS.

a breed away from its traditional type. Wise genetic management decisions assure the persistence of traditional type as well as the birth of viable, healthy calves.

The advantage of "single gene" traits is that modern technology allows these genes to be tracked and managed effectively. As long as carriers are not mated together, no undesired affected offspring will be born. This is a constructive use of the technology. A potentially destructive use is to remove all carriers from reproduction. Few breeds can sustain that loss if the goal is long-term breed viability. As with most of technology, testing for single genes is "value neutral" and the outcome depends entirely on how it is used. It is important to note that once an allele has been removed from a breed, it is gone for good and cannot be recovered (Figure 7.9). This includes genes that might be out of favor today, but tomorrow find a renewed and favorable demand. In most cases, effective breed conservation should at least attempt to save the entire breed package.

Genetic testing for single-gene disease traits has become especially strongly adopted by dog breeders of many breeds. Most dog breeds have at least a few diseases related to single genes, and breeders logically have a real desire to eliminate the production of disease-prone puppies. In many breeds this has led to a breeder culture where animals for reproduction are all tested, and all carriers are eliminated. This can have very negative long-term consequences because it drastically reduces the reproducing population of the breed, and takes away much more genetic variation than the single, identifiable, disease genes. A second consequence is more subtle. As animals are eliminated for carrying identifiable genes, it has also happened that the survivors carry genes that are in fact deleterious but for which there is no test, or no previous knowledge of the syndrome they cause. The newly encountered disease then becomes a widespread problem, all as a consequence of overeager use of testing and removal for the other genes encountered earlier.

Most individual animals have at least a few deleterious genes. One estimate is that they each have at least four or five. This means that effective management relies less on a "test and cull" mentality, and more on developing ways to manage the genes for successful outcomes.

Similar tactics of genetic selection based on single genes have been used in sheep breeding for control of the degenerative neurologic disease, scrapie. This disease has a profound genetic link, and the approach of most European countries, and some states within the USA, is to insist that all breeding rams have resistant genotypes. In some breeds, such as those in the longwool group, this is relatively easy because most sheep already have resistant genotypes. In other breeds, including many highly adapted breeds, resistant genotypes are reasonably rare. In those breeds the result of genetically based selection programs is to remove many rams (and many bloodlines) from the male lines of several breeds.

To muddle the issue further, at least some evidence has emerged that sheep of scrapie-resistant genotypes can harbor the scrapie agent but simply not show evidence of disease. This apparent absence of disease is actually due to prolonged incubation periods rather than true freedom from the scrapie agent. The agent can then express itself as disease when it connects with a genetically susceptible animal. To assure freedom from the agent, some countries have favored the approach that all imported sheep must be from susceptible genotypes without evidence of disease. By this mechanism they are assured of not bringing in the agent. In the USA, the approach varies breed-by-breed, and state-by-state, but the regulatory environment could change and may eventually be dictated by government edict. As a further complication, there are several strains of scrapie. If all sheep are selected to be of the same resistant genotype, all could be susceptible to another strain of scrapie. Hopefully, all sides of this complex issue will be weighed before strict regulations are established. The important lesson is that achieving uniformity for this, or other traits, often comes with a risk of a negative outcome that only becomes evident much later.

A troubling example of genetic testing and breed maintenance is the hyperkalemic periodic paralysis (HYPP) or the "Impressive Syndrome" trait of horses. This is due to a dominant gene, and results in heavily muscled horses. Unfortunately, some homozygotes occasionally collapse and can die. While Quarter Horse breeders have been diligent to quickly identify and reduce the incidence of most lethal traits, this one has persisted in the breed. A major reason for its persistence is that many HYPP horses are consistent halter class winners. To correct this problem it is essential that the show ring and the breed association rules speak with one voice on the issue of genetic flaws. Both should diligently assure that animals with flaws do not meet with increased demand, for in that situation it will be impossible to reduce or eliminate the flaws even in the presence of genetic testing. Market demand ultimately will dictate the fate of genetic defects, and in nearly all cases the best situation is for the defect to have a market penalty. Situations in which the reverse is true, such as HYPP, make selection against the defect difficult.

The key point is that selection programs based mostly on single genes can have devastating and unforeseen effects on a breed and its future viability. It has also often been the case that the initial "absolute truth" of a genetic situation in animals has later proven to be much hazier than initially thought, with the consequence that early attempts at wise genetic management have been proven to be just the opposite. Genetic uniformity can have devastating effects, as evidenced by the Irish Potato Famine where the uniformity of the potato varieties led to the collapse of this important crop as one disease eliminated production of the single variety that had been so extensively planted.

7.5 Polygenic Traits

Problems caused by multiple genes at multiple genetic locations are a bit more difficult to manage than those related to single genes. Polygenic traits, especially those related to diseases, can never be completely ignored, even in an early phase of a rescue project. Caution must still be used, though, to avoid "throwing the baby out with the bathwater." These situations are complicated and need to be tailored to each individual situation. As a result, no blanket recommendation is realistic. In situations where affected animals come

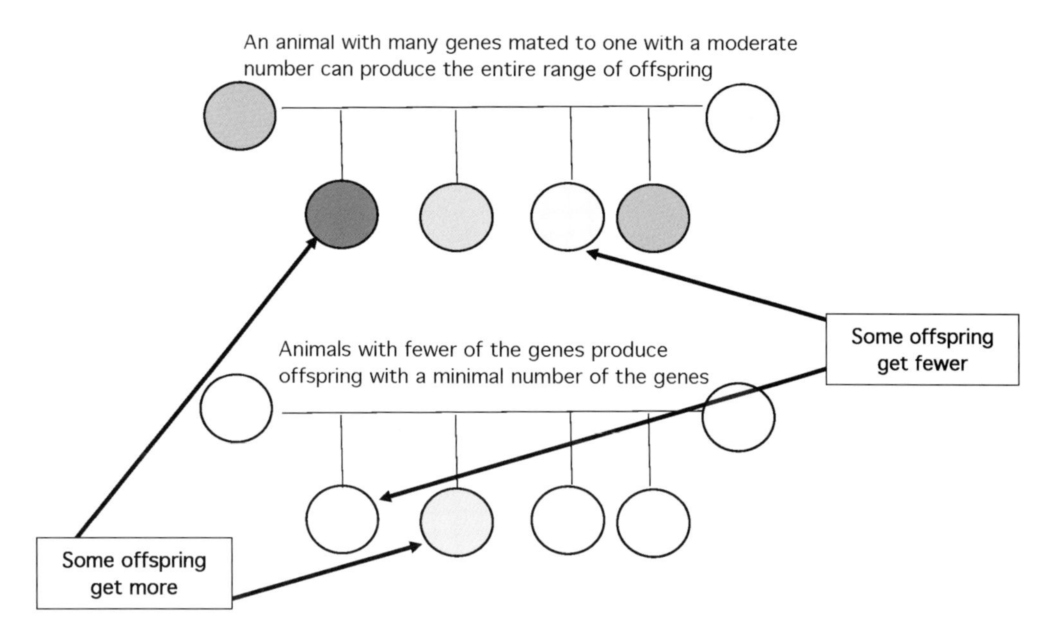

Figure 7.10 Polygenic traits can be imagined as shaded circles, with darker circles representing animals that have relatively more of the alleles that influence the trait and paler circles representing animals with fewer of those alleles. Each animal can contribute different amounts of the shading (alleles), but never any more than it has to offer. Taking the contribution of any animal to zero is unrealistic in most situations. The greater the number of alleles present (the darker color), the more likely it is that they will be passed along to offspring. Some offspring get more of the alleles, some get fewer. The process is one that is dictated by chance and probabilities. Figure by DPS.

from well-represented bloodlines, those animals affected with a deleterious polygenic trait should likely be removed from further reproduction, along with their parents, offspring, and siblings. These animals are all likely to have several of the alleles that contribute to the condition. In contrast, it might be necessary to continue to use the parents of an affected animal if they come from otherwise unrepresented bloodlines. They must be used cautiously, though, with an eye toward diminishing the occurrence of the deleterious trait while retaining as much as possible of the other important genetic variation they bear (Figure 7.10).

CHAPTER 8

Evaluating Individual Animals

Selection decisions are based on the evaluation of animals with regard to their relative desirability. This involves a whole range of options, ranging from the free hand of nature for feral animals to the very constrained world of industrial poultry. The key concept remains constant: excellence is rewarded with an opportunity to pass along genes to the next generation. The critical issue is how excellence is defined because this shapes the final result. Basically, "what you want is what you get."

Animals need to be evaluated in order for breeders to know which ones are performing well and which ones are performing poorly. Performance covers a wide range of structural, functional, and behavioral traits. Evaluation of animal performance needs to be put into the context of the genetic structure of populations. However, without adequate performance any breed is perched very precariously for long-term survival, so selection based on performance should never be ignored. Evaluating all of these aspects in a comprehensive and wise manner is a tall challenge. Demand for a breed is a major part of breed security, and demand depends on performance.

Testing the performance of one animal against others is a common way to assist breeders as they try to make wise breeding decisions. An ideal performance test cleanly and clearly ranks animals as to their productive potential. This can include any of a host of strategies, each of which has strengths and each of which is subject to misuse that can damage the population. Options for testing include competitive shows and performance trials that directly test various traits of interest.

Unfortunately, performance testing easily leads to the conclusion that one single animal is best. While the members of any breed vary in their ability and potential for performance across a wide range of traits, no single animal excels in all aspects of performance. Inclusion of a range of animals, each with different potential for a wide variety of traits, is more likely to lead to a successful breed than a philosophy that picks out only a few animals that are stellar performers for only a very few traits.

8.1 Competitive Shows

Competitive showing is a very common way of evaluating animals against one another. Competitive shows have long been a major activity of breed associations, and most of the stimulus to develop breed associations in the 1800s and 1900s revolved around the competitive showing of livestock, poultry, and dogs. Showing of animals has both negative and positive consequences for breeds. These tend to be accentuated in the case of rare breeds.

Positive aspects of competitive shows include public exposure and the potential for new breeder recruitment. This is especially true if showing is seen to be fair, fun, and constructive. Another positive aspect of showing is that the placement of animals in rank order of quality can guide breeders as they make breeding decisions. Showing and judging can have a profound impact on keeping the breed type intact, but only if show ring evaluation emphasizes those specific traits that make up breed type. This can be especially beneficial for educating new or young breeders. Many associations have specific programs that target young members, and these can be an effective way to generate enthusiasm within the next generation to stay active in a breed.

Competitive showing does have several potential negative consequences for breeds and breeders. One basic limitation is that the show only evaluates the animals that actually attend the show, and it only evaluates them on that one occasion. Showing therefore cannot ever be comprehensive over an entire breed, nor can it be a good comprehensive evaluation of animals over time.

Another potential problem with showing is that judges often tend to evaluate multiple breeds by a single mental picture of excellence. This can easily take a breed away from its traditional type. A single target for excellence across breeds ignores or blurs distinctive breed-specific traits that are so critical in maintaining breeds as unique genetic populations. Judges can also easily damage breeds by ignoring off-type characteristics in animals placed well up in the winnings. Changing type can be a result of show ring and judging fads, and is detrimental to a breed and its genetic integrity. Many breeds have seen profound changes in breed type after decades of being evaluated by judges who are poorly informed of the unique characteristics of various individual breeds.

Competitive showing has an inherent tendency to select extremes as the ideal. Favorable placement of extreme animals drives selection toward those chosen extremes and away from moderate and balanced animals that may well prove to be more functionally useful. An unfortunate aspect of the show ring is that anyone, including trained judges, tends to be favorably drawn to an extreme animal as a "first impression" response. This is easiest to appreciate in dog shows (Figure 8.1). In toy breeds the smallest dog makes the first exceptional impression, while in large breeds the largest dog often does. The result has been, for many breeds, that small breeds continually become smaller and large breeds continually become larger. This is frequently to the detriment of overall balance, function, and soundness.

Show ring wins easily translate into significant monetary earnings as well as bragging rights. This opens the door for a "win at any cost" mentality that can be very damaging to breeder integrity and to the breed itself. The show ring can end up dictating most breed policies for these breeds. When this occurs, other weighty aspects of breed biology and

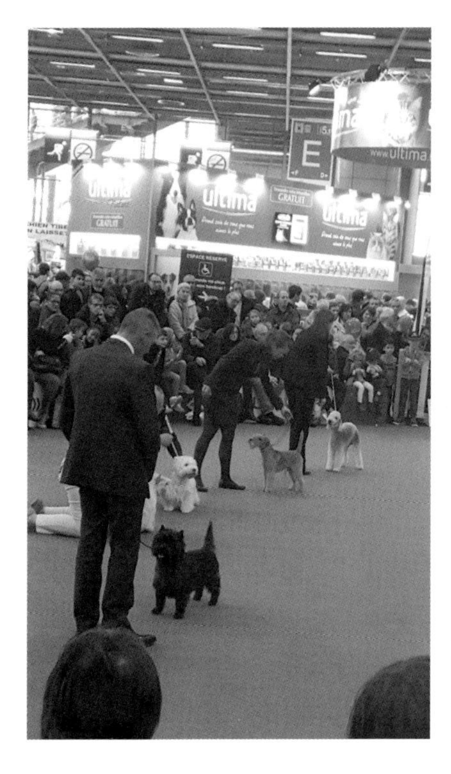

Figure 8.1 Show ring placements can either help breeds remain true to breed type, or can lead to selection for extremes of size or other characteristics. Photo by JB.

maintenance can be ignored to the long-term detriment of the breed. While any breed is made up of individual animals, it is a subtle concept that those individuals all must be evaluated relative to their potential contribution back to the breed as a gene pool.

An example of the show ring subverting breed integrity occurred within the Texas Longhorn cattle breed when some registries emphasized horn length, color, and size over longevity, production, and hardy adaptation. Some breeders, as a reaction to this trend, have gone back to deliberately favoring the traditional type. Similarly, Guernsey cattle breeders chased a trend for larger cattle for several years, only to discover that the traditional moderate size was more durable and productive over a longer lifespan, and therefore should be greatly treasured (Figure 8.2). Many sheep breeds have developed divergent lines that include some destined for the show ring, and others tailored for production of meat and wool. At times, these lines diverge so much that the two types can barely be recognized as coming from the same breed. This poses a real problem in breed management because neither one fits the production goals demanded of the other, despite their both going under the same name.

Competitive shows, therefore, have real strengths and real weaknesses when seen in the light of maintaining and promoting breeds of any species. The final balance of these depends on how breed associations use shows and manage the outcomes. They are "value neutral" in and of themselves, with the final result resting entirely on how they are actually accomplished.

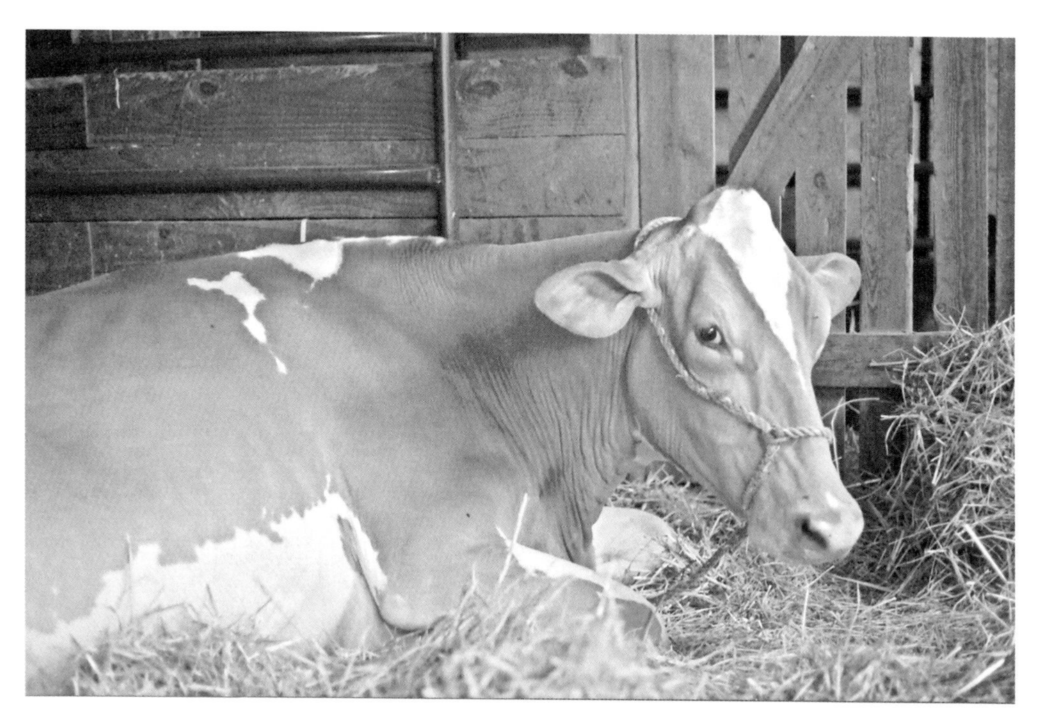

Figure 8.2 Guernsey cattle breeders returned to the original moderate size of the breed after pursuing larger cattle for several years. Photo by JB.

8.2 Card Grading

Card grading is an alternative to traditional showing, and this procedure has some real advantages. It accentuates some of the strengths of competitive showing and diminishes many of the potential negatives. In card grading, each animal that is presented is individually evaluated for how well it fits the breed standard (Figure 8.3). Card grading began in the UK as an attempt to make sense out of huge classes of poultry that were presented for evaluation and competition at some of the larger poultry shows. Detailed ranking of the birds was simply impossible due to the numbers of birds presented. Following card grading's success in managing poultry evaluation, it was further developed for livestock breeds by the Rare Breeds Survival Trust in the UK, as well as The Livestock Conservancy in the USA. Card grading has evolved into a system that offers many benefits to offset the potential negatives in traditional competitive showing.

Card grading evaluates each animal individually by comparing it to the ideal of the breed standard. This contrasts with competitive showing in which the animals are evaluated one against another. Card grading is usually performed by three judges to avoid a tie. The group of judges evaluates each animal in the absence of the owner or handler. The judges examine the animal by a hands-on evaluation, and ideally also have it walk freely up and down an alleyway. Watching the animals move is very important for all breeds, but can be tricky to manage for poultry evaluations. The animals are placed into categories: excellent breeding stock (blue card), good breeding stock (red card), acceptable breeding stock (yellow card),

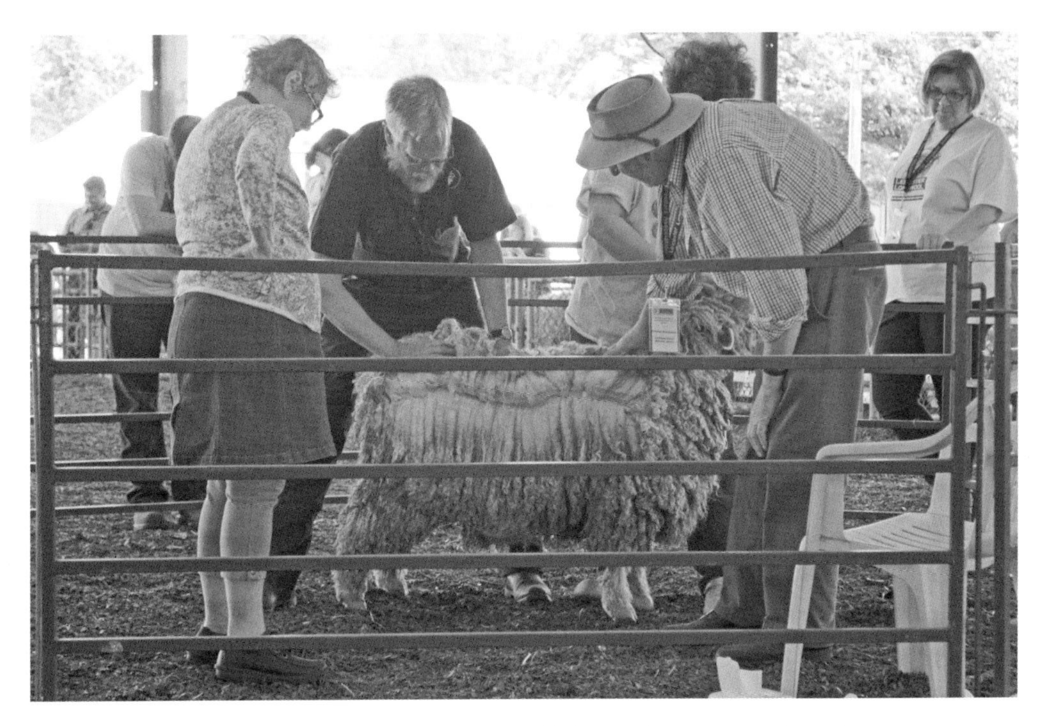

Figure 8.3 The Leicester Longwool breeders in the USA have long used card grading as an evaluation and education tool. Photo by Alison Martin.

and unacceptable for breeding (white card). In the UK, the colors are reversed for the first two categories so that a red card indicates excellent breeding stock while a blue card is given for good breeding stock.

Card grading has significant advantages over competitive showing. Each animal that qualifies for evaluation on the basis of the appropriate documentation (registration and identification requirements) is given a card reflecting its overall quality with respect to the breed standard. No specific proportions of the categories are set, so that it is possible to have all animals receive blue cards at a given event or for all to receive white cards. The usual result is a handful of blue cards, relatively higher numbers of red cards, and then varying numbers of yellow and white cards, depending on how selective the breeders were in bringing animals to the event. The general trend over the years is that the higher categories (blue and red) become better represented than the lower ones. This is a consequence of breeders becoming better educated and increasingly capable of evaluating their animals with respect to the breed standard. Breeders then leave the potential white-card animals at home rather than bringing them for public evaluation. In this regard, card grading does a great job in educating breeders about being selective and breeding to the standard.

Card grading sends a very powerful signal to breeders that no single animal is best. This is important, for it allows novices to realize that each animal in a group of several of the same card grade has a specific array of strengths and weaknesses. These variable animals can all be of value to the breed because each fits into it in its own unique way. Card grading also educates breeders to the concept that not all animals have equal value to a specific breeding program. Each animal, even a superior one, has unique strengths and weaknesses. Once the elements of card grading are understood, breeders can apply this same evaluation technique to their animals at home when selecting breeding stock. This helps them to pair the weaknesses of one animal with the strengths of another one.

Card grading can be accompanied by an open and public "reasons session" in which the judges indicate just exactly why a specific level of card was given to an individual animal. This is an especially powerful mechanism for breeder education. Judges can comment concerning the difference between a yellow-card animal that is weak overall, versus a yellow-card animal with a single major flaw in an otherwise exceptionally good and strong animal. This can alert breeders that each animal must be evaluated individually, for each has a different and appropriate role in the breeding structure of a herd or breed. In this example, an "overall weak" yellow-card animal probably has little or no use in most breeding programs. In contrast, a "single major fault" yellow-card animal may well be beneficial in a herd in which the one fault of this animal is matched by strength in the other animals in the herd.

A compromise between card grading and competitive showing has developed at some shows. The animals are card graded first, and then all of the blue-card animals are ushered into the ring for a more traditional competitive show among those superior animals. This tends to satisfy the breeders' desire for a competitive show with one first-place animal, while at the same time giving the nod to the strengths of the card grading system. The idea that no single animal is best for all breeding programs can still be communicated to the audience, and this is a very important aspect of card grading.

A step back from formal card grading is the sort of evaluation any breeder can do with animals that are in a single herd. Some evaluation procedures, used especially in poultry, were developed early in the 1900s that correlated physical traits with production characteristics. These evaluation techniques are seeing a renewed adoption by modern breeders, and the result has been a quick improvement of production parameters with a maintained adherence to breed standards. The techniques have produced excellent birds that do well in both the farmyard and shows. The procedures involve a detailed hands-on assessment of various body characteristics such as depth of keel, width of body, and the set and location of pelvic bones. An interesting detail is that the head conformation is important, because this nearly always carries through to the other body regions. A weak head betrays a great deal of information, as does a strong one (Figure 8.4).

8.3 Non-Competitive Exhibition

Exhibition, in contrast to showing, may well not involve any competitive aspect but may instead emphasize contact with the public and opportunity for the educational exchange of information. Many opportunities for exhibition and education are similar to those for competitive showing. Exhibitions can occur at fairs and stock shows, as well as nature centers, museums, historic sites, schools, and other public education venues. Breeder members of associations frequently work together to display and distribute educational materials such as photo albums and breed literature stall-side in the exhibition barns. These materials can

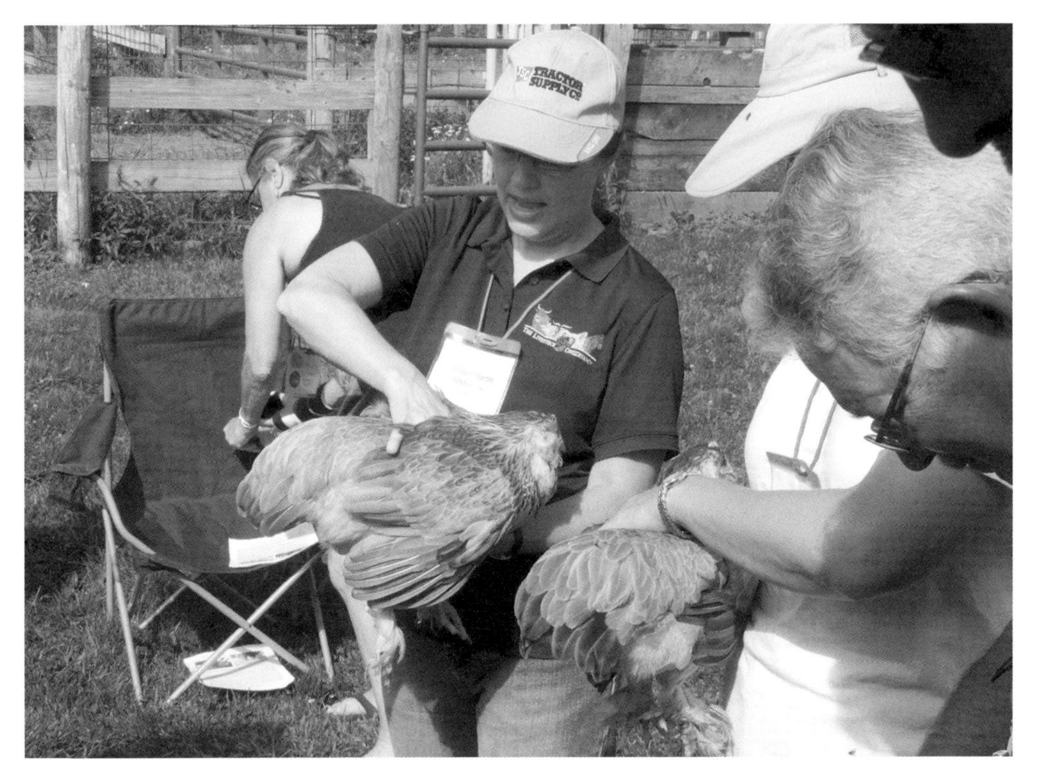

Figure 8.4 Hands-on evaluation of birds for selection into breeding flocks can be useful in improving production in backyard situations. Photo by DPS.

be helpful in promoting the organization and its educational resources to those visiting the exhibit and expressing interest in the breed.

A handful of breed associations have banned competitive showing and rely instead on exhibitions to disseminate information about the production characteristics of their breed rather than the visual characteristics. This strategy has been adopted specifically to minimize the potentially damaging aspects of competitive showing.

8.4 Performance Testing

Competitive showing is one way to evaluate animals, and card grading is another. Exhibition does not really have a component of performance evaluation. Showing and card grading have advantages, but one real disadvantage is that they only evaluate animals on a single occasion. Longer time frames are useful for most traits, and indeed many traits cannot be fully evaluated by anything other than good record keeping over relatively long stretches of time. Many methods of performance testing try to bring the element of greater accuracy to animal evaluation. The purpose of performance testing or performance evaluation is to gain evidence of the relative productive potential of individual animals within a group.

It is important to carefully determine the specific trait that is being measured. "Fast horses" is one trait, but different types of evaluations can lead to a very different final product. For example, today's racing Quarter Horses are sprinters over about a quarter of a mile. This is, after all, how the breed got its name. The final horse that is produced from the selection environment imposed by this evaluation is very different from a Thoroughbred that races over a longer distance of about a mile. Even within the Thoroughbred breed, the type has changed over the centuries because original races tended to be over four miles in contrast to today's shorter races. Both of these breeds contrast markedly from the Argentine Criollo that is raced over many miles and over several consecutive days. Each of these competitions places different demands on the horses, and the genetic responses to those demands yield distinct final products.

Performance testing can be done in a variety of different ways depending on the specific traits that are targeted for evaluation. Some of these are easy to measure early in life, while others, such as carcass traits or progeny performance, can only be measured later. It is common for breeders who are interested in traits with later expression to try to find other related traits or indicators that can be measured earlier in life so that the breeding decisions do not have to be put off until full expression of the trait. This strategy has some very real weaknesses as well as strengths.

The main advantage of using predictive testing rather than actual performance is that the selection decisions can be made earlier in an animal's life. This allows for selection to proceed at a more rapid pace. A major weakness is that the predictive data vary in their correlation to actual performance. The ideal situation is 100% correlation of the predictive data with the final actual performance, but this is never achieved. The inaccuracy of the prediction has to be weighed against the cost of waiting for the more accurate actual performance to be recorded.

Several traits have DNA probes that can measure productive potential; however, these have an important weakness. Different populations can solve identical selection challenges in very different ways. For example, various breeds use very different genetic pathways to achieve the single goal of prolific sheep. Booroola Merinos and Thoka Icelandics use a single allele. Finn and Romanov sheep use polygenic variation. Border Leicesters use yet another genetic mechanism. The key here is that DNA tests for most traits usually assume that "an" answer is "the only" answer. If selection is then based on that one DNA mechanism, it runs the very real risk of eliminating the others that might have been equally or more useful in the long run.

How performance is measured is very important, and varies over a wide range depending on the technology and support that are available. Some approaches are very technical, such as DNA probes. Others are highly developed and rely on massive data collection and evaluation. Others are less technical, but entirely appropriate for some situations. Some might be as simple as weighing animals periodically. Even simple measurements must be well planned and executed so that the measures are truly comparable from one animal to another.

Most evaluation measures involve traits with obvious and immediate commercial return, such as growth rate or milk production. Several cattle, sheep, and goat breeds, for example, participate in growth-rate trials where candidate males are brought to a central location and managed under similar conditions so that their rates of growth can be directly compared to one another. This has the advantage of making the environment as uniform as possible, so that variations such as feeding protocols can be eliminated as one source of different performance levels. A century ago similar methods were in place for comparing the egg production of various chicken flocks and breeds. These have long been made irrelevant by the role of the large commercial producers of chicken eggs.

For most traits it is possible to devise an evaluation scheme so that individuals can be compared. This is easiest on a single property or with a single herd, but the results cannot usually be applied on a broader scale. Analysis that works across various herds and locations takes more development and thought but can be made to work. Most of these require cooperation among breeders to assure that similar genetic material is present across the various sites. That strategy greatly increases the ability to dissect out the influences of genetics, management, and environment.

Other schemes involve on-farm evaluation, such as that for milk production. Most of this is accomplished through the Dairy Herd Improvement Association (DHIA). Farmers cooperate with one another, and with designated technicians, to periodically measure the milk production of individual cows and take samples for the analysis of milk components such as fat and protein. These results are then used to help individual farmers constructively manage their own herds, and also to compare related animals across different herds. These schemes are key to some genetic evaluations. The system works well in dairy cattle because the use of artificial insemination puts related cows in many different environments. Comparing genetic lines across environments allows very accurate genetic predictions of performance capacity to be made.

Cattle milk production can be evaluated in many different ways, and each has advantages in different situations. Milk production can be predicted by using the advanced analysis of specific genomic (DNA) information. It can also be measured directly, with the results being entered into the DHIA system. These two methods require different levels of support, but both require resources beyond what an individual breeder has available.

A rather elegant, but low-tech, system was once used in Nicaragua for the Criollo Lechero breed (Figure 8.5). These cattle were hand-milked in a farming situation with minimal infrastructure. Every milker used a standard bucket that held two liters (slightly over two quarts). Cows that failed to fill a bucket twice a day were culled. Cows that succeeded in filling two buckets twice a day were candidates for producing bulls that were used in the herd. Successful cows, though, could only provide one bull and not more, which provided for good genetic management of the herd and avoided inbreeding. This was a powerful yet simple solution to performance testing and its relationship to selection for production as well as population structure. The methods used were also possible in a situation with very limited infrastructure or technical support.

8.4.1 Adaptation

Traits of adaptation are difficult to evaluate but are vitally important to many breeds. Adaptation is the ability of animals to survive and produce in compromised environments (Figure 8.6). For many breeds this is an essential component of their history and their usefulness. Icelander Dr. Stefan Adalsteinsson referred to many breeds as having "the genetic heritage of survival" to capture this important concept. Maintaining adaptation is sometimes a very tall order. This is especially true for some breeds as they move from a landrace

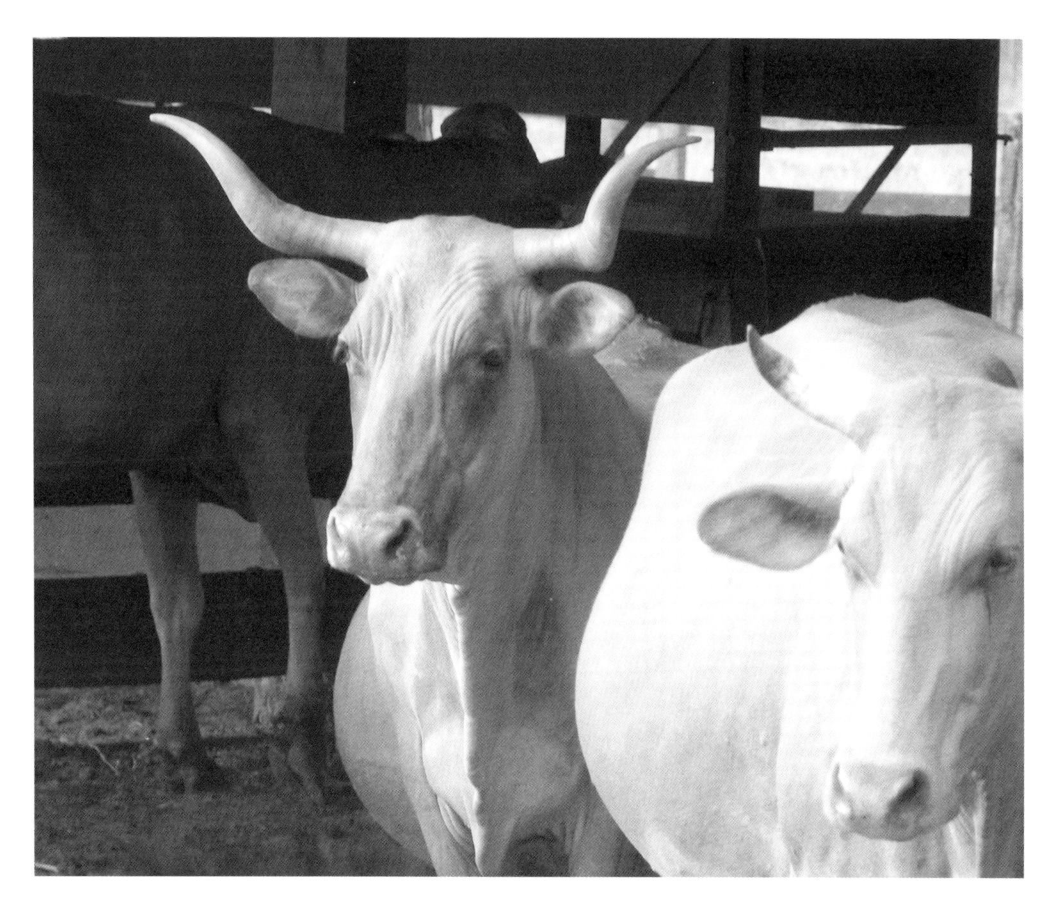

Figure 8.5 Criollo Lechero cattle are an important genetic resource throughout the Americas for their milk production and tropical adaptation. Photo by DPS.

situation to one based on the standardized breed model. When a landrace breed becomes popular, it tends to move from being a local resource to more of a national resource. It is common for increasing demand for the breed to be followed by increasing price. With that comes an increasing incentive to concentrate on production and eye appeal rather than on survivability in compromised environments.

Selection in favor of adaptation requires that the environment be managed to demonstrate differences in levels of adaptation. This translates into allowing some of the animals to demonstrate a lack of adaptation and to cull on this basis. Such a system allows some animals to fail. This can be frustrating or distasteful to breeders who are more comfortable providing a supportive environment that favors maximal opportunity for all animals to be productive. This situation also raises a moral dilemma as to the extent to which management should be "hands off" in order to allow adaptation to express itself. When treatments and resources exist to counter nutritional or infectious challenges, it is ethically questionable to forego their use, even though using these inputs may well mask differences in adaptation. This is especially true for the rarest of breeds for which health inputs such as vaccines may be the difference between short-term survival and extinction.

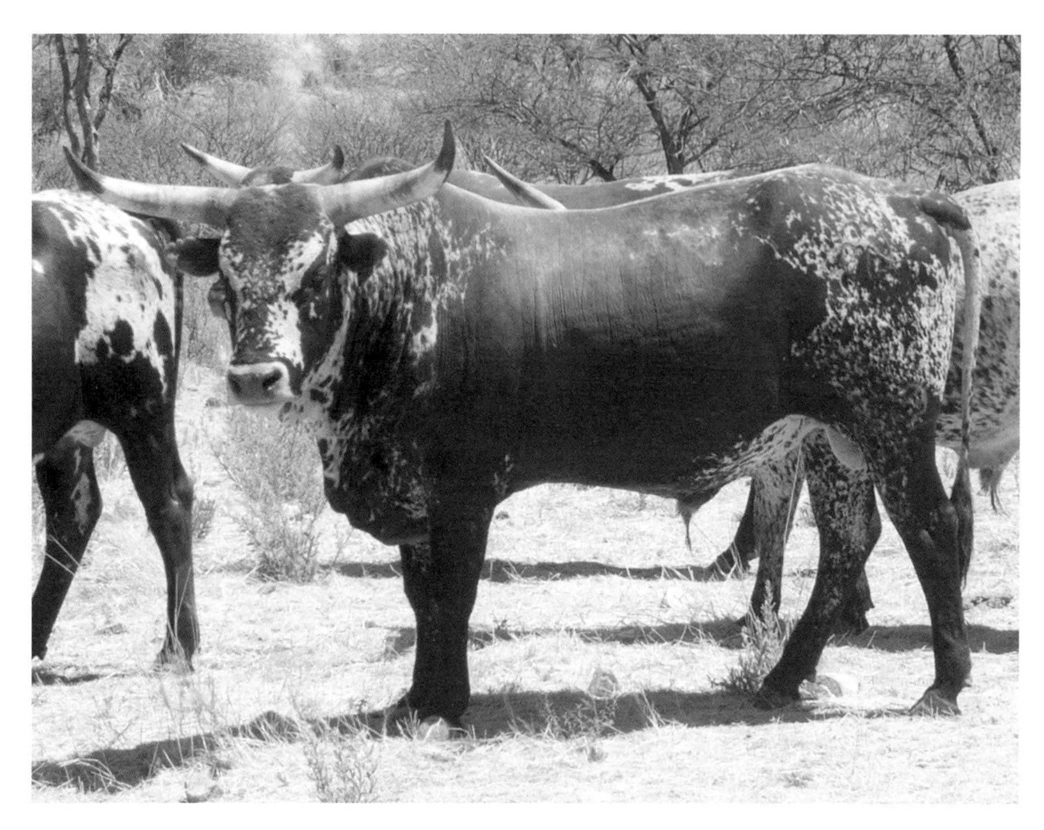

Figure 8.6 Nguni cattle in Africa are selected for adaptation (including surviving leopards!) but also for production. The result is a breed that fits well in its environment. Photo by DPS.

For example, the Tennessee Myotonic (or Fainting) goat is reputed to have some resistance to gastrointestinal parasites. This is an important trait in the breed that will only gain in importance in the future. To assure that parasite resistance remains present in the breed, breeders must not deworm every goat at three-week intervals, but instead must allow the worms to build up and infect the susceptible goats, and then select those that resist the effects of the worms as breeding stock. In most situations the result is that some goats will be wormy and relatively poor-doers, demonstrating which of the goats are worm-resistant and remain productive in the presence of worms. This situation presents both economic and ethical problems. Fortunately, in this case, the development of strategic deworming tactics for the most troublesome parasite, the barber pole worm, has produced amazing results. The evaluation of animals is based on the level of anemia (and thereby worm load). This has allowed selection for parasite resistance to proceed without allowing losses from parasitism to occur because animals with heavier worm loads can be dewormed before they are compromised. The key here is that breeders interested in parasite resistance need to be diligent to act on the information of relative anemia so that replacement stock is kept from the most resistant animals. Breeders should be eager to track the performance of their goats with respect to parasite resistance, so that future generations can benefit from decreased reliance on deworming chemicals.

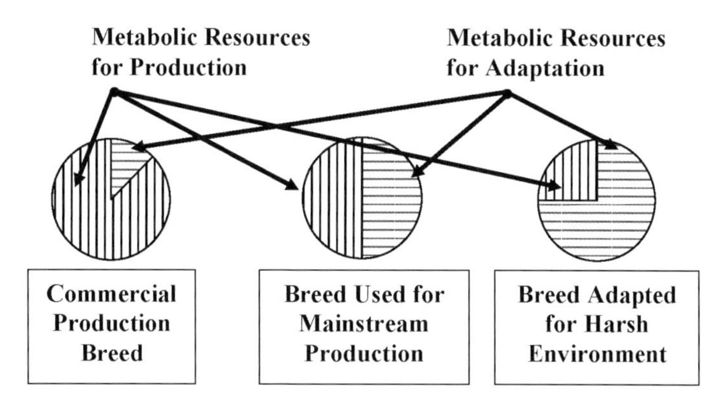

Figure 8.7 Different breeds partition their metabolic resources with varying emphasis on production or resistance, and this depends on their past selection environment. Figure by DPS.

The issue of selection for adaptation is nowhere near certain in the minds of breeders and researchers. To what extent any breed can have maximum resistance and maximum production is very much an undecided question (Figure 8.7). Some evidence points to the concept that animals have limited metabolic resources at their disposal, and so they must "choose" where to put those. Adaptation is one slot for these resources; production is another. While it may not be as simple as that, this approach does seem to have some merit. Breeders may well have to decide on the relative importance of adaptation and production for their own systems and their own breeds. A low-input adapted breed will likely never equal the production levels of individual animals of an industrial strain in a high-input system. What is lost in productivity is compensated for by lower inputs such as housing, dewormers, refined rations, antibiotic support, and veterinary interventions during births or at other times.

Some breeds have undergone very rapid transformation from adapted, rugged animals to smoother, productive ones. The show ring and exhibition lines of Texas Longhorns have certainly done this, and breeders of other breeds may well be tempted to take their breeds down this same road. The type of these breeds changes in response to a change in the selection environment from one of compromised deprivation to a life of ease and plenty. This change modifies the genetic resource forged by that original environment, and risks its loss. These issues have no easy answers, yet they must be considered in order to arrive at some sort of meaningful philosophy of genetic resource conservation.

Some breeders have managed to select for adaptation, as well as for production, and have produced some interesting and useful genetic resources in the process. Over a span of multiple decades, Robert Kensing of Menard, Texas, took the original local Spanish goats (60 lb females) and selected them from within the breed with no crossbreeding to produce females that were 150 lb at maturity. At that size he noted less adaptation to the rugged west Texas conditions, and so he relaxed selection for size and ended up with 125 lb females that were fertile and productive as well as adapted. These females were able to use the rough browse of the environment to raise kids without supplementation of other feedstuffs. It is possible to have adaptation and production in some combination, but it takes very wise and dedicated breeders to assure that the drive for production does not leave adaptation out of the equation.

It is a relatively frequent observation that animals of adapted breeds tend to be smaller than those of the more production-oriented breeds. This is likely related to the idea that the animals have to partition the resources available and shunt them either to adaptation or to production, with the consequence that it is impossible to have animals that are both highly adapted as well as maximally productive. The balance point between adaptation and production varies from breed to breed and environment to environment. Temperate lush environments easily move the balance toward production, while harsh deserts or humid tropical environments move that balance more toward adaptation. Indeed, many of the dwarf breeds hail from very compromised situations where they are highly valued for their ability to survive and remain at least somewhat productive.

8.4.2 Temperament and Behavior

Temperament is strongly heritable and a very important target of selection, but it can be very difficult to evaluate across a range of different individual settings. This is important for several species where breeding stock is likely to be moved from one setting to another.

Competitions provide one way of evaluating temperament and behavior, especially in dog breeds. These usually take the form of field trials but can also be accomplished by events such as obedience trials or other performance-related competitions. The extent to which these become truly competitive, with one "top dog," can become a weakness rather than a strength of the system. Competitions tend to select extremes, and extremes are not always best for day-to-day work. Some obedience dogs are very highly strung and quick, as well as being compliant and biddable. This behavioral package provides for great performance in an obedience trial but can be exhausting to an owner in a home setting. A quick and driven field-trial bird dog may likewise not be the best choice for a hunter interested in a more leisurely weekend outing.

Validating temperament objectively is notoriously difficult, although various tests have been developed for dogs. These can help to match puppies to buyers and assure a decent fit. Temperament and behavior are profoundly influenced by the environment and management that the dog receives. This is especially important for breeds such as the livestock guardians, where the final product is about half genetic potential and half environment (Figure 8.8). Each of those halves has complete veto power over the final product, and each can lead to complete failure, even when the other half of the equation is excellent. The final successful product in this case is a complicated combination of temperament, ability, and structural soundness. Measuring these in any meaningful way is challenging.

Putting together effective evaluation schemes for temperament and behavior can require intricate and inventive methods for demonstrating an animal's ability. One successful example is the Chilean style of rodeo (Figure 8.9). This involves only a single event where pairs of horses work a steer up to a barrier and then pin the steer. The event requires a great deal of training because it is usually done at a lateral canter. It also requires a very calm, biddable horse. The youngest horses in competition are usually no younger than about ten years old due to the advanced training that is required. This one event selects for soundness, trainability, longevity, and athletic ability all at once.

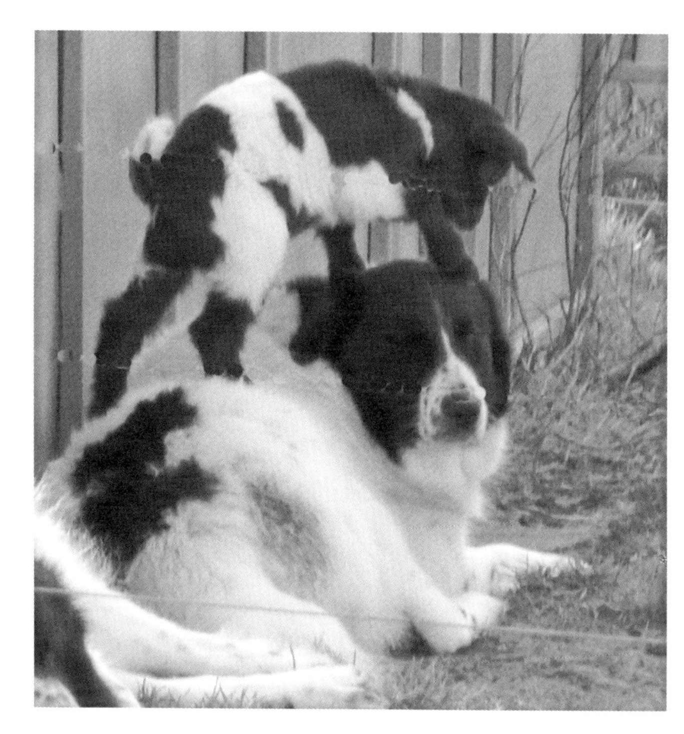

Figure 8.8 Successful livestock guardian dogs require the right genetics as well as the right environment and training. Photo by DPS.

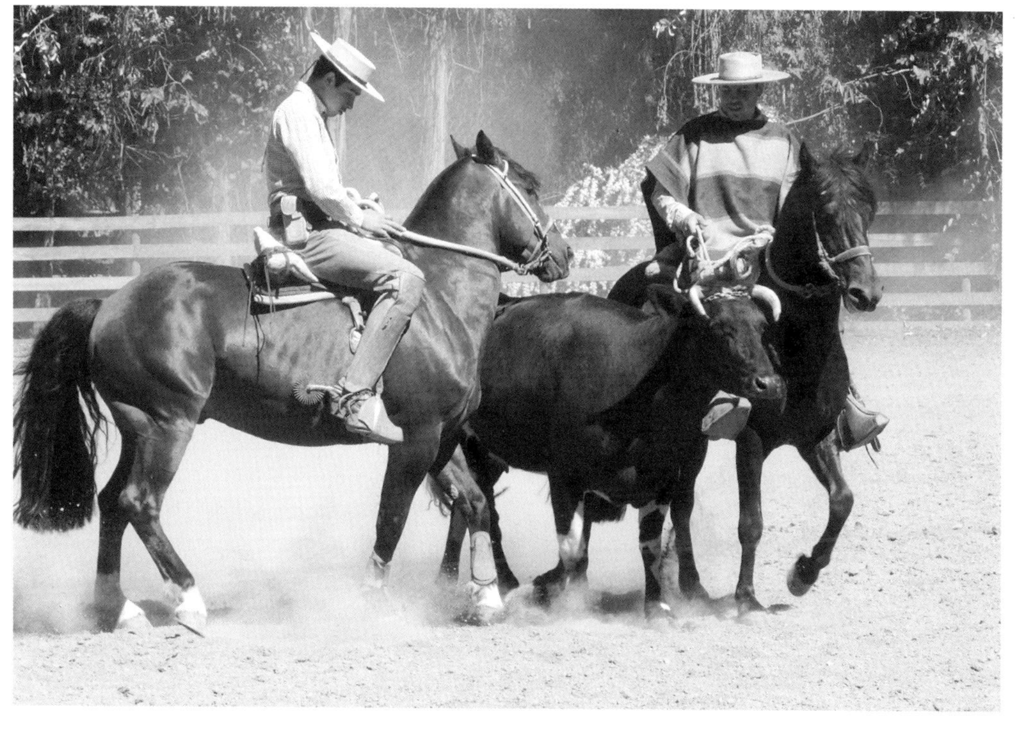

Figure 8.9 Chilean horses destined for rodeo work are trained for several years before they master the skills needed. Photo by DPS.

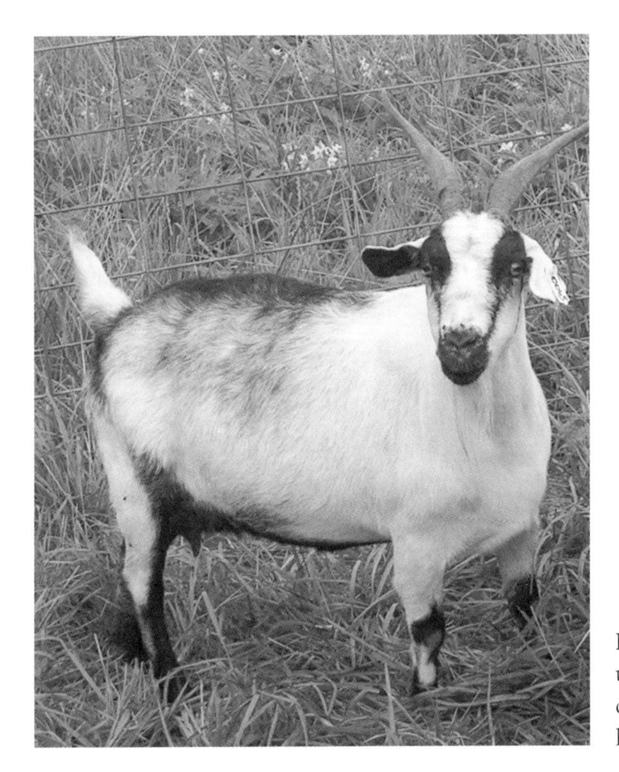

Figure 8.10 This Myotonic doe kidded up until she was 17 years old, and her daughters likewise led long, productive lives. Photo by DPS.

8.4.3 Longevity

Longevity is a convenient way to loosely measure a host of traits. It is an indirect measure of productive potential as a long-lived animal has generally been retained in a herd because of its utility at some level. Longevity also measures adaptation because poorly adapted animals simply fail to survive to old ages. At some level it also measures temperament and behavior, because dangerous or difficult animals are usually ushered out of the population earlier than their more compliant herd mates. As a single trait, longevity has a great deal of utility, and for many breeds in many settings it therefore makes good sense to use this trait for selection.

Longevity has another subtle advantage. When animals are long-lived, they are able, at least potentially, to contribute more offspring to a herd as replacements when compared to a short-lived animal. This opens up opportunities for breeders to make selection decisions based on a host of traits other than simple survival. Breeders with long-lived animals can select out replacement animals that boost other traits because they are not faced with needing to recruit simply to replace animals lost due to premature age-related declines or disease.

The obvious detraction is the length of time over which longevity takes to express itself (Figure 8.10). This slows down the rate of genetic progress, although this has to be weighed up against the very real fact that the progress is surer and more accurate. A second and more subtle disadvantage is that as animals age, the quality of their offspring can deteriorate. The last few parturitions of a truly ancient animal are likely to result in young that do not quite reach her own potential, nor the potential of her earlier offspring.

8.4.4 Comprehensive Strategies

Performance evaluation can shape breed populations in ways that are not intuitive and that can be counterproductive. Selection goals must therefore be carefully formulated, and evaluations must be creatively tailored to meet the final desired ends. Evaluation and selection based only on the phenotypic excellence of individual animals can lead to large, fast-growing animals that are poorly adapted and short lived. Evaluation and selection based only on longevity can lead to small animals that produce poorly but that attain maturity relatively quickly.

Balancing individual animal productivity and longevity takes creative thought and creative practices. One way to accomplish both is to evaluate performance as a series of steps along the way. This is especially important for the evaluation of males destined for wide use in reproduction. A useful first step is to eliminate all candidate young animals except those that had mature dams with proven performance in fertility and longevity. This, in most herds, should provide a group of animals which can then be further evaluated on their own growth rate and size.

This strategy does slow genetic gain from a theoretical maximum; however, it increases the security of the genetics and makes mistakes less likely. It is a good compromise that avoids ignoring any of the main factors in herd-based profitability: fertility, longevity, and individual performance for commodities such as meat or milk.

Agropecuaria Florestal in Venezuela developed a practical and successful comprehensive selection program that required minimal record keeping for their 40,000 head of cattle from three zebu breeds (Guzerat, Nelore, and Brahman) and one Criollo breed (Romo Sinuano) along with crosses among them. Their program is just one example among many of the way that creative thought can lead to powerful yet practical solutions. The key to their evaluation program was that each cow was branded with her birth year and an individual number. The selection program centered on female reproductive performance, so at the appropriate age for cows to wean a first calf, those cows that failed received an "X" brand on their back. No cow was allowed a second "X." Over a few decades this system yielded good results, with some individual cows in each herd managing to achieve no "X" brands while living up into their teens. This is phenomenal for zebu breeds in the tropics, and is a good example of an easy and practical identification and record method that provided for good progress in selection without the need for extensive or complicated record systems. Under this scheme the average cow size declined while the total weight of cattle sold increased (Figure 8.11).

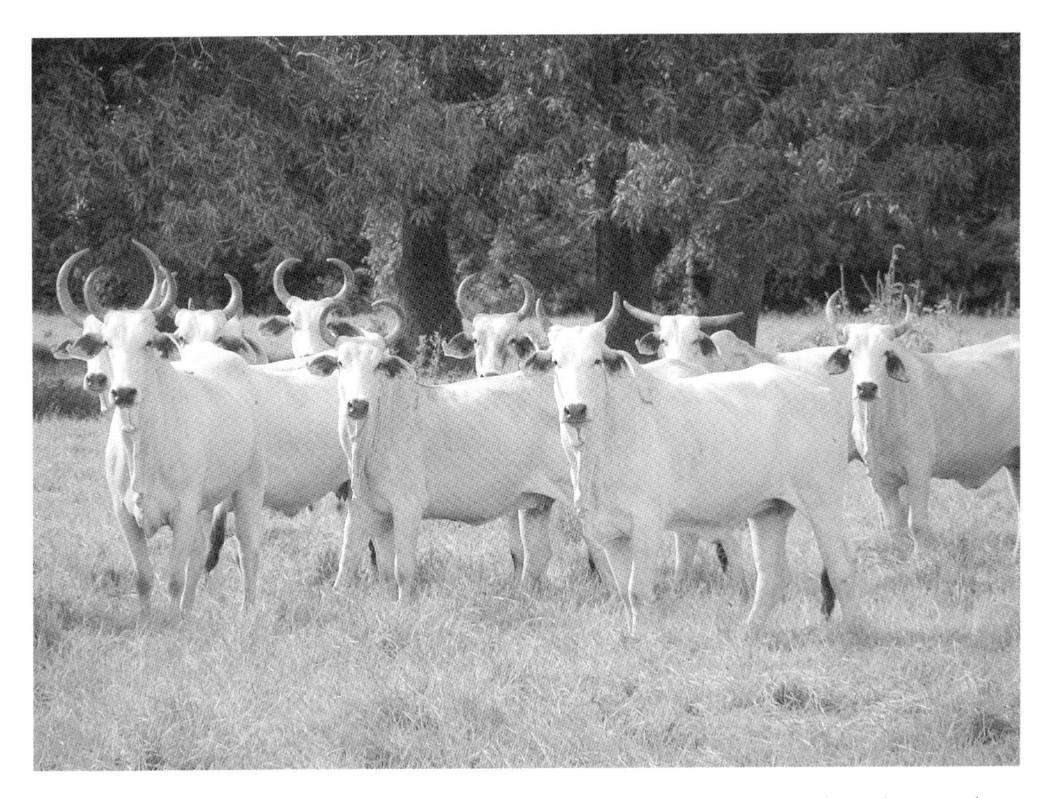

Figure 8.11 Agropecuaria Florestal made great progress in animal productivity through years of selection under a practical evaluation scheme. Photo by DPS.

CHAPTER 9

Practical Aspects of Genetic Management

9.1 Selection of Animals for Reproduction

Consideration of breed type, performance, and selection issues leads to the question of exactly which animals should be used for reproduction, and which should be culled. The goal for most breeders of purebred livestock is the constant improvement of their stock for specific goals while staying within the constraints of breed type and purpose (Figure 9.1).

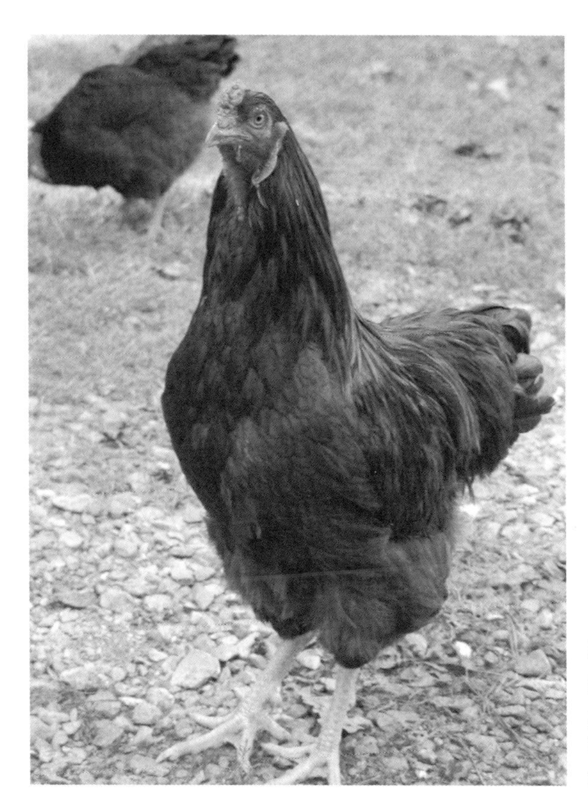

Figure 9.1 Selection of Buckeye chickens for breed type as well as production potential has resulted in birds useful in the barnyard as well as successful in the show ring. Photo by JB.

Most successful animal breeders have "eye," which is a fairly intuitive sense that recognizes which matings will work and which will be less successful. This somewhat conflicts with a more quantitative and statistical approach that has been followed by scientific animal breeders over the last several decades. Although both approaches have merit, the "eye of the breeder" approach has produced excellence in performance as well as in eye appeal and continues to do so. Most breeds benefit from a combination of both approaches.

It is important to remember that the breeds we have today were nearly all developed before the establishment of the modern genetics and statistical tools that aid in the selection of animals. While these later developments can all help, they only build upon a base laid by the true geniuses that gave the world these breeds in the first place. Their approach, intuitive and subjective though it often was, gave us these breeds and still has a powerful role to play in their conservation and continuation.

9.2 Pairing of Animals within Purebred Breeds

The specific manner in which males and females are brought together varies greatly across breeds and situations. Choices include individual pairing, group mating, and multi-sire systems. Mating systems have important consequences for pedigree maintenance, and most purebred breeders put great importance on pedigrees. A pedigree is an account of the ancestry of an animal and identifies specific individuals as sire, dam, grandsire, and so on. That is, pedigrees link an individual animal to specific ancestors. Pedigrees are of great value in establishing the kinship of animals within a breed so that inbreeding can be monitored. Pedigrees are useful when choosing mates for the next generation, regardless of which specific breeding strategy is deemed appropriate.

Individual pairing is the mating of one male and one female at a time. In most situations this is typical for horses, donkeys, swine, dairy goats, rabbits, and dogs (Figure 9.2). Most are matings done in hand, where the animals are haltered and controlled, and they are never turned out as a breeding group. In most of these species, individual pairing meets little resistance, although some stallions are notoriously choosy about mates, and individual dogs can also be choosy.

Individual pairing is also characteristic of geese, which form such strong pair bonds that matings will invariably be between bonded pairs, even if the geese are run in groups of multiple pairs or multiple trios of birds (Figure 9.3). One strategy for managing geese is to pair (or trio) them for their first breeding year and then put them in larger groups in subsequent years. The geese still mate in the original pairs or trios, but the larger groups are usually easier to manage. Putting them into groups results in no loss of pedigree information as long as each egg is identified as to which specific goose produced it. Most ganders in a trio have a primary and secondary mate, and as the years progress, they often begin to ignore the secondary mate so that her fertility may fall. Diligent breeders pay attention to this so that productivity can be monitored and maintained. Goose pairs can be disrupted so that geese can be paired with different mates. This usually requires pairing a goose with a new single gander and assuring that the previous mate is out of range of both sight and sound.

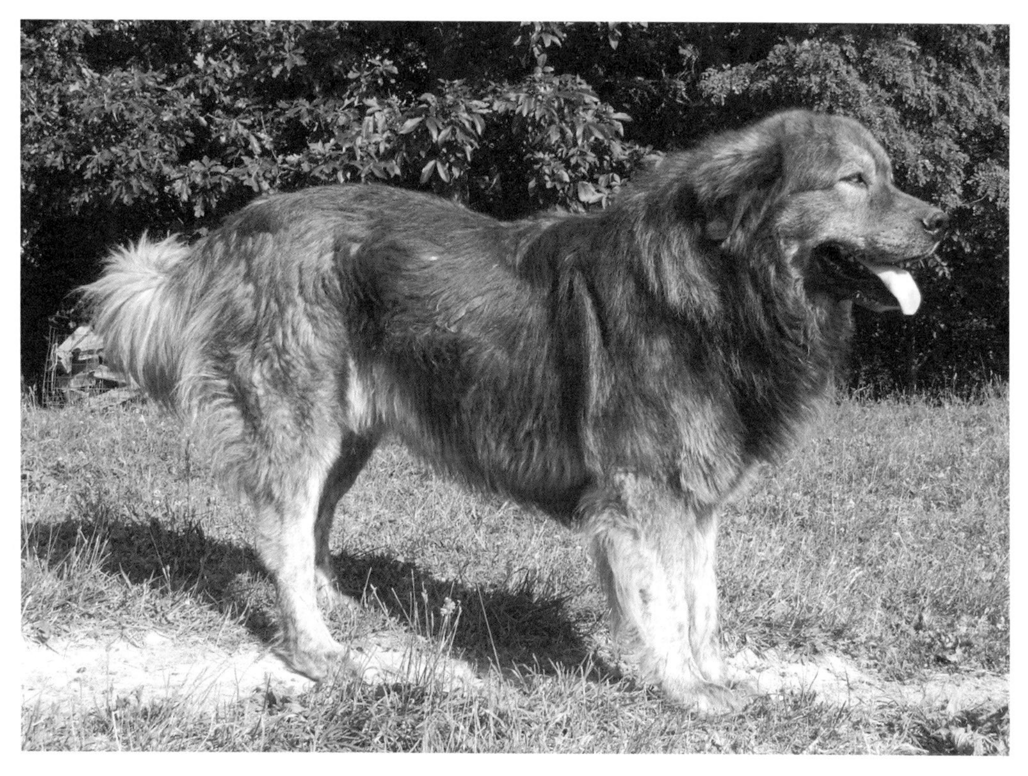

Figure 9.2 Purebred dog matings are nearly always single-pair matings. Photo by JB.

For most domesticated species, single-sire group matings are more commonly used than individual pairings, with one male used to mate with a group of several females. The sex ratio depends on the species, and can be as high as one male to fifty females (sheep, goats) or as few as one or two females (geese). For pedigree management, some producers use different males sequentially over a group, keeping track of the dates that each male is in the herd so that accurate pedigree information is maintained as the offspring arrive. In most species there is little problem in changing males. An exception is the hen turkey, which can resist these changes. Introducing a new tom into a group of hens should ideally be done months ahead of the time when hatching eggs are likely to be collected to allow the hens the time needed to accept the new tom. Horses also have a period of social readjustment after switching the stallion within a group.

Both individual and single-sire group mating methods can provide accurate pedigree information based on good record keeping. With these two systems, it is not necessary to resort to the expense of DNA testing to assign parentage, although some breed associations still require this as an additional verification of registry information. The high regard given to pedigrees by most animal breeders needs to be viewed from the perspective of breed history. Many breeds of conservation interest originated as landraces, and these tend to be among the most phenotypically variable and regionally adapted genetic resources. Mating of landrace animals in traditional settings was and still is commonly accomplished in multi-sire herds. Therefore, accurate pedigrees on the sire's side are not possible unless breeders

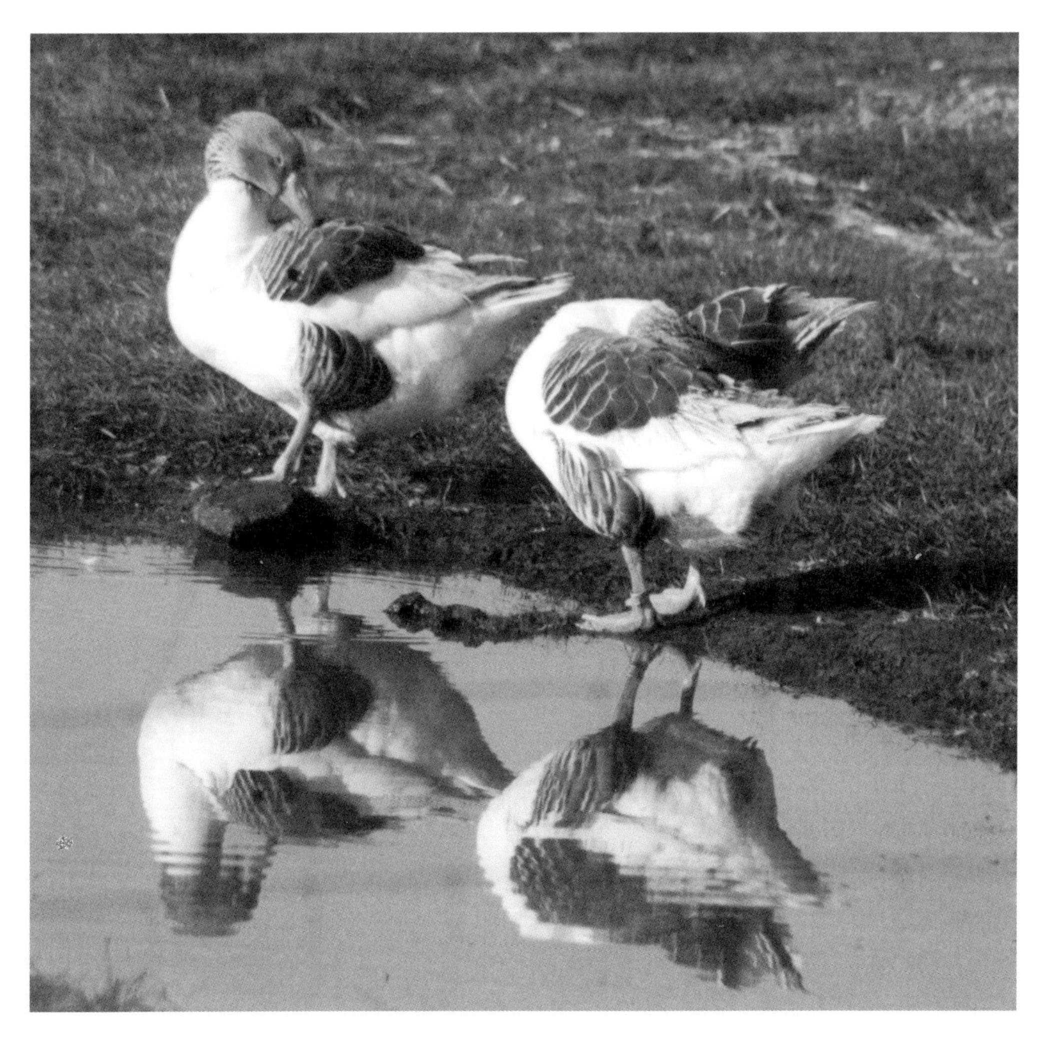

Figure 9.3 Pomeranian geese, as all geese, tend to form tightly bonded pairs that remain devoted to one another for years. Photo by DPS.

resort to DNA typing or blood typing. Such documentation is generally only worthwhile in species with high individual monetary value such as cattle and horses. It is not economical for animals having relatively low individual monetary value, such as chickens, turkeys, and ducks, as well as most sheep and goats. Rabbits, dogs, and swine avoid this issue because these species rarely use multi-sire mating systems.

For many adapted breeds, and even for several of the more highly selected production breeds, multi-sire herds can offer real advantages for breed maintenance. The multi-sire tactic for breed maintenance should not be dismissed simply because it negates the possibility of pedigrees. At a minimum, multi-sire herds put selection pressure on male competition and fitness for survival. This can be especially important in primitive and adapted breeds, where competition is the only means to assure that the fittest are indeed surviving and reproducing (Figure 9.4).

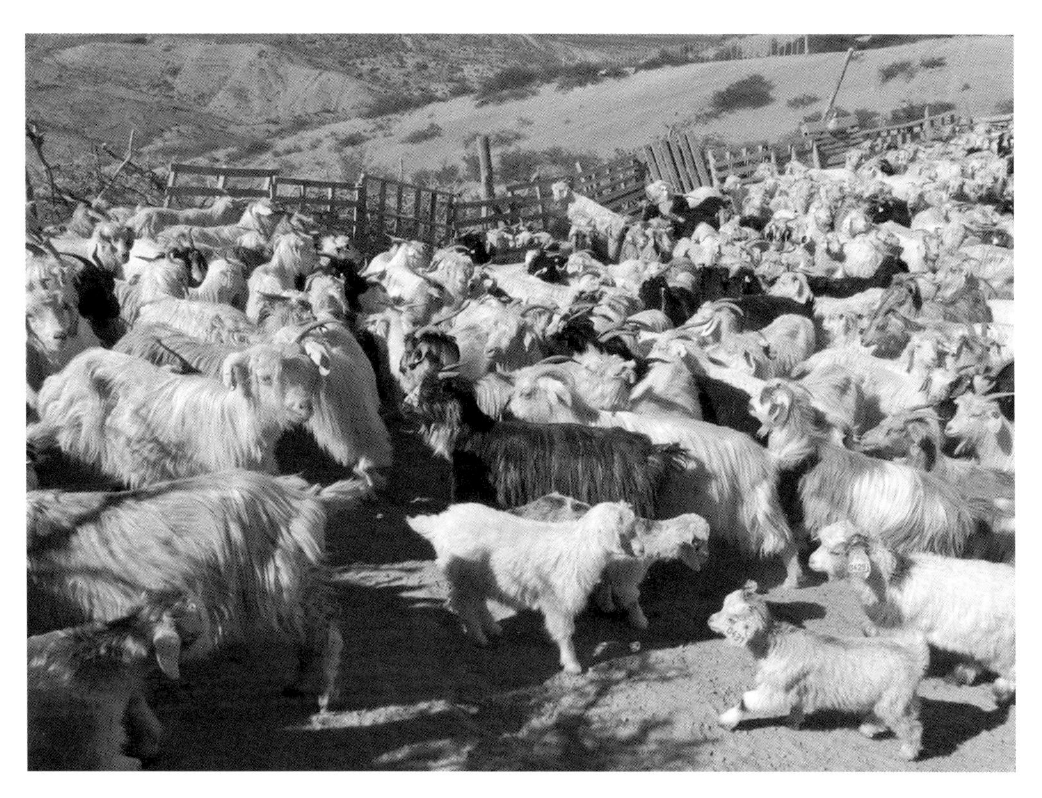

Figure 9.4 Traditional management of Chivo Neuquino goats in Argentina involves herds of hundreds, managed with multiple sires so that individual pedigrees are not available. This management does not diminish the purity, adaptation, and utility of the breed. Photo by DPS.

Some species, even if managed in multi-sire situations, can have accurate pedigree information. Depending on numbers and range, for example, horses tend to form relatively stable harems, and running multiple stallions on a single range has been a strategy long used by breeders of Choctaw and other Colonial Spanish horses. By noting the harem membership, it is possible to identify which stallions sire which foals, although it is well known that some mares do travel to visit stallions other than their harem stallion. As a result, harem affiliation is not completely accurate as a predictor of paternity. Other species form harems poorly, so that this strategy does not work for cattle, sheep, or goats.

It is possible to gain some benefits from multi-sire mating systems without completely losing the benefits of pedigrees. One strategy is to assure that the sires in the herd at any one time are all of the same bloodline. While pedigrees would not be available on the offspring, their status as being of one bloodline, or another, would be available. This information could be very helpful in managing genetic diversity across the herd or breed. An example of this is using a group of three Baylis strain bulls in a Pineywoods cattle herd, followed by a group of three Carter strain bulls. The rotation of the bulls as a group provides certainty that the calves have a certain strain of sire, and this helps to place the calves into genetic groups. A further refinement would be to always use groups of males that are half-siblings to one another, because then at least 75% of each calf pedigree would be known (dam, and paternal grandsire).

Another strategy that allows use of multiple males without losing pedigree information is to use males sequentially in the herd, one at a time. This can be unrealistic in large herds or on large ranges, but does work to provide accurate pedigree information. If males can be used sequentially, then the pedigree of only a few individuals that are born during transitions may be difficult to identify. Allowing for a break between males can circumvent this problem. For example, a large group of doe goats could have an individual buck in with them for a week, then none for a day or two, then a second buck for two weeks, none for a day or two, and finally a third buck for two weeks. The result is a five-week kidding period during which the kids come from three different sires and all kids are accurately identified as to sire based on their birth dates. The advantage of this approach is that multiple pastures are not needed; the disadvantage is that no specific doe is guaranteed to mate to the buck most preferred for her.

Multi-sire matings were once typical of many landraces, and worked well when breed numbers were in the thousands and individual herds were large (Figure 9.5). In today's situation, most multi-sire systems come with some significant negatives. While it is true that formal pedigrees were rarely kept during the development of landraces, it is also true

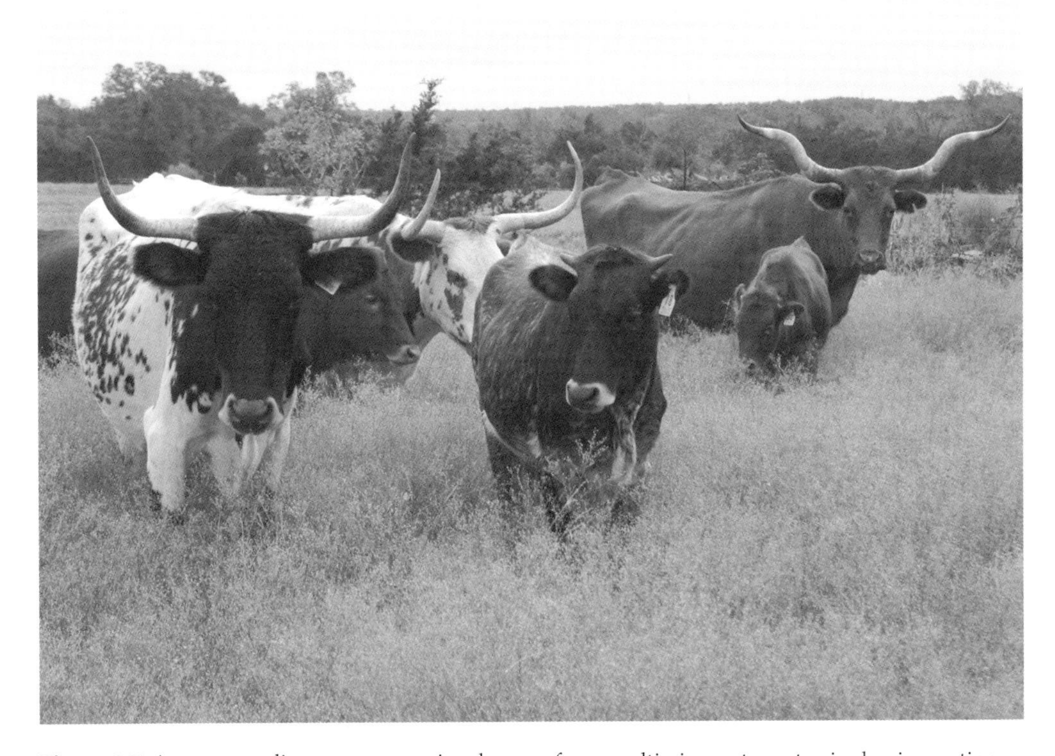

Figure 9.5 Accurate pedigrees may require changes from multi-sire systems to single-sire mating. Texas Longhorn cattle were once mostly managed in multi-sire herds, but are now nearly all in single-sire situations. Photo by JB.

that the huge herd sizes (hundreds or even thousands) assured a wide range of genetic variability. In that situation the genetic variation was high enough that pedigrees would have added little assurance to the long-term viability of the population. Today there are few herds with that huge traditional size, with the exception of some herds of Spanish goats in Texas. Despite the fact that some of these traditionally numerous landraces have dwindled to rarity, the management technique of multi-sire herds has not changed. However, for most herds of landrace livestock it has become increasingly important to carefully monitor inbreeding and founder contribution, and this requires accurate pedigree information. In populations with small population sizes, accurate pedigrees can be almost essential in managing the population's structure, and unfortunately accurate pedigrees are only poorly available in multi-sire situations. In situations where multi-sire matings must be accomplished it is a great boon to conservation to assure that pedigrees be established by DNA validation. A less accurate approach is to assure that the sires are half-brothers or at least of the same family line. When multiple sires come from widely divergent families, the resulting offspring fit poorly into planned conservation programs.

9.3 Strategic Selection of Specific Mates

Mating strategies that target improvement of livestock take the form of balancing weaknesses with strengths. For example, the weaknesses of one parent (set of hocks, for example) might be balanced by a mate with stronger, truer hock conformation. Or a productive and useful animal with an off-type ear could be mated to a mate with a more typical ear to try to correct the breed-specific fault while maintaining production. Note well that only rarely is a fault corrected by mating to the opposite fault. Such a strategy is usually very disappointing. An animal with sickle hocks is rarely corrected by mating to a post-legged animal, but is rather more likely to be corrected by one with a sound set of hocks. The balancing of weaknesses with the ideal is a much surer path to success than is attempting to balance one weakness with another opposing weakness.

Not every mating in every herd has the same goal or tactic, even though the obvious and intended outcome is a next generation. Understanding that the animals in the next generation might have different destinies helps breeders to shape their herds by planning which animals will contribute in which specific ways. Each animal within a single herd has a different importance in respect to its genetics, productivity, conformation, and contribution to the genetic structure of the population. For dogs, temperament and working ability can be added to this list as important key components for the success of individual dogs as well as for the utility of the breed.

In a very real sense, each animal in a herd has its own role and potential. Realizing this is key to making genetic progress at the population level. Likewise, each animal and each mating have different importance to the overall breed. For example, the single remaining female of a unique foundation strain needs to be used much more strategically than a female of a more numerous composite herd even if they are otherwise similar for conformation and production levels. Likewise, the sole remaining male of a rare strain might be allowed minor faults to a greater degree than the male of a common strain in order to assure that the positive attributes of the rare strain are not irretrievably lost.

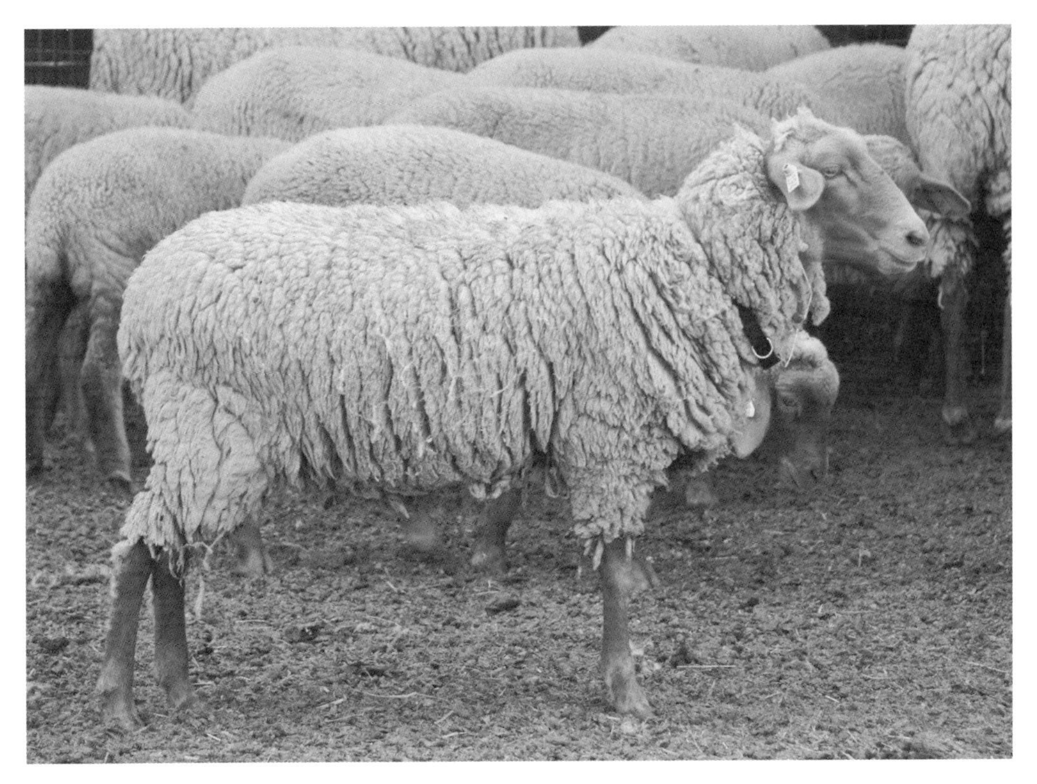

Figure 9.6 Well-conformed and productive animals with strong breed type are the goal of all breeding programs. This Tunis ewe is productive and has strong traditional breed type. Photo by JB.

Each mating should have the goal of improvement and genetic strength, and each should also be evaluated as to how the offspring, both male and female, will fit into the population as potential breeding animals. A typey and strong female, for example, can be mated to a typey and strong male to produce both male and female offspring that see wide use. The same female, mated to a somewhat weaker male, may provide female offspring to be used for specific purposes, but not to produce males that are to see wide use. One reason for such matings might be to balance bloodline representation in a herd. While not all such offspring may see wide use, each nonetheless carries with it expectations for at least some constructive use (Figure 9.6). Especially for rare breeds, specific matings should always consider the quality of the animals as well as their pedigree background. In some situations one or the other of these factors can be the most compelling, and there is no set rule to establishing which of these is more important in any specific situation.

9.4 Strategic Use of Coefficients of Inbreeding

In many breeds it has become fashionable for breeders to pay close attention to the coefficient of inbreeding. This is a measure of the level of inbreeding behind an animal. It is computed from the position of the ancestors that occur on both the dam's and sire's side of the pedigree, and many computer programs are available that do this handily. It is an important measure, but needs to be put into a broader context than simply stating that high coefficients are always bad.

Inbreeding has potential dangers, but it also has very real and constructive advantages in some situations. The real threat usually arises in situations where all animals in a herd, or in a breed, are related back to the same few individuals and so inbreeding cannot be avoided. In this regard, the concept of kinship is as important as the coefficient of inbreeding. Kinship measures the potential coefficient of inbreeding that would be present in an offspring produced by mating two individual animals. It is a sort of "future inbreeding coefficient," and is very useful because it looks at the relationship of potential mates. Kinship can be computed in proposed matings. It can also be computed for an individual animal and a group, or across larger populations. When done for an individual animal (a potential sire) across an entire group (a herd of females) the result gives a range of values. Some of those values might be quite high (inbred matings) and others might be all the way down to zero (outbred matings). Knowing the range of values helps to assess just how broad the genetic variation is in a population.

As with most of life, the devil is in the details, and simple solutions tend to overlook the real complexity that lies below the surface. One increasingly common recommendation is to simply avoid mating animals that produce a relatively high coefficient of inbreeding in the offspring. That level varies, but is often 10% or so. This sounds harmless, and even potentially good. In small populations, though, a constant drive to minimize inbreeding coefficients has the outcome that the minimally related animals are constantly mated to one another. Over several generations this tactic essentially uses up those unrelated matings. This happens because unrelated animals are preferentially brought together. The eventual result is that all animals become related to one another and at that point completely unrelated mating strategies are no longer available. This is subtle, and is not necessarily an outcome that is obvious to most breeders.

Kinship, and coefficients of inbreeding, must therefore be used wisely and with forethought as to how various strategies are going to play out over several generations into the future. A very high inbreeding coefficient in an individual animal is not necessarily bad as long as animals with no kinship are available. Those matings can then take the inbreeding coefficient back down to zero, which opens up many more options for the future use of those animals. In that regard, paying close attention to kinship might be more useful, if more difficult, than focusing on the much easier coefficient of inbreeding.

9.5 Use of Estimated Breeding Values

In many commercial breeds it is common to have statistically derived estimates of the genetic worth of individual breeding animals. These are known by different names in different species and in different breeds, but common ones include estimated breeding value (EBV) and estimated progeny difference (EPD). These estimates are derived from the performance of the relatives and progeny of the animals being evaluated. The techniques usually involve the measurement of commercially important traits including growth rates, milk production, and reproduction. A repeatability score is usually associated with each EPD which reflects the accuracy of the estimation. The higher the number of family members measured (especially offspring), the higher the repeatability on any individual animal that is evaluated. The repeatability can be a very important guide to the expected outcome of matings, and is usually highest for old, proven sires that have seen wide use.

The EPD values are calculated against breed averages, and are in the units in which the trait is measured. For example, in sheep it is possible to generate EPDs for the prolificacy of a ram's daughters. These might run from 0 (breed average) to –0.3 (daughters producing 0.3 lambs below the breed average) or +0.5 (daughters producing about half a lamb more than the breed average). The way in which this information is used is up to the breeder. If the breed is relatively prolific, it might well be that in some situations the best bet is the ram with the EPD of –0.3, because the goal might be to reduce the number of triplets and quadruplets. In contrast, a different farm with different goals might well want to use the +0.5 ram, because the farm and management can successfully manage and benefit from all those extra lambs.

A second example might be birth weights, in pounds (lb). EPD values of 0 (breed average), +1 (1 lb heavier at birth), and –0.5 (0.5 lb lighter at birth) could all be used to advantage in different situations. A producer with lambs that are too light at birth would opt for the ram with a positive score, while a different breeder might be experiencing birthing problems from lambs that are too large and might therefore use the ram with a negative value. In herds where certain traits are at an acceptable level, using EPD-rated sires with values of 0 may be an informed and targeted decision.

The EPD statistics have great value and can be calculated for a number of traits, depending on what the breeders choose as important targets of selection programs. In production herds the underlying philosophy is usually one of improvement, which might not always be appropriate if the goal is to maintain animals adapted to harsh environments. Improvement means change, and not all changes are desirable in all situations, including changes to population structure that may diminish the value of a rare breed as a genetic resource.

9.6 Breeding Goals for Various Sorts of Breeders

Breeders vary in philosophy and goals, but they can be grouped into various categories depending on their interest in purebred breeding, and their overall priority for selection for different general traits. For some traits, positive selection is needed to enhance the trait. For other traits such as defects, selection against the trait is needed so that it diminishes in the population. Some traits are neutral and experience no selection at all in either direction. This is true across all species. These differences are outlined in Table 9.1.

Table 9.1 Emphasis of different aspects of animal traits by different types of system.

Type of system	Breed purity	Production level	Longevity	Adaptation	Fertility	Mothering ability
Conservation	+++	++	++	+++	+++	+++
Exhibition	0	+	0	0	0	0
Commercial	+	+++	+	+	+++	+++
Dairy	++	+++	+	+	+++	–

It is important to recognize that none of these general philosophies is inherently wrong, but they are indeed different because each emphasizes different aspects of selection. Over long periods of time they can each take a breed in a very different direction. In some situations, such as the commercial production of an end product, the emphasis can result in many breeds becoming very similar one to another. Understanding the relative importance of these different targets of selection, along with the breeding strategies to achieve them, can have profound consequences to the genetics of a breed.

Conservation breeders have an especially challenging and important role because they need to be attentive to breed purity, as well as to animal performance and breed type. The goals for conservation breeders are long term, even though the short-term economic viability of the project can never be ignored. Short-term failures make long-term success meaningless.

In contrast, exhibition breeders can have more of a short-term outlook. Producing the next show-winner is the goal. While many exhibition breeders do have long-term goals and long-term breeding programs, the emphasis on overall type of the animals is paramount. Exhibition type usually includes breed type to an extent, but often a more homogeneous show type shared across breeds, like body size, can eclipse a breed-specific emphasis. This is true in many species and is blurring the identity of pure breeds.

An example of the consequences of selection comes from dairy breeds. While details vary from species to species, the general trend for most dairy animals is toward fecundity (high prolificacy) and away from mothering ability. This seems paradoxical, but good dairy animals need to be willing (or eager) for humans to take the milk that was originally destined for their own offspring. Especially in goats and sheep, selection for fecundity over many generations assures lots of milk, while selection for weak maternal protectiveness and bonding assures that the animals can be easily milked. As a result, many of the dairy breeds of sheep and goats tend to have relatively large litters, but are then perfectly content to walk off and let a human caretaker manage them. They have very low maternal ability.

In contrast, it is also possible to have situations where a very high maternal ability is a negative instead of a positive trait. Some does of meat goat breeds have very high maternal ability. Some of these does start this behavior a day before their own kids are born, and are perfectly happy to steal another doe's kid and provide it with the colostrum destined for her own. This can upset herd dynamics, and can compromise kid survival even though a casual glance would have suggested that the more maternal ability, the better. As with most of life, a balance is often the ideal spot to achieve.

The key lesson is that the intricacies of each system impose certain selection pressures, and over several generations these can change the genetic resource used to satisfy the demands of the system. A close look at the system can tease out these details, and the results can be important as meaningful conservation programs are instituted. Conservation works best when its goals are congruent with the other goals of the system.

9.7 Poultry Breeds and Breeders

Poultry breeders have unique approaches. It is especially important for conservation breeders to be aware of the wide range of outlooks and philosophies among poultry breeders

Table 9.2 Emphasis on different traits by various classes of poultry breeders.

Breeder class	Breed purity	Breed type traits	Longevity/ adaptation	Production	Reproduction/ broodiness
Conservation	+++	++	++	++	++
Institution	+++	0	0	+	+ to 0
Exhibition	0 to +	+++	0 to +	0	0 to +
Hatchery	0 to +	+	0	++	–
Homesteader	++	0 to +	++	++	++
Industrial	0	0	0	+++	–

(Table 9.2). Most breeds of poultry have breeders in each breeder class, and their wide array of selection goals and environments can make the resulting birds very different from one another even though they go by the same breed name and have a similar or identical appearance. As a result, customers must choose the source of their birds carefully in order to assure that their breeding goals are compatible with that breeder's goals.

Conservation breeders of poultry are few and far between, and they face challenges that breeders of mammalian livestock do not. Most conservation breeders need to pay attention to a wide range of traits. This makes their task especially challenging. One challenge is locating sources of purebred birds that are selected for productivity and survival in their specific system.

Institutional poultry breeders are usually academic institutions that maintain reference flocks of various sorts. These populations tend to be several decades old and are maintained as purebreds. However, selection for breed type is usually lax. The main target of selection in most institutional populations is for purity, with some attention to production. Other traits take second place. Most of these flocks are reproduced on an annual cycle, with subsequent elimination of the previous generation of birds. Consequently, longevity is irrelevant.

Commercial hatcheries face a peculiar array of challenges. They need to produce day-old chicks in high numbers to satisfy market demand. There is usually at least some attention to breed purity and breed type, with type slightly outranking purity in the narrow sense. Longevity is usually not valued because in some situations the breeder populations are depopulated annually as an aid to disease control. This precludes any selection for longevity. Egg production is valued, and this is true for all breeds whether primary egg layers, meat birds, or exhibition birds. Targeting egg production thus tugs against any allowance for hens to go broody because broody hens quit laying eggs. Few hatcheries can incorporate good broody behavior into their selection scheme.

In contrast, homestead breeders, or those interested in other aspects of low-input sustainable systems, might place a great deal of value on a hen's ability to brood eggs and raise chicks on her own. For some breeds, such as Dorkings, the wide variety of breeders, with a wide variety of environments, has resulted in some quite different populations all within a single breed (Figure 9.7). Dorkings for homesteads go broody in the summer, and are noted for winter egg production. In at least some commercial hatcheries, Dorkings have experienced selection against broodiness to maximize egg (and chick) production.

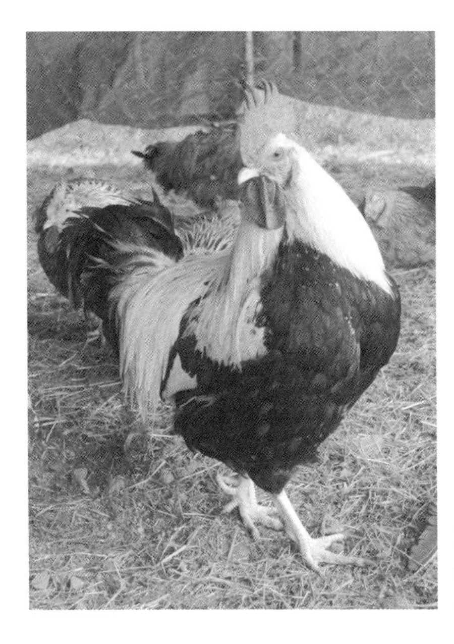

Figure 9.7 Strains of Dorking chickens have become quite variable functionally, depending on the selection environment of the breeding stock. Photo by JB.

This pattern is repeated throughout many breeds, which can be a perplexing dilemma for breeders interested in sourcing purebred seed stock with certain qualities.

Exhibition breeders have the goal of winning shows. This demands individual birds that closely match the breed standard, but this is not necessarily limited to purebred birds. While some exhibition breeders do work exclusively with purebred birds, others resort to specific combinations or crosses to produce their birds. Some breeders do not sell day-olds because their strategy is to cull out the nonqualifying birds from a very mixed brood of variable backgrounds. This strategy provides show-winning birds, but it does little to advance purebred breed conservation.

Commercial breeders focus nearly entirely on production levels. Traits of adaptation, broodiness, and maternal ability are likely to be ignored at best, and are often actively penalized due to the system in which the birds live and produce. Broodiness and maternal ability are detrimental if the goal is the maximum production of eggs to be artificially incubated.

The level of culling to achieve success in exhibitions or commercial production is important, and these two systems usually demand a high level of culling. This requires adequate numbers of birds. Having large numbers of birds available requires a relatively high rate of egg production.

The point of this discussion is that each different system needs different birds. Each is legitimate in its own way, but each is different. When a single breed is used in these different systems, the resulting selection pressures take the breed in very different directions. When those birds are given the same breed name, it can be very confusing for buyers interested in a specific bird for a specific purpose. The birds are the product of their selection environment, and this varies. Breeders should be aware of the selection criteria used to produce birds they purchase so that their new birds are appropriate for their management environment.

CHAPTER 10

Assisted Reproduction Techniques

Advances in this modern era make it possible to assist reproduction beyond that which would be possible by strictly natural means, and can boost the participation of individual animals to very high levels. Many uses of these powerful techniques can be either quite effective and constructive, or truly dangerous and destructive. They are, in a very real sense, "value neutral," and the eventual outcome depends entirely on how they are used.

10.1 Artificial Insemination

Artificial insemination is the oldest of the assisted reproduction techniques. It has been a major tool for advancing the production levels of poultry and dairy cattle. Artificial insemination, at least in mammals, removes the need for a male to be maintained by each individual breeder. This one advantage can be important both logistically and for management concerns. This is especially true for dairy cattle, where the bulls of some breeds are dangerous to be around on a day-to-day basis. Eliminating the bull eliminates a significant hazard. In a subtle way, relying on artificial insemination in dairy cattle has also removed most of the selection pressure for gentle temperament in bulls, because their management is relegated to specialists, meaning few people need to deal with them.

Artificial insemination works to make the contributions of an individual male go beyond what would naturally be possible. One possible outcome is to advance a healthy population structure. A more common outcome is to dramatically increase rates of selection. Fewer and fewer males of exceptional production potential are used more and more widely. These few males thereby rapidly swamp and replace the genetic diversity in a breed. This is the main threat from artificial insemination. The use of only a few males, especially over several generations, drastically reduces genetic variation to the point that inbreeding depression becomes a real threat.

The different species vary in their success rates with each step of artificial insemination. It is most routinely used in cattle, followed fairly closely by horses. Goats are also routinely collected and inseminated successfully, although the extension and freezing of semen do present a few hurdles. Swine breeders also routinely use artificial insemination, although

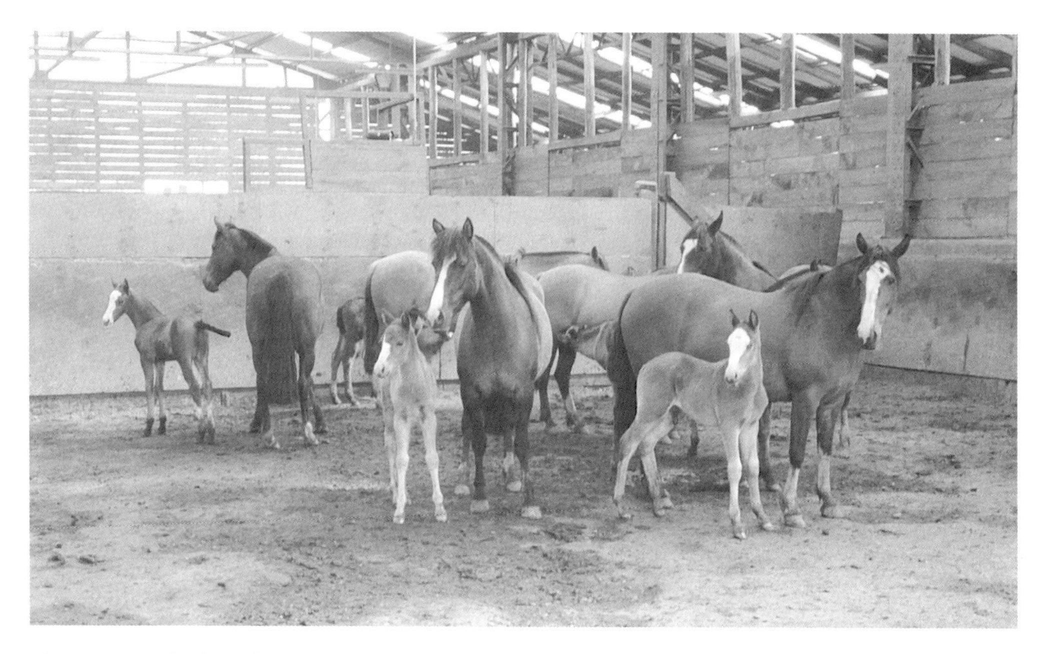

Figure 10.1 The breeders of the Caballo Chileno rely extensively on artificial insemination. Photo by DPS.

more often with fresh semen than with frozen. Sheep have few barriers on the male side, but important ones on the female side that are inherent in the anatomy of the ewe's reproductive tract. Overcoming these barriers requires surgical inseminations, so artificial insemination is unlikely to ever become routine. Dog reproduction is seeing an increasing reliance on artificial insemination. Some dog breeds have seen dramatic increases in the use of popular sires. Poultry are problematic. The use of freshly collected semen is routine, and is indeed the normal practice now for industrial birds. The use of frozen semen is nearly impossible, so the use of artificial insemination in poultry only reduces the number of males and does not completely eliminate the need to house and care for them.

Some breeds have experienced huge reductions of genetic variation through the use of artificial insemination. Holstein bulls can easily sire tens of thousands of calves. As the calves mature and are tested (either by mating or by genomics) only a few of them see wide use. After even a few generations the genetic influence of these few will prevail throughout the entire breed.

Other breeds of dairy cattle also use artificial insemination extensively, including Ayrshire, Guernsey, and Jersey cattle. A few horse breeds, such as the American Standardbred, Caballo Chileno, and to a lesser extent Warmbloods and the American Quarter Horse, also use this technique (Figure 10.1). Some horse breeds, such as the Thoroughbred, completely ban artificial insemination, largely as a tactic for enhancing the economic value of breeding males within the breed by assuring that many of them see use in reproduction.

Managing the risk of genetic loss that can come with artificial insemination can be fraught with political overtones. To some extent, "genetic loss" can be considered one of the legitimate goals of selection as less productive lines are removed. If taken to extremes this loss can imperil the survival of a population. Successfully managing the risk is therefore important. One possible solution in rare breeds is to mandate that no one sire can produce over 5% of the offspring that are produced in any one year. This is a much better strategy than completely banning artificial insemination because it allows for the positive uses of artificial insemination while also limiting the potential negatives. The level of 5% as a cap on production can in fact be imposed on any breed and any sire, whether this is achieved by artificial insemination or by natural service. This rule would not be accepted readily by those breeders who own the outstanding or most popular males, but it does serve the long-term interests of the breed itself.

Artificial insemination has consequences besides the immediate goal of enhancing the genetic contribution of the few desired sires. The technique of artificial insemination is itself a test of genetic material. Animals, whether the male donating the semen or the female receiving it, have different potential for success. Success in artificial insemination therefore becomes a trait that undergoes selection along with all the other traits that are evaluated in animals. An animal that succeeds well in natural service does not necessarily succeed well in artificial insemination. This sounds harmless, and can even seem trivial in the light of the many decades of success of dairy cattle breeders using this technique. The success in dairy cattle breeding has been achieved with frozen semen, which puts yet another layer of complexity onto the endeavor: the semen from some bulls freezes well, from others it does not.

At the tail-end of many decades of successful artificial insemination of dairy cattle it is easy to forget that the early days of this technology saw a higher rate of failure among bulls than is currently the case. This is a result of the removal of the failed genetics from the breeding population. In the early days this was a slow process, but it still worked to largely eliminate their genomes from the breed. The earlier cattle included variation in levels of success for every stage of artificial insemination; the descendant contemporary cattle have eliminated genetic variation for all except those animals that can succeed in the system.

Other breeds, and especially rare breeds, run a risk as they newly adopt artificial insemination, especially if they are using frozen semen. The risk is that some males of some lines simply cannot reproduce well by that procedure, and their genomes will be lost to the breed. Each step in the cascade that leads to a successful artificial insemination becomes a potential site of veto for participation in the breed: semen collection, semen extension, semen freezing, semen thawing, the introduction of semen into receptive females, and the successful conception of an embryo.

Breeds vary, which is a basic reason for worrying about their conservation in the first place. One way they vary is in this whole cascade of events. Recent experience with the use of frozen semen in both Large Black and Gloucestershire Old Spots hogs has revealed that these breeds do not respond in the same way as the more common commercial swine breeds (Figure 10.2). Techniques for success have had to be developed by trial and error, and these are not always available for all rare breeds. Success depends on both breeders and researchers being interested in the problem.

Artificial insemination, if widely used, removes specific selection pressures from the entire equation of animal breeding. This is another example of a "value neutral" phenomenon that is neither "always bad" nor "always good." Poultry breeding provides a useful example

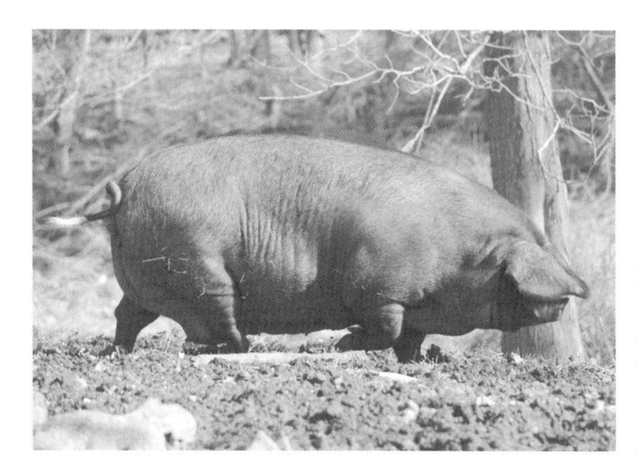

Figure 10.2 Large Black sows respond differently to artificial insemination than the commonly used commercial breeds. Adjusting procedures has led to successful conception and pregnancy. Photo by JB.

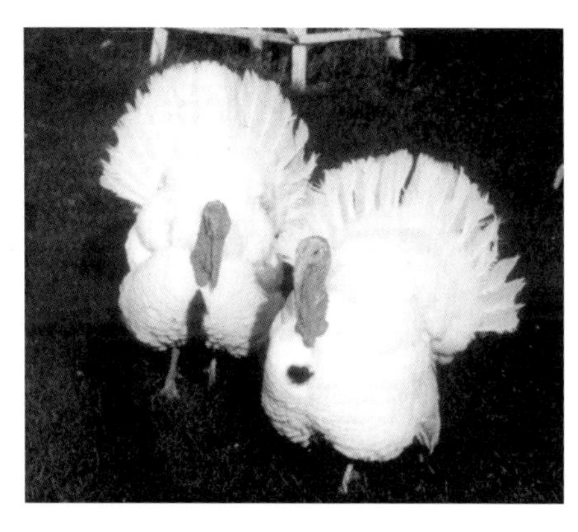

Figure 10.3 Artificial insemination allows industrial poultry selection to go to extremes. Photo by DPS.

here. Industrial stocks of both turkeys and broiler chickens have long been reproduced by artificial insemination. This has reduced the number of males used in reproduction, which automatically increases the degree of selection that is possible for production traits. A more subtle consequence is that artificial insemination increases the overall fertility of the flock because every female is deliberately inseminated, and none are missed as might well be the case where a male plays favorites among the females. This uncoupling of selection from behavior likely has minimal consequences, but this is an example of a change in selection environment having potential side effects.

A more important consequence of artificial insemination in meat birds has been the possibility of selection for extremes of phenotype that include incredibly massive breasts (Figure 10.3). These birds are exquisitely productive, but only in an industrial situation. Their conformation makes it impossible for them to reproduce naturally, and they have become dependent on artificial insemination for any hope of a next generation. They also cannot walk all that well, which limits the range of environments in which they will succeed. This is an extreme example, but is a useful one because it shows the potential consequences if a selection procedure becomes uncoupled from environmental constraints. In this example, the environment for industrial poultry imposes minimal constraints on natural reproduction and environmental adaptation. The result is that genetic resources of both turkeys and broilers cannot be readily put into environments other than the one for which they were designed. They have become the ultimate specialists, and have done so through extreme selection for production that is uncoupled from broader environmental constraints. This has only been possible through the technology of artificial insemination.

These negatives, though, do not mean that artificial insemination has no positive value. It has a wide variety of very helpful and constructive uses in the management of rare breeds. It allows the genetic material of old, founder, or geographically isolated animals to see broader use than might otherwise be possible. It can salvage the genetic potential of males that become injured or lost to accident. Strategic use of such males can be essential to balance out founder contributions in rare breeds. Artificial insemination makes their use available over broader geographic areas than would be possible due to limitations of transport impeded by distance or regulatory issues.

10.2 Embryo Transfer

Embryo transfer is a more recent development than artificial insemination, and has a greater number of technological hurdles that must be cleared. Cattle, once again, have led the success with embryo transfer, followed closely by the other ruminants (goats and sheep), and now also increasingly by horses. Swine and dogs have lagged behind due to various complexities of reproduction in species that bear litters (Figure 10.4).

Embryo transfer usually involves superovulation so that multiple oocytes are shed by the dam, fertilized (almost invariably by artificial insemination), and then at an appropriate

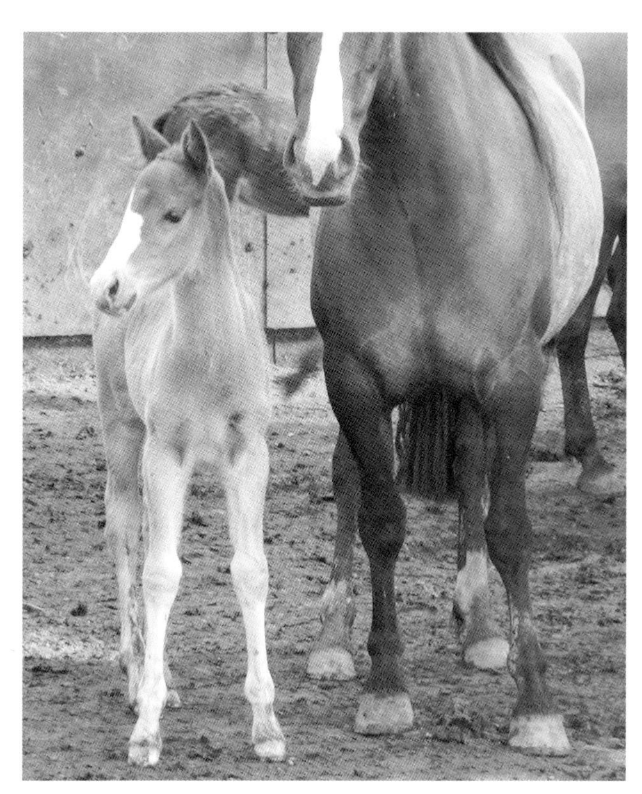

Figure 10.4 Transfer of embryos from mares in competition to surrogate mares provides opportunities for evaluating the performance of the donor mare while also assuring her contributions to the next generation. Photo by DPS.

early stage these are transferred into surrogate dams that carry the fetuses to term. It is readily apparent that this radically increases the number of offspring possible from a single female. As is true of artificial insemination, embryo transfer is "value neutral." It can easily lead to overrepresentation of the genetic influence of some animals at the expense of others. Alternatively, it can be used to assure a good representation of underrepresented genetics that might otherwise drift to extinction.

It is important to realize that the whole process of superovulation and embryo transfer has a number of steps, each one of which serves as a site at which selection occurs. Some females respond well, others do not. It is tempting to view success in superovulation and embryo transfer as a useful and accurate measure of inherent fertility and fecundity, but this is not the case. Success in embryo transfer and success in natural reproduction are two independent traits, so success in one cannot be correlated with success in the other. If embryo transfer is used extensively over multiple generations it becomes a major point of genetic selection for success in the procedure itself, which has potential negative consequences if not managed carefully.

10.3 In Vitro Fertilization

In vitro fertilization ratchets the whole procedure of assisted reproductive technology up yet another notch. In this case oocytes are harvested (either directly from an ovary or from a superovulation event). These oocytes are then matched up with semen, often by directly injecting a sperm nucleus into the oocyte. It is readily apparent that this is a complicated procedure, with many steps, all of which must succeed in order to achieve a good outcome. This procedure is yet to become widespread, but is being perfected in multiple species and may one day be more widely available.

10.4 Cloning

Cloning is the process of putting a nucleus of one animal into an oocyte of another in an attempt to recreate the donor of the nucleus. This process has had an uneven track record. The early success with Dolly the sheep generated a great deal of enthusiasm, although the actual success rate was fairly low and several of the successful births provided animals with orthopedic or other problems that precluded their having long, comfortable, and productive lives. It is a procedure still in its infancy. Most of the interest in cloning centers around two main areas. One of these is to multiply animals of vastly superior production capability. This brings with it the potential problem inherent in all of the assisted reproduction technologies: a rapid decline in genetic variability. A population made up only of clones will have no real avenue to a genetically viable future. A second intriguing use centers on the production of pharmaceutical or industrial agents. Insulin and proteins related to control of hemophilia are among these targets. These are generally produced by genetically modified animals, and this whole endeavor is very much outside the arena of breed management and breed conservation.

An important use of cloning has emerged through the fact that it works well to produce piglets. Cloning of pigs has been undertaken in a wide variety of settings, especially with

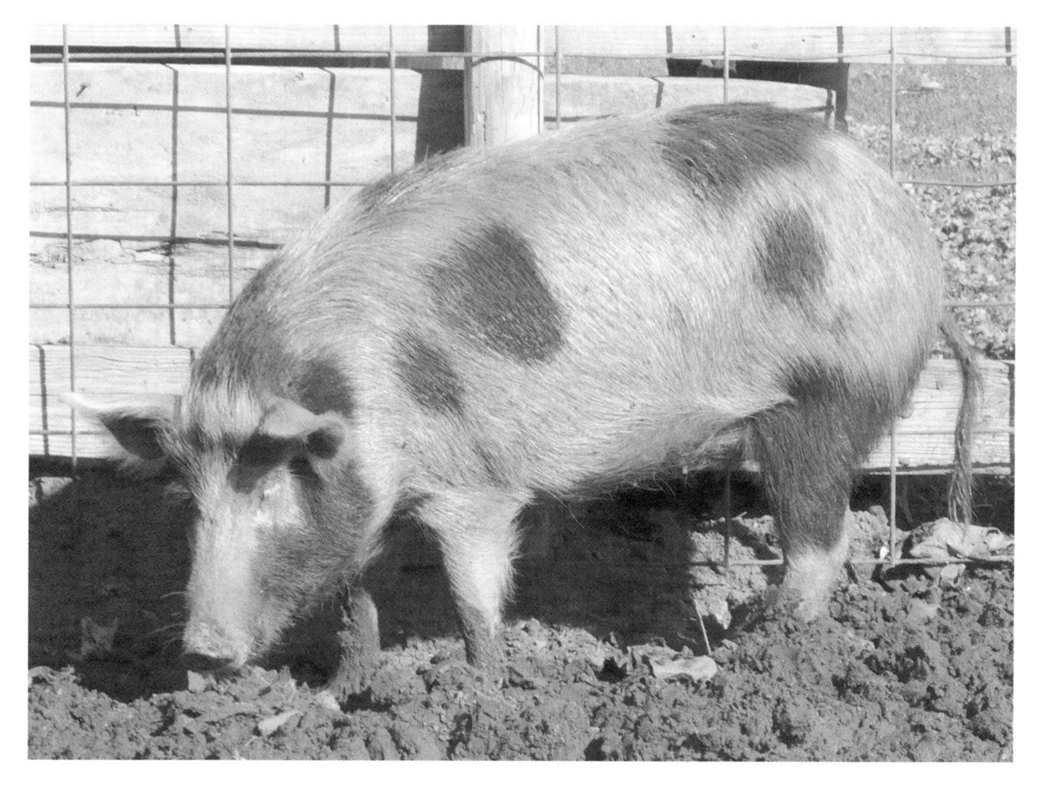

Figure 10.5 Cloning offers great potential for rescuing endangered populations of feral swine such as the Ossabaw hog. Photo by DPS.

genetically manipulated piglets used either in biomedical research or in the production of certain drugs. Another emerging use of cloning in swine is the potential to reconstitute rare breeds from a store of frozen material. This opens up exciting potential to freeze a baseline of genetic material from endangered populations, such as some isolated island feral hogs, and then reconstitute them so that their unique genetics are not lost. This technique provides a useful way around the very real difficulty of trapping and removing live feral animals in most environments. It may also serve as a very powerful way to conserve swine genetic resources that harbor certain diseases that can be eliminated by the cloning procedure (Figure 10.5).

10.5 Cryopreservation

Cryopreservation of breeds, also called cryoconservation, is the long-term freezing of semen, oocytes, embryos, or other tissues. This strategy is increasingly in vogue as a long-term insurance policy to guard against the loss of all living members of a breed. The goal is to be able to reconstitute the breed from the frozen store in the event of a catastrophe. This aspect of saving a frozen store demands that the sampling of the breed be complete in order to restore the complete breed in the event that it is lost as a living population. It is often a component of programs of both artificial insemination and embryo transfer.

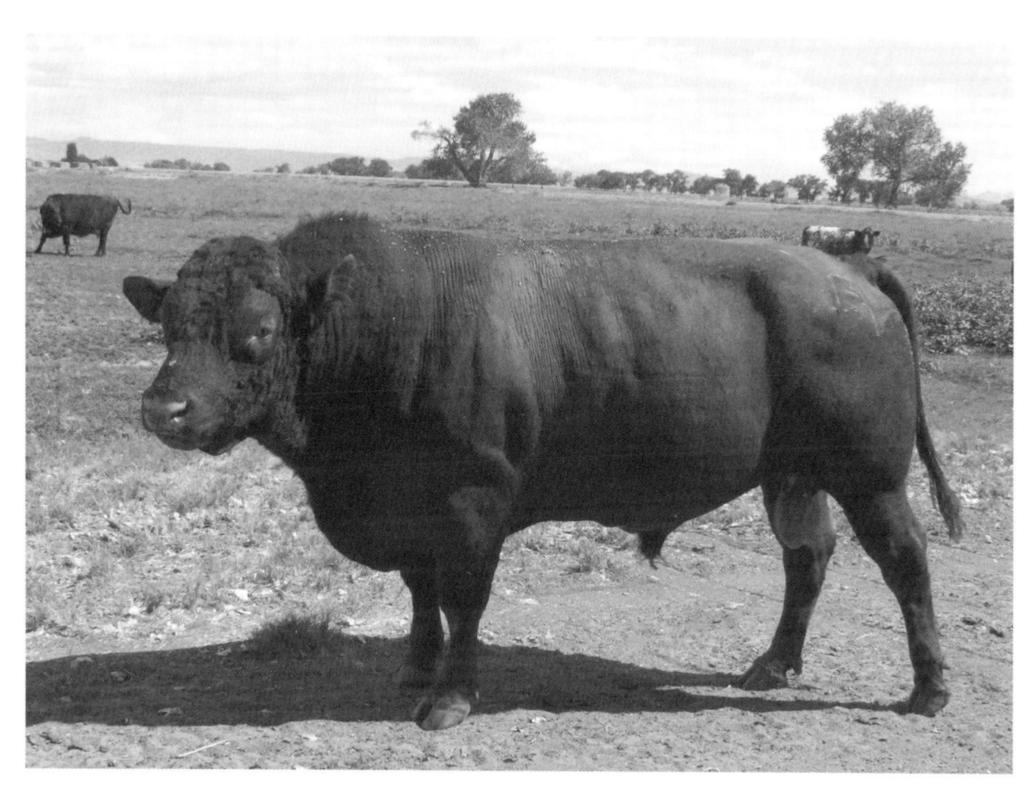

Figure 10.6 Dairy Shorthorns have benefitted from calves produced by semen stored decades ago. Photo by JB.

Cryopreservation is a very useful adjunct to the breed management and breed conservation systems that are based on living animals out on farms. This is because the frozen store can provide access to past animals should their contributions wane at some point. Their genetic influence can be reintroduced into the living breed, and can help to reinvigorate genetic diversity that may have been lost.

A few examples demonstrate the power of such a store. Dairy Shorthorns have become very rare internationally (Figure 10.6). Even though the breed is present in several different countries, in each individual country the cattle tend to be related to one another. This results in most matings being inbred to some extent. By using semen frozen long ago it has been possible to regain access to bloodlines that either have become rare or are extinct today. This brings renewed vigor to today's Dairy Shorthorns. A similar situation is true of many breeds, where the tendency has been to lose variation over time. In this situation the frozen store is a vital part of the living breed.

Some experts suggest that the frozen store might be the best way to conserve genetic diversity, while others prefer to emphasize that a living breed has advantages. One advantage to maintaining living animals is their constant exposure to the contemporary environment, so that selection can be ongoing for survival even as the environment changes. A second advantage of living breeds is that they are easily available and therefore not easily forgotten as options for people to select for their own ongoing use. In most situations a positive conservation outcome can be best achieved by combining good cryopreservation programs along with strong genetic management of living populations. The two approaches ideally work hand-in-hand for effective breed maintenance.

Cryopreservation of birds has seen interesting developments recently. The freezing of semen is notoriously difficult for most bird species and the freezing of oocytes would mean the freezing of large bird eggs, which is an impossible task. A technique developed fairly recently takes the gonadal ridge of a day-old hatchling and freezes it appropriately. This tissue can then be introduced into a day-old hatchling which has had its own gonadal ridge removed. A percentage of the recipients will have successfully taken the transplant to develop into a functioning testis or ovary. This technique, while exciting, has so far proven to be fairly fickle. It works in some instances, and fails in others. At least some evidence points to widely different rates of success from breed to breed. With a lack of experience across a wider variety of breeds it is a fairly risky bet to rely on this technique for ensuring the future of all genetic resources of poultry.

10.5.1 Selection of Samples and Numbers to Conserve

The selection of animals to target for cryopreservation is an important issue if the technique is to be successful. Animals should be selected so that the entire breadth of the breed's diversity is preserved. Efforts should avoid freezing only the highly selected and popular animals. Likewise, limiting the frozen store to those animals most easily available is also unwise because it excludes too much genetic variation. The final strategy for sampling should vary from breed to breed, but should always assure access to rare bloodlines because these are so important for the genetic diversity they have.

The numerical target for cryopreservation strategies varies depending on the final goal. If the goal is to be able to reconstitute the breed in the event of extinction of live animals, then saving as much genetic variation as possible is wise because that is the only way to allow reconstitution of the entire breed. While "more is always better," this is an unrealistic target because "more" eventually means the entire breed. Freezing is expensive due to the costs of sourcing the animals, accessing the samples, and maintaining these samples over long periods. The expense tends to impose a certain degree of leanness on the process, with the goal being the freezing of as few animals as possible while still obtaining a reasonably complete sampling.

Targeting the specific animals to use for a frozen store can rely on different strategies. One strategy is random sampling. The random sample is attractive for theoretical reasons, because statistics can guide the numbers needed for a reasonably complete representation of a breed. A random sampling protocol is the underlying assumption for most cryopreservation strategies. The assumption behind random sampling is that it will accomplish a reasonably complete sampling. However, this is often untrue due to the fact that rare bloodlines are inherently more difficult to find and access for such efforts. Rare bloodlines are also the ones most likely to be overlooked by a random sampling protocol. Random sampling tends to overemphasize more common bloodlines.

An alternative to the random sample is to target specific animals for inclusion based on phenotype and pedigree. This strategy assures better inclusion of rare variants within the population. When combined with the numerical aspects that are suggested by the theory

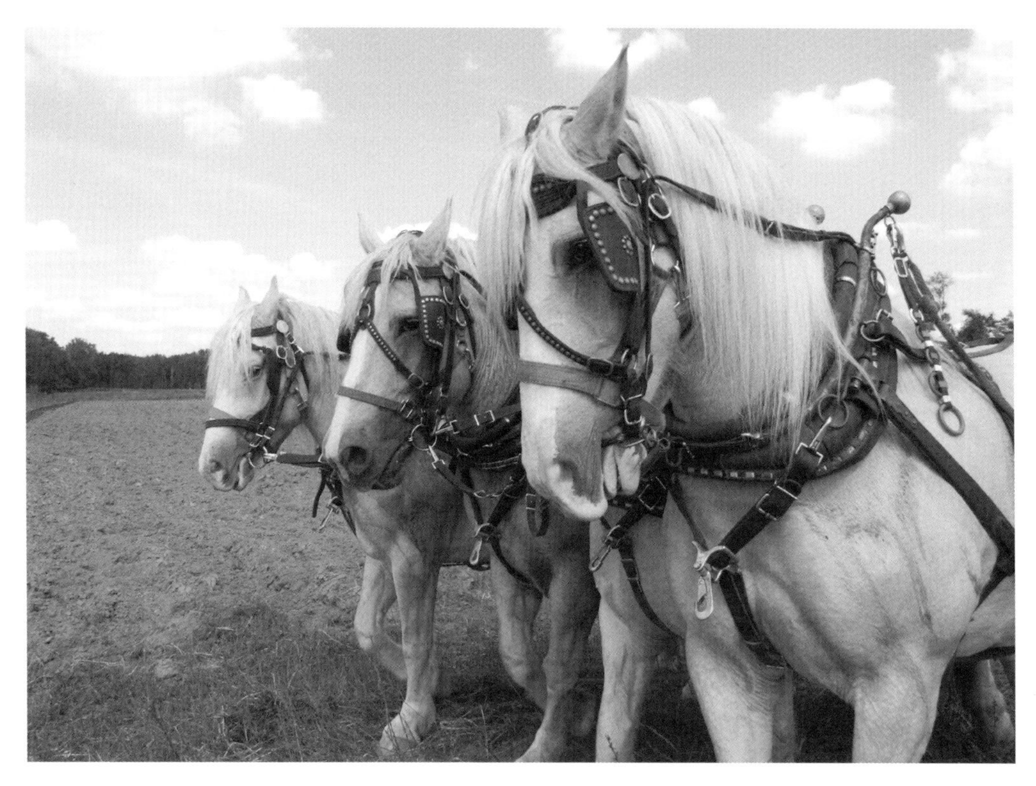

Figure 10.7 Some breeds, such as the American Cream Draft Horse, have such low numbers of breeding males that the entire breed falls short of cryopreservation recommendations. Photo by JB.

driving the random sampling, the final sampling is much more likely to be more complete than one which is driven by numbers or random selection alone. In many cases it is possible and wise to specifically target the collection of samples to include animals with either rare pedigrees or with rare genetic variants. There is little sense in duplicating the freezing of multiple examples of common variants while a strategy of deliberate inclusion of rare animals or traits increases the chances of the complete sampling of a breed's genetic heritage.

Genetic theory influences recommendations for numbers to preserve. These vary from a low figure of 31 animals all the way up to 250 animals for some populations. To be sure that most of the genetic variants are included, a sample of 50 males is usually sufficient, while a sample of 100 is needed if the goal is to assure the inclusion of 87% of the variants. This is a very high target, and is likely to be unrealistic in many breeds. Some breeds lack that number of males in the entire breed (Figure 10.7)! The strategy of deliberately including the least related animals can help ensure broad sampling, even at the lower range of numbers of samples. The FAO recommends that, for most populations, saving semen from 25 unrelated males would save most genetic variation. This should be done along with saving the embryos from 25 matings that are unrelated to the frozen males as well as unrelated to one another. While some rare variants will be lost, the majority of the breed will be saved. In practice this can be difficult, especially if the individual identification of animals is relatively weak, because this makes assurance of the unrelated status of animals sampled an impossibility.

Semen is generally relatively cheap to freeze and store when compared to the price tag for embryos. This difference in cost can affect the final strategy that is adopted for a cryopreservation effort. New breakthroughs are always coming along, and some of these have proven to be very effective. Technology is advancing, and situations once considered nearly impossible can rapidly turn into ones that are routine.

Saving DNA from animals, rather than germ cells, is generally inexpensive. While current technology precludes any realistic use of the DNA to reconstitute animals, advances are always being made in cloning and other technologies. The low cost of saving such DNA makes it an attractive target for preservation efforts. This is usually done by freezing somatic cells such as skin cells or others. These can then be thawed and cultured for various uses later.

10.5.2 Sampling Standardized Breeds

Most standardized breeds are relatively easy to sample because the elite portion of most standardized breeds has a powerful influence on the remainder of the breed. It is therefore possible to sample the elite portion of these breeds broadly with fairly good assurance that this sample has encompassed the majority of genetic variation present in the breed. This approach does have at least some limitations because rare variants are likely to be missed, although these might be of arguable importance to most standardized breeds. In any case, a somewhat broader sampling should assure that even rare variants are included and is a strategy that can be added in for most standardized breeds.

Sampling dog breeds presents specific challenges because the temptation is to sample only dogs that are show-winners, or that otherwise meet the breed standard perfectly. For many breeds this may be too narrow a sample if the goal is to eventually reconstitute the breed as a genetically viable population. A broad sample is always better than a narrow one, but finding and accessing dogs that have not been promoted in competition can be difficult.

10.5.3 Sampling Landraces

Landraces present different challenges because they generally lack a tiered population structure. Landraces are much more likely to be made of a host of isolated herds within the main breed (Figure 10.8). Complete sampling of landraces should always be the goal, but

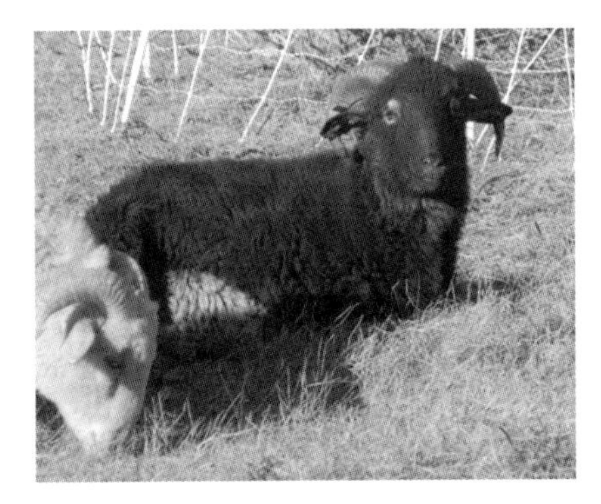

Figure 10.8 Landraces, such as Navajo-Churro sheep, are challenging to sample because of the need to include isolated bloodlines. Photo by DPS.

this is inherently difficult because it requires deep familiarity with the population structure of the breed so that candidate animals can be located, and samples can be preserved. A complete sample requires that each bloodline within the landrace should have at least one sample, and perhaps more if pedigree or phenotype suggests further variation.

With most breeds, whether standardized or landrace, the initial sampling is likely to be fairly simple because common bloodlines are easy to locate and easy to sample. The more difficult task is to assure that rare bloodlines, and in some cases rare individual animals, are located and have been cryopreserved in order to be sure that their genetics can contribute to the breed in the future. This is especially challenging in landraces where the rarer bloodlines are usually in the most peripheral circumstances. Even if they can be identified, the next step of actually sampling them presents real hurdles.

It is also important to target the sampling of rare visible variants in landraces because they are visible indicators of underlying variation. For example, a complete sampling of Navajo-Churro rams should include various colors, as well as polled, two-horned, and four-horned varieties. Guinea dwarf Pineywoods bulls should be targeted along with full-sized bulls, and in this breed the few polled bulls should also be sampled. Many other breeds have similar examples of rare variants that should be specifically targeted for inclusion.

10.5.4 Sampling Feral Populations

Feral populations present yet other problems, not least of which is obtaining the material that is targeted for cryopreservation. Free-ranging animals are nearly always in rugged situations, and are wary and wild by definition. Feral animals tend to cooperate poorly with efforts to take samples for cryopreservation! However, feral populations that are genetic resources should be sampled and preserved as broadly as possible. One tactic to accomplish this is to sample as broad a geographic representation as is possible. With island populations this could well mean that different portions of the island are deliberately sampled. In addition, the sampling should target the full range of phenotypes, with the one stipulation that any animals that are obviously crossbred should not be sampled. After removing these from consideration the remaining animals should be evaluated with an eye to identifying and sampling the ones that are outliers for the usual phenotype, while not ignoring the common phenotypes.

The frozen store of feral animals can be especially important for long-term conservation because many of these populations are targeted for removal from their current ranges. As success develops with eradication efforts, the animals are either eliminated completely or are removed to captive management. Once their free-living status is changed, the entire selection environment in which the breed lives has changed, and with this comes inevitable genetic changes. The frozen store, if complete, can assure that the original genetics are not lost. Fortunately, technologies for the preservation of semen and oocytes from recently dead animals are advancing. This provides an opportunity for good sampling of populations targeted for elimination.

CHAPTER 11

Animal Identification

It is important to appreciate that the culture and practice of identifying animals varies widely from place to place, time to time, and breed to breed. Individual animal identification is nearly essential to the success of selection programs because performance has to be linked to specific individual animals. Accurate individual identification is assumed in most selection schemes regardless of where in the world they occur and is an important part of selection programs. This identification is a necessary part of breeding programs for rare breeds where population management and wise mating practices are essential in achieving success and aiding conservation (Figure 11.1).

Accurate identification of individual animals contrasts starkly with some historic situations, especially those involving hundreds or thousands of animals. Extensive range situations could often succeed with minimal identification of individual animals, especially where performance was monitored only barely or not at all. In such situations the animals are allowed to run with multiple breeding males. The large numbers of animals included assure minimal inbreeding across the entire population, resulting in minimal risk of inbreeding depression as a genetic dead end. Inbreeding in such situations presents a minimal threat, but it is also important to note that most performance-related selection is unattainable.

The tradition of minimal identification of individual animals persisted until quite recently in many areas. A very good example of this is seen in some foundation herds of Pineywoods cattle that numbered into the several hundreds of cattle up until the 1960s. While owners might have used an earmark, this only indicated ownership and not the individual identity of each animal. This tradition persists to some degree through to today, but the problem is that the numbers of cattle in a herd are now much reduced. Each herd is now more likely to have multiples of ten cattle rather than the multiples of hundreds that were typical a century ago. This increases the risk of inbreeding that was negligible in the past into something that is nearly unavoidable now. Today, cattle must be individually identified and wisely managed for mating.

The easiest and most successful identification of individual animals is typical of larger animals, and then becomes less and less distinct as animal size and individual value goes

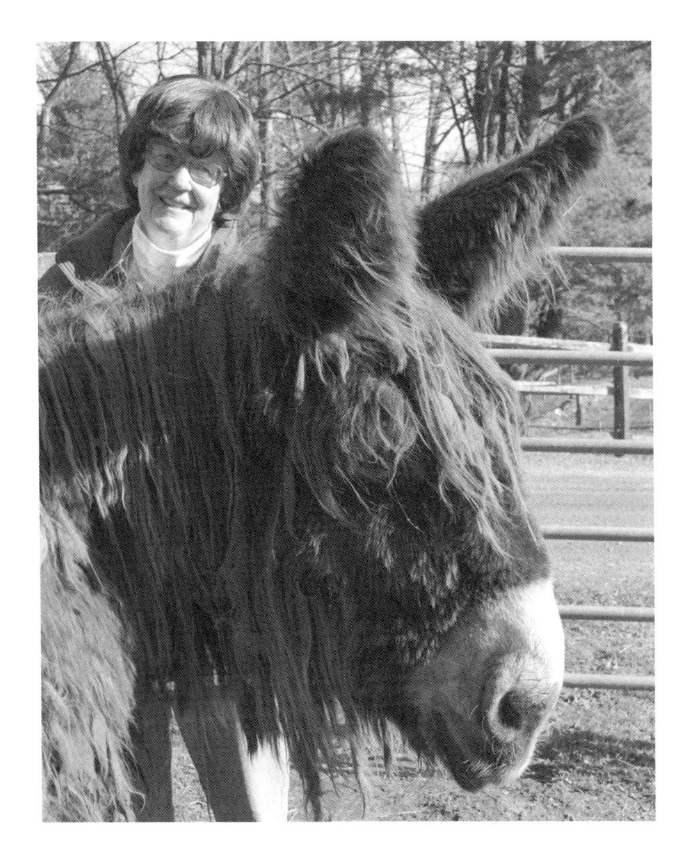

Figure 11.1 Debbie Hamilton's care and attention to detailed animal identification assured that her important Poitou donkey breeding program survived her own life. Photo by JB.

down. Horses are nearly always identified as individuals, even in breeds that are uniform for color. This identification is usually linked to registrations, and can involve color, markings, hair whorls, brands, tattoos, or microchips.

Cattle, likewise, are usually individually identified for registration purposes. This is especially important in breeds that are uniformly colored. Cattle breeders often resort to ear tags for identification, or occasionally to number brands (Figure 11.2).

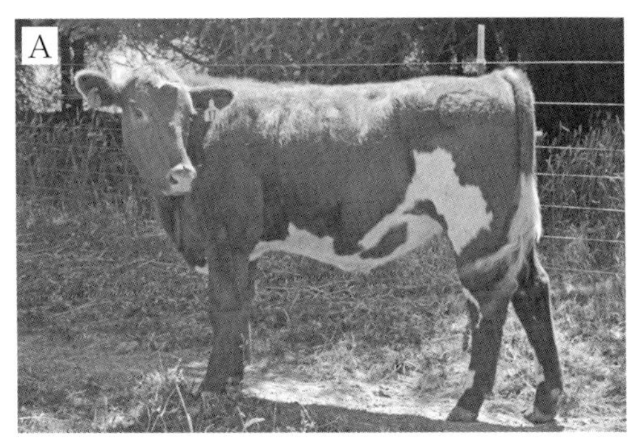

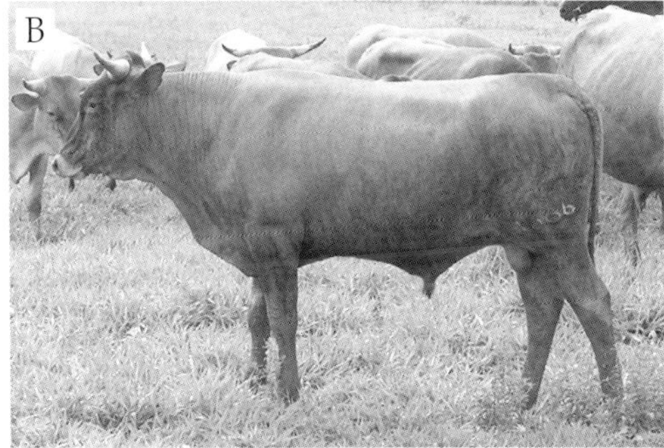

Figure 11.2 Ear tags and brands are long-established means of cattle identification. Ear tags are more likely to be used in breeds such as the Shorthorn (A), while branding is traditional for the Criollo Saavedreño (B). Photo A by JB, B by DPS.

Hogs are likewise generally known to their breeders and owners as individuals rather than as groups. This is variably accomplished through ear notches, ear tags, or occasionally tattoos. Sheep and goat identification varies from situation to situation. Many farms manage individual identification quite easily with ear tags and tattoos. More extensive operations with huge populations might not have record-keeping systems that are robust enough to provide for linking each individual to its record or to an identifying ear tag, even though such tags are increasingly required in order to sell animals through market channels. One problem with ear tags in sheep and goats is the propensity of the animals to lose them. One solution to that problem has been to double-tag with identical information in each ear. Animals rarely lose both tags at the same time.

Microchips are becoming more and more popular as a way to identify animals. They have the advantage of each bearing a unique identification number. Significant drawbacks include that they are invisible, and they also require a specific electronic reader in order for an observer to know the animal's identity. An animal that is in fact identified could easily be considered as not identified simply because the scanner was not available, and the microchip is invisible to external inspection.

Agropecuaria Florestal in Venezuela developed a practical identification system that works successfully to help manage their huge herds of extensively ranging cattle. At one point their herds numbered about 40,000 head of cattle. The key to their identification procedure involved branding each cow with an individual number as well as her year of birth. A glance rapidly indicated the cow's identity and age. Cows that failed to wean a calf received an "X" brand on their backs, which linked identification with performance.

Easy systems can also be devised for sheep and goats in range situations. The goal is to somehow identify superior performance on the one hand and substandard performance on the other. In most situations, identifying superiority (successfully raising twins, for example) by ear notches may be a solution. If notching the superior animals is objectionable, then the strategy can be reversed to notch the poorest performers to identify them for culling. A system of notches that identifies the most prolific females that also raise their offspring well can assure that they are identified, and that their offspring are selectively retained for breeding. An important detail is that the notch or other identifier needs to permanently follow the superior animals along. For example, in some compromised years it may not be possible to save replacements from the superior animal because they need to be sold in order to generate revenue. A few years later, though, it may well be possible to retain offspring from those animals that performed so excellently in compromised years. A permanent way to identify those individuals is essential.

Identifying animals for selection programs is only one of several important reasons for accurate animal identification. Identification is also essential if animals are not to be lost to the breed in the event of the untimely demise of an owner or other lapses. The breeding programs for Lipizzaner horses were successfully reconstructed after World War II because their branding protocols allowed for the identification and recovery of horses after the conflict was over.

A convenient way to identify animals in large groups is to "name" them by numbers. The farm name can go first (and should, if the producer is proud of them), then a number that codes year and order of birth. The Sponenberg farm is Beechkeld, and the naming system labels the 45th kid born in 2012 as "Beechkeld 1245," which is the number on the goat's ear tag. This quickly reveals age, identity, and relative order of birth within a year.

Ear tags numbered in this system or one similar to it work well in most large species. Horses and donkeys tend to be individually recognizable so that ear tags are rarely if ever used for them. Cattle can be branded with their number as an alternative to tags, and this is done in many parts of the world quite effectively. This numeric strategy helps to identify the animal as to source farm, age, and relative age within the year cohort. Animals can be evaluated for growth rate and maturity across the herd by knowing their number. In cases where a "real" name is needed, that can be added after the farm and number, so "Beechkeld 0755 Dendra" is a goat that warranted a name, but it is still easy to know that she was born in 2007 toward the end of the kidding season. By putting the number on ear tags, and keeping a reasonably current herd list, anyone can match animals to identities (and registrations) even in the absence of the owner. This becomes important if the owner meets an untimely demise.

Individual identification of birds in poultry breeds is rare except in pedigreed flocks of exhibition birds (Figure 11.3). Conservation-minded hatcheries also do an exceptional job of the individual identification of birds, which allows pedigree breeding. The identification for birds can be based on small bands in the web of the wing, toe punches, or leg bands. While most other livestock can have an age estimation based on teeth, this is impossible for birds. In situations where birds are kept for multiple years it helps greatly to be

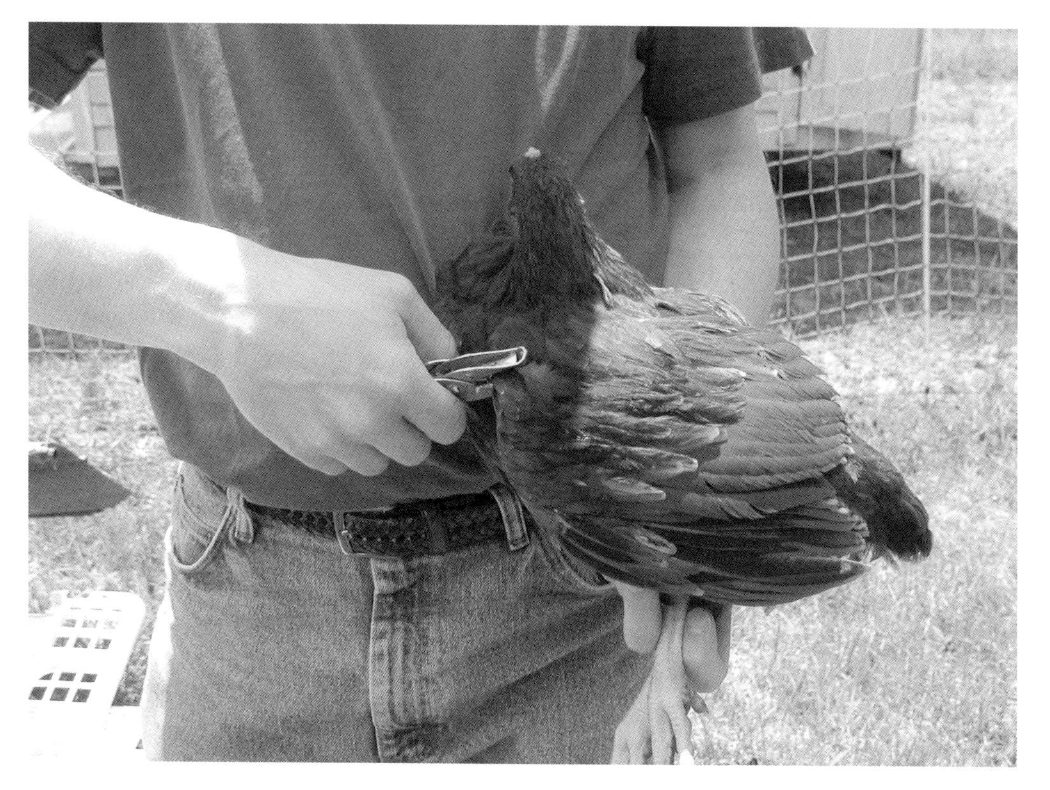

Figure 11.3 Wing bands that are numbered can easily and effectively identify poultry. Photo by JB.

able to identify birds as to the year they were hatched, so that ages can be tracked against productivity.

Animal identification is not only important at the individual herd level, but is also essential at the registry level. Multiple horror stories can be told of genetically important animals, or whole herds, being lost to a breed due to inadequate identification. At the level of the registry, it is also wise for there to be multiple copies of the registry herd book. This is especially easy to do in today's digital age. This assures that valuable information is not subject to loss in a house fire or other disaster, or by the failure of a single computer. It also helps to guarantee the continuity of information if people die, drop out, or suddenly quit for other reasons.

CHAPTER 12

Population Analysis

Analysis of the various details of a breed or a subpopulation of a breed is helpful in providing basic data that can be used for effective management decisions. This can be a daunting task, and fortunately a wide variety of tools are available to help. Many of these tools are available through breed associations, and they are easiest to use in that setting. However, they can also be used effectively in the absence of a breed association or registry. The tools can be tailored for breeds, bloodlines, or strains. Each tool has its own level of complexity and need for technical support. Each requires attention to detail, which is always a key component of successful breed management.

The tools used in a detailed breed analysis include a census, DNA studies, and an evaluation of pedigrees and relationships. Each of these reveals different information and is therefore useful in its own way. However, they are strongest when all three are used in combination. The census is usually the first step because it does not rely on laboratory tests or data manipulation. DNA studies require considerable technical and logistical support, but provide important insights into the genetic makeup of the population. Evaluation of pedigrees and relationships is essentially a herd book analysis. In situations where a herd book is not available, a fairly robust analysis can still be undertaken based on census information. Herd book analysis gives a snapshot of the breed at a specific moment in time, and can be used to suggest ways to move forward. This is especially true when the goal is to find specific animals or bloodlines that should be used to their full potential in order to not risk losing underrepresented genetics. Both DNA studies and herd book analysis can be essential for very small populations, and fortunately they are also easiest for them because the low numbers make the detailed assessment more practical. Small population sizes make it easier to devise detailed action plans which tend to be especially urgently needed for breed rescues. Pairing the data from DNA studies with that gathered from pedigree analysis greatly helps conservation breeders to develop targeted breeding plans. Both of these assume some sort of prior census data.

Before embarking on an analysis of a population's genetic structure, it is important to reflect on the nearly random way in which genetic material flows through generations. The details of this flow affect the reliability of inferences made from the various techniques.

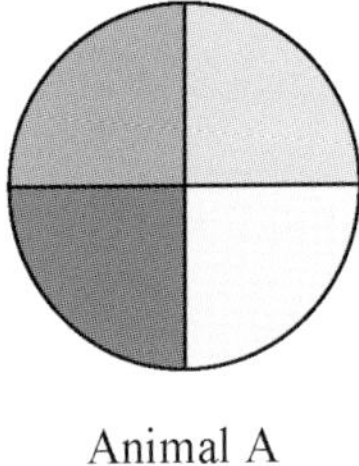

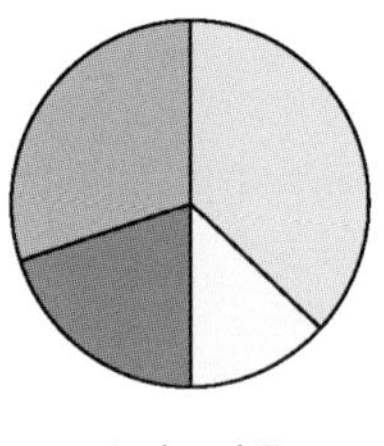

Figure 12.1 Pedigrees predict that each grandparent contributes exactly 25% of an animal's genome, as depicted for animal A. Paternal grandparents are in dark greys and maternal grandparents in lighter greys. DNA directly documents that many animals have somewhat greater amounts of genetic material from specific individual grandparents, and correspondingly less from others, as depicted for animal B. Figure by DPS.

Commonly held assumptions associated with the techniques for breed analysis can be incomplete to varying degrees, and are even wrong in some instances. Understanding how genes flow from one generation to the next is important in order to take full advantage of the strengths of these analyses while minimizing the risks imposed by their weaknesses.

Every animal gets half of its genetic makeup from its sire and half from its dam. However, this consistently uniform sampling is often not true for generations further back than parents. Pedigree analysis assumes that the genetic sampling that occurs from generation to generation is consistently and evenly random, leading to the outcome that each ancestor in the same generation of the pedigree is represented equally to the others in that same generation. This assumption is often incorrect, even if it is useful in most circumstances because it does reflect the average situation.

The 50% contribution that each parent makes to an offspring involves randomly sampling its own parents, which become the grandparents of the offspring. Under the assumption of equal sampling, each grandparent should contribute 25% of the final genetics of a grand offspring (Figure 12.1). An exact 50% contribution of each parent of a breeding animal is unlikely in most cases due to the way that random sampling actually works out in practice. Grandparents that end up contributing less (or more) than their expected final 25% affect the genetic material that is available down the line, and this disproportional contribution easily compounds from generation to generation. Assuming equal representation of distant ancestors is nearly always incorrect to some degree or another, DNA techniques, in contrast to pedigree analysis, more adequately reveal what has actually occurred because they accurately indicate situations where the sampling of distant ancestors has not been equal. Both pedigree and DNA analyses can be useful, but they each need to be appreciated for both their strengths and weaknesses. The key detail is that while every animal is 50% its sire and 50% its dam, ancestors that are further back may well not have contributed equally.

12.1 *Census*

The first useful tool is a proper census of the population, whether this be done for an entire breed, a bloodline, or a herd. This census ideally includes an accurate count of all animals

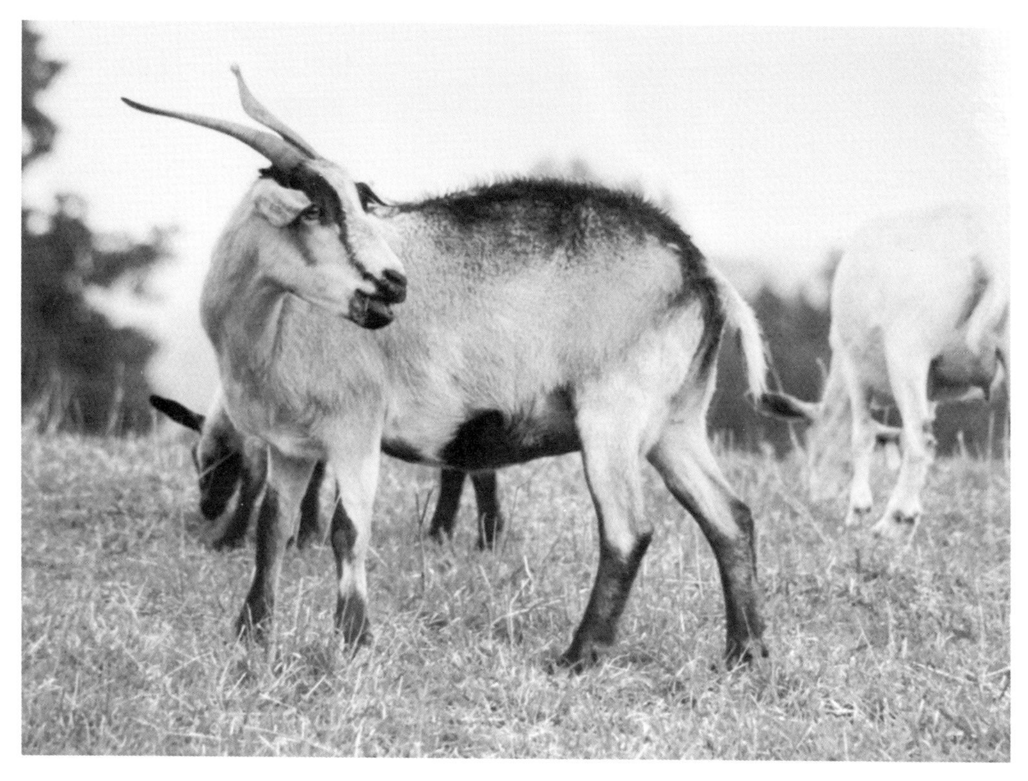

Figure 12.2 A good census documents each animal by sex, age, and location. It helps to identify animals, such as this Myotonic doe that is the last of her isolated bloodline. Photo by DPS.

available for reproduction, along with the age and location of each one (Figure 12.2). A complete census should accurately reflect births and deaths or other removals from the reproducing population. Examples of other removals include stallions that are gelded, animals that are sold for slaughter, or animals that die from other causes. In some populations this level of census is difficult to achieve, especially if a breed association is not functioning all that well. Of course, breeds without functioning associations are the most likely to be facing rescue crises, which in turn ramps up the odds that complete census data will not be available.

Monitoring the census of a breed is an important registry function for all breeds. Census is especially important for rare breeds because of the considerable risk of rapid and serious numeric depletion or loss of individual bloodlines. Trends must be monitored as an ongoing process in order to avoid surprises that come from sudden, unanticipated changes. The census should be monitored in a few different ways in order to capture information that is most helpful for breed management.

12.1.1 Numbers of Animals

One relatively easy way to monitor the census is to simply monitor annual trends of registrations. This is usually easy, and provides a direct and useful measure of purebred recruitment. It has several advantages as a convenient single measure of a breed's numerical health. The number of new registrations counts those animals that are most likely to contribute to the next purebred generation, and overlooks those that are unlikely to contribute. The number of registrations is almost always much easier to obtain than a complete count of every individual animal living at any one time.

Registration figures have advantages over other measures such as total number of breeding animals. This is especially true for breeds that are largely used for crossbreeding because many adult animals may not contribute to purebred replacement. Counting only adult breeding animals in such breeds will overestimate the level of purebred breeding. Counting all adult animals is also time consuming, and in most cases is likely to be woefully incomplete. Purebred replacement of horse breeds is especially likely to be vastly overestimated by counting only adult animals capable of reproduction (stallions and mares) because many mares are deliberately kept out of reproduction and are only used for athletic performance or as companion animals. Registration figures neatly and efficiently get around most of these problems by cleanly reflecting purebred breeding activity, despite the potential drawback that not all animals that are registered will themselves go on to participate in purebred breeding. Such animals were, however, registered as purebreds, and this in and of itself reflects the relative level of purebred breeding that is going on within a breed community.

A general tendency for nearly all species of production animals is that breeders of most breeds generally only register those animals that they are likely to use themselves or to sell as purebred breeding stock to other breeders. This works well to assure that registrations are a reasonably accurate reflection of the numbers of animals that are destined for reproduction within the breed. A few species deviate from this norm in different ways that affect the relationship of the registered population to the unregistered population. Many rabbit breeders only register rabbits that are likely to be shown. This is done because rabbits must be registered to compete in sanctioned shows. The result is that only a small percentage of purebred rabbits are documented in registry systems. Non-breeding animals of most breeds within most species are the least likely to be registered, with the important exceptions of horses and dogs.

An important issue is whether any incompleteness in registration results in a loss of information that impedes its practical use. Eliminating non-reproducing animals from registry records tends to reveal the level of pure breeding more accurately within the breed than would be reflected by the registration of every animal produced. Incomplete registration of purebreds indicates that culling is occurring, which means that breeders are being selective. This is generally good for any pure breed, because not every purebred offspring offers genetic excellence to the breed.

While the usual trend with registration numbers is to somewhat underestimate the total production of purebred offspring, breeders of some rare breeds tend to register all or nearly all of the young that are produced, and then cull some of them before reproduction. When this tendency is widespread within a breed it results in registration numbers that overestimate the actual purebred recruitment into the breed. Familiarity with the specific situation in each breed is necessary to correct for this tendency.

For many rare breeds, a simple count of annual registrations is not sufficient to monitor the genetic status of a breed, despite the convenience of this measure. More detailed analyses are important for some breeds, including the numbers of animals within the various distinct

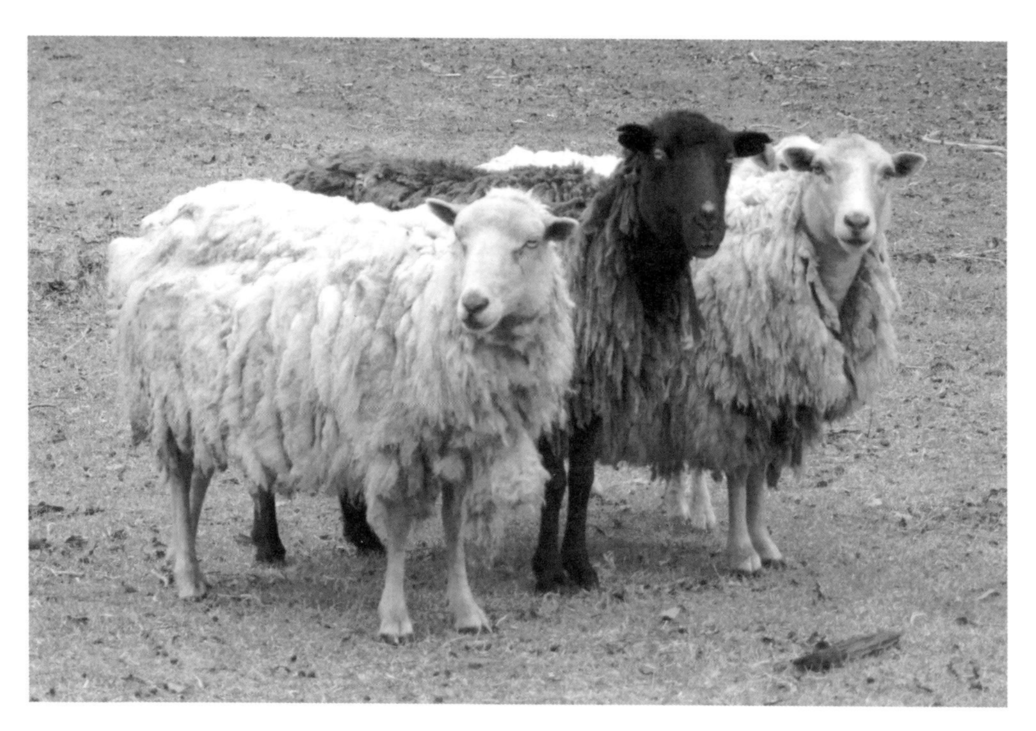

Figure 12.3 Landrace breeds, such as Gulf Coast sheep, often have unregistered purebred populations much larger than is represented by the registries. Photo by JB.

bloodlines or families of the breed. This can be an arduous task, but computerization of registry records can be a great help. If bloodlines are linked to pedigree information, then automated analyses are possible and tedious analysis by hand can be avoided.

Relying on registry records to reflect the total living population of registered animals has a few inherent problems. Many factors within a registry sometimes tend to either overestimate or underestimate the living population of registered animals, let alone the entire population of the breed that includes both registered and unregistered animals. Breeders usually do not relay information to the association concerning animals that are removed from the population, whether by death, or by sale to situations in which they will not be used for purebred production. Relying on registry records for a total count is therefore generally inaccurate and overestimates the actual census of animals that are actively participating in purebred breeding, although this varies from breed to breed.

Another situation in which registry records can easily give an inaccurate estimate of a breed is commonly encountered in landrace or local breeds where the registered populations are nearly always smaller than the actual population (Figure 12.3). Landraces with reasonably open herd books are especially likely to undercount animals, and it becomes nearly impossible to get an accurate estimate of breed populations. This situation is true for a handful of standardized breeds as well, but generally to a much smaller degree. For breeds with closed herd books, the issue diminishes for the registered population because entering new individuals of unregistered background into the registered population is difficult or impossible. The status of the breed as a registered population versus a functional agricultural entity that includes both registered and unregistered purebred animals can be important and is often overlooked. Exceptions where standardized breeds are underreported are important, and include some dairy cattle breeds as well as commercial breeder sows where registration documentation is seldom used. If the registered population excludes significant numbers of purebred animals, then the association is not fully accomplishing its mission to monitor and conserve the breed.

While census figures can rely on annual registrations in populations that are indeed registered, this is obviously impossible in unregistered populations. Poultry, specifically, are not individually registered by any association, and keeping track of numerical trends in poultry breeds is consequently very difficult. Surveys of a few key breeders and seasonal hatcheries can be very helpful. Surveys are notoriously easy to disregard and many fail to be returned, and telephone interviews are often required to get information on population numbers of poultry breeds. Poultry present another challenge because many breeds have small but potentially important populations that reside in isolated situations. These are likely to be overlooked by any census technique. Poultry census has an inherent tendency to focus mainly on large hatcheries or very engaged private breeders. This does have the advantage of targeting the very segment of the breeders that is most likely to heavily influence the breed's status by being the usual source of breeding stock. As a practical issue, poultry census work does establish the "worst case scenario" reasonably well by consistently underestimating total numbers.

Poultry present another challenge because it is difficult to sort through the relative importance and quality of breeding groups (Figure 12.4). Not only is the numeric assessment

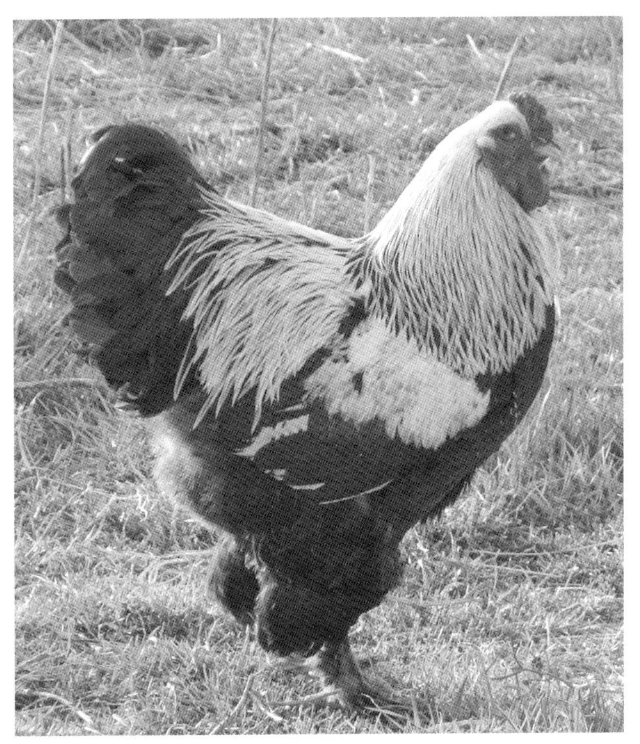

Figure 12.4 Census of poultry breeds and varieties, such as this Dark Brahma, is notoriously complicated because numbers, genetic status, and breeding practices should all be included. Photo by DPS.

important, but it is also important to have some idea of which populations are being bred to the standard, which are being selected for production characteristics, and which are pure-bred from a base of the original founding genetics. These more qualitative aspects are very difficult to assess by anything other than a site visit, and this is impossible in all but a very few situations. As a result, the census work for most poultry is difficult and has inherent inaccuracies. While details may be less finely focused than those for livestock, it remains true that census figures, whatever their drawbacks and inaccuracies, give a very good idea of the relative status of breeds. Even a flawed census is especially good at pointing to those breeds in critical need of conservation attention.

Rabbit breed registration issues lie somewhere between larger farm animals and poultry. Registration is required for any animals entered into competitive showing. This ensures that show animals will be registered, but gives no clear indication of the number of either the reproducing population or the total population, and therefore significantly underestimates the population of rabbit breeds.

In some situations, full counts of living animals are possible. Even in this situation it is important to realize that the timing of the count influences the results. Most species have seasonal fluctuations in numbers due to the production of young and their sale through commercial channels. The sheep breeders in Iceland neatly get around this complication by only counting adults that are overwintered. This strategy effectively removes from the census the young of the year that are destined for slaughter, and only reflects the animals retained for breeding.

12.1.2 *Monitoring Bloodlines, Strains, and Families*

Monitoring and managing the population structure within a breed involves keeping track of bloodlines, strains, or families within the breed. Each of those terms basically covers the same general concept: a portion of the breed more related to itself than to other portions of the breed (Figure 12.5).

Several different strategies can be used to monitor bloodlines. One strategy uses registration data to track the bloodline contributions of every animal registered. This can be done automatically through databases, although few registry software packages currently offer this. It is still possible to accomplish this task, but it usually requires a separate tracking system that computes bloodline percentages directly from parental information. This is easiest in young registries because founders can be categorized by bloodline. In older registries containing data from centuries of backlog, it is usually too cumbersome to go

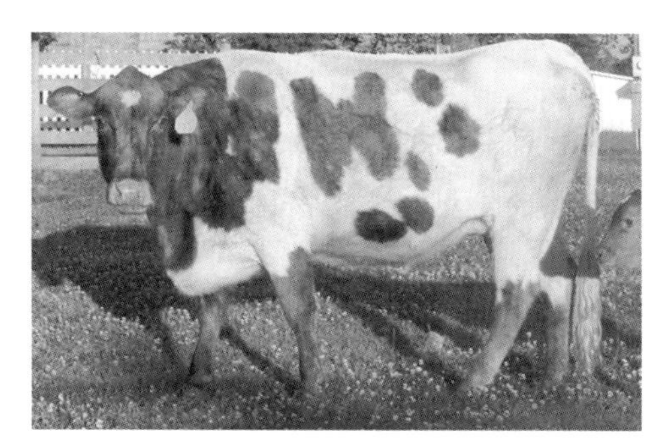

Figure 12.5 Rare strains within breeds, such as this polled Palmer-Dunn Pineywoods cow, need special attention when a breed census is performed. Photo by DPS.

back and categorize founders. In these situations a more recent start date can be used to accomplish the same purpose.

While tracking bloodlines can be done automatically with databases, it is also possible to accomplish the same goal using other methods. One strategy is to sort through the registered animals by sire and grandsire, grouping them by related animals. This is usually done by someone who is familiar with the animals of the breed because names and relationships will be familiar, and the task can be more easily accomplished by an informed person. The analysis can quickly show which sires are less well represented, and which ones are becoming overrepresented. While few breed registries can dictate specific matings, it is still possible to alert the breeder community when certain lines are becoming very rare. The hope is that breeders then act to correct the situation. The results of bloodline analysis can also help to target the cryopreservation of specific animals with rare genetic backgrounds. This can focus on rare bloodlines so that even if they become lost to the living breed, their influence can be retained through the use of the frozen store.

Results of these analyses reveal the relative status and influence of different families within the breed, which can help to target inquiries into why the levels of breeding activity differ for different animals or groups. If the difference is due to quality, then no action is required. If the difference is due to promotion, and some good animals are being overlooked, then the association and the breeders can take action to assure that good lines that are underrepresented are targeted for expansion before they are lost.

12.1.3 Monitoring Health Issues

The monitoring of breed health includes multiple aspects. One of these is the general genetic status of the breed. This involves calculating the level of inbreeding, the availability of sublines, and other related issues. These issues are all addressed in detail in other chapters due to their complex but important character. A second aspect is specific genetic-related diseases or traits that might be present in a breed. A third is the general health and vitality of the animals of the breed and how that affects the breed, its breeding, and its use.

Congenital defects include any defect present at birth. This is important because the definition does not imply a genetic cause. While many congenital defects are genetic in origin, many others occur due to viral or environmental causes. Conversely, some genetic defects are not noticeable at birth but become evident later. Examples include metabolic storage diseases, or the recently important bovine leukocyte adhesion defect (BLAD) the consequences of which only surface later in life and are not present at birth (Figure 12.6).

It is wise for breed associations to track congenital defects that are currently documented as genetic, as well as newly emerging ones. This forward-looking approach allows associations to quickly identify and develop a strategy for managing all defects. Developing a reporting method for defects is no easy task. The most successful methods are those that are employed by the most populous dairy cattle breeds. These provide for a description of the defect as well as for pedigree information. The reason these work so well in dairy cattle breeds is that calves are nearly always conceived by artificial insemination, so owners of dams have no vested interest in protecting the sire's reputation. Instead they have every incentive to quickly uncover any genetic weaknesses that may be present.

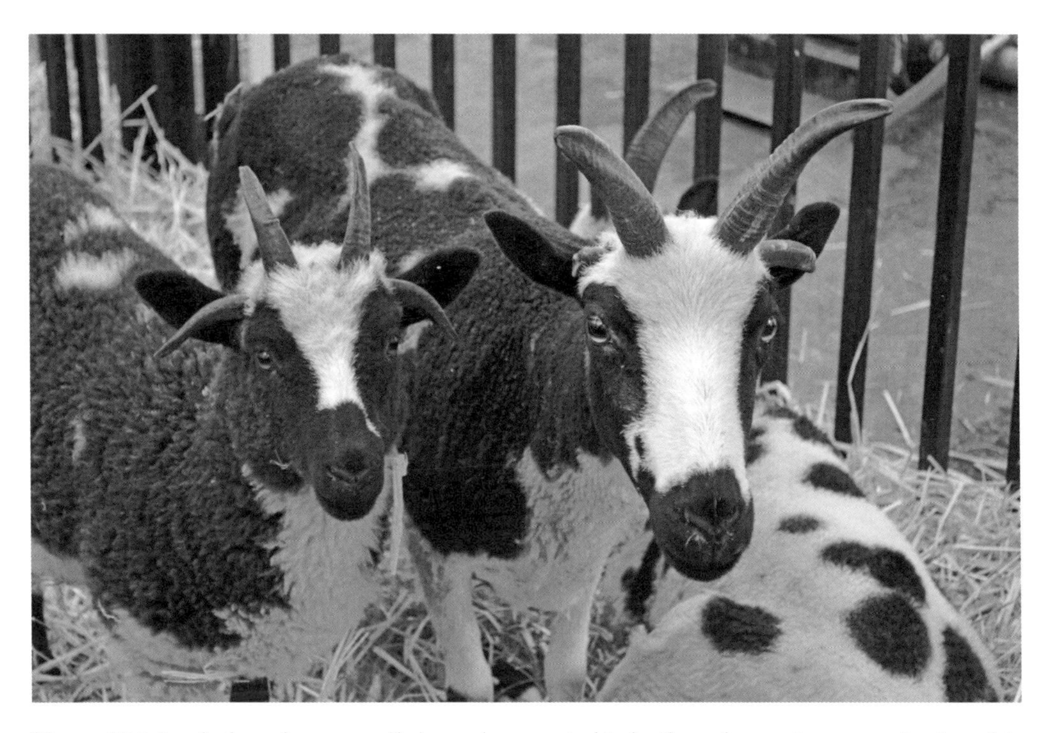

Figure 12.6 Jacob sheep have recently been documented to be the only spontaneous animal model for the devastating human Tay-Sachs disease. This metabolic defect is genetic, but its effects are not present at birth. Photo by JB.

The situation in most other breeds is opposite that of dairy cattle breeds because breeders generally have a direct economic stake in the reputation of the sires involved in producing defective offspring. Silence is a more likely response than full disclosure of faults. No strategy can completely eliminate this incentive, but a few tactics can help reduce it. One useful option is to make reporting anonymous and avoid a link with pedigree information. The benefit of this is that the association can then keep tabs on the overall incidence rates of various defects. If a specific defect begins to increase, then steps can be taken to educate breeders, investigate the cause of the defect, and potentially develop or employ a test for carriers if the defect is proven genetic.

Levelheaded and fair policies toward genetic defects are tough to formulate, but are essential if success is to be achieved in discovering defects and reducing their rate of occurrence. Fairly strict measures are appropriate for populous breeds. These might include elimination of all carriers, or requiring that males be certified free of a given defect that might be common in the breed. For rare breeds, this approach can be problematic, because the elimination of breeding stock takes away the entire genome of carriers and not just the one offending gene. The approach of testing and then rapidly culling to remove a defect has proven paradoxically detrimental in many breeds due to the subsequent loss of genetic diversity.

For traits such as *junctional epidermolysis bullosa*, a lethal skin defect of Belgian and American Cream horses, it becomes a little more difficult to make simple decisions

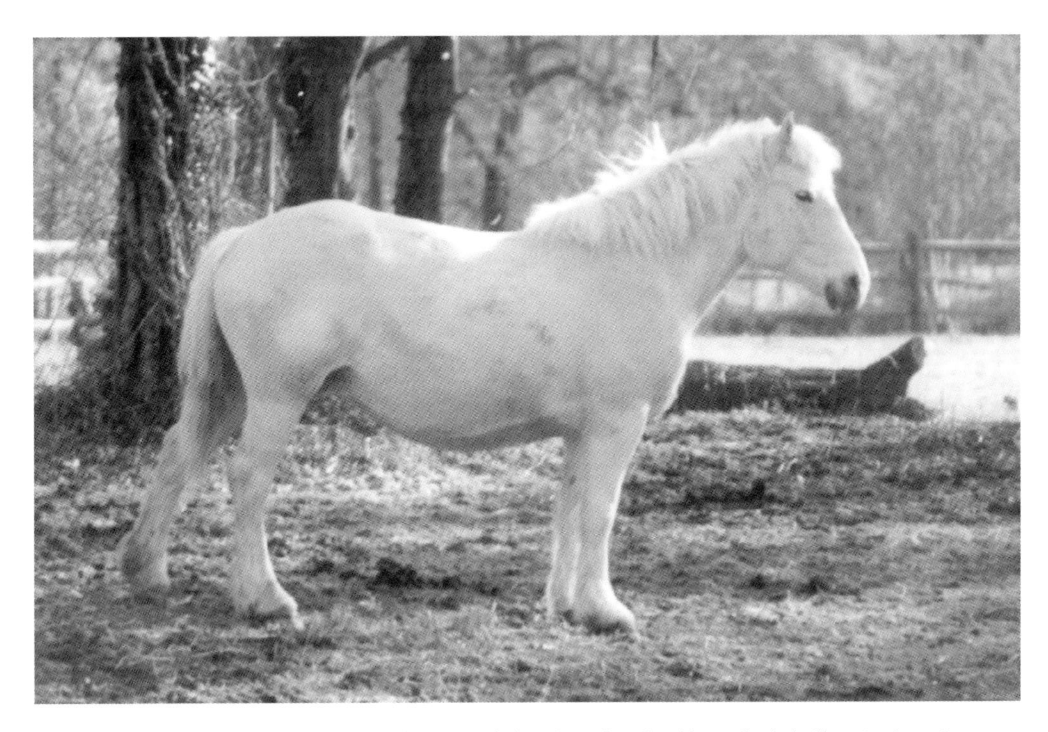

Figure 12.7 Managing the congenital genetic defect *junctional epidermolysis bullosa* in American Creams requires testing to assure that carriers are not mated together. Photo by DPS.

(Figure 12.7). This defect is recessive, and is lethal to foals. Carriers can be identified by a DNA test. If all carriers are eliminated from reproduction, a rare breed such as the American Cream moves ever closer to extinction through the loss of breeding animals and genetic variability. An alternative strategy is to insist that all stallions be tested, and the results be made public. Carrier stallions can (and should) be mated to non-carrier mares to produce replacements, with the eventual goal of generating sons that are not carriers so that the bloodlines are not lost but the offending single gene is. This can take several generations to accomplish, but breeders should all be encouraged to move toward that goal while preserving the genetic integrity of the breed by not discarding carriers too hastily.

Discovering which defects are present in rare breeds can be a great challenge. Most published accounts of genetic defects appear in veterinary or genetics journals, which have historically not been widely available to the general public because their cost prohibited all but large university and research libraries from subscribing. The present situation with open-source publishing has fortunately made information much more widely available. One drawback that remains is that once a defect is described in any one breed it is unlikely to appear again in publications because reports that only document the occurrence in an additional breed are unlikely to be accepted for publication. This phenomenon results in the literature tending to underreport the breed incidences of defects. The best strategy to circumvent this problem is for breed associations to be forward-looking and to carefully document information on the various genetic and other defects that have been found in the breed, and then make that information widely available.

12.2 DNA Analysis

DNA studies can be based on a wide range of techniques: microsatellites, single nucleotide polymorphisms (SNPs), whole genome sequencing, mitochondrial DNA analysis (maternal), or Y chromosomal DNA analysis (paternal). Each of these techniques yields slightly different information, but by combining them it is possible to gain a detailed and accurate snapshot of a population's genetic structure and its relationships with other populations. The portions of a pedigree that are probed by these techniques are illustrated in Figure 12.8. Most of the DNA techniques provide an assessment of the current genetic situation within a breed, but they unfortunately can have limited utility in planning out specific future directions for a breed's genetic management unless they are linked to a detailed census or herd book analysis. The various approaches are different, and they achieve maximum benefit when used together.

Each of these DNA techniques has value, and each has strengths that the others do not. The history of development of these genetic technologies can be considered to have started with blood typing techniques, which are based on protein polymorphisms rather than DNA. One advantage of blood typing technology was the presence of breed-specific "private" variants that could quickly and accurately detect past influences from foundation

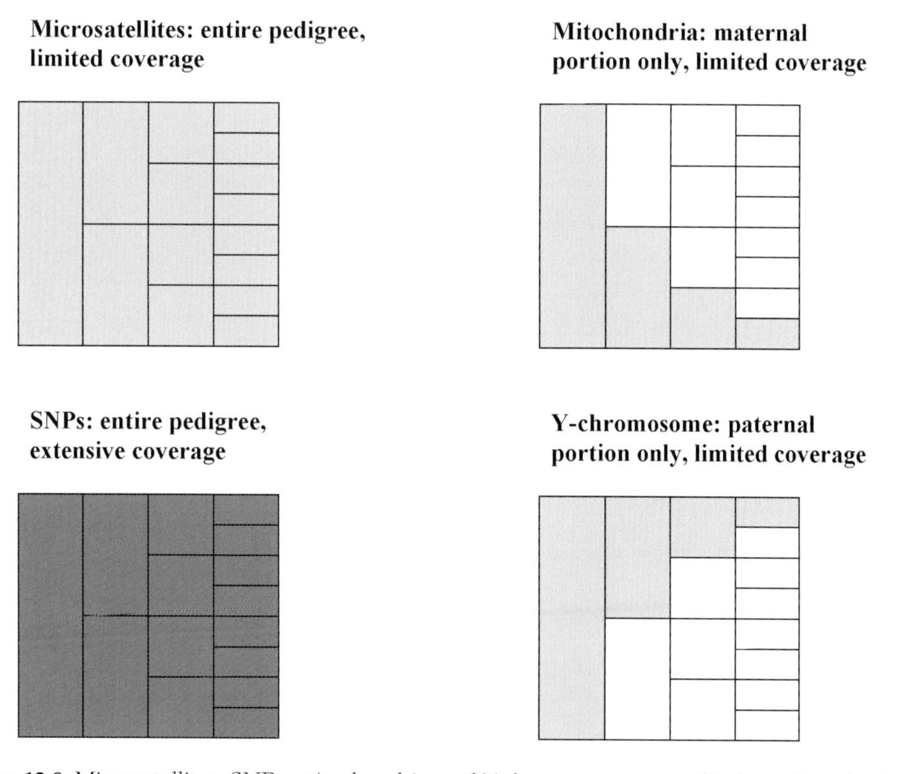

Figure 12.8 Microsatellites, SNPs, mitochondria, and Y chromosomes reveal information about different parts of the pedigree. The specific technique used depends on the information that is being sought. Figure by DPS.

animals or from introgression events. Techniques based on DNA polymorphisms were developed after blood typing. These started with microsatellites, moved to SNPs, and finally now include whole-genome sequencing. Each step along the way brings more information and more data, but at each step it is also true that unique pieces of information from previous techniques tend to be lost and unavailable. Some of those were especially useful in managing breeds as genetic resources because they included breed-specific variants that the later techniques could not detect.

Regardless of the technique used, the specific animals included in the tested sample of the breed population have a huge influence on the results. Unfortunately, targeted and wise sampling is all too rare. This is usually due to poor planning or inadequate care in the selection of the specific animals to include. Ideal sampling of a breed needs to include a complete and representative cross-section of the breed's bloodlines, including sampling of animals from each available bloodline and especially those animals that are least related. Bias in sample selection can skew results if rare bloodlines fail to make it into the analysis. It is equally true that inclusion of bloodlines with introgression from other breeds can easily skew results and conclusions. Careful sample selection is therefore an essential detail for accuracy of interpretation and should ideally involve people with detailed knowledge of the population structure of the breed. These are most likely to be long-time breeders, but other experts should also usually be included.

A more common and unfortunate approach is the use of a "convenience" sample based entirely on samples from those animals that are easiest to access. Another common approach is random selection, but this also has the disadvantage of tending to exclude animals from lineages that are rare in the breed. Both of these approaches assume that genetic variants are evenly distributed throughout the breed, and are therefore unlikely to detect variants that occur only in some herds and not in others whether due to founder effects, selection, or genetic drift. Rare bloodlines are most likely to be sources of genetic variation that might be needed for long-term breed viability, and therefore it is wise to include them by especially targeting their sampling.

Incomplete sampling is very common in genetic studies. Despite this, the conclusions of most studies assume that either random or complete sampling has occurred and that these have comprehensively sampled the entire breed and its genetic variability. Interpretations tend to assume broad and complete sampling when in fact sampling is likely to have been restricted to only common bloodlines or easily accessible animals. It is always more powerful to have a sampling strategy that encompasses the entire genetic variability of a breed. This is best accomplished by paying close attention to bloodlines, geographic origins, and distributions of animals. In the case of numerically small breeds, every effort should be made to include all animals because such an approach very neatly gets around the problem of inadequate sampling.

12.2.1 DNA: Microsatellites

Microsatellites are repetitive strings of genetic information that are scattered throughout genomes. They do not actually code for proteins but are based on repeated sequences of a few of the base pairs of DNA. Microsatellites are sometimes called "tandem repeats" reflecting their character of repetitive short elements. They are assumed to not be the target

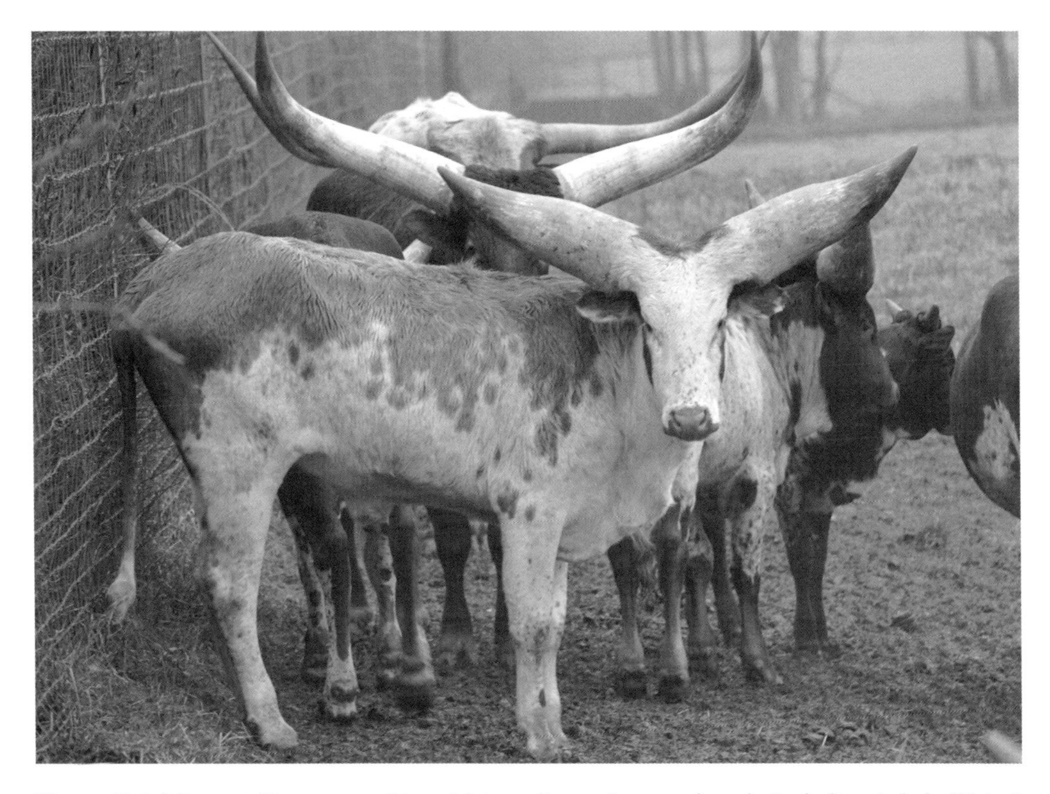

Figure 12.9 Microsatellites are used to validate pedigrees in many breeds, including Ankole-Watusi cattle. Photo by JB.

of any selective pressure that would affect the frequency of protein-coding genes. Instead, they pass from generation to generation as somewhat passive passengers within the DNA. The result is that microsatellite DNA reflects population genetic processes such as foundation, inbreeding, and genetic drift. Microsatellite evaluation is widely used in many breeds for validation of parentage before animal registration (Figure 12.9).

The specific DNA sequence that is repeated varies from microsatellite locus to microsatellite locus. One example of a microsatellite is GA, GA, GA. A second is GTACGT, GTACGT, GTACGT. The different alleles, or length variants, within the locus refer to the number of repeats, so that $[GA]_{98}$ is allele 98, and has 98 consecutive repeats of GA. In contrast, $[GA]_{103}$ is allele 103 for this locus, with 103 repeats of the GA sequence. Similarly, $[GTACGT]_{50}$ is allele 50 for this microsatellite, while $[GTACGT]_{64}$ is allele 64.

The number of repeats of an allele is fairly stable, but not invariably so. A new allele forms when the number of repeats increases or decreases. This happens frequently enough that in large data sets the appearance of a new allele can be expected rather than surprising. This is important because such an occurrence does not necessarily mean that outside genetic material has been introduced into the population. Instead, a new variant reflects the relatively low but inherent instability of microsatellite systems. In fact, microsatellites are useful genetic markers because the alleles do vary because of a tendency for a rate of mutational change that alters the numbers of repeats. In that sense, the very utility of

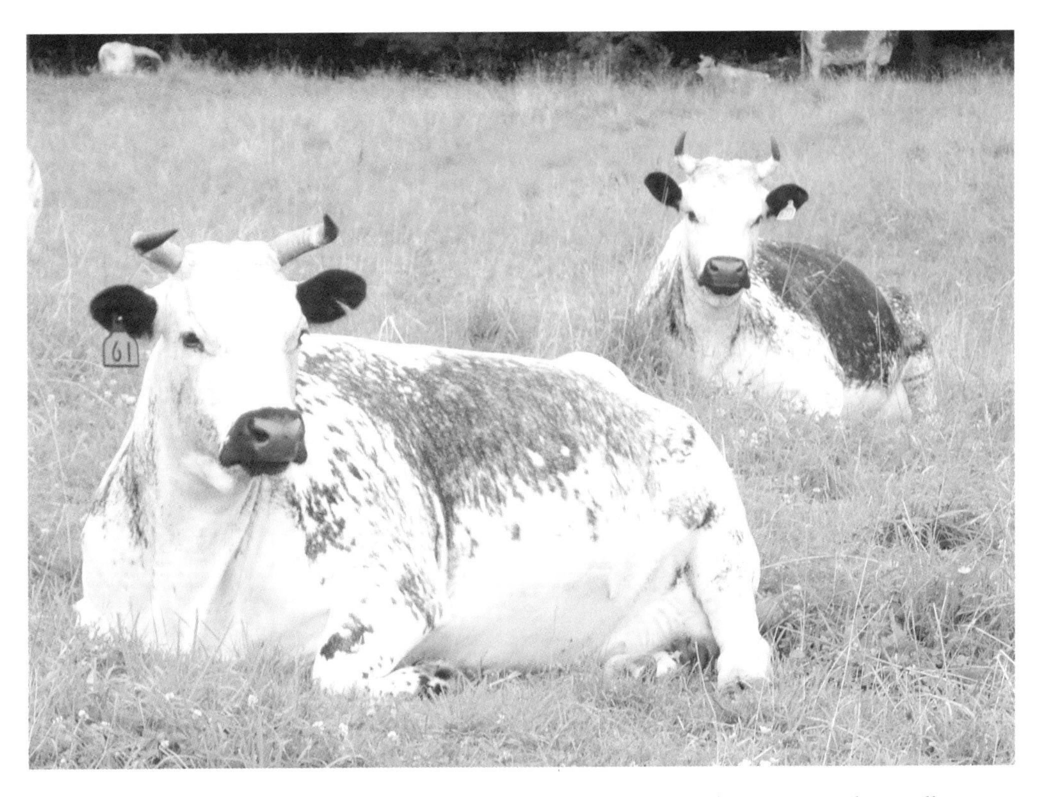

Figure 12.10 Blood typing technology and SNP analysis were key to documenting the small foundation and unique genetic status of Randall Lineback cattle. Photo by DPS.

microsatellites in genetic studies is based on ongoing low levels of mutational change. This generates new allelic variation and, while not routine, it does occur frequently enough that it becomes an important consideration during data analyses. Not every new allele in a population is evidence of crossbreeding, and this is an important detail.

Microsatellites occur frequently on all chromosomes, and specific sets of these variable markers have been designated for study within each livestock species. These sets have been carefully chosen to assure broad coverage of the genome. The sets are standardized internationally so that findings in one breed or one investigation can be easily compared to those in others. Studies based on DNA microsatellites have long been common techniques for breed genetic analysis in the peer-reviewed literature. This is currently changing as newer single nucleotide polymorphism (SNP) technology becomes less expensive. It is likely that SNP technology will be replaced by genome-wide sequencing at some point. The technology of DNA analysis is still emerging and becoming more and more detailed. It remains true, though, that genetic studies based on earlier techniques, including older blood typing analyses, remain valid and very useful even if some of the older techniques are no longer available to investigators (Figure 12.10).

The results of microsatellite DNA analysis are most usefully used as a snapshot of the genetic composition of the breed at the time of sampling. This includes the identity and frequency of each distinct microsatellite variant at each of the loci tested. The results can be used to evaluate a host of genetic measures of variation. They can also be used to compare the breed of interest to other breeds, or to compare subpopulations within the breed. These comparisons can involve several different analyses.

One potential use of microsatellites is to create a profile of variants acceptable within the breed. This is especially tempting in the case of landraces because it can be an important and effective strategy in assuring the relative purity of the genetic resource when used as a tool to screen candidates for inclusion. However, this is only a valid strategy if it is based on a broad and complete initial sample because it is essential to capture and validate all of the diversity within the breed for profiles that will be used for this purpose. Especially in landraces, isolated subpopulations or herds are likely to have unique variants due to founder effect or genetic drift. These can easily be excluded from future consideration if left out of the initial sampling. The danger is that legitimate variation in an isolated pocket of the breed can be inadvertently left out of the initial sample and therefore remains undocumented. Such a profile can then be used to erroneously omit those variants from the ones accepted as typical of the breed. After the initial omission, future breed investigations can all too easily reject animals with those variants, even though their exclusion was based on insufficiently broad sampling at the outset.

The utility of microsatellites for the determination of inclusion or exclusion in a breed varies with the sort of breed involved, and with the breed's history. Breeds with a small foundation and strict isolation, such as Randall Lineback cattle, San Clemente goats, and Arapawa Island goats, are very likely to be successfully analyzed and managed with microsatellite profiles. Breeds with broader foundations are unlikely to be as successfully characterized. Likewise, populations with weak levels of isolation are unlikely to ever develop the limited variation that allows microsatellites to serve as an effective tool for inclusion or exclusion of animals into the breed. Also challenging are breeds, such as the Spanish goat, that are still in relatively early stages of discovery. Such breeds are unlikely to have a complete catalog of microsatellite variants because new ones can be expected from each new purebred herd that is encountered.

One analysis that is often based on microsatellite data is accomplished using a computer program called STRUCTURE. This analysis is helpful in ferreting out details of foundation influences and breed relationships and relies on the accurate identification of animals and assignment to various populations (breed or bloodline). The structure technique is used to validate the genetics behind a designated subdivision. It works less well to impose subdivisions onto an otherwise undesignated population. In other words, this analysis validates classifications such as bloodlines or breeds that are suspected on the basis of origin or type but is less effective at pulling these out of what is assumed to be a uniform mixture.

Structure analysis can help guide conservation decisions. One study involving hundreds of cattle breeds from around the world was specifically designed to investigate relationships within Criollo cattle from the Americas (Figure 12.11). In one of the iterations, seven foundation influences were assumed to account for all cattle variation. That is, seven distinct origins for cattle: Spain, Portugal, Northern Europe, Africa, Asia, Britain, and Criollo. The result of this analysis revealed that several of the Criollo breeds from the Americas did indeed have a strong representation of the Criollo root, which was surprisingly rare and nearly extinct in Europe despite the historic European origin of the Criollos. This result

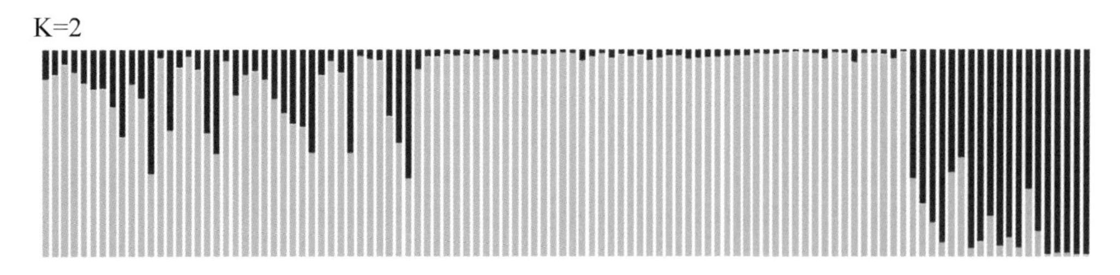

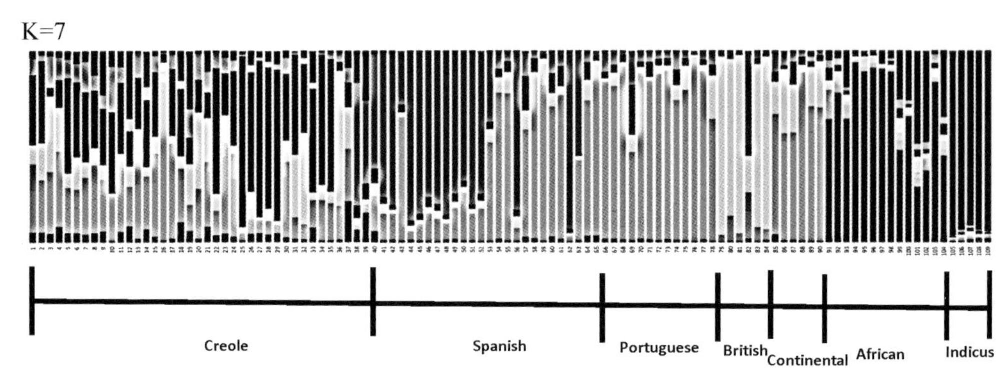

Figure 12.11 Structure diagrams are complicated, but reveal a lot of information. These two diagrams are from a study of microsatellites from 109 breeds of cattle from various regions. Each vertical bar is one breed, split by geographic origin: Criollo (from the Americas), Spanish, Portuguese, Continental European, British, African, and *Bos indicus* zebu breeds from South Asia. The bars are arranged consistently from top to bottom: black (zebu), dark grey (Spanish), black (Criollo), white (British), medium grey (Portuguese), light medium grey (Continental), and dark grey (African). At the level of K=2, the breeds are assumed to have only two origins. The breeds neatly reflect genetic influences represented by a dark grey bar from India and Africa, and a light grey bar from Europe. K=7 assumes seven different origins. The grey shades do not fully convey the complexity, but the general idea still comes through. The zebu in this case is black and at the top of the bars. This influence shows up in Indian-derived breeds, as well as in a few breeds in the Americas that are known to have this influence. The darkest grey influence designates an African origin largely limited to African breeds, and persisting in the Americas through influences from the Azores and Canary Islands. Continental European influences are medium-light grey and persist in Spanish breeds from northern Spain. Portuguese influences are medium grey, and are limited to Portuguese breeds, a few Spanish breeds, and several Criollo breeds. Spanish influences are a darker grey, and are strongest in breeds from Southern Spain. The black segment, toward the middle of the bars, is the influence from the Criollo origin. This influence is only common in the Americas, persisting as a minor influence in a few breeds from Spain and Portugal. This reflects the importance of conserving these Criollo breeds. Through some accident of history they have retained a genetic influence that is now nearly extinct in Europe. Source: Ginja, C., Gama, L.T., Cortés, O. et al. (2019) The genetic ancestry of American Creole cattle inferred from uniparental and autosomal genetic markers. https://www.nature.com/articles/s41598-019-47636-0 (Date accessed 12/12/2020).

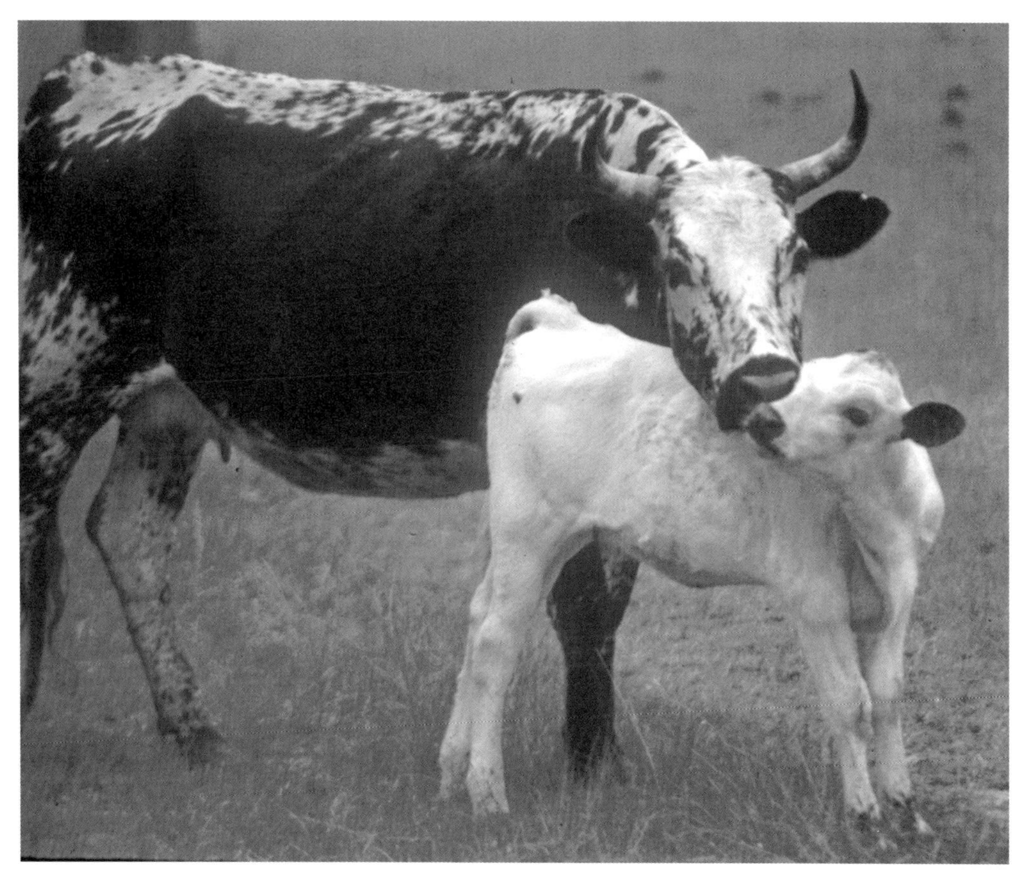

Figure 12.12 Pineywoods cattle have a small contribution of the unique Criollo foundation, but still lack heavy influence of British or zebu breeds that are otherwise common in the region.
Photo by DPS.

helps drive conservation because it alerts scientists and breeders to the importance of this group of breeds for their unique genetic variation that is missing from breeds that hail from all other parts of the world.

Structure analysis can yield subtle results that warrant careful interpretation. In the example of the study outlined in Figure 12.11 the Texas Longhorn (bar 1) and Florida Cracker cattle (bar 2) show very strong origins within the Criollo group. Surprisingly, Pineywoods cattle do not (bar 3) (Figure 12.12). This result raises the question of whether Pineywoods are indeed a true genetic breed or instead a composite of variable influences. Fortunately, an analysis that set the number of foundation populations to 41 instead of 7 indicated that most Pineywoods cattle share a common origin, so they are indeed a distinct breed, just one with a fairly weak Criollo root. Other influences, including Continental and Spanish, are important to the Pineywoods, along with a minority influence from British breeds consistent with the history of the breed. These results, along with history and geography, help to establish the Pineywoods breed as an important conservation priority, despite their being peripheral to the other Criollo breeds.

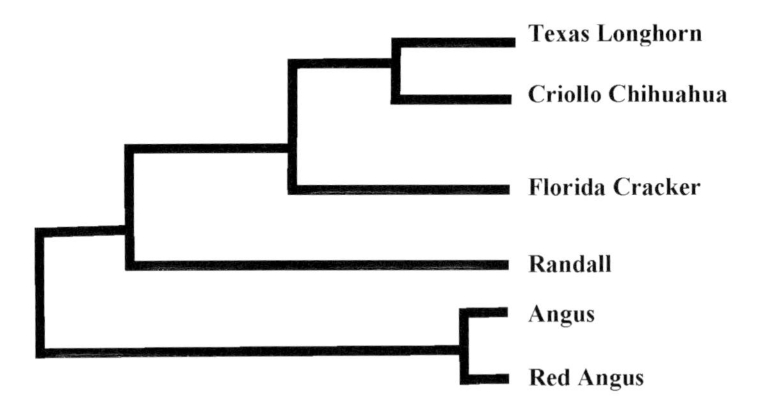

Figure 12.13 Dendrograms are a branching tree that captures the sequential separation of breeds by time and genetic distance. Branches that are longer, and further to the left, occurred earlier than shorter branches to the right. Greater genetic distance between breeds is separated by longer lines. Figure by DPS.

Dendrograms and other distance plots can be derived from microsatellite data. These help to illustrate breed relationships. The results, as always, depend on the original sample selection, so deliberate and broad sampling is always best. This sort of analysis shows how the various breeds branch off over time. For example, zebu cattle branch off early from humpless European cattle, while Angus and Red Angus branch from one another only recently (Figure 12.13).

Microsatellite data analysis can include several aspects. Each yields different information about the sample and the population. These same measures are used for some of the other DNA techniques. These are generated by software packages that can analyze the data collected from the microsatellite genotyping technique. Each of these measures reveals specific information about the population.

- Number of animals typed (N). Sample size is just a straightforward total of the number of animals studied. Larger and more broadly selected samples are the most likely to accurately represent the whole breed. Smaller samples can skew results due to statistical phenomena.
- Observed heterozygosity (H_o). This is a measure of the number of heterozygous loci within the animals that were studied. Values range from 0 (no heterozygous loci) to 1 (all loci are heterozygous). H_o is an indicator of loss of diversity. Populations with low diversity are less heterozygous and have a lower H_o than those with greater diversity. Observed heterozygosity can also indicate levels of inbreeding, especially when compared to expectations of the Hardy-Weinberg equilibrium that would arise from random mating. When homozygotes are overrepresented compared to Hardy-Weinberg statistics, inbreeding is present in different isolated pockets of the breed.
- Expected heterozygosity (H_e). This measure is slightly different than observed heterozygosity. It is the theoretical expectation of levels of heterozygosity based on the allelic diversity and frequency of alleles at the various loci. Values range from

0 (no heterozygous loci) to 1 (all loci are heterozygous). A high figure indicates high levels of genetic diversity. Comparisons of this more theoretical statistic with observed heterozygosity are important. An H_o that is lower than H_e signals that inbreeding is occurring in the breed, whether only in portions of it or across the whole breed. This situation does not necessarily reflect a reduction in overall genetic diversity, but does indicate that it is packaged differently than would be true with a more even mixing within the breed. H_o is rarely higher than H_e, but this can indicate sampling error or fairly deliberate outbreeding. A notably high H_o coupled with a low H_e is also rare, and often indicates genetic introgression from other breeds.

- Within-breed inbreeding coefficient (F_{is}). This is calculated as 1 (H_o/H_e). Positive values indicate inbreeding, zero or negative values indicate no inbreeding.
- Effective number of alleles (A_e). This is the number of alleles of equal frequency (0.5 and 0.5) that it would take to generate the expected heterozygosity that is computed for the breed. This is a theoretical number that makes comparisons meaningful across different breeds with different sample sizes.
- Number of alleles (N_a). This is the total number of microsatellite variants found across all loci that were tested in the population. This is the actual number, rather than the more theoretical figure of the "effective number."
- Mean number of alleles (*MNA*). This is the average number of alleles across all the loci tested. This reflects the overall genetic diversity within the population. Higher numbers indicate greater diversity, lower numbers indicate less diversity. This figure often reflects the history of the breed. Numerically small breeds with a single foundation source characteristically have a relatively low *MNA*, while those that descend from several different bloodlines tend to have a higher *MNA*.
- Rare alleles (*RARE*). Rare alleles are identified in some microsatellite panels. These are the alleles that occur at a frequency of 0.05 (5%) or less, and are most likely to be lost due to genetic drift. Animals with such alleles need special monitoring to assure that their rare variants are not lost.

12.2.2 DNA: Single Nucleotide Polymorphisms (SNPs)

A newer technology that evaluates single nucleotide polymorphisms is currently eclipsing the studies based on microsatellites. This technique directly measures changes in the specific DNA nucleotide at specific locations in the genome. The information from SNP studies depends somewhat on the size of the chip used (the actual number of SNP loci). All of the different levels that come from the different size chips usually result in a robust level of detail. While microsatellite studies might include up to 20 or 30 loci, SNP analysis routinely includes thousands or tens of thousands of loci. SNP studies generally yield much more detail than microsatellite studies, although the two are not interchangeable and each have unique strengths. Currently the cost of analyzing SNPs is rapidly decreasing, and this technology is consequently seeing ever-increasing levels of use. SNPs involve a heftier chunk of the genome than is possible for microsatellite studies, and as a result they can be useful in selecting breeding animals for genetic diversity. The specific genetic loci are at least somewhat less well documented than those used in microsatellite analysis, so the assumption that the loci are neutral to selection pressure does not hold true across

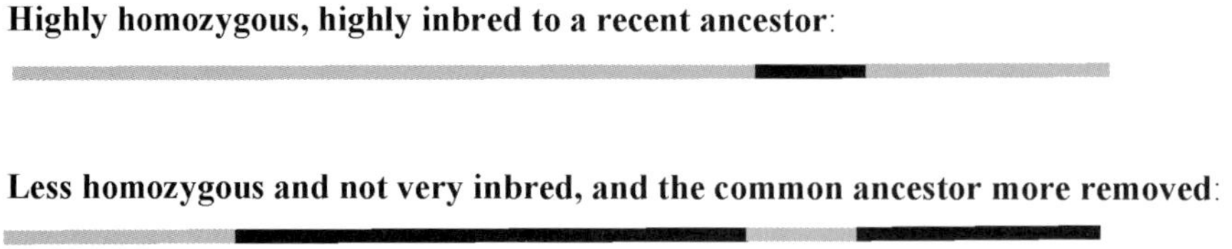

Highly homozygous, highly inbred to a recent ancestor:

Less homozygous and not very inbred, and the common ancestor more removed:

Figure 12.14 SNP runs of homozygosity indicate which portions of a pair of chromosomes have identical genetic information. These areas are longer and more frequent in animals that are inbred back to a recent ancestor. The grey lengths are the portions of homologous chromosomes that are homozygous. Figure by DPS.

all of them because some are related to genes subject to selection for production or other traits.

In addition to the sorts of analyses that are similar to those outlined above for microsatellites, it is possible to evaluate "runs of homozygosity (ROH)" in the SNP data because the loci are keyed to specific locations on specific chromosomes. The consequence of inbreeding is homozygosity, so ROH can be used as a direct measure of actual levels of inbreeding. This contrasts with the more theoretical levels that are computed from pedigree data. The result of ROH analysis from SNPs is an accurate and useful glimpse into levels of inbreeding. They are also the most accurate data for managing rare, as well as overrepresented, genetics of any breed. In addition, the ROH analysis can yield insights into the time frame of inbreeding. Recent inbreeding results in longer ROH, while inbreeding further back in the ancestry has the result of shorter ROH due to the recombination within chromosomes that occurs with each generation (Figure 12.14). The ROH analysis does not require accurate pedigree information because it directly measures the consequences of inbreeding in the genome. In many situations this is a very real strength that overcomes the significant hurdles that arise when evaluating populations with poor pedigree documentation.

More recent advances in SNP analysis can provide data for breed relationship analyses. Such analyses are still being developed. They require high levels of sampling and data in order to fully replace the relatively robust data sets available with microsatellites. The power of these studies varies a great deal depending on the species involved because the history of breed formation varies so much in the different species. While breed formation in all species depends on founders, isolation, and selection, the relative role of each of these differs species to species. This affects the interrelationships of breeds.

12.2.3 DNA: Mitochondria

Studies based on DNA from mitochondria are limited to only the maternal side of inheritance because mitochondria are only passed along from dam to offspring and not from sire to offspring. Over several generations this equates to "tail female" portions of the pedigree. These studies have limited power as a snapshot of the present state of the breed but can reveal a great deal about foundation events. It is easy to overinterpret these, although when used appropriately they are very powerful.

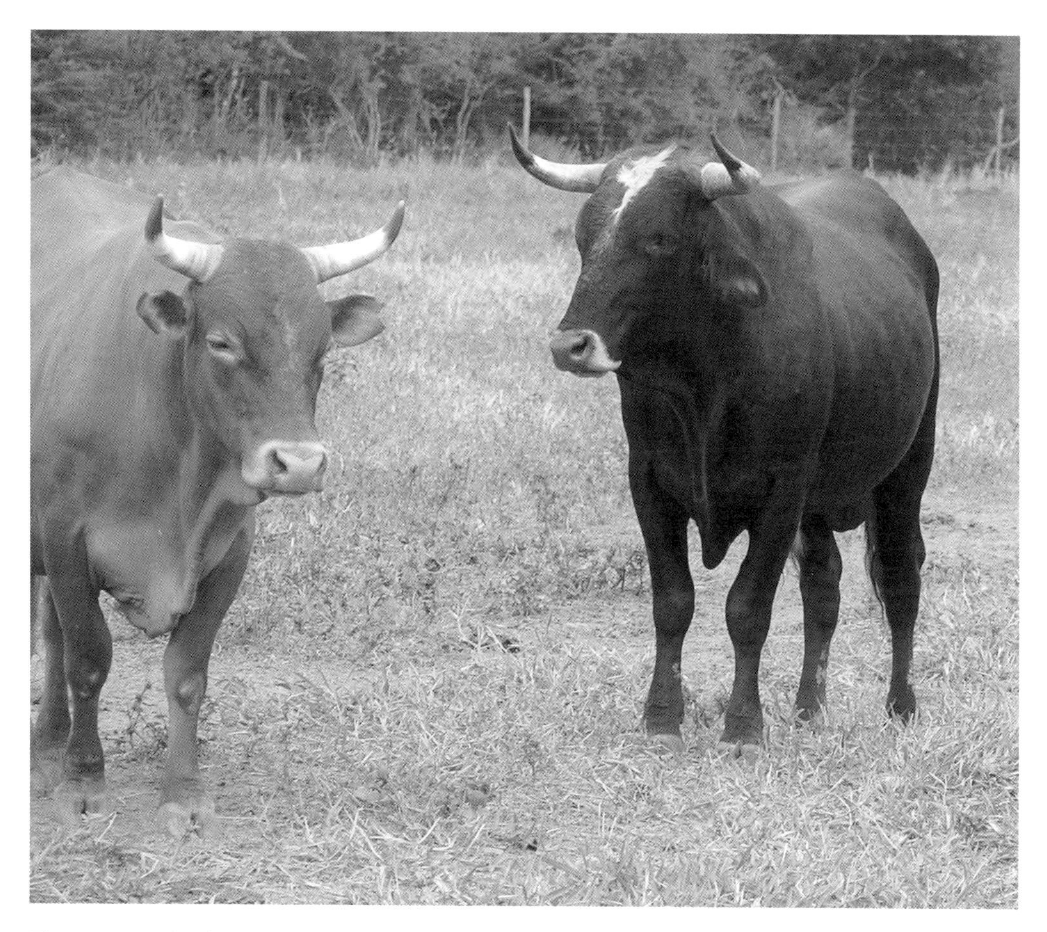

Figure 12.15 Studies of Y chromosomes have been especially useful in analyzing Criollo breeds such as the Criollo Yacumeño. Photo by DPS.

12.2.4 DNA: Y Chromosomes

The results based on DNA variation in Y chromosomes mirror that of the mitochondrial studies but instead produce information about the "tail male" portion of the pedigree. In mammals, the Y chromosome is passed along from sire to sons and never to daughters. This information can be useful for sorting out foundation events and introgression events. For example, in cattle the types of Y chromosomes split out into Northern European, Southern European, African, or South Asian groups. Tracking these chromosomes through different breeds can demonstrate the influence of bulls from these regions into cattle populations such as the Criollo breeds of the Americas or the zebu and sanga breeds of Africa (Figure 12.15).

12.2.5 Other Uses of DNA Technology

One common application of DNA testing is for validation of parentage. Many registries, especially for cattle, horses, and alpacas, require the validation of sire and dam for every animal registered. This serves as a useful check on pedigree accuracy, but it is helpful to

Table 12.1 Each horse has different variants, up to two per locus. The variants each have a standard abbreviation. Foals must get one of each pair of variants from its sire, and one of each pair from its dam. If the foal's variants do not match up to the parents, then either the sire or dam is eliminated as a candidate in the pedigree. In this example, two different loci do not match for foal three, which effectively rules out mutation as a cause. The dam, in this case, has been eliminated as a parent of foal three, because that foal has two loci that lack her variants.

	Locus 1	Locus 2	Locus 3	Locus 4	Locus 5	Locus 6	Locus 7
Sire	AA	BC	DD	EF	GG	HI	JJ
Dam	KL	MM	NO	PP	QR	SS	TU
Foal 1	AK	BM	DN	EP	GQ	IS	JT
Foal 2	AL	CM	DO	FP	GR	IS	JU
Foal 3 *(dam does not match)*	AK	BM	DW	FP	GQ	IV	JT

keep in mind that not all errors are due to fraud. A certain percentage of the errors creep in from non-fraudulent mistakes in record keeping.

Parentage testing relies on either microsatellites or SNPs. The key to either one is that each animal can have only up to two variants per locus, one from the sire and one from the dam. Every offspring must only have variants that are present in the parents. In the case of both microsatellites and SNPs, this works well most of the time. It is important to remember that these genetic systems are variable and serve as useful markers because they are subject to a low level of mutation. While rare, a new variant does occasionally appear in the offspring that is not present in the parents. Table 12.1 is a brief explanation of how the theory plays out in practice. With an adequate number of loci sampled, such rare variants do not preclude successful parentage assignment.

A view of parentage testing can be expanded to include evaluation across breeds, usually with the hope of discovering the breed (or breeds) from which a candidate animal descends. This approach summarizes the variants at different loci that occur in a specific breed. One method is to simply include all variants, with candidate animals then being compared against this list for either inclusion or exclusion. That approach fails to work for populous breeds in many species, because most breeds have a wide array of variants at each locus. When this is the case, it is still possible to evaluate candidates by considering not only the variants, but also their frequencies, in different breeds.

This technique for evaluating breed influences is generally accurate. It can also suggest some very spurious inferences. This is especially true when a valid member of a breed just happens to end up with multiple rare variants at different loci. Some species, such as horses, are also noteworthy for being highly variable and also for the breeds having a relatively recent history of isolation from an originally very diverse population. This can lead to results for candidate horses that are not very congruent with either history or phenotype. A major drawback of this approach is that it does use averages as a sort of expectation. Because horses are so mixed up, the averages can be misleading. Only rarely do breed-specific variants occur, but when they are present, they make this approach much more accurate. Even when they are present, the breed-specific status refers to the presence

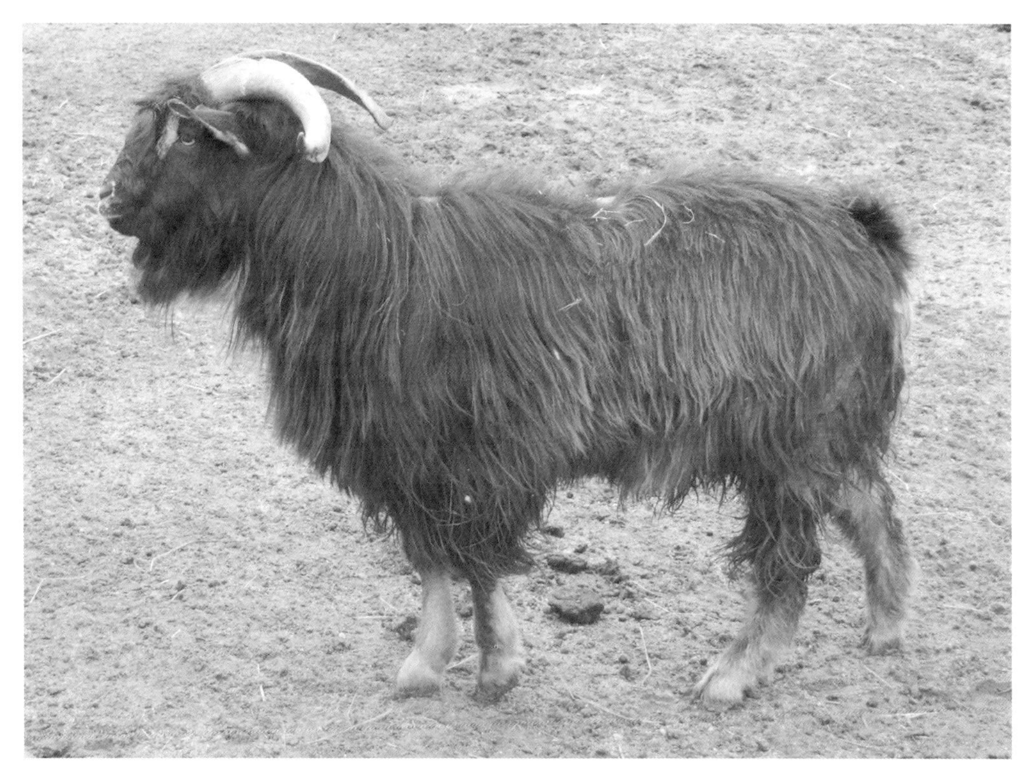

Figure 12.16 Arapawa goats have a low level of genetic variation, so DNA analysis is very accurate at determining whether a goat is indeed an Arapawa or not. Photo by JB.

of that variant in only that breed, but even then, the variants usually only occur in a small minority of the animals of the breed. Despite the many limitations of using these techniques to identify breed of origin, the process can and does succeed when considered across broad populations. However, individual exceptions to the accuracy are relatively common.

The evaluation of candidate animals proceeds more accurately in rare breeds with a small founder population and long isolation. This is due to relatively low levels of genetic variation within most breeds with this history (Figure 12.16). If the original data set is to be used as a major hurdle for inclusion or exclusion of candidate animals, it is essential that it includes as broad a representative sample of the breed as is possible. Especially for landraces with small herds that have long been isolated, it is easily possible for newly discovered herds to have variants that were lacking in the original sample. Discarding those animals solely on the basis of DNA results risks the loss of animals that could greatly contribute to breed survival. The DNA approach is powerful, but must always be included in the context of a complete analysis that also includes history and phenotype.

In dogs, especially mixed-breed dogs, DNA technology is increasingly used to uncover the contributions of different breeds into the final hybridized product. This technique is of limited use in conservation breeding of purebreds, but is commonly sought by many owners of dogs that are not purebred. The technique relies on the breeds having different frequencies of SNPs, and for these to be passed along relatively intact in long stretches on different chromosomes. This works well when the hybrids have recent purebred ancestors but works less well when those purebred ancestors are further back.

12.3 Pedigree-Based Analyses

DNA studies are useful for a glimpse at genetic diversity and can indicate the overall need for directed conservation action. They usually do not indicate which specific actions need to be taken for conservation. However, the results from individual animals can indicate which specific animals can offer the greatest contribution for genetic diversity as well as for trueness to breed origin. For detailed decision-making on conservation strategies, a pedigree-based approach is usually needed alongside the DNA results. Both DNA and pedigree approaches have their strengths and weaknesses, but they are especially powerful when used together. In some situations, the DNA approaches are simply unavailable, and pedigree analysis is all that is possible despite its limitations. Pedigree-based analysis can take different forms.

12.3.1 Pedigree-Based Inbreeding Coefficients

Inbreeding is the mating of related animals and identical ancestors occurring on both the sire's side and the dam's side (Figure 12.17). Inbreeding coefficients reveal the relative degree of inbreeding, and can be fairly easily calculated for individual pedigreed animals. This can be done using a variety of software packages that work with most pedigree databases. The number of generations to be used in the calculation can be set at a specific number. Genetic theory proposes that recent inbreeding is more of a threat to viability than inbreeding that occurs further back in a pedigree. This is due to the possibility of recombination through chromosomal crossover events as the generations proceed. As a result, it might be useful to include both a five-generation and a ten-generation inbreeding coefficient for each animal. These calculations are often, but not always, different from the direct measurement that can be had by the ROH analysis done on SNPs. Pedigree evaluations often yield a higher value of inbreeding than ROH analysis. In that sense, pedigree analysis tends to represent

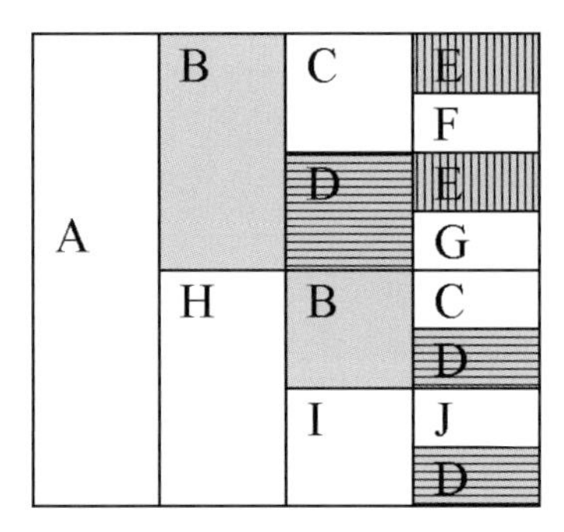

Figure 12.17 Inbreeding is revealed when a single ancestor appears in multiple places on a pedigree on both the sire's and dam's side. Animal A is inbred back to ancestor B as well as independently to ancestor D. While B is inbred to E, through both C and D, A is not, because E only occurs on the sire's side of the pedigree. Figure by DPS.

the "worst case" situation, which turns out to be useful for genetic management even if not always entirely accurate.

Average inbreeding values can be computed for the breed. Alternatively, the entire range of values can be noted. The average value is a useful benchmark, even though it fails to capture whether the inbreeding that occurs in the breed is all back to one specific ancestor, or whether the inbreeding is occurring in different directions within different subpopulations of the breed. In the latter case the high coefficients can be taken back down by crossing between the various lines, while in the former case this is impossible. The range of values is also useful because it helps to target the most inbred individuals as well as the most outbred. Breeding strategies can then be tailored for these animals to achieve decently balanced levels as the generations proceed.

12.3.2 Pedigree-Based Kinship Levels

Kinship is the level of relationship of a specific animal to another specific animal. Put another way, this is a prediction of the level of inbreeding in a theoretical offspring between two animals. Depending on the power of the analysis, this can be expanded to include an average of one individual (potential sire, for example) to a group of potential mates, or even to the entire breed. This analysis is useful in teasing out some of the details that are glossed over in the more generic inbreeding coefficient techniques because it is possible to evaluate relationships back to specific individual animals. In this way the kinship analysis can compensate for weaknesses in a more generic analysis of levels of inbreeding because it considers the specific individuals involved as sources of inbreeding.

It is wise to do two different kinship analyses. One is the kinship of an individual to the rest of the overall breed. The second is to calculate the kinship of an individual to all potential mates, one to one. These two pieces of information are different, and the second analysis is usually lacking because it is time consuming. The first (kinship to entire breed) reveals a general level of relationship. The second, because it is individual, can greatly help in figuring out the lowest and the highest kinships to other specific individuals. If kinship is zero or low in some cases, then outbreeding is possible if mating is carefully planned. If all of the pairwise levels are moderate or high, then different levels of inbreeding are all that is possible for that specific individual animal.

Kinship can also be evaluated by using the ROH technique and comparing homozygous regions of one animal with those of another animal. This is a more accurate analysis than the pedigree-based approach because it directly compares the issue of concern, which is homozygosity arising through relatedness. It is, however, a much more tedious exercise and must be aided by computer technology.

12.3.3 Foundation Bloodline Analysis

The mechanics of an analytical snapshot of a breed vary, especially depending on the relative length of time that registration has occurred for the breed. For relatively recently registered breeds (landraces and local breeds, usually), the analysis can begin by computing the percentage contribution of each founder in each living animal. It is then possible to rank individuals from highest to lowest contribution from an individual founder. This helps to identify individuals with the highest influence and also with the lowest influence. In the

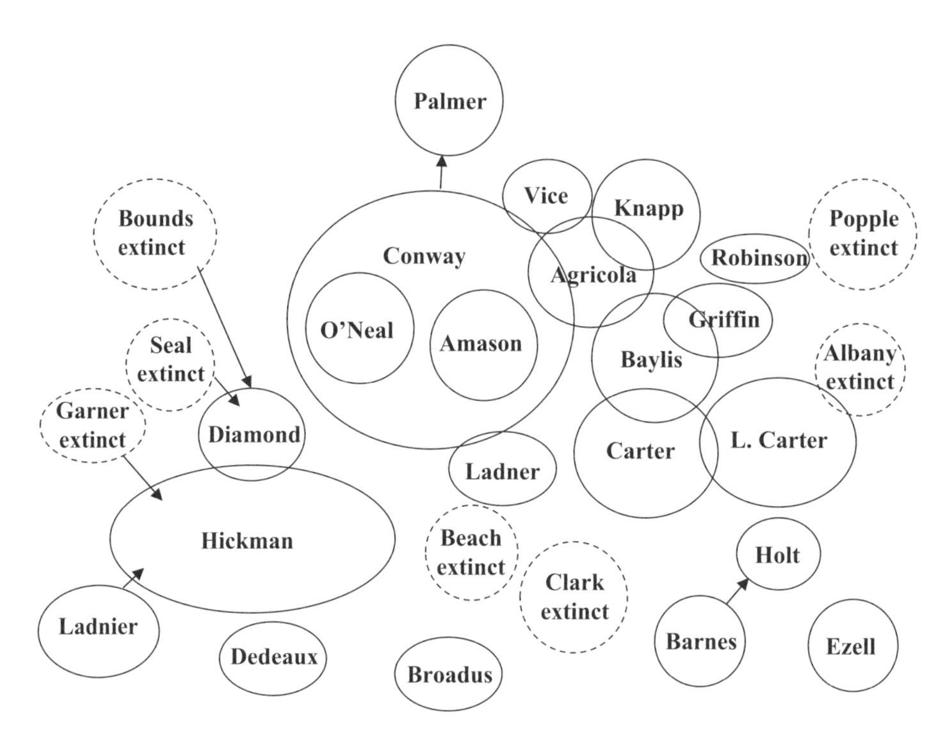

Figure 12.18 Foundation bloodlines in a breed can be complicated and intricate. These are the foundation bloodlines of the Pineywoods cattle breed. Some stand alone with minimal outside influences (Dedeaux, Broadus, Barnes). Others form groups with mutual contact and overlap (for example, Baylis, Griffin, Carter, and Luther Carter). Some, like Conway, have influenced several. Others, like Diamond, have influences from several extinct lines. Figure by DPS.

case of founders that are generally underrepresented, this helps to target those animals most capable of balancing the contributions of those founders. Alternatively, in the case of overrepresented (bottleneck) founders, the analysis can demonstrate which animals are lowest in contribution and identify candidates for balancing out founder contributions that might swamp the genetics of the breed.

Analysis of founder contribution can be derived using a database approach. The efficacy of this approach varies breed to breed. In breeds with a small number of founders (20 or fewer), this analysis can be based on each individual founder animal. Most breeds will have more than 20 founders, and in these cases a more realistic strategy is to group the founders into founding bloodlines by some logical system. This grouping is usually done on the basis of farm of origin or breeder of origin, or in some cases geographic origin or time of contribution. For this strategy to succeed, each founder is designated into a bloodline. Details of one approach to doing this are outlined in Appendix 2.

A few examples might illustrate how this works. In the Randall Lineback cattle breed, all cattle descend from 12 original founders. For this breed it is easily possible to track the contributions of each founder down through the generations. In Pineywoods cattle the number of founders is too high for that approach, but the founders all come from old established and isolated family herds (Figure 12.18). In this case, all founder cattle (those

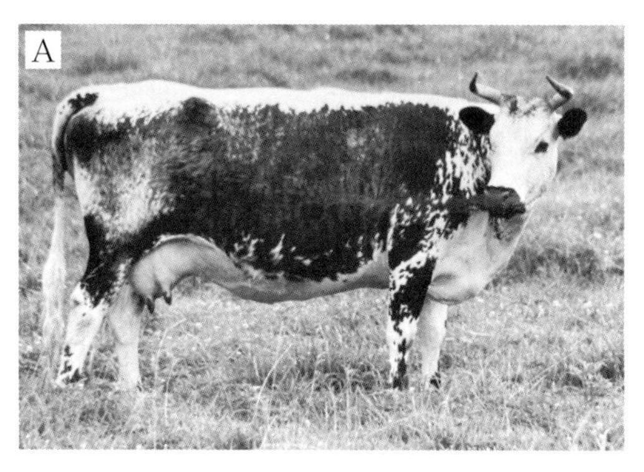

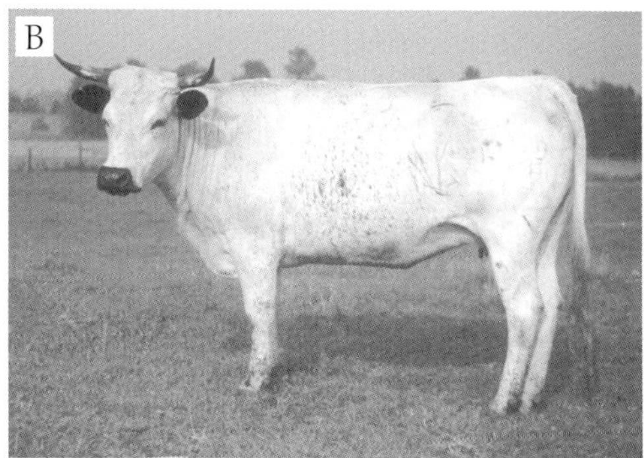

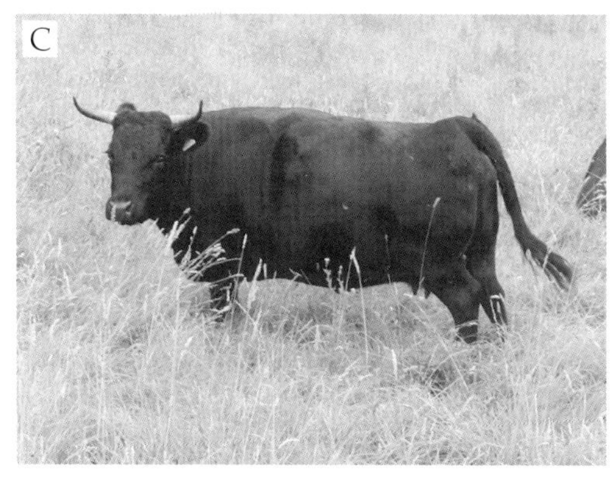

Figure 12.19 Foundation bloodlines, or individual founders, can be essential in managing the genetics of many rare breeds. The significance and interaction of these varies breed to breed, so that strategies that might work well for Randall Lineback cattle (A) are a poor match for Pineywoods (B), which are an equally poor match for Dexters (C). Photos by DPS.

without registered sire and dam) from Bura Conway's herds are designated as "100% Conway bloodline," and similarly for other traditional family herds. These influences can then be tracked through the generations.

Dexter cattle in the USA present yet another situation (Figure 12.19). The original cattle that founded the breed in the USA came from three origins: Irish, English, or untraced American. These can each stand as founding strains, to which are added several others: English imports after 1920, the Woodmagic herd in England, grades, Colorado from a herd with lapsed pedigrees, specific influences from three different imported bulls, and a rare "other" category. This approach yields a total of 11 threads to follow through the generations, each of which is distinct enough to help in the genetic management of the breed and to guide breeders as they make informed decisions in keeping with their own breeding philosophy. The assignment of foundation influences must be individually tailored to the needs of the breed under consideration.

12.3.4 *Popular (or Rare) Sires (or Dams)*

Evaluating for popular, as well as rare, sires and dams can help breeders to balance genetic influences across a breed to maximize the breed's genetic health. This analysis can be done by evaluating the last 20, 50, or however many years are appropriate for the species or breed. The registry database can be searched to count the number of times an animal appears as sire, grandsire, or great grandsire. Details of a way to do this are outlined in Appendix 3.

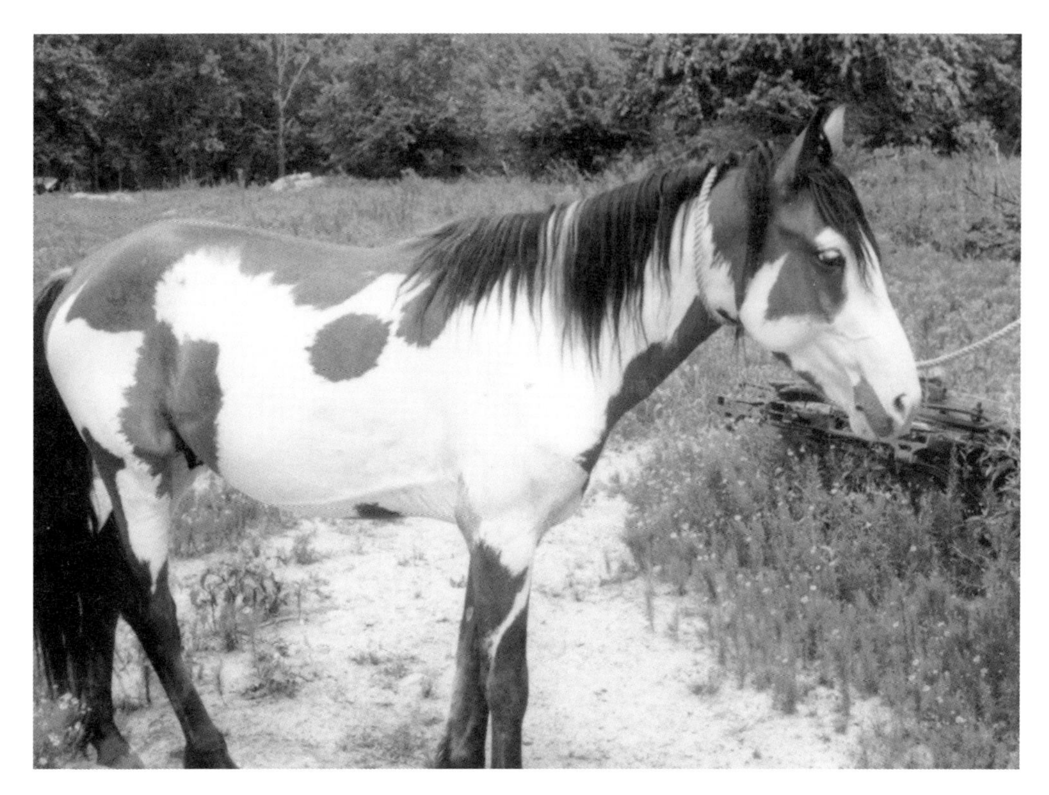

Figure 12.20 Most Choctaw horses now have this stallion, Chief of the Choctaws, somewhere in their pedigree. Photo by DPS.

The final results of this analysis are the abilities to find rare sires or dams and to know which sires and dams are most common (Figure 12.20). For example, once the more popular influences are documented, it should be possible to search for animals lacking those influences in an effort to capture genetic diversity more adequately. This must always be done with the recognition that some animals that are underrepresented have achieved that status for good reason: unsoundness or defect. But, in many breeds, perfectly sound and typical animals are underrepresented because they are in situations where they are simply overlooked as having excellent potential for the breed and its future. It is these animals that can hold the key to breed survival. This is not to detract in any way from more widely distributed bloodlines, though, because these have often achieved their popularity for good reasons.

12.4 Summary

The various investigations based on census, DNA analysis, and pedigree analysis each provide different pieces of information that can be woven together to give an accurate snapshot of a breed's current status. In addition, they can help to chart out future strategies to assure that a breed has maximum chances for survival. Several of the DNA analyses (microsatellite and SNPs especially) can provide a wealth of information about the current genetic makeup

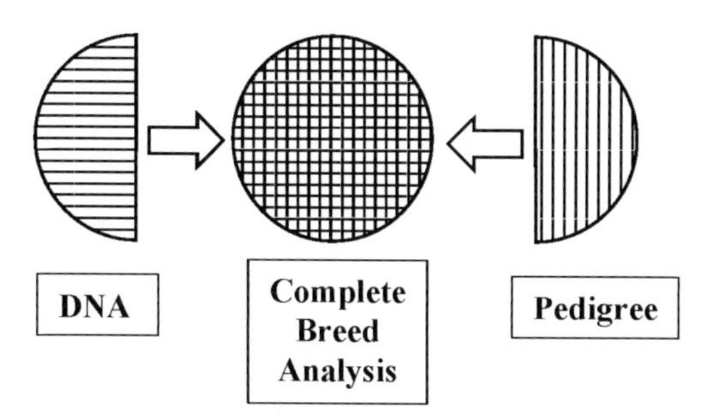

Figure 12.21 Accurate and complete breed analysis ideally involves both DNA and pedigree analysis. Only by putting these two together can an effective breed strategy be developed. Figure by DPS.

of a breed as well as its relationship to other breeds. Other DNA techniques (mitochondria and Y chromosome) can provide information about breed history. If there is inappropriate or inadequate sampling, each of these analyses will be limited or will yield a poor representation of the breed. With proper sampling the true genetic health of the population can be estimated, and a realistic current evaluation of the breed's genetic status can be made. DNA analyses alone cannot provide the specific information necessary to craft breeding plans for the animals. These can be provided by analysis of individual kinship values, founder percentages, and the relative contributions of individual sires and dams. Used together, these two types of analysis (DNA and pedigree) offer a powerful toolkit for the development of effective conservation breeding plans (Figure 12.21).

CHAPTER 13

Maintaining Breeds for Long-Term Success

Successful strategies for breed management always support purebred breeding within the breed's gene pool. Long-term management of the genetics of populations is basically the management of inbreeding in order to assure that benefits accrue from its positive aspects while avoiding the risks that can arise from its negative aspects. The long-term management of inbreeding assures that outcrosses are available for every animal within the population. "Population" in this case can mean a single herd or an entire breed. Inbreeding (and the depression it can bring) is most likely to occur when it becomes inevitable as the only option within a breed or herd. This happens when all animals are related. Inbreeding can be managed by outcrossing occasionally to unrelated animals, with the stipulation that these be from within the same breed. Crossing to an unrelated animal immediately takes the level of inbreeding for that offspring back to zero. Managing breeding programs to assure that this is possible over the long term is challenging and requires attention to a host of details. This chapter delves into more generic ways this can be accomplished. Chapter 14 outlines specific templates that can be used for this purpose.

A general consideration is to understand where most genetic variation lies within the breed or herd of interest. The most usual reservoirs are older females, but this is not universally true. In some breeds the most significant variation is present in males, often from semen that was frozen several years ago. In other breeds, significant variation lies in small, isolated subpopulations. Strategies need to be sensitive to the specific situation encountered with the target population. Population structure, along with the dynamics of how animals move through the population during their lifetime, affects inbreeding levels and the strategies used for its management.

13.1 Genetic Bottlenecks

Genetic bottlenecks occur when only a few individuals of a breed remain. The original, larger population narrows to only a few animals. Bottlenecks are a drastic form of overrepresentation of specific animals. These individuals then become the founders for the entire future of the breed. The bottleneck concept can be important in deciding the fate of

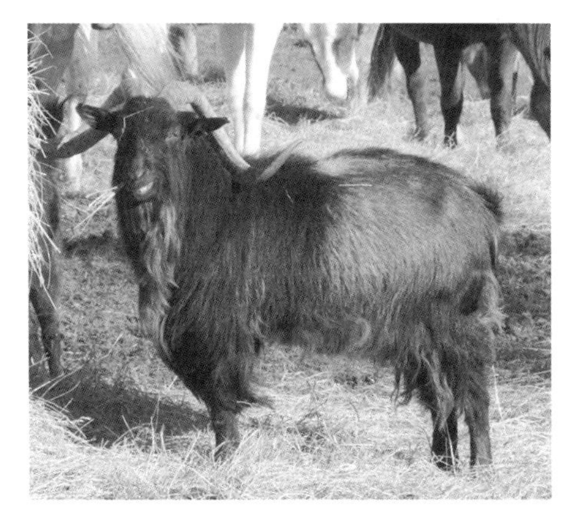

Figure 13.1 San Clemente goats have gone through successive genetic bottlenecks: the original foundation of the island population, and then those few island-caught individuals that reproduced after capture. Goats have been eradicated from the island, eliminating the prospect of ongoing recruitment. Photo by DPS.

breeds. For example, some breeds such as the Texas Longhorn and the Colonial Spanish horse once had populations which numbered in the millions. These populations then crashed to several hundreds, and the current registries were founded on still fewer individuals. The contemporary breed population goes back only to those few individual animals that actually founded the current registered populations, so the bottleneck that they represent now provides the total genetic variation in the entire breed (Figure 13.1).

Bottlenecks reduce genetic variation, and they often constrain viability of the breed. A short bottleneck happens when a single constricted generation of low numbers is followed by rapid expansion. This is much less harmful than a long bottleneck that lasts for several generations. Long bottlenecks, especially when only a few males are used for several generations in a row, are especially damaging because they drastically reduce genetic variation. Cloning a few individuals to rescue an endangered breed, such as occurred with the Enderby Island cattle, is a sort of ultimate bottleneck and greatly reduces genetic variation.

In any breed or herd, using only one breeding male constrains the next crop of offspring to be half-siblings. The result over several years can be to severely limit genetic variation. This worked in some situations to provide serviceable, viable, and productive breeds such as Conway Pineywoods cattle, KaraKitan Karakachan dogs, and Farceur American Belgian horses. These success stories can lull breeders into thinking that bottlenecks are of no consequence, but in most populations this breeding practice eventually leads to inbreeding depression and failure of the population. Bottlenecks must be managed carefully so that purebred outcrosses are always available.

The misuse of assisted reproductive technologies can lead to bottlenecks. These technologies are most commonly used to provide wider access to an outstanding individual than would be possible through natural reproduction, which results in an overrepresentation of that outstanding individual. Alternatively, these technologies can be used wisely for targeted goals that can be very helpful in providing genetically sound and viable structures for rare breeds. For example, semen and embryos can be saved from foundation animals so that their genomes are present for future use. Going back and occasionally using semen stored from long-dead ancestors in a contemporary breed can also lengthen generation intervals. Additionally, important and genetically underrepresented females can be superovulated in order to assure their broader contribution to the breed (Figure 13.2).

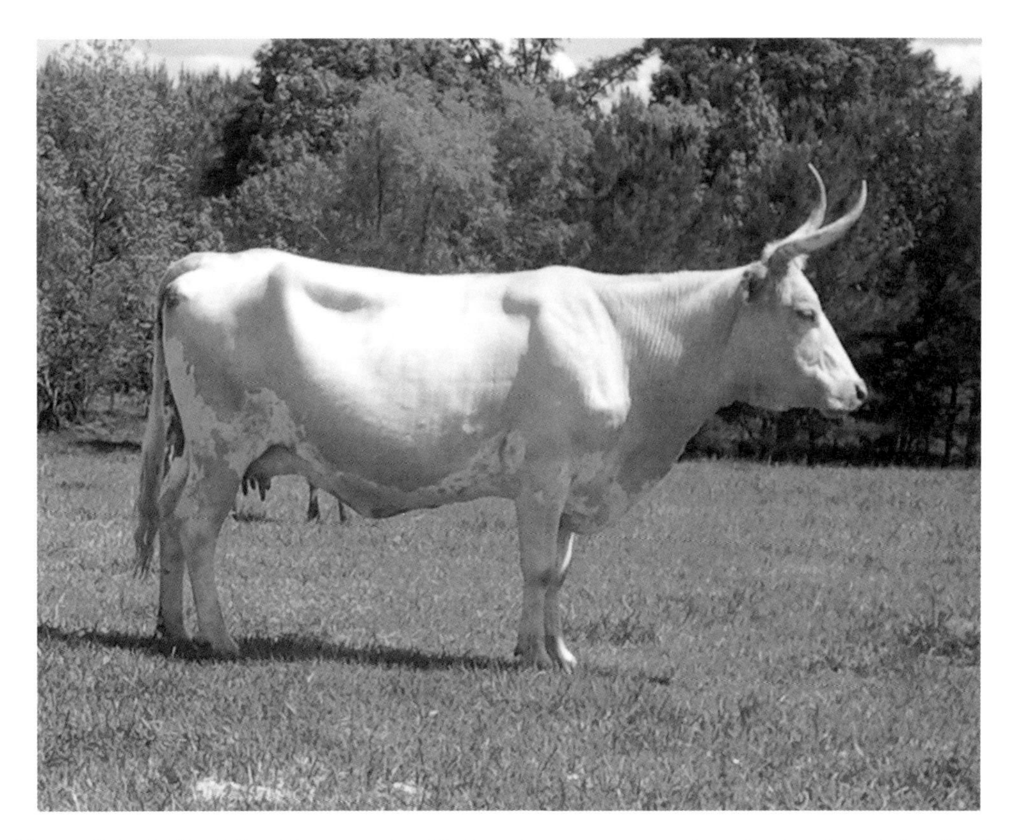

Figure 13.2 Griffin Yellow Pineywoods cattle have increased in numbers due to a targeted artificial insemination and embryo transfer program. This has benefitted the entire Pineywoods breed. Photo by Jess Brown, Cowpen Creek.

13.2 Monitoring Effective Population Size

Effective population size is a relative measure of the number of truly different genetic individuals in a population. For example, a group of ten full siblings represent a lower number of genetic individuals than a group of ten unrelated animals do because the genetic variation is much lower in the family group than in the non-family group.

Some breed associations place great value in estimates of effective population size for their breed as a rough measure of its genetic health and the degree of genetic variation. Effective population size can be a useful estimate of future inbreeding trends because low effective size indicates a future in which all animals will be related and therefore all matings will be inbred. Effective population size is related to specific expectations in the increase in inbreeding coefficient per generation.

Effective population size is most simply expressed as:

$$\frac{1}{\text{effective population size}} = \left[\frac{1}{4 \times \text{number of males}} + \frac{1}{4 \times \text{number of females}}\right]$$

The numbers of males and females in the formula are the numbers of reproducing males and females. The mathematics of this can be overwhelming, but the core of the idea is that the least numerous sex tends to determine the effective population size. For most livestock and dog breeds this means males. The most obvious consequence of this, if effective population size is to be boosted, is that effective conservation breeding usually involves using more males than would be absolutely necessary if the only consideration were the number of females a male can manage to successfully mate with. Genetic consequences dictate a different answer for the number of males that should be used when compared to the number required by husbandry considerations.

A population of 50 animals could include 40 females and 10 males, which gives an effective population size of 32. If the population included 25 males and 25 females, then the effective population size would be 50. Constraining the population to have a relatively higher number of males dramatically raises the effective population size. The effective population size is markedly affected by different sex ratios, as illustrated in Table 13.1. If the total population size is kept constant, then more equal sex ratios lead to greater effective population sizes. In most situations with livestock, poultry, and dogs, an even sex ratio is unrealistic. Geese are an exception to this rule because they so strongly prefer monogamy.

Two additional important points about effective population size are presented in Table 13.2. One is the outcome of using different numbers of males on a constant number of females. As the number of males becomes fewer, the effective population size goes down rapidly. The second is the effect of increasing the numbers of females mated to only one

Table 13.1 Effective population sizes relative to proportions of males and females in populations of fixed size. Reducing the number of males dramatically reduces the effective population size.

Number of males	Number of females	Effective population size
25	25	50
10	40	32
5	45	18
1	49	4

Table 13.2 Consequences of sex ratio and population census on effective population size. When low numbers of males are used, even dramatic increases in numbers of females have minimal effect in increasing effective population size.

Number of males	Number of females	Total population	Effective population size	Increase in inbreeding coefficient per generation
30	30	60	60	0.82%
9	30	39	27.6	1.8%
3	30	33	10.9	4.6%
1	30	31	3.87	12.9%
1	60	61	3.934	12.7%
1	90	91	3.96	12.6%

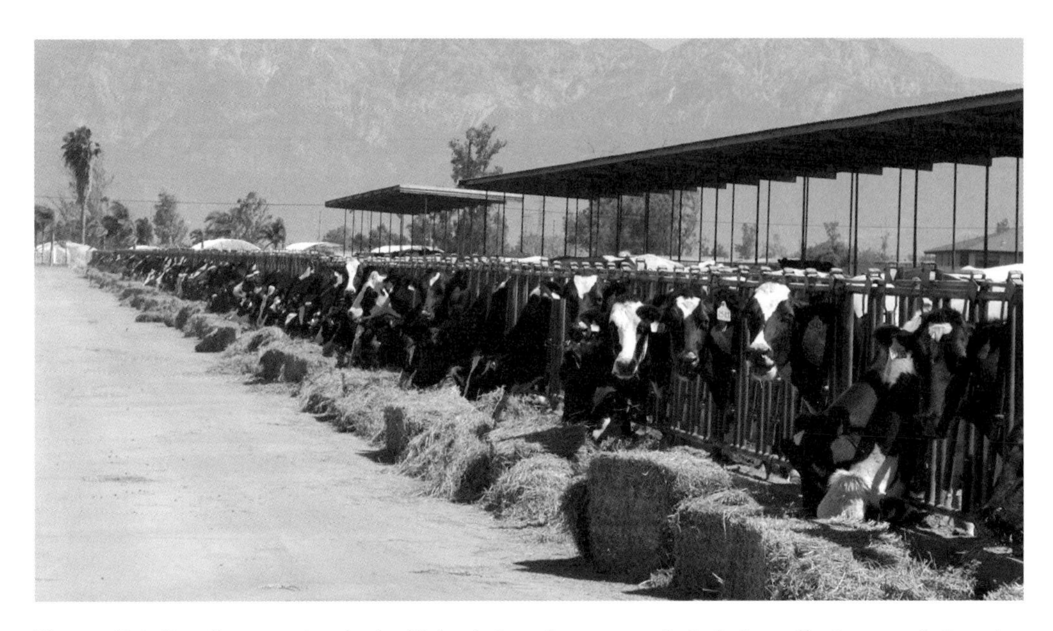

Figure 13.3 Breeding practices in the Holstein breed assure a relatively low effective population size despite a huge numerical census for the breed. Photo by JB.

male. Raising the number of females even two- and three-fold in that situation does very little to increase effective population size. The lesson here is that sex ratios for effective breed management need to be carefully considered, and they usually involve using more males than might seem logical for strictly reproductive purposes. These figures have profound implications for more common breeds, too. The Holstein dairy breed, for example, has bulls that produce 10,000 calves a year, which definitely pushes the effective population size in a downward direction and decreases genetic variation.

The equation given above for effective population size is oversimplified, and a longer but more accurate equation includes the time interval from parent to offspring for each sex, as well as the degree of relationship between animals. These are important issues for effective population size, but are difficult to account for in most situations. Internationally popular breeds such as Holstein cattle (Figure 13.3) have relatively low effective population sizes due to widespread use of artificial insemination with semen from bulls that are related to one another. In this breed, and others in similar situations, the effective population size tends to decrease over time. This limited effective population size makes significant inbreeding impossible to avoid, with the result that viability and reproduction can suffer despite the breed's huge actual census of individual animals.

Effective population size is generally lower than the census would suggest. Any shared ancestry among breeding partners (especially in recent generations) takes that number even lower. For rare breeds, the effective breeding population size is almost always much smaller than the outright census. Unfortunately for the breeders of rare breeds, it is impossible to easily capture all of the information for an accurate determination of effective population size. The level of detail needed to arrive at an accurate answer is overwhelming. The simplified equation is useful in highlighting the importance of sex ratio, especially in rare breeds, but it is important to note that the number generated by this result is likely to be a relatively optimistic one. True effective population size is generally even lower than the figure predicted by the simplified equation.

Effective population size is a more critical factor for breed survival in rare breeds than it is for breeds with large populations, because inbreeding in rare breeds is more likely to be widespread throughout the entire population. The principles of effective population size are a compelling reason to keep track of different bloodlines within rare breeds so that breeders can assure that outcrosses are available to each and every animal in the breed. No specific guidelines can be offered to suggest a ratio between census and effective population size, as this is a complicated biological concept and oversimplifying it leads to a false sense of security about the true genetic composition of purebred populations. Breeders should monitor their breeds closely to assure that outcrosses are available within the breed. They should also be diligent to keep different bloodlines viable and secure as insurance against future needs.

13.3 Generation Interval

Generation interval refers to the average age of parents at the time their offspring are born. It is not the age of the parents at the time of the first offspring, but is instead the average age of all parents and for all offspring. As a result it is a difficult computation for many populations. A simplified example is that if sows and boars are used to produce only a single litter, then the generation interval is about a year. If, in contrast, sows are kept up to seven years and boars for five, then the generation interval goes up to about three and a half years for the population. This assumes an even distribution of ages up to the maximum age.

Selection programs to promote genetic improvement generally favor a short generation interval. This allows breeders to maximize genetic gains per year, for (ideally) each generation should be genetically superior to preceding generations if selection is indeed successful. Decreasing the interval between generations should therefore hasten genetic improvement. It is true, though, that genetic superiority may not always result in production superiority. For example, a genetically superior two-year-old dairy cow is unlikely to produce as much milk as a somewhat more genetically average six-year-old dairy cow because the six-year-old is benefitting from being able to produce at her mature potential. In this situation the increased production potential coming from genetic gain can only be fully realized in the milk pail if the cows are kept to maturity. This, of course, increases the generation interval.

For many rare breeds, and especially for adapted ones, the generation interval may well need to be kept longer than is typical for industrial breeds (Figure 13.4). One reason for this is that older parents have demonstrated their adaptability and production success over longer time periods than younger ones have. They are therefore safer bets for having the genetic strength desired in an adapted breed than younger parents that are less well proven in the environment. In addition, especially in small populations, increases in inbreeding are related to generation interval. Keeping the generation interval as high as possible is one tactic used to minimize a dramatic annual accumulation of inbreeding, because any

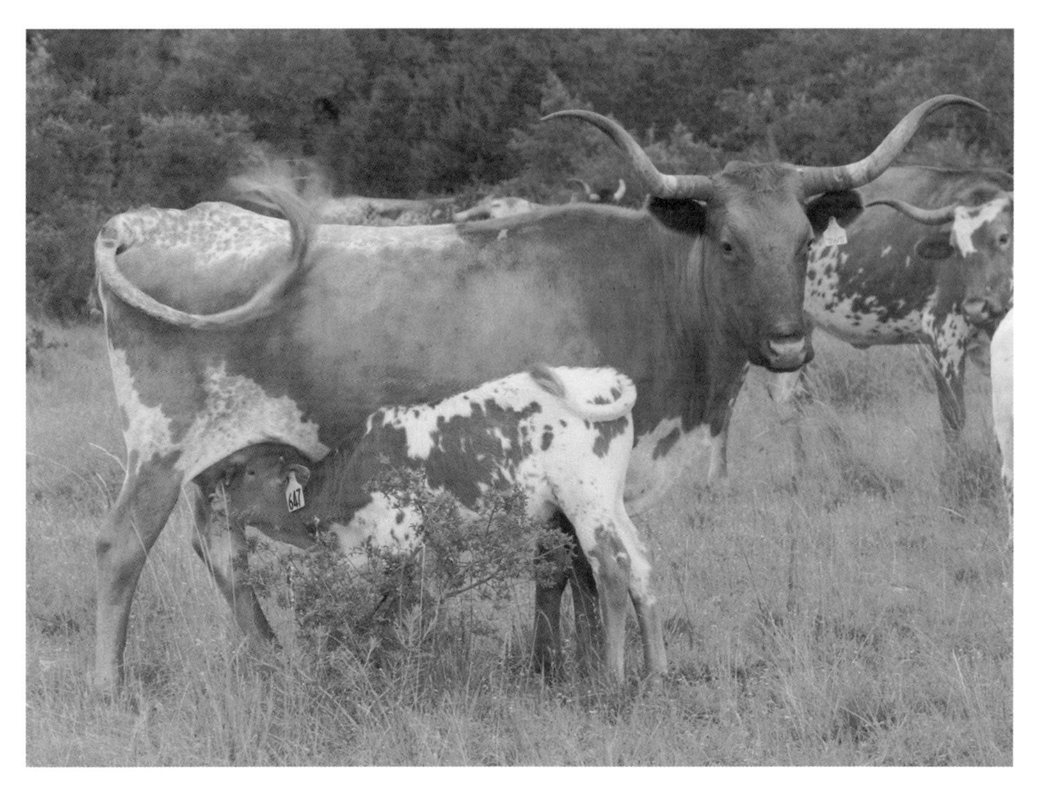

Figure 13.4 Many heritage breeds, such as Texas Longhorn cattle, have longevity as one of their strengths. This increases the generation interval and makes breeding animal replacement much more sustainable in many farming systems. Photo by DPS.

inbreeding accrues over a much longer period of years. The generation interval stretches out from the use of older animals.

Especially in the case of foundation animals, the wisest plan is to use them until they are no longer reproducing (Figure 13.5). This increases the opportunity for them to contribute their entire genome to the breed. Exceptions to this rule are important, and include situations in which a few founders in a small breed may swamp the entire breed by becoming bottlenecks if all replacements are saved only from these few. In that instance it is best to balance the contributions of all population members through tightly constrained breeding programs. Longevity of production has several advantages in nearly every situation. Not least among these is the fact that a long-lived animal has a higher number of offspring from which to select a replacement, so that selection can act among a greater number of candidates.

Males are much more likely to overcontribute their genetic influence than females are if the males are kept actively breeding for long careers. This is because they produce more offspring than females. A relatively common practice in many rare breeds or rare strains is for herds to use a single sire for multiple years, replacing him with a son, and continuing this practice for several generations in a row. Randall cattle and Conway Pineywoods cattle both have this history (Figure 13.6). The initial result of using the male is the production

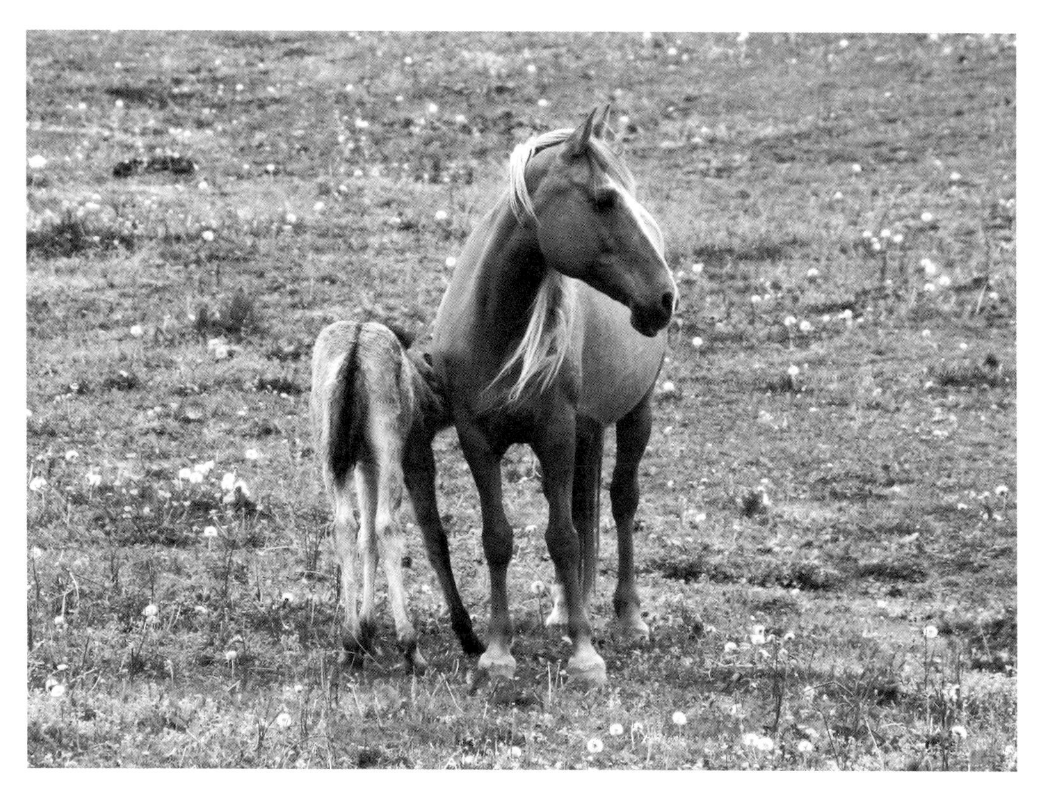

Figure 13.5 Milton's Chickasaw Penny continues to produce foals into her late twenties. She is a good example of the longevity of Choctaw mares, demonstrating the adaptability and strength of the breed. Photo by JB.

of daughters and sons. Retaining daughters in the herd leads to sire-daughter matings along with those to the original founder females. If the male lasts a long time, then he is likely to be mated to his granddaughters that were produced by daughters. When a son eventually replaces him, this son is related to the entire herd. The cycle continues with ever-increasing relationship among all animals in the herd as the years and generations progress.

Several cycles of this sort of breeding, over decades, assure that all animals in the population are very closely related. This situation can be exacerbated with the widespread use of artificial insemination. One tactic to avoid the males becoming a genetic bottleneck is to replace the males relatively rapidly, while maintaining the females for as many years as is practical. Keeping both sexes for long reproductive lives tends to lead to a genetic bottleneck, but a drastic reduction in the reproductive lives of both sexes likewise tends to lead to a constricted genetic pool due to a very short generation interval. Having one sex at a short interval and the other at a very long interval is a good compromise for the long-term genetic health of the population. In most situations it is more practical for the longer breeding careers to be devoted to the females, and the shorter ones to the males. Males, due to their ability to produce more offspring in a year, still contribute appropriately even if this is for a short interval of time.

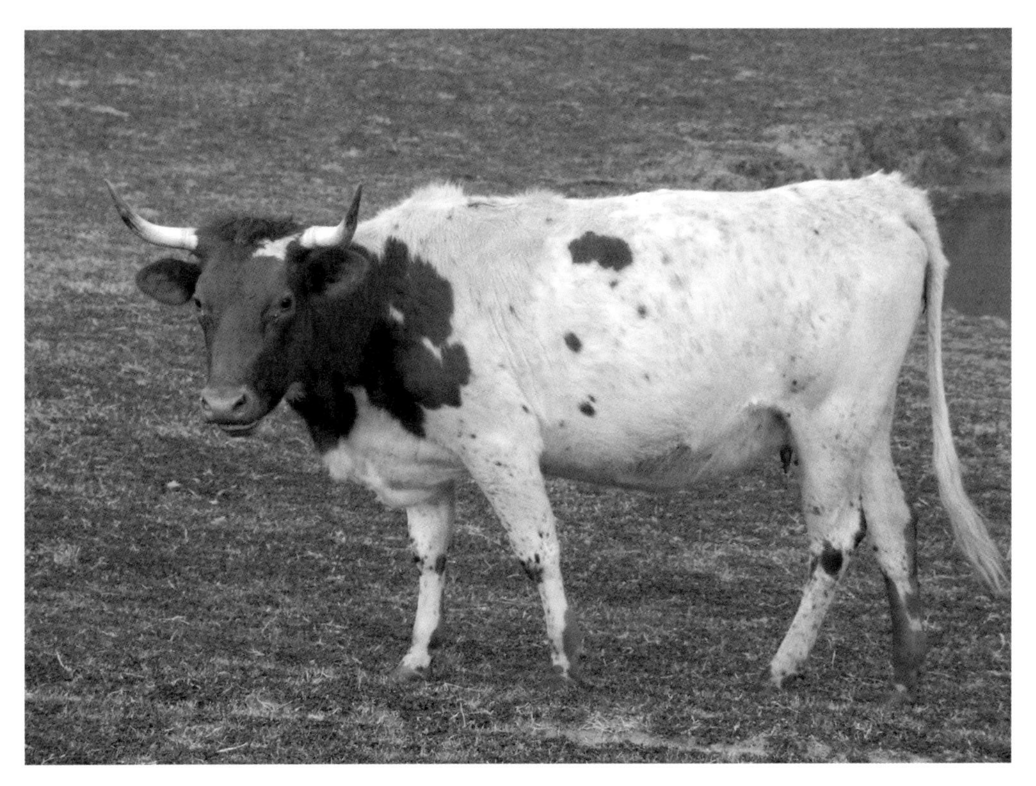

Figure 13.6 Conway Pineywoods cattle are all descended from a herd that used bulls for long reproductive careers, assuring a degree of linebreeding across all animals in this strain. Photo by JB.

13.4 Inbreeding and Loss of Diversity

Inbreeding has several important consequences. One is inbreeding depression, which refers to the decline in vigor of inbred animals as compared to outbred animals. Inbreeding usually diminishes the overall vigor of the resulting animals, as well as their reproductive success. This occurs at variable rates in different populations so that the practical significance of this phenomenon varies. Exceptions to the general rule do occur, but they are just that: exceptions. Focusing on those successful examples overlooks the overwhelming long-term risk that uncontrolled inbreeding often brings to a population.

A second and important consequence of inbreeding in small populations occurs when it combines with genetic drift and selection to reduce genetic variation. The end result can strengthen and accentuate predictability. As animals become more genetically uniform, they also tend to become more similar in looks and performance. Predictability is the hallmark of pure breeds, and so this can be a good consequence of reduction of genetic variability. The downside is that genetic variability is essential not only for population health, but also for providing the raw material for selection and improvement. Highly inbred populations may lack sufficient variability for selection efforts to make any progress in production levels.

Even though some lines of some breeds withstand inbreeding very well, inbreeding depression is a widespread and well-documented phenomenon. All breeders should

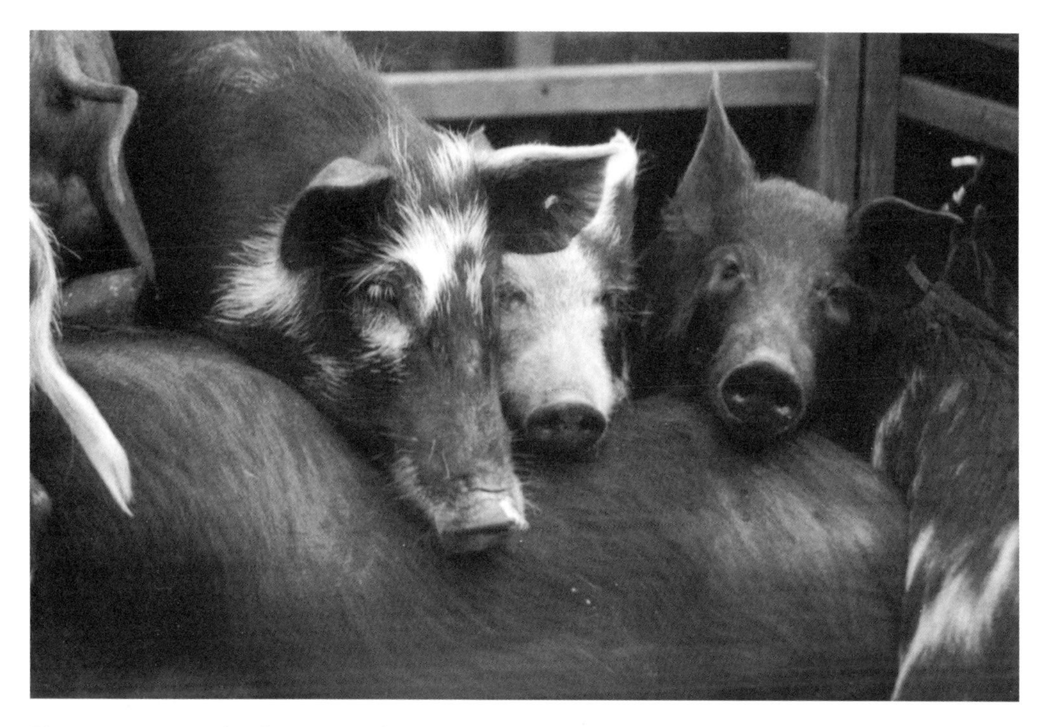

Figure 13.7 Animals of some populations can all become related to one another without close attention to pedigrees and mating choices. Ossabaw hogs of some herds have become interrelated, and this can only be countered by introducing unrelated hogs from other herds. Photo by DPS.

manage their populations to assure that the consequences of inbreeding can be avoided in the long term, by making sure that every animal within the breed has an outcross available. This strategy assures that a "back door" escape is available to the breed should inbreeding depression become evident. The situation most to be avoided is the one in which all animals within a breed or herd are closely related to one another so that inbreeding becomes inevitable (Figure 13.7). This is a common trap for rare breeds when attempts are made to "change the ram" every year by cross-country trading. This strategy results in all flocks becoming related through all having sequentially used the same males, and it therefore becomes impossible to correct for inbreeding depression should it manifest itself in the breed.

Genetic variability and genetic uniformity play tug of war. Populations at one extreme are so variable that they are completely unpredictable as to type and production. Populations at the other extreme are so uniform that vigor diminishes, and genetic selection is impossible because all animals within the population are so similar to one another. Most breeds lie between these extremes and must be managed so that the benefits of predictability are not lost to diminished vigor on the one hand, and enhanced vigor is not gained at the expense of low predictability on the other hand.

13.5 Monitoring Inbreeding

Monitoring the generational increase in inbreeding is important for small, isolated populations such as rare breeds. Monitoring inbreeding is relatively easy if database registry software is used to track registrations and pedigrees. Any other approach is likely to be too time consuming to be practical for most registries and associations, even though traditional breeders do have a phenomenal ability to keep details of breeding and relationships in their heads. While not strictly a generation-to-generation evaluation, a more practical approach is to compute breed-wide inbreeding coefficients annually. These can determine a breed-wide trend. In addition, an overall range of inbreeding coefficients can also be computed.

More difficult to assess than an overall breed-wide average is the status of the degree of inbreeding within the various individuals of the breed taken one by one. If animals in one year are highly inbred, but the inbreeding is not all to the same individuals within the breed, then it is possible to lower the inbreeding coefficient in subsequent years by selectively mating to unrelated animals. In contrast, if all of the animals are inbred to the same individuals, then such corrective measures are impossible. As a consequence, the specific character of the inbreeding is of as much concern as the overall degree of inbreeding. If the inbreeding is occurring in different directions (to different individuals) then the breed is less precariously perched than if the inbreeding is all occurring to the same few individuals across the entire breed (Figure 13.8). The degree of inbreeding across the breed as well as

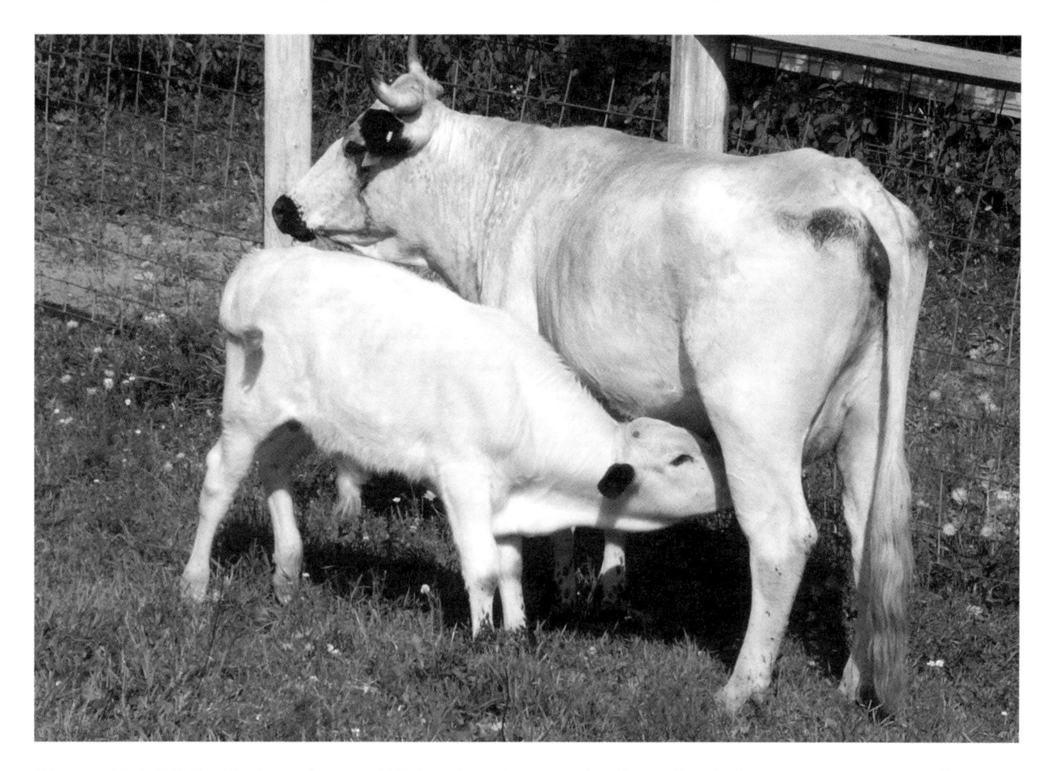

Figure 13.8 White Park cattle are all inbred, and managing breeding is important to assure that whatever genetic distance remains in the breed can be maintained on into the future. Photo by DPS.

the degree in individual animals are both important. To track this detail most effectively, it is necessary to evaluate the degree of inbreeding with respect to several different founders instead of using a single average across the entire breed.

Analyses of the finer points of the degree and direction of inbreeding are more difficult to obtain than overall degrees of inbreeding across the entire breed. Some databases will allow analyses to compute overall relatedness (kinship) to specific individuals. These techniques are usually used when breeders are planning to purchase a new breeding animal, so that the new animal can be compared to the existing herd to determine the inbreeding consequences. These approaches can be used more broadly to determine the overall relatedness of a breed to a few key individual animals that may be swamping the breed's genetics. Not only is the overall degree of kinship to those individuals important, but also a more detailed individual-by-individual analysis to assess the range of kinship should be considered. An example is to consider two hypothetical situations where the overall degree of kinship to a specific individual (usually male) is 25%. In one situation the range of kinship across individuals is 20–75%, so all animals are related to the individual in question. In the second situation the kinship has a range of 0–50%. In this second situation, outcrosses are still available because unrelated animals are in the population. In the first case, they are not available, and the breed has hit a true bottleneck with regard to that individual animal because all matings must now be linebred to that individual.

A current trend in many breeds is to simply constrain all matings to avoid producing a high coefficient of inbreeding in the offspring. This sounds wise at first glance, but can easily lead to a few unanticipated consequences. This is especially true in small populations. A strategy of breeding that constantly pairs animals to produce minimal coefficients of inbreeding in offspring ends up pairing the least related animals. The offspring is then related to both of those previously unrelated animals. If this is pursued over several generations, the result is to essentially use up the pool of unrelated animals and to provide younger generations related to all of them. The least related are constantly incorporated into the general pool until all animals are related. At that point, all matings are related, and all will result in an inbreeding coefficient of some size.

It is wiser, but more difficult, to be sure to inbreed and outbreed sequentially. This can be managed so that the inbreeding stages do not result in all that extreme a coefficient of inbreeding, while at the same time assuring that at least some potential mates in the population are minimally related.

13.6 *Inbreeding within Individual Herds*

Degrees of inbreeding levels are likely to be higher within an individual herd than they are across an entire breed. This is largely due to the use of relatively few males in any herd, with retention of breeding stock from a single or only a few sires or outstanding dams. Over several generations of closed-herd breeding this strategy can lead to fairly significant inbreeding within a herd. This can be one of the sources of the uniformity that is usually desired in a herd, but must be done with forethought.

In most breeds, inbreeding within a single herd is little threat to the overall genetic health of the breed. This is true because other herds are either being outbred or are being inbred to different individuals. As long as the inbreeding is not the result of the same few individuals across the entire breed, then the breed is relatively safe and does not risk the loss of much genetic variation. The reason for this is that one inbred line can be linecrossed to a second unrelated inbred line, and all of the inbreeding that is built up vanishes in the next (linecrossed) generation. A backcross to either parental line will assure that inbreeding is once again occurring, so wisdom and close management are needed if the goal is continued assurance that outcrosses are available to every animal in the breed.

13.7 *Inbreeding within Breeds*

Inbreeding is much more problematic when it is uniformly distributed across an entire breed rather than within separate herds. When inbreeding is uniform at the breed level it is nearly impossible to avoid its negative consequences. If all breeders pursue the same successful bloodlines and individual animals, then the result is that the entire breed is being inbred in the same direction. This can be visualized as a circle with the tension at the boundary all being directed into the same middle point, which is usually a popular individual animal or bloodline (Figure 13.9). Over several generations the circle, which represents the overall genetic variation in the breed, becomes smaller and smaller. Popular sires or bloodlines that expand at the expense of others in the breed are common culprits for significant inbreeding problems across entire breeds. It is especially dangerous to use uncontrolled artificial insemination, as the entire breed can be mated to a handful of related sires. Such a strategy accelerates the inbreeding that can occur.

The ever-contracting inbred circle can be contrasted to the situation in which different bloodlines within the breed are being bred in different directions and to different individual animals (Figure 13.10). In that situation the inward forces are subdivided into smaller circles

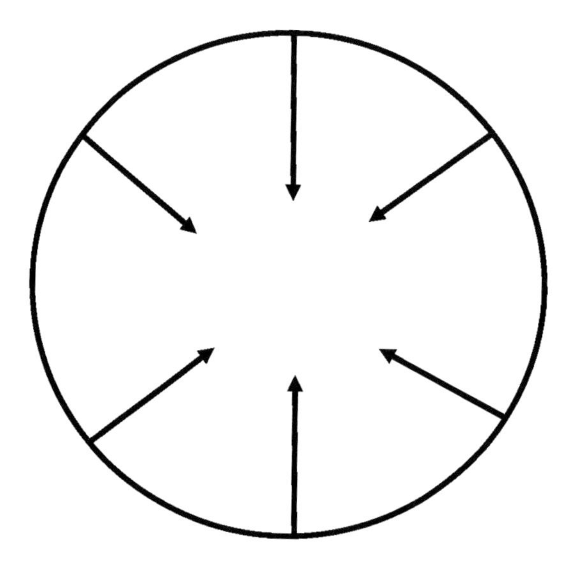

Figure 13.9 Inbreeding in a single direction across an entire breed yields a constricting gene pool for the entire breed. Figure by DPS.

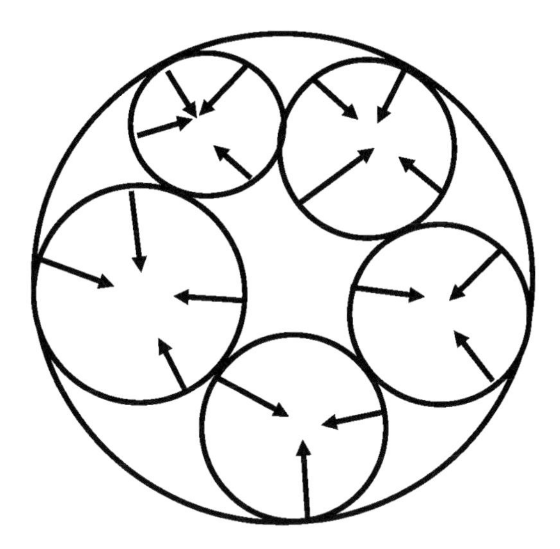

Figure 13.10 Inbreeding in various different directions by concentrating it in different herds can keep more genetic diversity in a breed than inbreeding all in one direction. Figure by DPS.

within the larger breed circle. The result is that the overall breed circle tends to maintain its original size without much loss. Genetic variation is maintained, and with it, breed health.

Strategies for managing inbreeding vary from breed to breed. At one extreme there is no control at all over inbreeding, nor strategies for managing it. Some dog breeds, and cattle breeds such as the Holstein, are among those that allow for breeding to be concentrated on a very few individuals. The result is unavoidable inbreeding, and some of these breeds are now reaping the unfortunate consequences of this as diminished vigor. The philosophy and practice of purebred breeding, as envisioned over the last two centuries, have not yet fashioned a good strategy for dealing with inbreeding in closed populations. Over the next few decades, breeders and associations need to address this issue if the genetic heritage of breeds is not to be lost through their attrition to extinction from lack of vigor.

Dog breeds provide very good lessons for the management of long-term purebred breeding. Due to their short generation interval, and the production of litters, their role in this grand experiment of purebred breeding is ahead of most other breeds in most other species (Figure 13.11). As the standardization and closure of breeding populations was initiated about a century ago, it began a process of isolation and therefore consistent, if gradual, diminution of genetic variation from generation to generation. How to manage this while preserving the very real advantages of purebred dogs is a challenge that will require creative thinking on the part of both breeders and breed associations.

Some breed associations may well choose to control inbreeding by limiting the number of offspring registered per animal per year, although few breed associations actually use this sort of control. This tactic can be especially important in breeds in which artificial insemination and embryo transfer are allowed. Putting a limit on the number of offspring an animal can produce in a year or a lifetime assures that no single animal swamps the entire breed. One useful benchmark is that in most breeds it is unwise for any sire to produce more than 5% of the offspring in any given year. This can be a very difficult step for a breed

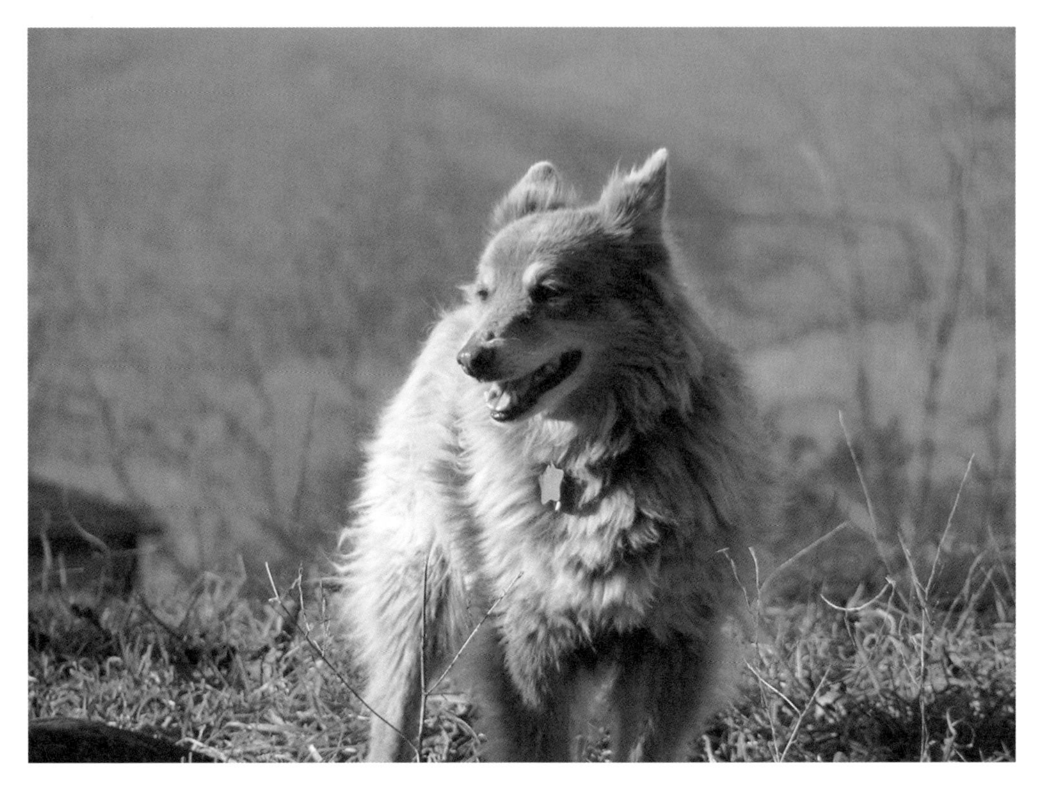

Figure 13.11 Kelpies are sheep herding dogs. Dog breeds run a risk of fairly high degrees of inbreeding due to repeated matings to popular individual sires. Photo by DPS.

association to take, as it pits the long-term survival of the breed against the short-term economic benefit for individual breeders who have popular animals.

Most breeds may be able to avoid the use of formal rules to manage inbreeding by educating breeders about the bloodlines within the breed and the need to keep these going into the future. A quick analysis by the breed registrar can usually reveal which lines are becoming rarer and which are in danger of swamping the breed. Alerting the membership to the status of the bloodlines can boost activity within the rarer bloodlines, especially if this is matched with long-term educational endeavors on the part of the breed association about the importance of bloodlines within a breed.

Noting the production record of sires that produce offspring can help breeders to analyze bloodlines and sire families. One way to do this is to count offspring and grand-offspring for all sires. This can be done either as a year-to-year analysis, or as a lifetime analysis. The results of the analysis keep track of the breeding activity for each animal, and when done by someone familiar with the breed it can be used to track the breeding success of entire families (Figure 13.12).

For rare breeds it is helpful to have a more detailed analysis that tracks the breeding status of different family lines, especially targeting those that have few animals or are lacking animals of one sex or the other. These underrepresented families can then be targeted to make sure that they reproduce, and that offspring are recruited into the breeding population

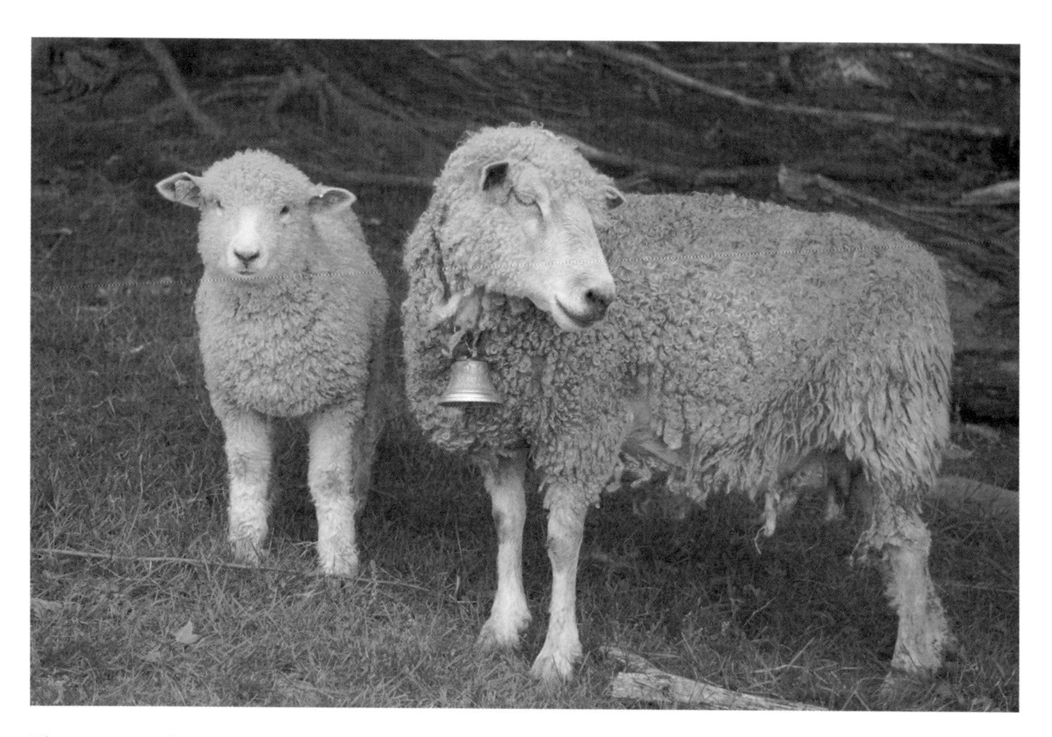

Figure 13.12 Leicester Longwool breeders have been diligent to closely track the influence of the various founders of the breed in the USA to assure broad representation within the breed. Photo by Kelly Miller, Hopping Acres.

of the breed. When accomplished over several bloodlines, this approach can help to assure that each animal within the breed has an unrelated potential mate. This contrasts with the situation in which all members of the breed are related to one another, with the result that inbreeding can never be avoided.

13.8 Combining Linebreeding and Linecrossing

One mechanism for population maintenance that can work well for a number of breeds uses the advantages of both linebreeding and linecrossing. Mating can be constrained so that following a linebred generation the animals are then linecrossed. By alternating the two mating strategies generation to generation it is possible to reap the benefits of each without experiencing too many of the negative aspects of either. Such a plan does require great attention to detail because matings must always consider the fate of the animals several generations into the future. A protocol for this strategy is detailed in Chapter 14.

Both inbreeding and outbreeding have a place in breed and herd maintenance. Making sense of all of the details of inbreeding and linebreeding can be perplexing, especially when these issues hit the barnyard and the breeding decisions that must be made by breeders. Associations can help their breeders by educating them concerning the lines within the breed and the importance of these for breed-wide genetic health.

Especially difficult is the very real possibility that short-term economic interest will place pressure on all breeders to go in a single breeding direction by trying to produce animals that fit current demand. In contrast, long-term breed viability requires that breeders maintain sufficient diversity for breed viability. Managing the tension of these two demands on breeders is a very important role of associations and breeder communities.

13.9 Inbreeding and Linebreeding to Expand Rare Genetics

Linebreeding has a few specific powerful benefits for many rare breed conservation programs. A major strength of inbreeding, and also linebreeding, is the fixation of traits in a given line of animals. This can be used to good advantage in several situations. Linebreeding is a power tool that must be used cautiously and safely to assure its benefits and avoid its potential risks. Targeted close linebreeding or inbreeding is an effective strategy that can correct the underrepresentation of the genetic influence of rare bloodlines or the specific founders of rare breeds. It can also enhance imported bloodlines that may have only come through a single sex of animal. This is usually through a male imported via semen, but occasionally involves a female of a rare bloodline.

Many rare breeds have some bloodlines that have dwindled down to a few individuals. In most cases these are females. This is especially likely to happen in breeds where females are widely used for crossbreeding, such as Florida Cracker and Pineywoods cattle. This is because the males of some lines were long ago replaced by the crossbreeding to bulls of other breeds, and consequently only females remain. The opposite situation, with only males remaining, does occur but much less frequently.

A strategy can be outlined for situations where a line has dwindled to a few females. As a practical issue these females are generally closely related to one another, all coming from the same bloodline. The first step is to mate the females to a purebred male, which must come from another line because no males are available from the targeted bloodline. This is by definition a linecross mating. For the next generation, a male offspring should be mated back to the original females (Figure 13.13). The result is a crop of young stock that is 75% the original line. These "75%" males can be used back on the original females, and the use of this strategy (young males, older foundation females) can continue until the older females cease being productive. The goal is to take genetic material that can only be used to a limited degree by virtue of being in female form, and generate males that can be used more widely to distribute the genetic material in these rare foundation bloodlines broadly throughout other portions of the breed. It is important to note that while these initial linecross (first generation) and linebred (succeeding generations) males are being produced, sisters are also being produced and these can be effectively used in other portions of a breeding program without endangering the critical role that the foundation females are playing. By this strategy, the older founder females are being used to increase numbers of animals. These animals make ever-increasing contributions of the rare founder genetics as the generations progress.

A similar strategy can be used with individual outstanding females of any breed, but this process is especially useful when used in rare breeds for bloodlines that are lacking males. Such a female can be mated back to her own sons to produce offspring (hopefully male)

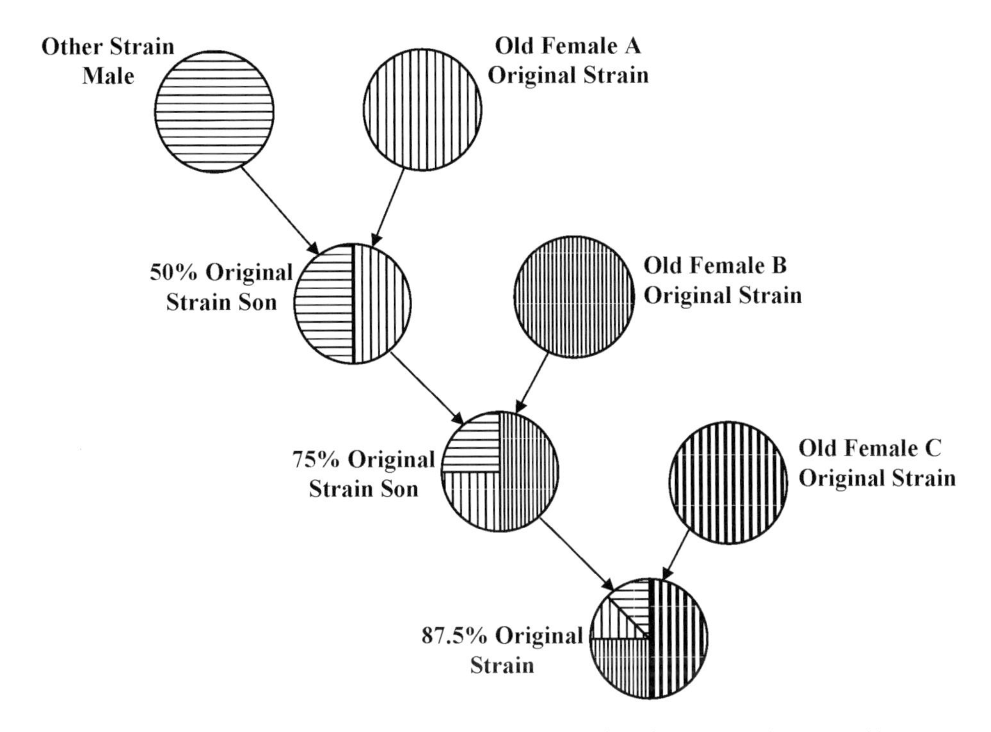

Figure 13.13 Rare bloodlines are often only represented by females, but can be rescued by a protocol that uses purebred, linecrossed sons of the females as a strategy to consolidate the genetic material of the original females. Figure by DPS.

that are 75% the influence of the original outstanding female. This has been done in many rare breed conservation programs with individual rare line females. Going back multiple generations to a single female can be successful, but this results in closer inbreeding than when a group of related animals is available so that sons of one female can be mated to other females rather than their own dam. As a consequence, this strategy of repeated mating back to young, related males cannot be used over several generations with a single female without running some risk of inbreeding depression. However, even with a single female it is usually a successful strategy for a generation or two, at which point the males produced can be linecrossed to other lines and thereby contribute widely to the breed in a way that the single female could not.

The key to success with this strategy is to use it only as a rescue strategy for a rare bloodline, or to limit its use to truly outstanding individuals. This strategy depends on the past efforts that long-term breeders of purebred livestock have made to assure the availability of truly excellent animals. Every breed benefits from having such breeders and such animals. It is the long-term dedication of individual breeders that provides these distinctive genetic packages that are so useful for others to build upon. Each breed and each generation within the breed needs breeders dedicated to safeguarding the genetic heritage and productive potential of the breed. In contrast, if this strategy is used on weak or average individuals, the risks of inbreeding depression outweigh the potential benefits of salvaging the genetic material.

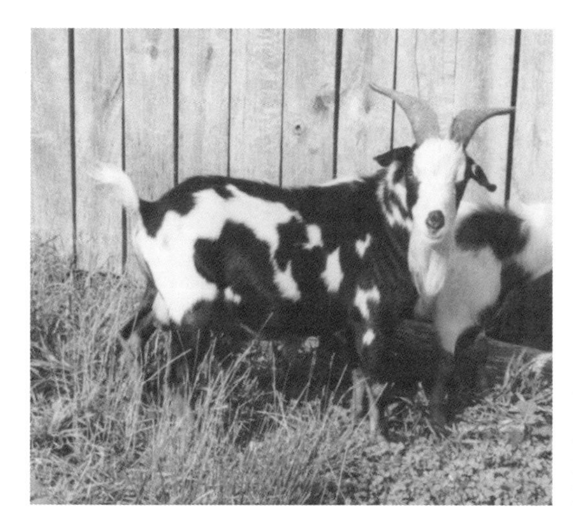

Figure 13.14 This Myotonic buck resulted from repeated linebreeding back to the same few remaining females of an old bloodline. Photo by DPS.

An example comes from Tennessee Myotonic goats. A 15-year-old, productive doe was mated to sons of her sisters, the result being 75% that one line. She produced a son from those matings, and was mated to him to produce a buck kid that was 87.5% the genetic influence of the original productive bloodline. This inbred buck never grew as big as his herd mates, but he consistently produced exceptional kids when he was used for linecross matings (Figure 13.14). This example shows both inbreeding depression (the inbred buck) and hybrid vigor (his kids). This illustrates that inbred animals are likely to outproduce their own performance when used for linecrossing. Managing both strategies long term is the challenge, for the goal should be production of animals that are both viable and predictable.

13.10 Managing Contributions of Individual Animals

It has already been stressed that every animal should have a potential linecross within the breed to assure the breed's genetic health. This requires attention and careful planning; otherwise all animals of a breed can become related to one another. This usually occurs through the overuse of individual excellent animals. For some breeds of livestock, and especially in breeds of dogs, certain individual animals have become overrepresented, to the extent that it is nearly impossible in some breeds to find linecrosses. When certain animals become overrepresented, other animals become underrepresented, and the breed risks losing their genetic contribution. When individuals become overrepresented, it means that the breed has lost variability, and could be in danger of losing the genetic variation essential for long-term survival.

One way that individual animals become overrepresented is through the "founder effect." Founder effect describes the phenomenon in which a population that descends from a few founders cannot contain any genetic variability that was not contained in those founders. Founder effect is very constricted when new herds are started with a few animals, and this is especially the case when only a single male is present in the newly established population. It is common for an original founder male to account for a great proportion of the genes of the resulting population, largely because he and then his sons tend to be

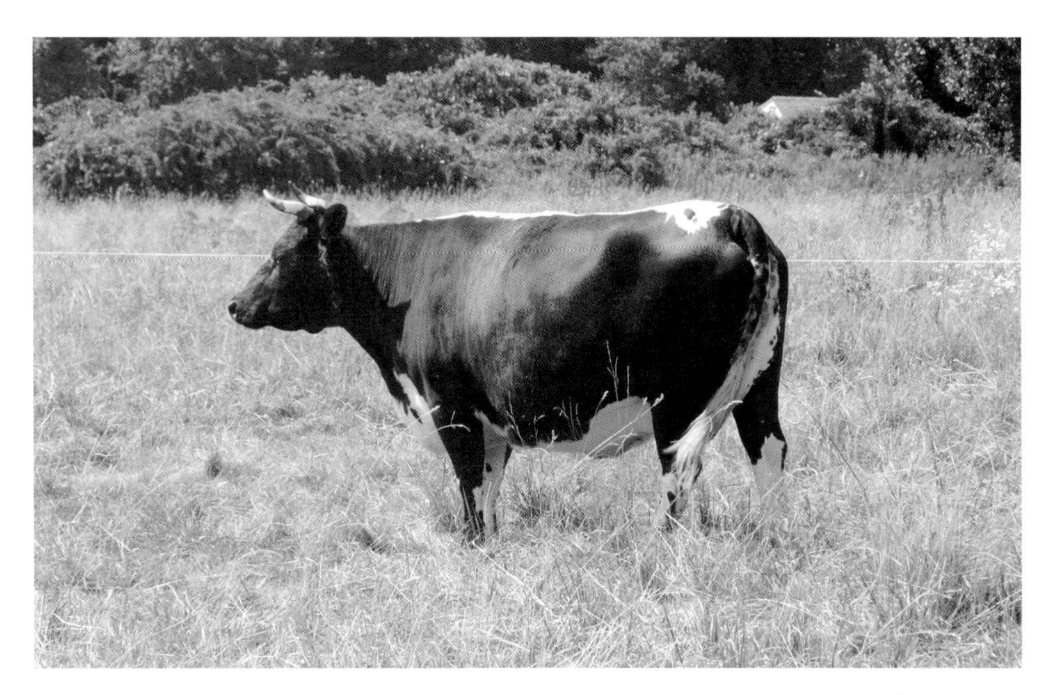

Figure 13.15 Randall Lineback cattle demonstrate the challenges of managing a handful of founders for long-term breed security. Photo by DPS.

used in the group for generation after generation. This is especially likely in traditional systems where a male becomes highly regarded by the owner and might well be used until he physically plays out. At this point he has usually swamped the population with his own offspring, and has also been mated to his own daughters, thereby increasing his genetic impact on the population all the more.

The Randall Lineback cattle breed provides an example of founder effect (Figure 13.15). This breed descends from a limited number of founders, all of which were closely related. Detailed pedigree records were, unfortunately, not available at the time of the breed rescue. The most optimistic analysis still has all cattle related to a single male, whose contribution to individuals of the breed ranges from 12% to 48% (Table 13.3). In this case it is impossible to avoid inbreeding to that one founder, though careful breeding management can assure that relatively low percentage cattle are always in the population. The low percentage cattle allow for the relatively high percentage cattle to be mated strategically to avoid further concentrating that one founder. The other founders in the Randall breed vary from 0–50% in their contribution to individual cattle. The variation in contribution allows for some distance in matings between cattle so that higher percentage cattle can be mated to lower percentage cattle for the various founders. If breeding during the rescue had not been carefully monitored it could easily have occurred that the contribution of certain founders would have been uniform across the breed, at which point all matings would be equally linebred.

Managing the contributions of the founders in the Randall Lineback breed has a few other interesting points. For example, founder 12 was not used widely, having been located years after the breed rescue was established and ongoing. This is a bull, and his contribution

Table 13.3 Management of percentage contributions of founder animals through breeding management of Randall cattle. "Founder 1" is the original bull, and can be seen to have had a profound influence on the breed. In the case of nearly every other founder, some individuals can be found with no influence of that founder, while others have a higher influence. This difference can be used to manage the degree of inbreeding out into the future.

Founder	Average % in cattle alive in 2005	Minimum % in cattle alive in 2005	Maximum % in cattle alive in 2005
1	33	12	48
2	16	0	50
3	15	2	25
4	5.7	0	38
5	7	0	25
6	4	0	50
7	5.9	0	25
8	2.5	0	19
9	4.6	0	25
10	2.4	0	13
11	2.1	0	25
12	1.5	0	50

to the breed is a minimal 1.5% overall. However, the highest influence of this founder in an individual animal is 50%, and this opens up real opportunities for using him widely (and wisely) to enhance his overall contribution to the breed. In contrast, founder 10, a cow, has a relatively low maximum contribution to any animal (13%) and therefore it is impossible to increase her influence more broadly across the herd because her influence does not predominate in any individual animal.

One successful strategy to avoid overrepresentation of a founder male is to use males for only one or two breeding seasons. In this way a foundation sire's sons are used on foundation females, instead of the original foundation sire being used on his own daughters. The resulting progeny are then only 25% his influence, rather than the 50% that his direct sons and daughters would be, and much less than the 75% that would result from mating him to his daughters. Though the son will also be mated to his sisters to result in 50% relationship to the original sire, this is still much lower than the 75% result of using the original sire on his daughters. The strategy of using males for a short time allows for the females to have a much higher proportionate effect in the population, and is a useful strategy for assuring more uniform genetic contributions of founders.

The strategy of using a successive series of younger males on original founder females has the added advantage that it can assure retention of the maximum amount of genetic variability present in those females (Figure 13.16). This is counter to the usual, and simple, strategy of using a single male for many years, and thereby replacing most founder genetic material with that from this single founder. If younger males are used on founder females, the balance of genetic material from all founders is more likely to be proportional. A very uniform balance of founder contributions is possible by this strategy when combined with careful record keeping and the selective retention of breeding animals from the founders with the least contribution to the herd.

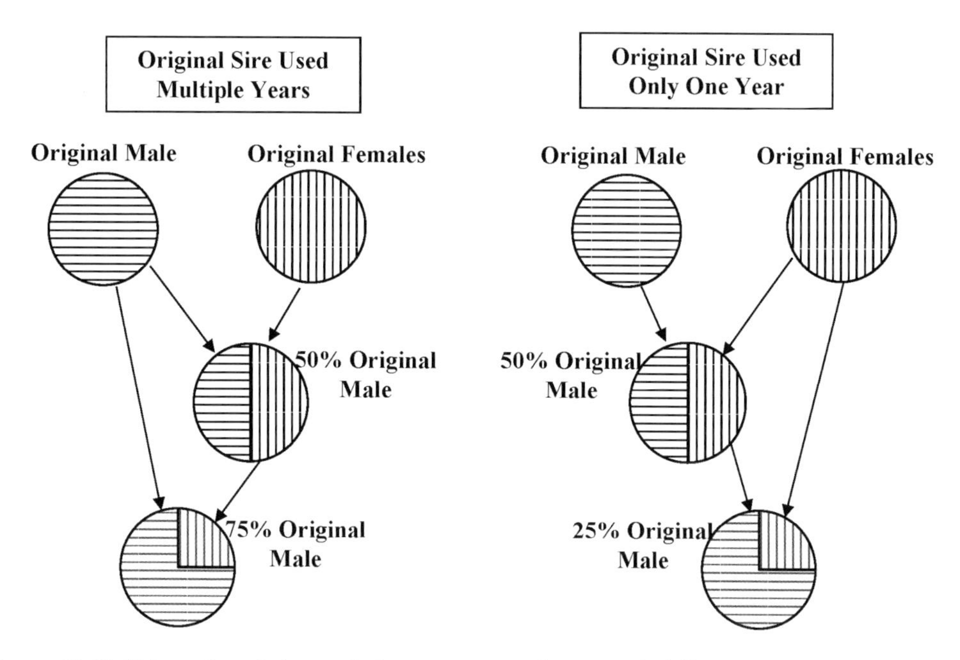

Figure 13.16 Using a foundation male for one or several years with different outcomes for the population. Figure by DPS.

In situations where multiple sires are used in a single year, or for a single generation, it is important to recruit replacements from each sire rather than from a single one of the sires (Figure 13.17). This assures that genetic diversity is retained. It can be tempting to deviate from this strategy when the sons of one sire are better than the others, but by constraining

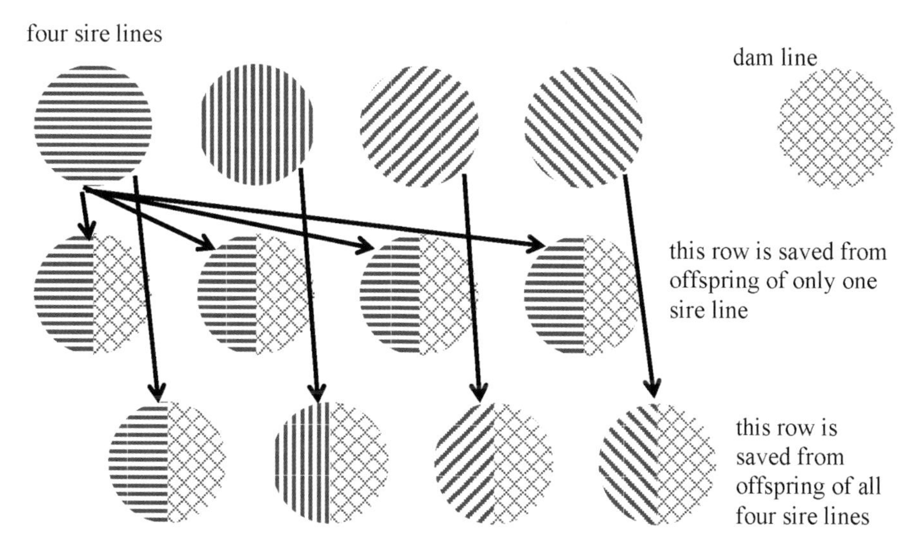

Figure 13.17 Consequences of selecting sons from only one sire or from multiple sires. The next generation is one half the sire's, one half the dam line that is used. Figure by DPS.

replacement males to be from all sires instead of only one, the result is to combine selection (select the best son!) with a genetic breadth that can lead to long-term success.

Another way that individuals become overrepresented is the "popular sire" phenomenon. The popularity of a given male may be such that many breeders use him, or his sons. This can easily swamp a breed, and is a major problem in some purebred dog populations. Show ring success is commonly the underlying reason for a sire's popularity. In many cases breeders have discovered only in later generations that a genetic problem has been identified with some such popular sires. By that time eliminating the problem has become a major logistical headache because of his influence throughout the breed. A much more secure path is to make slow progress by making certain that no single animal becomes overrepresented in a breed.

CHAPTER 14

Specific Plans for Maintenance Breeding

Many breeders find it useful to have a defined breeding protocol for planning matings, almost like a specific recipe for a delicious meal. Specific ways to manage breeding stock include several options, and some of them are explored in this chapter. No single breeding plan is a best fit for all situations. This is especially true with rare breeds. Different sizes of populations have different needs, and many breeds also have other issues such as differences in relative contributions of founder animals. These important details must not be ignored if long-term breed survival is the goal. For example, when a breed has rare founders or rare bloodlines, then special attention to these is warranted to assure that they contribute to the breed by a disproportionately large contribution. Otherwise their potential to contribute to the genetic viability of the breed will be quickly lost. Strategies for dealing with situations where imbalances need to be corrected are commonly encountered in rescue situations, and these are dealt with in Chapters 15 and 16. This chapter is devoted to the long-term maintenance of herds and breeds that already have stable numbers.

The details for maintenance breeding vary widely with individual breeds and herds, but it is possible to outline some of the more common approaches that succeed in conservation breeding systems. Breeders can then choose which one best fits their species and situation, or can adopt elements of several of them for a more tailor-made approach. No single one of these works well in all settings. Some very effective programs are based on a single element, while the success of others relies on a combination of elements.

14.1 "Regular" Conservation Breeding

This protocol was developed in response to the conservation needs of the Lazy Js herd of Yates Texas Longhorn cattle owned by Jeff Burhus, Jack Duren, and Phil Sponenberg (Figure 14.1). Even though originally designed for cattle, this plan can be adapted for other species. This protocol targeted ease of management, good cow longevity, and the constraints of maintaining a reasonably closed herd. An important goal was to make sure that all of the genetic variation needed to avoid inbreeding was available within the herd.

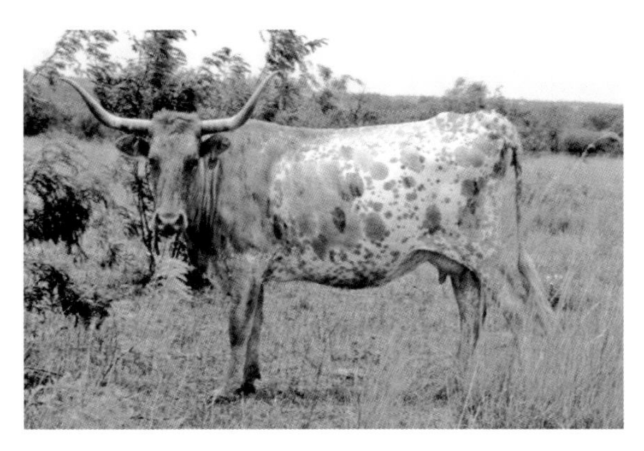

Figure 14.1 The original conservation breeding plan was developed to make the management of the Lazy Js herd of Yates Texas Longhorns as easy as possible, while also meeting production and conservation goals. Photo by DPS.

In this situation, bulls and cows from outside the herd were simply not readily available for this bloodline. In other situations, issues such as biosecurity may also offer compelling reasons to have a closed herd. Regardless of the reasons for maintaining a closed herd, the challenge is to manage isolation for many years while also assuring that inbreeding does not increase dramatically.

The mechanics of managing various species differ, and while this system was designed for the gestation length and age of maturity of Texas Longhorn cattle, it is readily adapted for any livestock species. The considerations for various species are outlined following a detailed presentation of the conservation protocols used for cattle. This conservation breeding protocol has various subtleties that address genetic management, but that also consider the practical aspects of managing cattle safely from day-to-day. Genetic goals, conservation goals, and practical constraints all contribute to the overall success of the program.

For long-term genetic management it is important to realize that one sex or the other needs to be turned over fairly quickly in order to avoid inbreeding. A herd of cows mated to the same bull for eight years churns out calves that are all half-siblings as a minimum, or are even more closely related when he is mated to his own daughters. That sort of breeding strategy drastically constrains future genetic variation, because a single bull ends up having a very disproportionate influence on the population as all younger animals are related to him. After using a bull for many years, his influence has swamped that of any other founders.

In most situations it will be practical to use a bull for a short period (usually a year) and then replace him. This helps genetic management, while also making herd management easy. It also diminishes the swamping of the genetic structure of the herd by a single animal and assures that young bulls are in the herd instead of older bulls. Younger bulls tend to present fewer headaches for the day-to-day management or the safety of personnel, facilities, and other animals. This manageability aspect varies across both species and breed, but in most species, it is generally true that younger males are easier to manage than are older ones (Figure 14.2).

The rapid turnover of bulls does have the disadvantage of the breeder never having the luxury of developing a truly outstanding mature herd sire and enjoying him for several years. This is not a trivial or merely sentimental drawback, because such animals can be a joy to produce and to manage. Producing them can be one of the important emotional as well

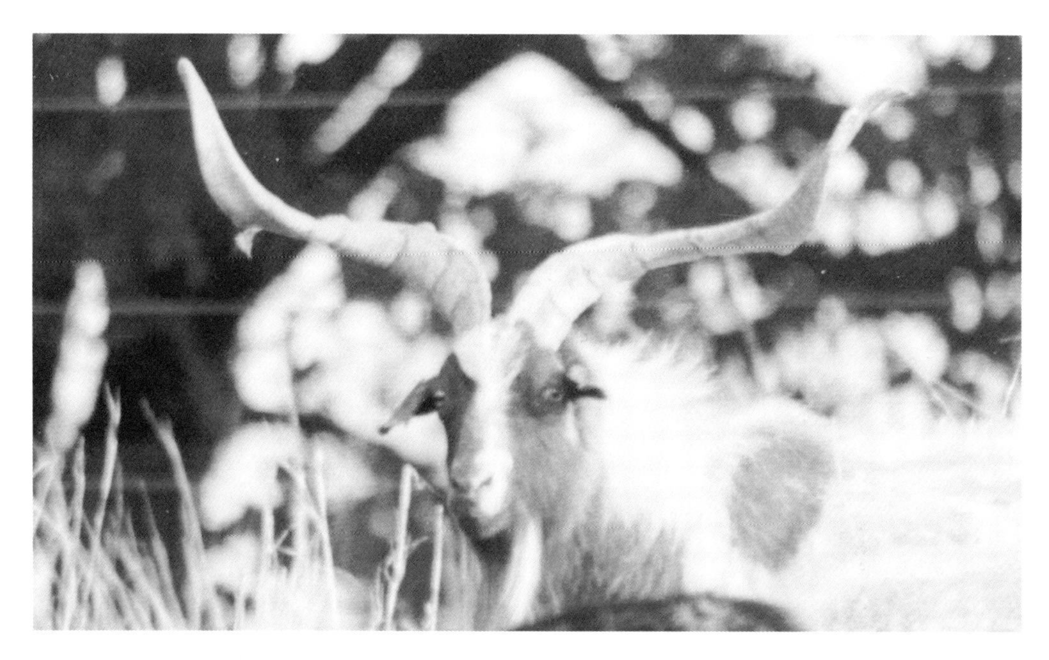

Figure 14.2 This mature Myotonic buck is magnificent, but developed a hobby at maturity: battering fences! Photo by DPS.

as economic paybacks for animal breeders. Unfortunately, issues of genetic management lead to the conclusion that keeping males for several years is a long-term mistake in most conservation situations.

The herd can be managed as a single unit, but within the herd individual animals have specific identities as to which bloodline they represent. The first step is to subdivide the population into three groups. Keep in mind that this is a subdivision by identity and not by separating the herd into different sub herds in different pastures. This division is most effectively done by bloodline or family affiliation, but other strategies could be used. The best strategy for subdivision reflects both the final numbers in each group and their genetic relationships. The issue of numbers is important because having relatively equal numbers in each group simplifies the practical management and recruitment of replacement animals into the subgroups. The issue of genetic relatedness is important. If the groups are as genetically distinct from one another as is possible, then the management of inbreeding becomes more straightforward.

The three subgroups are labeled "A," "B," and "C." In the ideal situation, the "A" animals will be related to one another and not to "B" and "C," and so on with each group. The subgroups can be based on herd of origin, or family relationships, or other ways to assure that each subgroup has some genetic difference from the remaining animals even if they all reside in the same herd.

In a single herd, the program works well when three lines of bulls are used sequentially in the herd. The bulls are used on the entire herd, each bull for one year. This fine detail also varies from situation to situation. The Lazy Js herd resided in Nursery, Texas, and so year-round calving was reasonable. Bulls could be left in for an entire year without risking

Table 14.1 Management of a small population by subdivision into three foundation bloodlines with sequential use of bulls over the entire herd. This is a complicated table with lots of details in it. This table illustrates how the genetic material reorganizes over time while still allowing both linebreeding and linecrossing.

Year	Bulls			Line membership of cows, with calves they produce						
	A	B	C	A	AB	AC	B	BC	C	ABC
1	Calves	In herd, mating	Yearlings	A	A	A	AB	ABC	AC	A, AB, or AC
2	Yearlings	Calves	In herd, mating	AB	B	ABC	B	B	BC	B, AB, or BC
3	In herd, mating	Yearlings	Calves	AC	ABC	C	BC	C	C	C, AC, or BC
4	Calves	In herd, mating	Yearlings	A	A	A	AB	ABC	AC	A, AB, or AC
5	Yearlings	Calves	In herd, mating	AB	B	ABC	B	B	BC	B, AB, or BC
6	In herd, mating	Yearlings	Calves	CA	ABC	C	BC	C	C	C, AC, or BC

the birth of calves in seasons of the year where calf survival would be in doubt. The recommendation of using each bull for only one year can stand even for other breeds in other climates where seasonal reproduction is more likely to be the norm.

Sequential use of the bulls of the various lines dictates where each bull is, and what he is doing, as illustrated in Table 14.1. If a Line A bull was used for mating the cows last year, then the calves born this year are Line A calves (or Line A crosses), growing at the sides of their mothers until they are weaned. The Line B bull is in the herd, mating the cows for next year's calves. The Line C bulls are yearlings from last year's calf crop which are weaned and growing. At the end of the year, the Line B bull is sold (his calves will be born next year), and the best Line C yearling is now a coming two-year-old and is put into the herd to mate the cows. The Line A calves have been weaned and are now yearlings, growing out to see which one is best. This strategy accomplishes the separation of genetics by time rather than by fences because each line is used in a different year. Keeping the herd as one unit can be a boon to general husbandry concerns because separate pastures are not needed.

The specifics of the program demand that animals be labeled with their bloodline identity. To do this, any animal that is over 76% one line should be designated as that line, regardless of the remaining 24% of the breeding. Similarly, any animal with at least 25% the breeding of a foundation line should also have that line included in its designation. So, an animal that is 50% A, 25% B, and 25% C could be labeled "ABC," while one that is 50% A, 44% B, and 6% C is simply "AB," and one that is 87% A and 13% B is simply "A." While these minority genetic influences can be important in some situations, they complicate record keeping beyond what is practical and have only minimal consequences for managing the protocol.

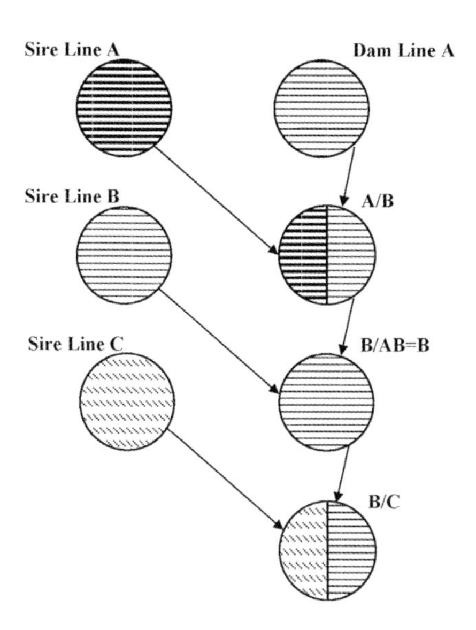

Figure 14.3 The use of linebred sires with varying lines of linebred and linecross dams can modulate the progression of the genetic material through generations. Figure by DPS.

The important detail in this management scheme is that the basic rules for line assignment allow the genetic material to move from linebred to linecrossed individuals, and then back into linebred individuals (Figure 14.3). So, for example, a linebred "A" dam mated to a linebred "B" sire produces a linecrossed "AB" offspring. This "AB" offspring, though linecrossed, can contribute linebred offspring to both the "A" line and "B" line following mating to sires from those lines. AB animals can also contribute linecrossed individuals following mating to a "C" line sire.

Rotation of sires through the entire herd assures that linecrossed and linebred animals are being produced every year. The system works well, and diversity is maximized in the long term if the replacement females include both linebred and linecrossed heifer calves. The bulls, in contrast, should always be linebred. This avoids the whole herd becoming a uniform mix of the three strains. In the case of female replacements it is important for breeders to assure retention in the herd of both linebred and linecrossed replacements every year. For example, failing to retain "AC" animals in year three could result in this category being lost (even if only temporarily) so that one portion of the distribution of the genetic material is missing. In addition, bull candidates should come from different dams to assure that no single maternal source of genetics becomes overrepresented in the herd.

Using linecross bulls could indeed work in some situations, but over the long term the use of linecross bulls is a strategy that actually increases the overall inbreeding more than the sequential use of linebred bulls from different lines does. This is not a trivial detail, because the linecross bulls may actually have a bit more "bloom" on them than the linebred bulls. Using linecrossed bulls only assures closer relationships across the entire herd in a few generations, ending up in a situation in which there is nowhere to go within the herd for linecrosses. If the goal is a closed, isolated herd, then using linecross bulls defeats success.

14.2 Variations on "Regular" Conservation Breeding

If the size of the herd warrants, it can be split into two or three breeding groups, each with a different bull. It is also possible for multiple breeders to cooperate, each having a distinct herd but periodically swapping bull calves. In either case it becomes possible to use multiple males in any given year, each on his own group of cows as a single-sire herd. If the herd has three strains in it, they should all participate in each sub herd. That way the bull calves produced in one herd can be used in the cooperating herd. So, the line A bull calves from the first herd could be used in the second herd, and the line A bull calves from the second herd could be used back in the first herd. By doing this with each strain each year, the level of relatedness of mates is kept low for many generations.

This multiple herd system is similar to the "kinship breeding" protocol used in the Netherlands by cattle breeders in organic production that excludes the use of artificial insemination or embryo transfer. Individual breeders use multiple bulls in single-sire groups. Each bull is used at a young age and only for one year. Bull replacements are kept from each group of half-siblings. Periodically, bulls are swapped among the collaborating breeders when they see a need for the enhancement of specific traits. Following the use of a newly introduced bull, his offspring are deliberately taken back to mates from within the herd. This limits the introduced genetic material to only 25% influence, preserving the distinctions between the various herds, while at the same time allowing for some degree of genetic exchange among them.

In some situations, mating is seasonal rather than year-round. In that case it can ease management for the herds to be split up for breeding, and then put back together as one large herd for the rest of the year. The goal is to maximize both the ease of management as well as the effective manipulation of the genetics of the population.

Some aspects of this system need to be carefully evaluated, with the option of deviations from it in situations where these serve conservation better than a rigid adherence to a set system. Endangered bloodlines are conserved more adequately if the uniqueness of the line is not diminished with the linecrosses, at least initially. This is usually true of old, distinctive lines that are walking a tightrope between being rare and at risk of extinction if numbers slip, but also numerically strong enough to have the genetic variation needed to go forward if numbers of the line are rapidly increased. In that case, the rare line itself can be sorted into three sublines, based on pedigrees, with the different sublines being managed as outlined above. This is especially wise in rescue situations, where it is best to manage the rescue for a few generations before putting the animals in a more generic conservation breeding program. Specific rescue protocols are outlined in Chapter 16.

In some breeds certain bloodlines may be diminished to very low numbers, below the level at which persistence in isolation is likely to succeed. In these cases it is practical to put the rare lines together with other similarly rare lines into a single composite line (Figure 14.4). The genetic material they offer is then not lost, and the use of linebred males and females assures that the influence of the line is not eroded over time. In contrast, if these "rare line" animals are stuck in with "common line" animals, then their genetic uniqueness will eventually get swallowed up and will be lost to the breed and to the future.

Using multiple sires in the herd is routine for some species, breeds, or management

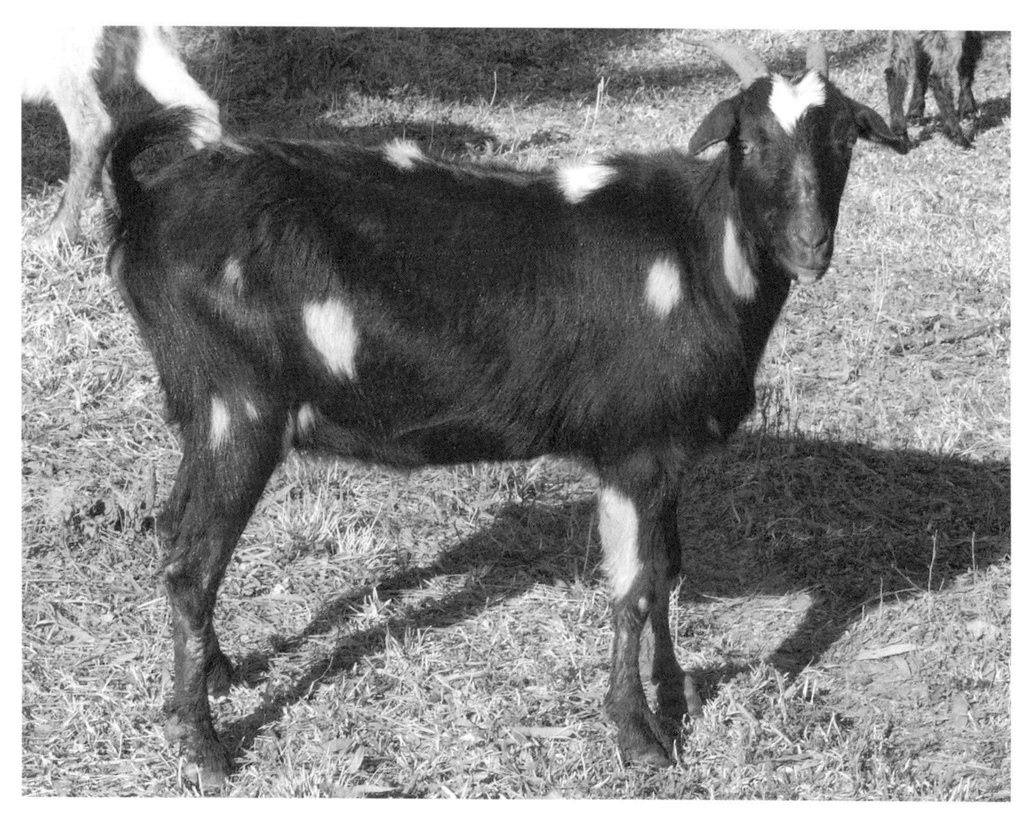

Figure 14.4 Spanish goats from the coastal islands of South Carolina hail from a few different herds, each with only a few animals. Blending these together allows for the maintenance of the unique genetic resource while also assuring long-term success in conservation. Photo by JB.

systems. This is especially true of cattle, sheep, and goats on extensive ranges, as well as chickens, ducks, and turkeys in nearly every situation. Using multiple sires can complicate the assignment of the offspring into the various lines within the herd. One strategy that allows for the use of multiple sire matings is to use groups of sires that are half-brothers from a single sire. This allows the breeder to know at least 75% of the pedigree of the resulting offspring (dam, and paternal grandsire), making it easier for the breeder to identify and manage the genetic material. The selection of the group of half-brothers can assure that they are all linebred representatives of their sire's line. Using a group of bulls each from a different line defeats this goal, and should generally be avoided.

14.2.1 Strategies for Tracking Animals to Manage Bloodlines

Animal inventories can easily become problematic, especially for owners of large populations. Owners should always keep a current inventory of animals in order to manage breeding decisions. This should include individual animal identity and bloodline. There are multiple ways to tackle this problem. One solution is to use computer-based spreadsheets, and this works successfully for many people. Spreadsheets can be manipulated in various ways, and some also allow trial matings to be conducted in order to see the potential results. Spreadsheets should include animal identification, bloodline percentages, age, and other details that might be important, such as the results of any genetic testing.

Another simple but elegant idea that links animals to bloodlines in a visual manner comes from Pam Hand and was published in the Barbados Blackbelly Sheep Association International newsletter, "*Blackbelly Banner*," in 2016. This involves using index cards to track animal identification. The front of each index card is used for the animal's identification, age, bloodline percentage, results of genetic testing, and any other details needed. The back of the card can have the animal's two-generation pedigree, or even more generations if that is helpful. Different bloodlines are assigned different colors of index cards. So, line A might be blue, line B pink, line C yellow, and so on for any additional bloodlines in the herd. The males and females can be separated either by using different colors, or by using the card horizontally for females and vertically for males. Each animal has its own card, and as animals leave the herd, their card can be removed. As young stock are born, a card can be generated for each one.

The deck of cards represents the entire population, and has the advantage of the breeder being able to arrange the individual cards on a table or other surface. This allows animals to be arranged in various ways to plan breeding groups. The technique also works well to put animals into "starter groups" for new breeders, because it provides a visual representation of the genetic variation going into the group. The technique permits a quick visual check on the degree of both linebreeding and linecrossing going on as the groups are put together in different ways.

14.2.2 *Small Populations with Single Males*

Some breeders have no options other than to have a relatively small population, and husbandry constraints dictate that these be mated as a single group. This is an especially common situation with sheep and goats. These species, and others that have a relatively short generation interval and a low age of maturity, can still be managed effectively for conservation even with this constraint.

In this situation a single male is used, and is replaced each year. To the extent possible, the replacement males should be selected from different dams, and ideally from the oldest dams. If the founder dams are unrelated, and if they have good longevity, this system can work as a closed population for several years. This strategy is charted in Table 14.2.

One negative aspect of this strategy is that females are routinely mated to close relatives. This is especially true for the younger females. Over a few years this means that all young stock are interrelated, and the only unrelated animals are the original founders. As a result, this strategy requires the occasional introduction of outside breeding animals and in most cases, these will be males.

14.2.3 *Managing Populations Where Males Have Long Careers*

Breeding programs where males are kept for long careers are more difficult to manage over the long term than programs where males are only used for a short time. The strategy of retaining males for long breeding careers is common in some species, notably horses and donkeys. The consequences need to be carefully considered in order for conservation to succeed (Figure 14.5).

Table 14.2 Management of a small population with mating to a single male. The example presented here is a single founding male (A), and six females (B, C, D, E, F, and G) that are unrelated, with B the oldest and G the youngest. Assumptions are that male replacements are always retained from a founder female rather than a younger female. This is unrealistic in many situations, and in that regard this table is the "best case" for genetic distance. It still demonstrates a gradual mixing of genetic material as the years progress. Eventually, outside genetics will need to be introduced, but this system can succeed for several years before that is necessary.

Year Breeding male	Results produced by each female					
	B	C	D	E	F	G
1 Male A	AB	AC	AD	AE	AF	AG
2 Male AB	B/A	C/AB	D/AB	E/AB	F/AB	G/AB
3 Male C/AB	B/AC	C/AB	D/ABC	E/ABC	F/ABC	G/ABC
4 Male D/ABC	B/ACD	C/ABD	D/ABC	E/ABCD	F/ABCD	G/ABCD
5 Male E/ABCD	B/ACDE	C/ABDE	D/ABDE	E/ABCD	F/ABCDE	G/ABCDE
6 Male F/ABCDE	B/ACDEF	C/ABDEF	D/ABCEF	E/ABCDF	F/ABCDE	G/ ABCDEF
7 Male G/ABCDEF	B/ ACDEFG	C/ ABDEFG	D/ ABCEFG	E/ ABCDFG	F/ ABCDEG	G/ ABCDEF

One problem with maintaining males for long careers is deciding when and how to select a replacement. This must be done judiciously so that a replacement is available should the male meet an untimely demise. However, male management (especially for stallions and jacks) can be problematic for many breeds and situations, so holding on to several extra young males is usually not an attractive option. The answer to this dilemma will need to be tailor-made to specific situations. At the very least the candidate young males should come from the rarest of the bloodlines involved, rather than dipping into the same common bloodlines repeatedly.

When males are kept for long careers, the fates of their daughters can also become problematic. They need to be moved to other herds or situations to avoid sire-daughter matings. This needs to be considered strategically. In a situation where a breeder manages multiple herds each with its own male, the solution is usually to move the young females along to the next group. The daughters of these young females can then be moved along in their own turn, and the result is that linebreeding is reduced to sire-granddaughter matings, or sire-great-granddaughter matings, which are much less inbred than the sire-daughter matings would have been.

Maintaining males for long breeding careers can succeed, especially for those species

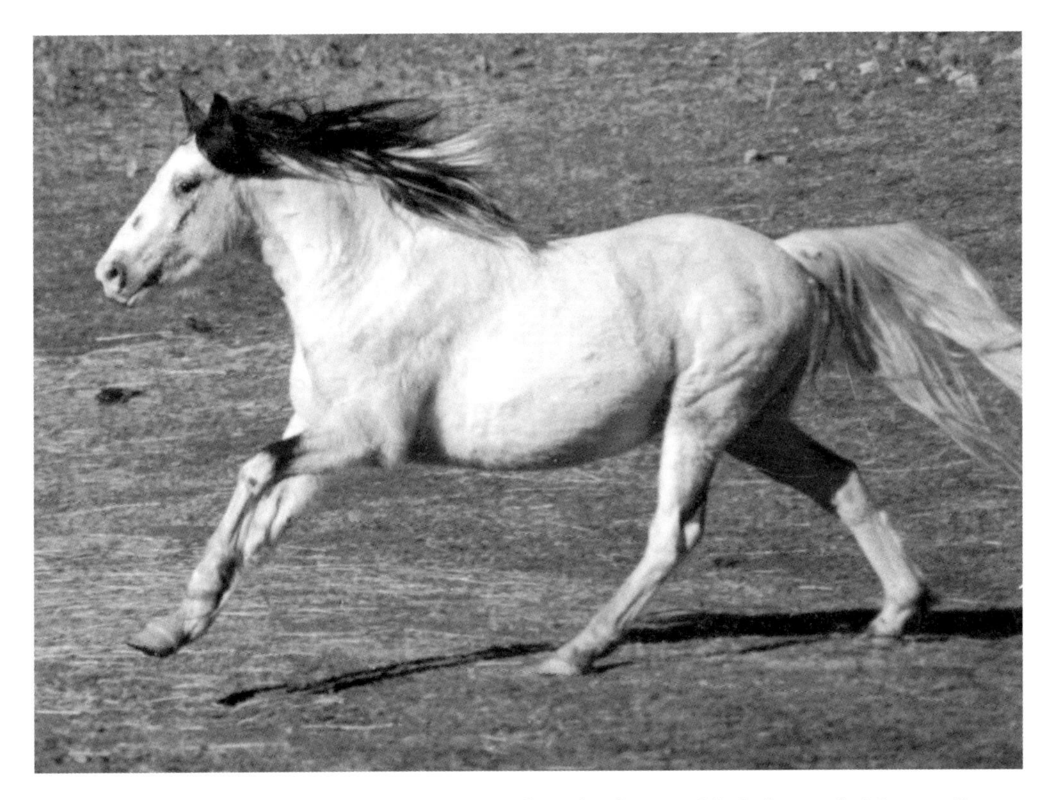

Figure 14.5 Beechkeld Icktinicki is a Choctaw stallion that has sired foals for nearly 30 years. By carefully managing his influence it has been possible to take advantage of his rare bloodlines yet not swamp the other bloodlines of the breed. Photo by DPS.

in which only few or moderate numbers of females are put to an individual male in most years. Horses, donkeys, and some poultry systems fit this model. This strategy also usually works best in situations where multiple breeders can cooperate, or a single breeder has the infrastructure to manage several different breeding groups concurrently.

14.3 Species Considerations for Conservation Breeding

The plans for conservation breeding work well with cattle, and were designed for them due to the husbandry advantages of using two-year-old bulls, the gestation length of cattle, and other factors specific for cattle. Each species has its own peculiar array of gestation length, age of maturity, and group husbandry issues, and these must be considered if success is to be achieved with this conservation breeding protocol.

14.3.1 Sheep and Goats

Sheep and goats are both managed in groups. Males and females of most breeds mature at or sometimes before a year old. Many breeds of both sheep and goats are seasonal breeders, meaning they mate in the autumn to produce young in the spring. Despite their five-month gestation period, it is still only possible to achieve one birth per female per year in many

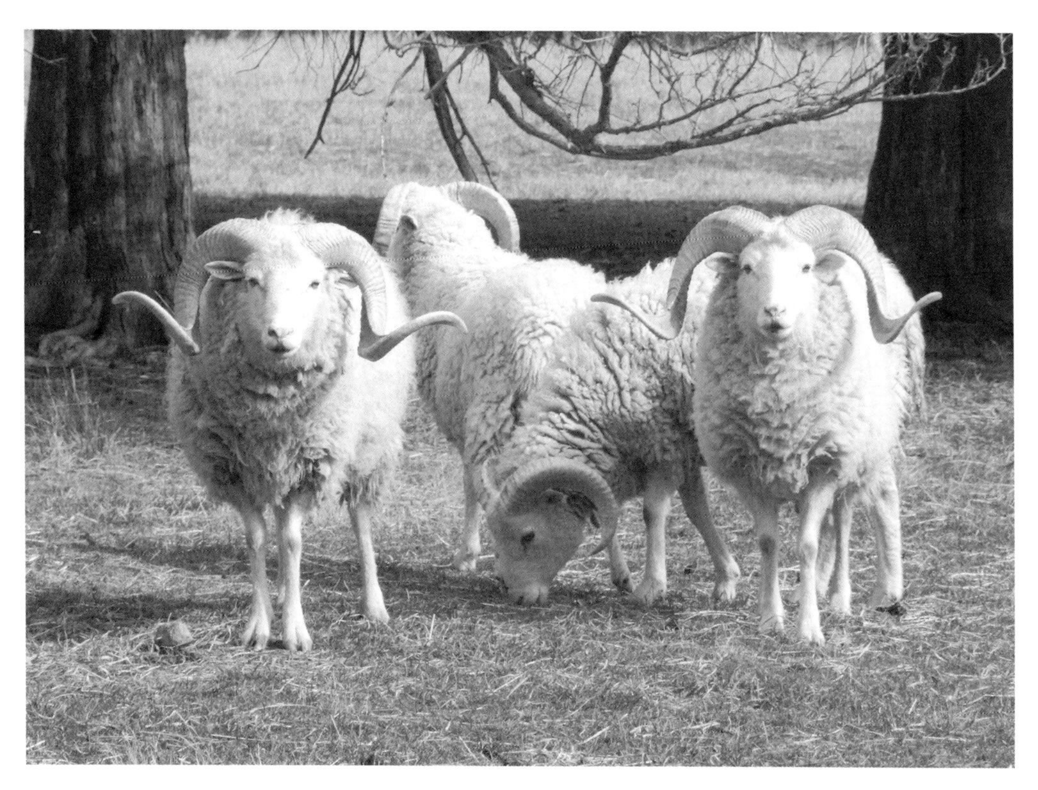

Figure 14.6 Gulf Coast sheep present several challenges to conservation breeding, including the early maturation of males, as well as multi-sire breeding. Photo by JB.

breeds. A positive attribute of both species is the relatively frequent occurrence of twins and even triplets, which can boost numbers rapidly, although prolificacy varies greatly from breed to breed.

The conservation breeding protocol hits a slight snag with sheep and goats when compared with cattle. For both sheep and goats it is usually convenient to use breeding males at 18 months old (their second autumn), rather than when they are 30 months old (their third autumn) (Figure 14.6). If the males are used at 18 months old, and if the group is run as a single unit, the result is that only two lines are going through the herd/flock instead of the three lines suggested for cattle. Basing the program on only two lines is unlikely to adequately avoid inbreeding after a few cycles of the protocol. For sheep and goats the conservation breeding protocol works better when the population is divided into two or more breeding groups. This ends up separating the male lines by physical space rather than time as is the case in the cattle protocol. If the population is mated in two different groups, each to an 18-month-old sire, the result is that two bloodlines go through each of two herds, resulting in a total of four bloodlines. This modification provides for good success, but requires sufficient infrastructure for the subdivision of breeding groups.

14.3.2 *Swine*

Swine vary greatly in general husbandry practices, from highly intensive confinement to free-range management. One huge advantage of swine is their production of litters. Most breeds also mature rapidly, so that mating at six or seven months old is reasonable in many situations. In addition, sows routinely produce two litters per year. Swine tend to be mated in smaller groups than cattle, sheep, or goats. It is also common practice in many herds to hand mate swine by individual pairs rather than as groups. Housing and managing multiple boars can be problematic, but is reasonable in most situations. Carefully planned individual matings are therefore more possible and practical with swine than for most ruminant species.

The conservation protocol can work well with swine, although it requires the maintenance of multiple males of distinct bloodlines. If a stand-alone conservation herd is managed, then numbers of sows will have to be adequate to represent different distinct bloodlines. For the long-term management of an isolated population this will require both linebred and linecrossed sows, increasing numbers even more. A fairly minimal approach would be the use of a sow from each of three bloodlines, and their crosses with one another. That works out to a minimum of six sows and three boars. The boars would be linebred A, B, C, and the sows would be linebred A, B, C, and linecross AB, AC, and BC. As with all breeding schemes, higher numbers work even better.

14.3.3 *Rabbits*

Rabbits reproduce like rabbits! This makes them a good match for conservation protocols and rescue protocols. They are housed individually, produce litters, mature rapidly, and are hand mated by pairs. Individual housing makes the maintenance of multiple males simpler than it is for other species, due to the relatively small space needed as well as the modest housing needs. The fact of litter production means that selection can be ongoing, and also means that expansion of a population is easily possible when needed. Rapid maturation helps the conservation protocols to succeed, because males of appropriate line composition can be easily produced, raised, and then used. Hand mating contributes to genetic management because each mating can be accomplished with specific goals in mind.

14.3.4 *Poultry*

At first glance, poultry seem to have several characteristics that would facilitate conservation. Poultry are generally prolific, and they mature rapidly. Longevity of reproduction is a problem, because egg production for all but geese tends to fall off rapidly with age. Birds that are even a few years old are problematic for assuring genetic contributions. Another practical obstacle is the lack of easy, rapid identification of individual birds in most situations. This makes accurate pedigrees impossible in those situations, which can defeat the strategies for conservation by thwarting the assignment of bloodline composition of recruits into the breeding population.

Ducks and chickens have advantages because the females and males are not too choosy about mates. This provides opportunities for the sequential use of males within a population, so that while individual pedigrees may not be known (unless breeders resort to trap-nesting), a general assignment to a group may be possible. Turkey hens are choosier, so rapid turnover of toms is unlikely to succeed. Geese have long productive lives and form lasting pair-bonds that are difficult to disrupt, bringing a host of challenges that are unique to this species.

The result of all these issues is that poultry generally fit poorly into the conservation protocol developed for cattle. Fortunately, other breeding schemes have proven successful for breed maintenance in poultry species. Many of these were developed specifically for poultry, and several are outlined in section 14.5 of this chapter.

14.3.5 Horses and Donkeys

Horses and donkeys mature slowly, so that they are initially mated only at three years of age or older. The training of animals for work or saddle use also contributes to the time investment in individual animals, so most animals that are destined for reproduction are kept in use for long breeding careers. Mating is seasonal, in the spring. Gestation is about a year for both, and the result is that the maximum expected reproductive rate is a single offspring each year. They are also rarely mated in large herds. For these reasons, horses and donkeys fit poorly into conservation breeding protocols (Figure 14.7).

Any breeding protocol for horses and donkeys needs to be tailored for their unique maturation and reproductive aspects. The goal of using multiple males still holds true and can be especially challenging depending on how stallions and jacks are managed. When these

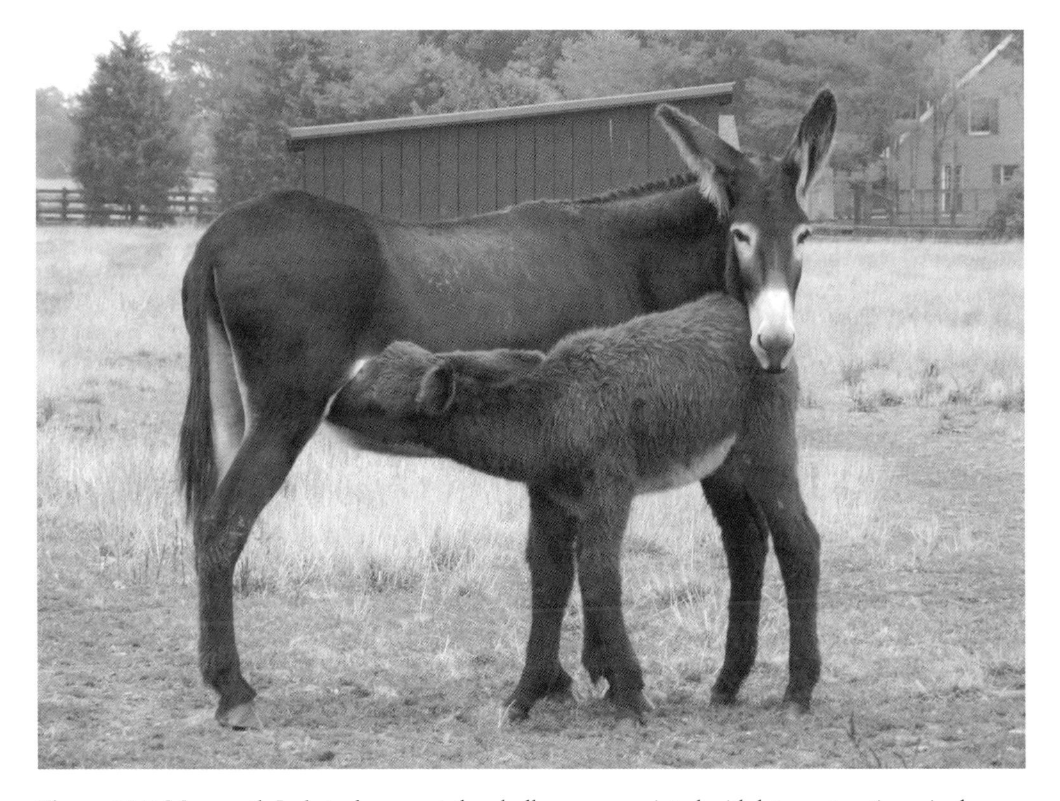

Figure 14.7 Mammoth Jackstock present the challenges associated with late maturation, single births, and long breeding careers for breeding jacks. Photo by JB.

species are managed in free-ranging herds, a further complication arises from the need to keep the breeding groups stable due to ease of management and social cohesion of groups. The result is that the females are repeatedly mated to the same stallion or jack. This eases management concerns, but it does not serve long-term conservation optimally to the extent that it constrains the genetic mixes that go to the next generation. Wherever possible the mares should produce foals to different mates, rather than always to the same mates.

The peculiarities of horses and donkeys assure that only large breeding programs can truly stand alone in isolation from others. The cooperation among breeders that is ideal for all species is nearly essential for the conservation breeding of horses and donkeys.

14.3.6 Dogs

Dogs, due to their being individually mated, also break the rules of the conservation breeding protocol. However, certain aspects can be adopted and used to good success. This is especially true if rare bloodlines need to be conserved and expanded. Dog breeders have the advantages of being able to individually mate each pair, and having litters of pups from which to select the next individuals for a breeding program. The latter is an especially important advantage when trying to expand the genetic influence of rare bloodlines.

14.4 Rotational Breeding or Spiral Breeding

Rotational breeding is also called spiral breeding, and is a commonly used strategy for many situations. The most common variant of this system designates the females into groups, usually containing four or so animals. Female offspring remain in the same group as their dams. Male offspring are moved on to the next group. The goal is to avoid the population going in only a single direction toward only one of the sublines. Recruiting breeding animals from all four groups solves this potential problem.

Gloucestershire Old Spots hog breeders use this system (Figure 14.8), with the groups designated by colors: green, blue, red, and black. Groups could also be labeled by numbers or letters. If the starting point is four groups, then these can be labeled A, B, C, and D. The same considerations that succeed for the conservation breeding protocol can be used for establishing these groups, with both pedigree and number considerations affecting the final grouping. Females are retained in their birth group, while males are advanced to the next group as shown in Figure 14.9.

The genetic consequences of rotational breeding are subtle and can be confusing. It is possible to chart these out in successive generations, under the assumption that the founding groups were distinct bloodlines: A, B, C, and D. The composition of the various groups progresses over multiple generations due to the movement of males and the retention of females. This is detailed in Table 14.3.

The first round of rotational mating has the males from one group going on to the next group, so the first generation of offspring would be the result of male A mating with females in group B, male B to females C, and so on. As a result, the youngsters in the second generation of group A would be 50% A and 50% D, because group A received a male from D.

The details of blending the genetic material over several generations can get complicated, but if considered step-by-step, the general pattern emerges. One detail is that the

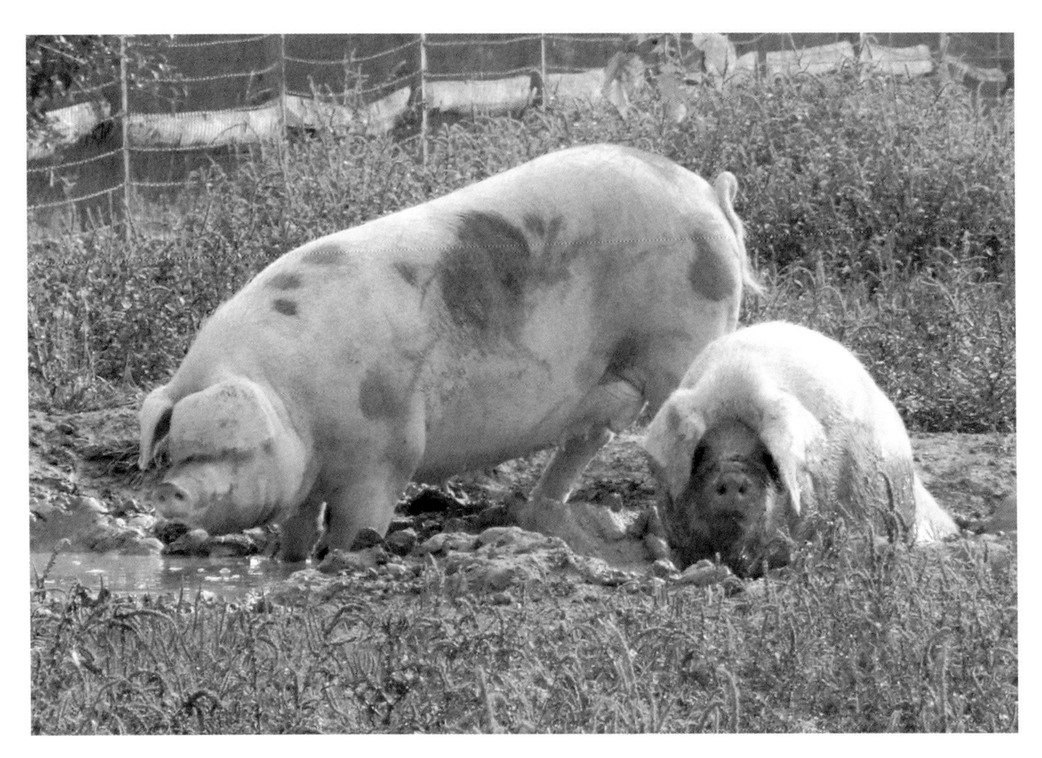

Figure 14.8 Breeders of Gloucestershire Old Spots hogs have used rotational breeding successfully for many generations. Photo by JB.

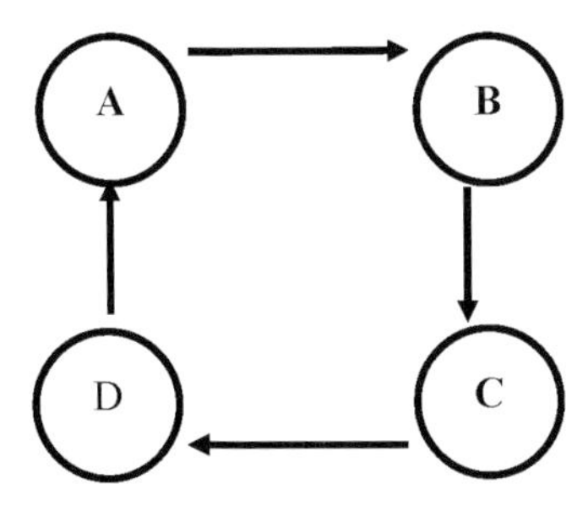

Figure 14.9 Rotational, or spiral, breeding is easily charted. Female offspring are retained in their birth group, while male offspring are used in the next group. Figure by DPS.

breeding groups begin to have genetically mixed female members even though they start as one single line. This occurs because females are retained in the group over multiple production cycles, each having received a different male over the generations. In the beginning, each group consists of founder females. If these are kept in production for multiple years (as is common) then the oldest females will retain the genetic material from one of the original founder strains unmixed. Their female descendants, though, each have a combination of various founder strains. The specific blend depends on the generation of male that is used.

Table 14.3 Tracking the percentage bloodlines in a rotational breeding plan can be daunting if pursued over several generations. This table is simplified and only shows the results of mating animals which both come from the same generation. If animals of different generations are mated, the results vary. This table therefore reflects the "maximally mixed" situation, which is the "worst case" result because each generation results in lineages becoming mixed with one another rather than remaining distinct. Even though the genetic material becomes mixed, this strategy can work over several generations, especially when combined with effective selection for productivity and viability.

Generation	A	B	C	D
1	100% A	100% B	100% C	100% D
2	50% A	50% A	50% B	50% C
	50% D	50% B	50% C	50% D
3	25% A	50% A	25% A	0% A
	0% B	25% B	50% B	25% B
	25% C	0% C	25% C	50% C
	50% D	25% D	0% D	25% D
4	12.5% A	37.5% A	37.5% A	12.5% A
	12.5% B	12.5% B	37.5% B	37.5% B
	37.5% C	12.5% C	12.5% C	37.5% C
	37.5% D	37.5% D	12.5% D	12.5% D
5	12.5% A	25% A	37.5% A	25% A
	25% B	12.5% B	25% B	37.5% B
	37.5% C	25% C	12.5% C	25% C
	25% D	12.5% D	25% D	12.5% D
6	18.75% A	18.75% A	31.25% A	31.25% A
	31.25% B	18.75% B	18.75% B	31.25% B
	31.25% C	31.25% C	18.75% C	18.75% C
	18.75% D	31.25% D	31.25% D	18.75% D
7	25% A	18.75% A	25% A	31.25% A
	31.25% B	25% B	18.75% B	25% B
	25% C	31.25% C	25% C	18.75% C
	18.75% D	25% D	31.25% D	25% D

As the generations proceed the relative contributions become a bit more tedious to tease out, especially if multiple generations of females are retained in the same group. While the details over the entire group become overwhelming, it is possible to figure out the specific ancestral influences that would be present in animals produced in any given generation of one of the groups. One way to chart this out is to assume that in each generation the males come from the youngest females. While this might not always be the case, it works well for a demonstration of the extent to which rotational breeding can blend the genetic material in a population. In the fifth generation, the sire of animals produced in the second group is ABBCBCCDBCCDCDDA, the dam is BCCDCDDACDDADAAB. While this is daunting, each letter represents 6.25% of the breeding of the animal. By summing up the contributions to the offspring, this "fifth generation, second group" animal would be 18.8% the influence of original group A, 18.8% the influence of original group B, 31.3% the influence of original group C, and 31.3% the influence of original group D. Table 14.3 tracks the bloodline components of the latest generation produced each year, realizing that this is the "worst case" situation and ignoring the actual percentages of influence produced by the older females in the group. The older females retain a higher percentage influence of the original bloodlines, while the younger ones successively become more and more mixed.

An interesting detail is that the genetic influence of the original group actually declines within the group that bears the same label. The animals of the most recent generation maximally reflect this trend. The genetic material of each group is not lost, but tends to move on to the other groups. A second detail is that over multiple generations the eventual mix of genetic material from the foundation stock becomes relatively evenly distributed. This is true even after relatively few generations. The curious fact is that the influence of the original founders of a group does remain a minority influence in the youngest animals in that group after a few generations.

When coupled with selection for vitality and production this breeding management protocol is likely to maintain a sufficient genetic distance among the groups, and to work as a long-term strategy for population management. A potential problem is the long-term tendency for a relatively even mixture of the founding lines across the entire population. With that even mixture comes the inability to avoid inbreeding, because eventually all animals within the population are related to one another, even if that relationship is distant. This is countered, at least somewhat, by pushing that inbreeding back further into more distant generations. This gives genetic material more opportunity to reorganize, which should at least theoretically diminish some of the threats of inbreeding depression.

The greater the number of groups, the greater the number of generations before the uniform mixture becomes evident. This is likely of less concern in large populations of those species that have long generation intervals than it would be in small populations of species with a rapid turnover of generations. Rabbits, swine, and poultry have maturation rates that at least potentially allow the turnover of generations to be very rapid, even if most breeders do not maximally exploit this potential.

While this system can and does work for individual herds and flocks, it can also be modified to work with multiple cooperating breeders. Each breeder can pass along a select male to the next breeder, and this male can be inserted into the system by joining any specific one of the groups. This allows for a rapid introduction of new genetic material into one group, with a slow diffusion to the others that are more downstream. One good way to manage long-term genetic diversity with this system is to run it as two cooperating herds of four groups each. Each herd manages the rotations in isolation for four generations. The fifth generation sees an exchange of males from the four groups of one herd to the four groups of the other. The result over the first four generations is demonstrated in Figure 14.10.

Then in the fifth year, males from the ABCD groups go to the EFGH groups, and vice versa as shown in Figure 14.11. This modification provides for better maintenance of genetic

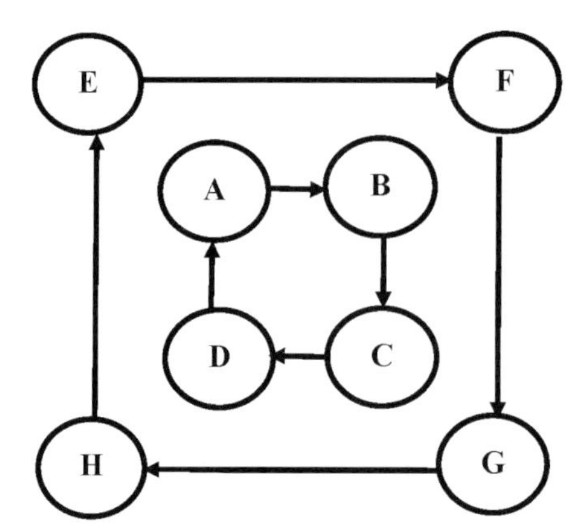

Figure 14.10 Rotational breeding can be varied by including more groups. This example has eight groups, working in cooperation with one another for periodic swaps of breeding stock.
Figure by DPS.

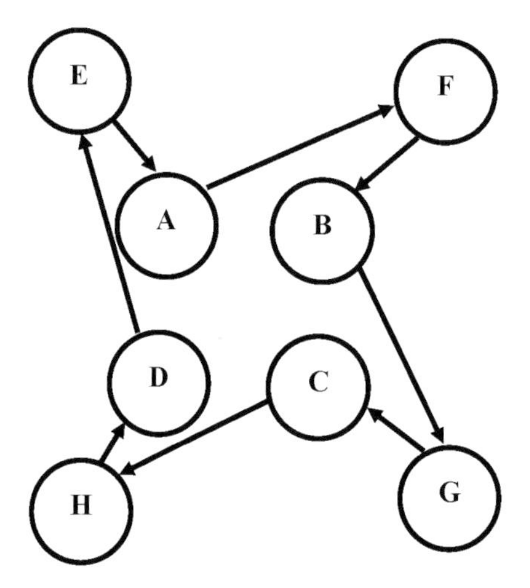

Figure 14.11 Cooperating herds can swap breeding animals every five generations or so.
Figure by DPS.

diversity over greater numbers of generations, because it collapses down on a uniform genetic mixture much more slowly.

14.5 Poultry Plans (except Geese!)

Poultry breeding presents several challenges. From the outset, geese are different. The tendency of geese to develop strong and exclusive pair-bonds means that they are usually mated as pairs. Geese should be mated in the anticipation that the entire production from any individual goose or gander is going to be limited to a single mate for its entire long productive life. Chickens and ducks are the least fussy about mates, while turkey hens can take months to accept a new tom (14.12). Conservation breeders cannot ignore these quirks!

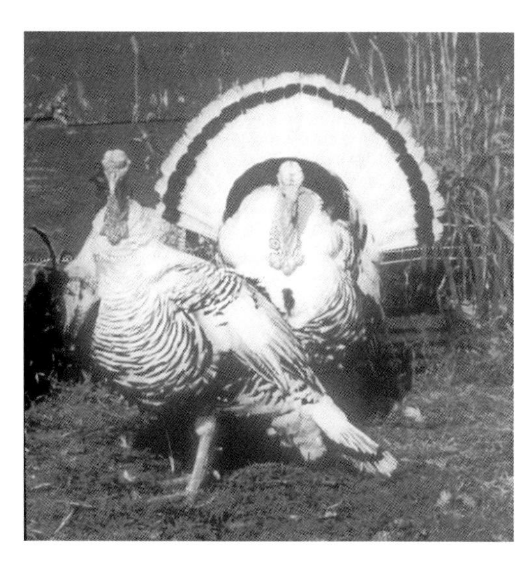

Figure 14.12 Turkey hens take time to adjust to new toms, and this needs to be considered when formulating breeding plans. Photo by DPS.

Unlike livestock, accurate pedigrees can be tedious for poultry because trap-nests must be used in order to match eggs with specific females. Breeders also need to carefully manage the time frame over which specific males are in the flock, because eggs can be fertilized by a mating that occurred up to a month previously. A strategy used by some exhibition and industrial breeders is to mate poultry in pairs or trios to ensure accurate pedigrees. The main detractor from this strategy is the need for separate housing and husbandry for each small group.

Poultry breeding plans go by various names. One common approach is the rotational breeding strategy outlined above. A variation is to use the males for two years, once within their own birth group, and the next time rotating on to the next birth group. This strategy results in inbreeding one year, linecrossing the next. As long as selection is occurring, it should produce sound vigorous birds for several generations before needing a boost from outside genetics.

Another potential variation on the rotational breeding plan outlined above involves five instead of four groups and uses breeder birds for only a single year. This is especially feasible with chickens and ducks, and usually with turkeys and rabbits. With these five groups, the females are retained in their group (so pullets from pen A stay in pen A) while the males are used "two pens down" so that A group cockerels go with C group pullets. This is outlined in Figure 14.13.

Importantly, by increasing the number of groups to five, and by rotating males two groups down instead of just one, the result is a much more uniform blend of the genetic material over time. This is illustrated in Table 14.4. While the details can be mind-numbing, the end result is that this scheme can be safely used on isolated populations a bit longer than the "four group" rotational breeding plan because high levels of inbreeding are avoided for a greater number of generations.

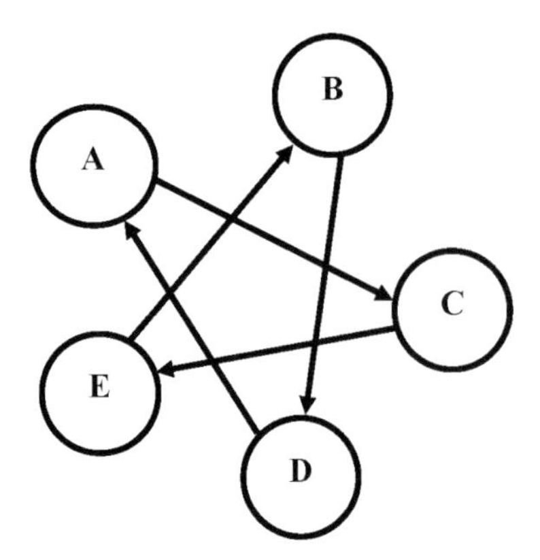

Figure 14.13 A variation of rotational breeding with five pens is a very effective approach for poultry breeding. Figure by DPS.

Table 14.4 Rotational, or spiral, breeding with five groups has advantages in the overall blend of genetic material.

Generation	A	B	C	D	E
1	100% A	100% B	100 % C	100% D	100% E
2	50% A 50%D	50% B 50%E	50%A 50%C	50% B 50% D	50% C 50% E
3	25% A 25% B 50% D	25% B 25% C 50% E	50% A 25% C 25% D	50% B 25% D 25% E	25% A 50% C 25% E
4	12.5% A 37.5% B 37.5% D 12.5% E	12.5% A 12.5% B 37.5% C 37.5% E	37.5% A 12.5% B 12.5% C 37.5% D	37.5% B 12.5% C 12.5% D 37.5% E	37.5% A 37.5% C 12.5% D 12.5% E
5	6.25% A 37.5% B 6.25% C 25% D 25% E	25% A 6.25% B 37.5% C 6.25% D 25% E	25% A 25% B 6.25% C 37.5% D 6.25% E	6.25% A 25% B 25% C 6.25% D 37.5% E	37.5% A 6.25% B 25% C 25% D 6.25% E
6	6.25% A 31.25% B 15.625% C 15.625% D 31.25% E	31.25% A 6.25% B 31.25% C 15.625% D 15.625% E	15.625% A 31.25% B 6.25% C 31.25% D 15.625% E	15.625% A 15.625% B 31.25% C 6.25% D 31.25% E	31.25% A 15.625% B 15.625% C 31.25% D 6.25% E
7	10.9375% A 23.4375% B 23.4375% C 10.9375% D 31.25% E	31.25% A 10.9375% B 23.4375% C 23.4375% D 10.9375% E	10.9375% A 31.25% B 10.9375% C 23.4375% D 23.4375% E	23.4375% A 10.9375% B 31.25% C 10.9375% D 23.4375% E	23.4375% A 23.4375% B 10.9375% C 31.25% D 10.9375% E

14.5.1 The Felch Method

A successful and popular method for poultry breeding was developed in the early 1900s by I.K. Felch. This is a fairly complicated way to manage a single founding male with a group of founding females. This system does work well to achieve concentration of the genetic influence of specific founders in some birds, while blending the genetics more evenly in others. When coupled with good selection the result can be a genetic pool that works well when linebred, as well as when linecrossed. This is illustrated in Figure 14.14.

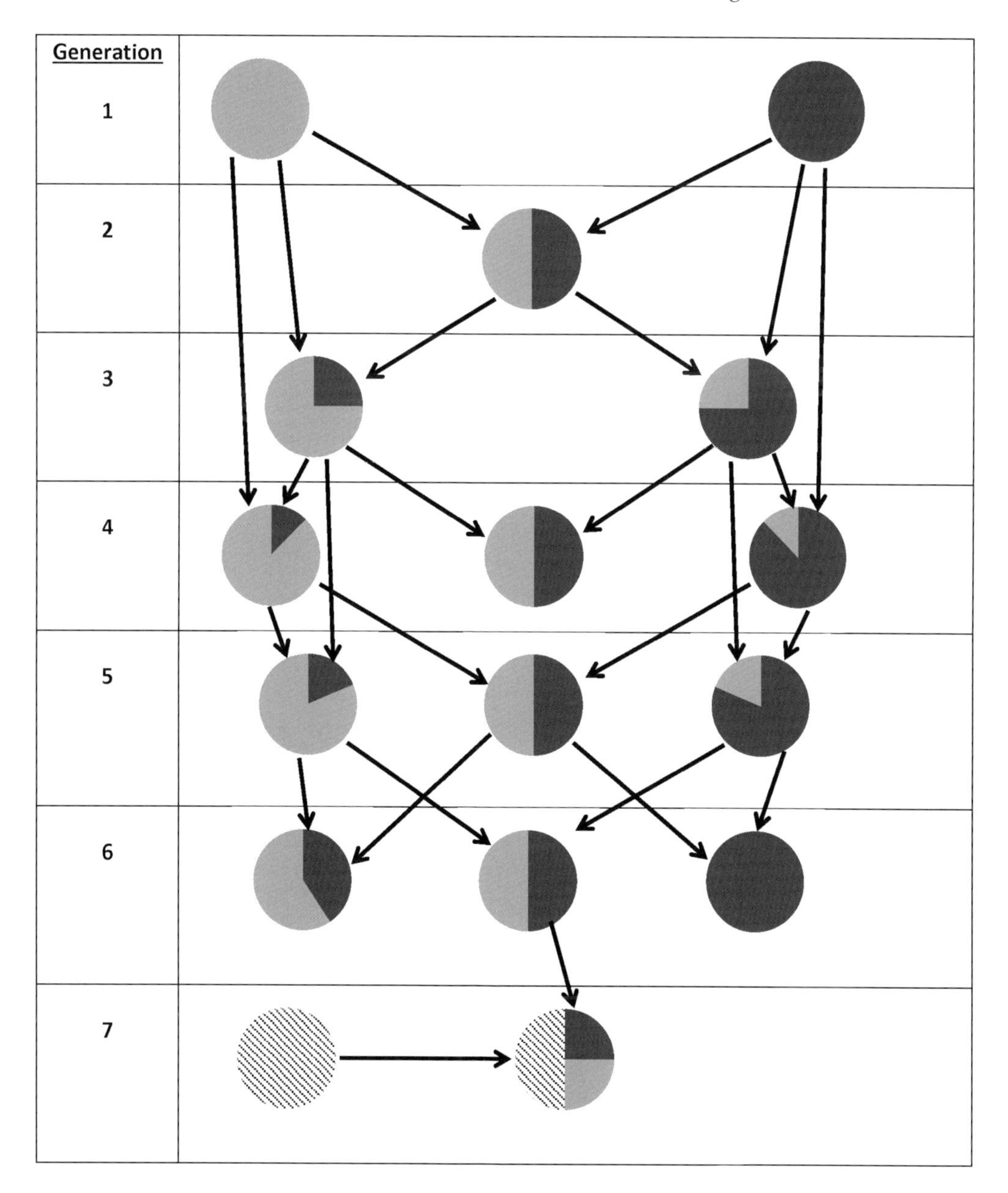

Figure 14.14 The Felch method has been tested over decades by chicken breeders. Figure by DPS.

The original male is from one bloodline, and is mated to the original female(s) that are of another line, producing the birds in the second generation. These are all 50% each the founder male and the founder females. These first-generation crosses are then mated back to parents to produce the third generation, which are either 75% the original male line, or 75% the original female line depending on the specific mating. These matings take the genetic material back toward a linebred situation with each parental strain. The basic principle from this point on is that the birds are deliberately mated to produce some birds that are 50% each line, and then other birds that are majority either the original male or female line. As the generations progress it becomes impossible to pull the birds too much into either parental generation, but it is always easy to recreate birds that are 50% each by mating the two extremes back together.

At some point (in Figure 14.14 this is the seventh generation), it is possible to add in new stock and to reinvigorate the results. Proceeding from the outcross in the same way as in the second generation provides for the infusion of new genetic material for vitality, while also pulling the population back toward the original stock. This assures a consistent influence of the original stock so that breeders can reap the results of their selection and predictability from the preceding generations. This can be especially important for show stocks that have been highly selected for perfection of form.

Some breeders have had great success with this approach, over decades or longer (Figure 14.15). While some genetic stocks will never need any addition of outside genetics, this is

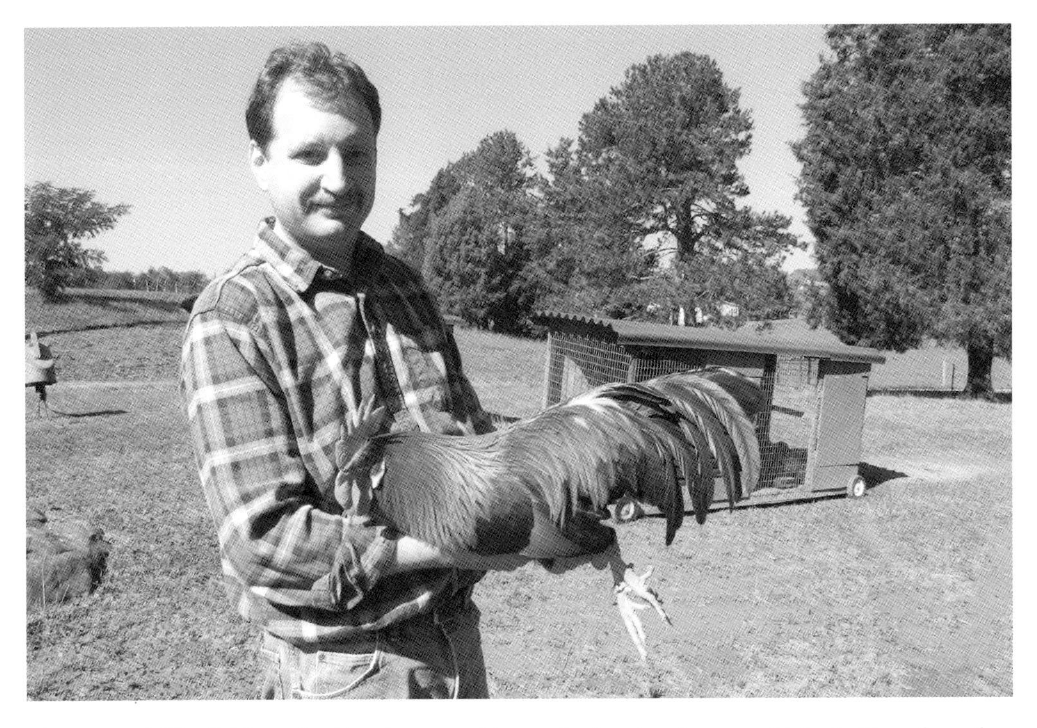

Figure 14.15 The Felch method has been used to good advantage by several talented breeders of purebred poultry. Don Schrider is a long-term breeder of a highly respected strain of Light Brown Leghorn chickens. Photo by JB.

not true in every situation. The astute breeder will be keeping an eye on overall quality, vitality, and reproductive fitness to be alert as to whether, or when, to add that outside influence back into their stock. This breeding protocol works best with species that are prolific, such as rabbits, chickens, ducks, and turkeys. They provide adequate offspring for good rates of selection for both performance and vitality at each step.

14.5.2 Sequential Rotation of Male Poultry

It is also possible to sequentially rotate males into a pen of females (especially for ducks or chickens), and in this manner recruit replacements from multiple males. If the eggs from each time slot are incubated separately (which they generally would be), then the chicks, ducklings, or poults can be leg-banded, wing-banded, or toe-punched in order to keep the various broods separate at maturity. Good record keeping is a must, and is made more difficult in poultry by their small size and the intricacies of the various identification systems. The broods should be separated by at least a week from the time males are changed, and ideally separated by one month because of prolonged residual fertility of sperm in poultry species.

14.5.3 Only Two Lines Available: Poultry, Swine, and Rabbits

Many poultry, swine, and rabbit breeders have limited space, and in some situations, it is realistic to keep only two males and several females. In this situation the genetic material can still be managed to keep a relatively isolated population for several generations. This can be seen as a modification of the Felch method outlined above, which requires three pens or groups in some generations.

The diagram for the Felch method can be used, remembering that instead of "male only" and "female only" founding strains, each includes both males and females. This modification of the Felch method can work well in poultry, swine, and rabbits, in part because these species produce multiple offspring in each production cycle. This provides the numbers of offspring that can be selected, so that type and vitality can be assured at each step.

14.5.4 "Double Mating" of Poultry

"Double mating" is a confusing term to people new to poultry breeding, and is not really a specific breeding plan. Some poultry breed standards are constructed such that the genetic stocks used to produce exhibition males are different from the ones used to produce exhibition females. This is mostly true of a few chicken breeds, but historically some duck breeds have also fit this situation. Barred Plymouth Rocks are a good example. The standard calls for similarly barred cocks and hens, and due to the sex linkage of the gene responsible for the pattern this is difficult or impossible to do with only a single breeding population (Figure 14.16).

In Barred Plymouth Rocks the well-marked males have two doses of the gene leading to the barring. Unfortunately, their female counterparts only have one dose, which leads them to be too dark by virtue of having thicker black bars and narrower light ones. In contrast, the males that go with well-marked females are too light because their light bars are too wide. The strategy of exhibition breeders is to have two separate breeding populations. These are called "cockerel breeders" and "pullet breeders." Each group, of course, has both

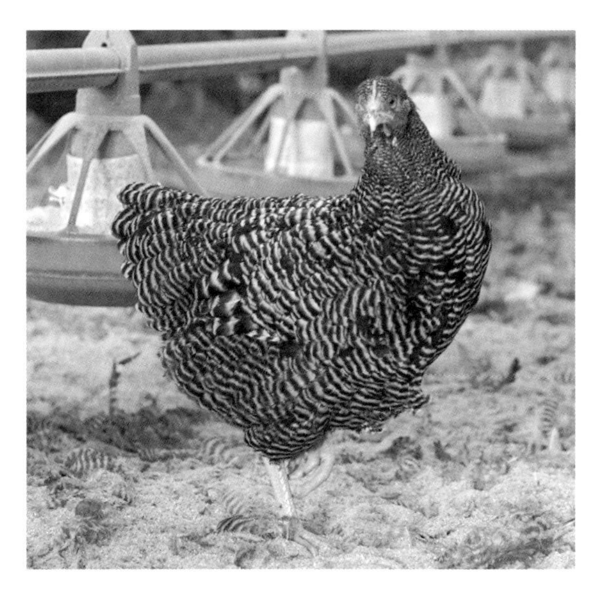

Figure 14.16 Production of well-marked Plymouth Rocks is a demanding task, and usually requires separate populations for the production of male and female show stock. Photo by JB.

cocks and hens. The "cockerel breeders" are used to produce the exhibition cockerels and cocks, and the pullets and hens of these strains are never used for exhibition. Similarly, the "pullet breeders" are used to produce exhibition pullets and hens, and the males are never used for exhibition. This has the peculiar result that the exhibition males and the exhibition females of these varieties are never mated together to produce the next generation of exhibition birds.

While double mating is not necessary for most varieties or breeds, it is a long-standing strategy for some of them. Breeders need to be aware of whether or not their selected project requires double mating, because it requires the maintenance of duplicate groups.

14.6 Trio Breeding Plan for Rabbits and Others

Rabbits (Figure 14.17), pigs, and exhibition poultry are often bred as trios of one male and two females. This is a common way for new breeders to start with a breed of these species. In most situations the trio will be a male and two unrelated females. Despite this narrow genetic base, it is possible to go several generations before needing an outcross, as outlined in Figure 14.18.

It is ideal to buy a trio of two mated females and a male. Each female brought in has already been mated to a male that is unrelated to the male of the trio. The optimal situation is for each female to have been mated to a male unrelated to the one mated to the other female. This serves to maximally diversify the founding genetic variation. With this start it is possible to breed the trio and descendants for several generations before needing outside genetic material. This is outlined in Figure 14.19.

In either case, the success of trio breeding depends on being able to save males from multiple litters, and to use these back on the foundation stock to manipulate the breeding so that relatively outbred matings are always available. If the original stock survives several years, it is possible to go back to them to increase the genetic distance between some of

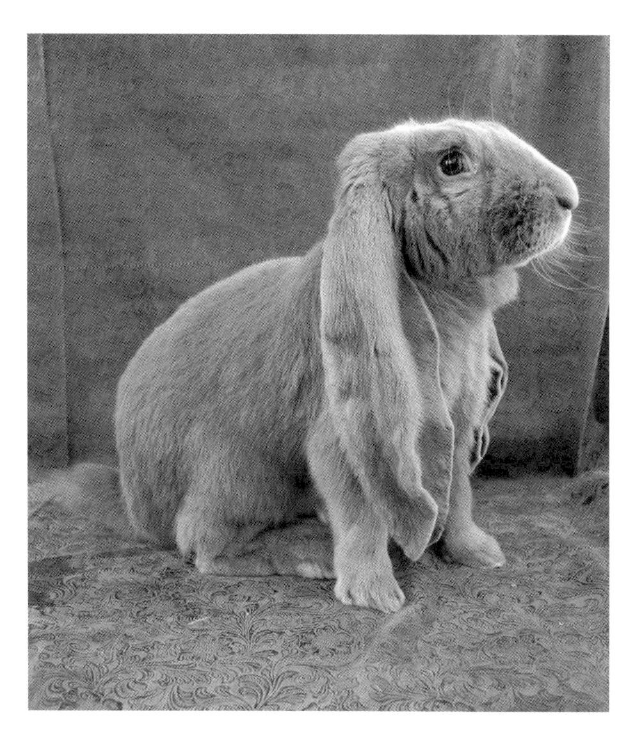

Figure 14.17 New breeders of rabbits commonly start with a trio of one male and two females. This English Lop buck would go to a breeder along with two does for a good start in a breeding program. Photo by JB.

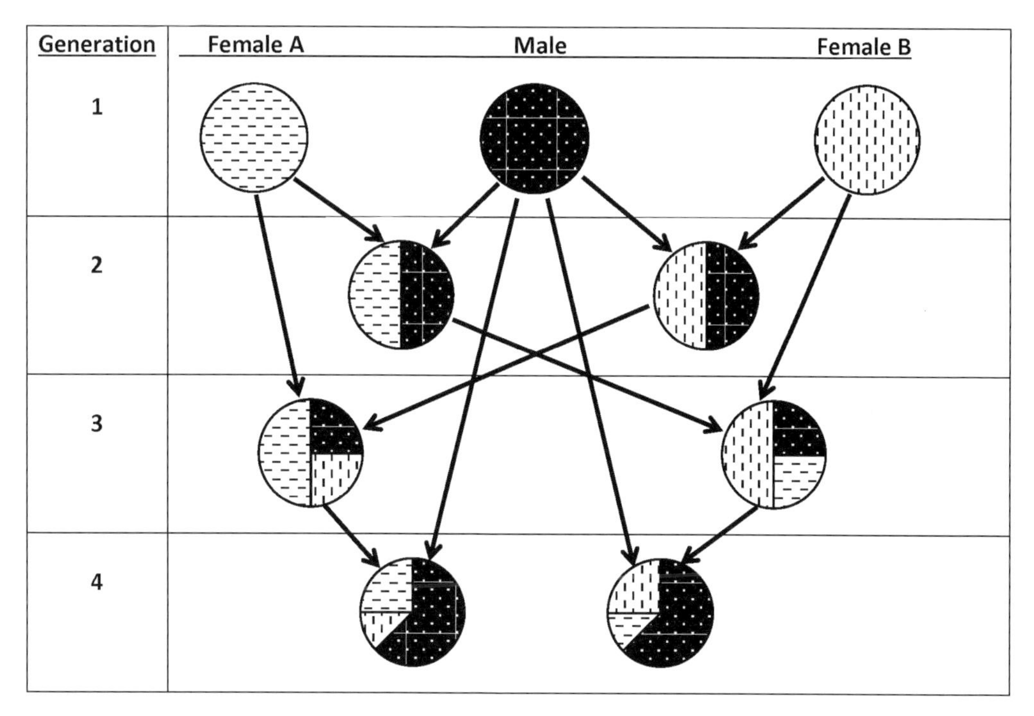

Figure 14.18 Trio breeding is fairly tightly constrained if the original two females and male are the only starting point. By mating young males back to foundation females, it is possible to increase the genetic distance a bit and continue on for a few more generations. Figure by DPS.

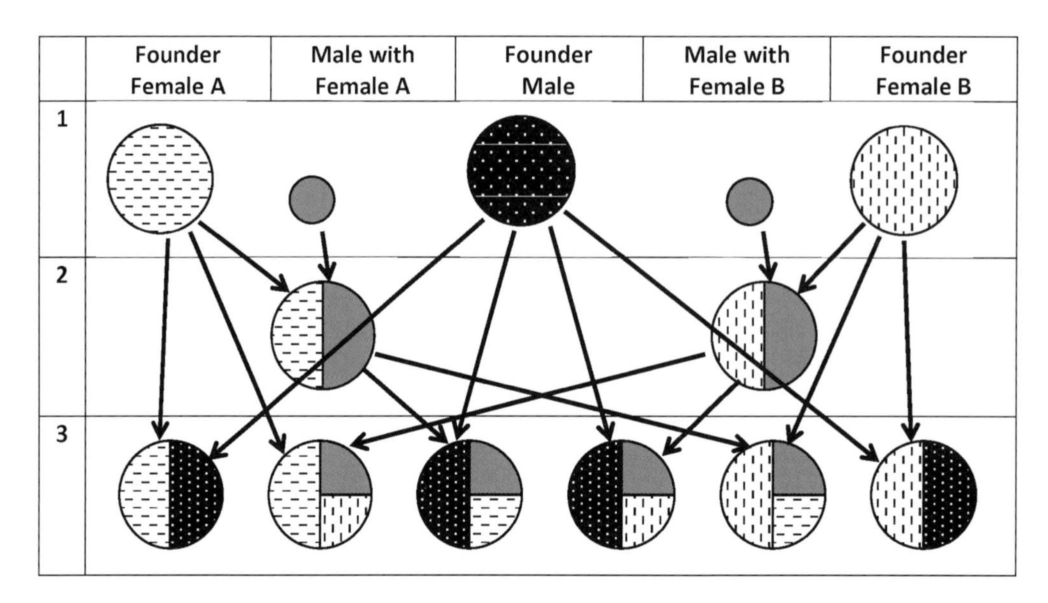

Figure 14.19 Trio breeding is strengthened by mating the two females prior to starting the population, and bringing them in pregnant. The resulting offspring provide relatively unrelated options for mating. Figure by DPS.

their descendants and those of the other founders. This opens up options for minimizing inbred matings. If the goal is to maintain an isolated population over the long term, then care must be taken to select a wide array of female replacements as the litters are produced.

Male replacements are more difficult. As soon as males are saved with contributions from all the lines, then every mating is a linebreeding. As long as the linebreeding is not too close this should work acceptably. Alternatively, each male would have a replacement somewhat linebred in his own bloodline, and this could be the basis of a start with the conservation breeding strategy outlined above for cattle. One way to do this is to mate sire to daughter, specifically to get a replacement male. This is likely to work as a "one off" strategy, but is not likely to succeed for repeated generations because inbreeding would rapidly increase to dangerous levels.

CHAPTER 15

Rescuing Small Populations: General Aspects

The recommendation that breed rescues should maintain genetic diversity seems almost too obvious to warrant mention. The details become important, though, and these play out in various ways depending on the challenges faced in each specific situation. Genetic diversity is needed for population viability, but tugs in the opposite direction from predictability and uniformity. In rescue situations it is important to first assure the conservation of maximum levels of diversity. Genetic diversity is nearly certain to decline rapidly unless specific actions are targeted to maximize it, and rescue protocols need to be tailored to recover the diversity wherever it lies (Figure 15.1). Genetic diversity can be located in different general sorts of animals depending on the specific situation. The most usual sites of most diversity are older females or frozen semen from long ago.

The importance of a healthy population structure is paramount in saving genetic diversity. Even numerous breeds, such as the Holstein, so widely used for dairy production, have suffered from losses of genetic diversity (Figure 15.2). In the Holstein, those losses have led to declines in overall health and immune function, even as milk yields have risen dramatically. The sad fact is that the declining health of a breed's animals can eventually negate any gain made in levels of production. It is essential, even in rescue situations, to keep in mind not only individual animals, but also the population as a whole. Added to these concerns is the entirety of the environment and production system into which the animals fit and function. Maintaining genetic diversity and a good genetic structure for the breed's population are key components of this comprehensive view. A comprehensive view is important even

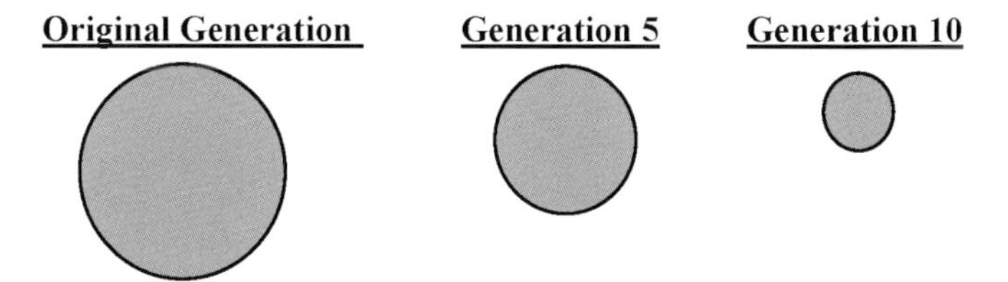

Figure 15.1 Maintaining genetic diversity is the main goal in a breed rescue. Without targeted efforts to maintain diversity it is nearly certain to decline over the generations. Figure by DPS.

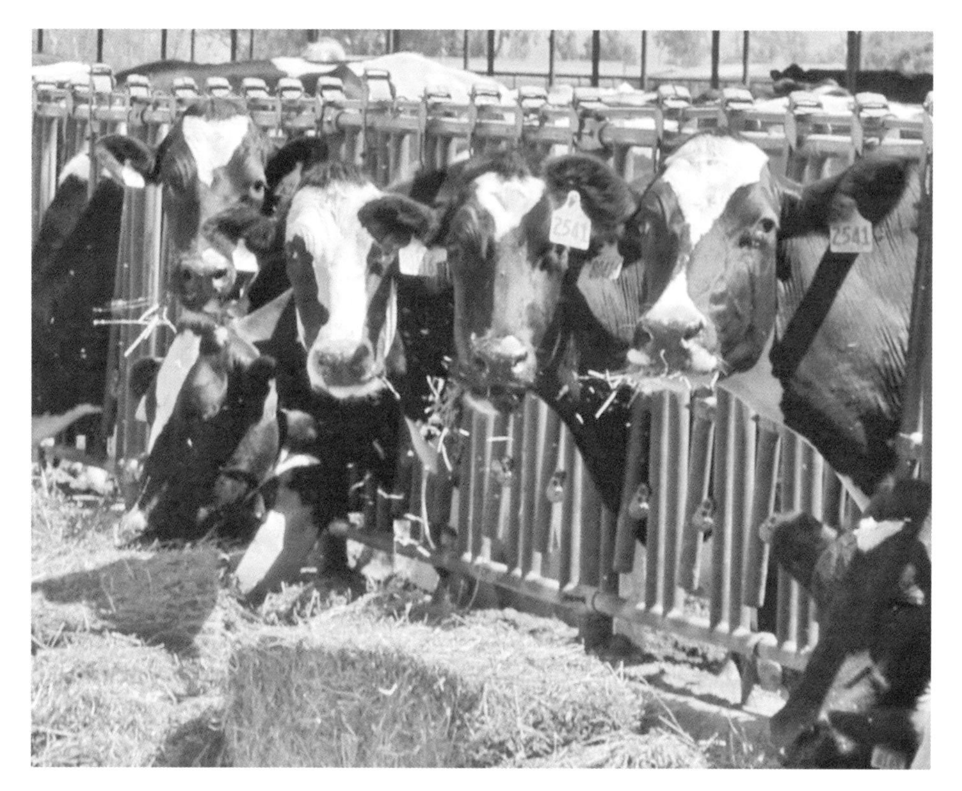

Figure 15.2 The Holstein breed has numbers in the millions, but has only limited genetic variation due to long-term breeding practices and a pursuit of production at the expense of the genetic structure of the breed. Photo by JB.

in the most numerous breeds, and is all the more pressing in rare ones. Genetic diversity and population structure become the primary concerns in rescue situations based on very low numbers.

Breeders need to emphasize population structure in any situation where population sizes are small. This sounds obvious, but diversity is sometimes ignored because it can work against selection for productivity. A successful rescue that leads to eventual numerical recovery of a breed will allow future selection to be successful for traits related to production. Basically, selection for production might have to take a back seat for a few generations. This assures that the breed population's genetic structure is in good shape, which makes selection that is oriented toward production possible for the long term. The goal is always long-term success, and in the early stages of a rescue the population's genetic structure ends up being more important than any immediate concern for production levels. Without sound population structures, a breed will collapse in on itself. If that happens, it precludes any future for the breed, at all, whether productive or not (Figure 15.3).

While selection for production can logically take a bit of a back seat to population structure in the early generations of a rescue, a few of the ways that genetics works make this complicated. Even if it is of somewhat secondary importance in the early stages of a rescue, genetic selection for production and overall vitality can never be completely ignored.

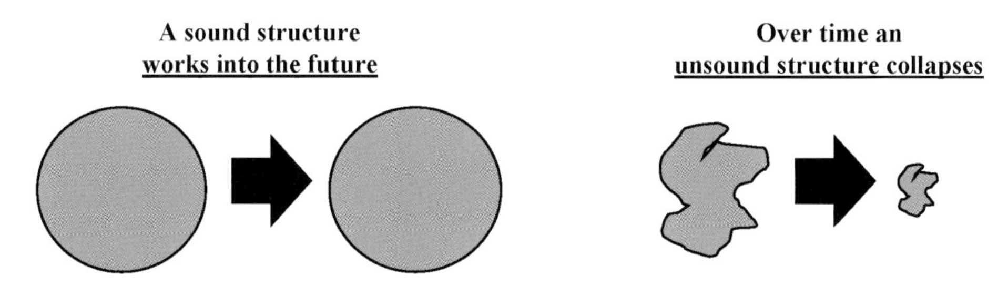

Figure 15.3 Assuring a sound genetic structure for a breed can assure the possibility of long-term selection for productivity. Ignoring the genetic structure of a breed can lead to insufficient genetic breadth to allow for maintaining production over the long term. Figure by DPS.

Exactly how much each of the different traits should be emphasized depends on how they are inherited. Some traits are easily manipulated, and action can be delayed to the future; others are more difficult to manage or eliminate once established in a population, and this type of trait can never be completely ignored even in the early stages of a rescue.

15.1 General Guiding Principles

The eventual goal of the rescue of a small population is to be able to achieve stable long-term management. This is a complicated endeavor, and strategies for success have been detailed in previous chapters. However, it remains challenging to know exactly what to do when very short-term actions are needed in order to rescue a numerically small population of animals. This chapter sets out the general principles involved in a rescue, and Chapter 16 delves into a specific set of recipes that can be followed in different situations in order to assure successful outcomes.

Each rare breed rescue comes with its own array of specific problems, but several general concepts run through all of them which provide a good framework for breed rescue work. Understanding these concepts empowers breeders to chart a successful course when confronted with a rare population (breed or bloodline) that faces immediate threat of loss.

Rescues, by their very nature, involve relatively few animals. Under the assumption that the animals are all purebred representatives of their breed, the main issue is how to use them most effectively. One general goal is to conserve as much genetic diversity as possible, because diminished diversity is a real threat to long-term breed viability. In order to do that, especially in small populations, accurate animal identification is essential (Figure 15.4). This step enables matings to be planned and tracked so that the influence of each of the original animals involved in the rescue can be as balanced as possible. The identification of individual animals may be quite difficult in feral or extensively raised landrace populations, but every effort must be made as the risk of loss that can come from the absence of good and accurate identification is high.

Another important general principle in the early phases of a rescue is that each specific mating and subsequent recruitment of the next generation into the breeding population should be determined by the population structure. This repeats the general rule of "population structure first, productivity second" for breed rescue. Establishing a secure and

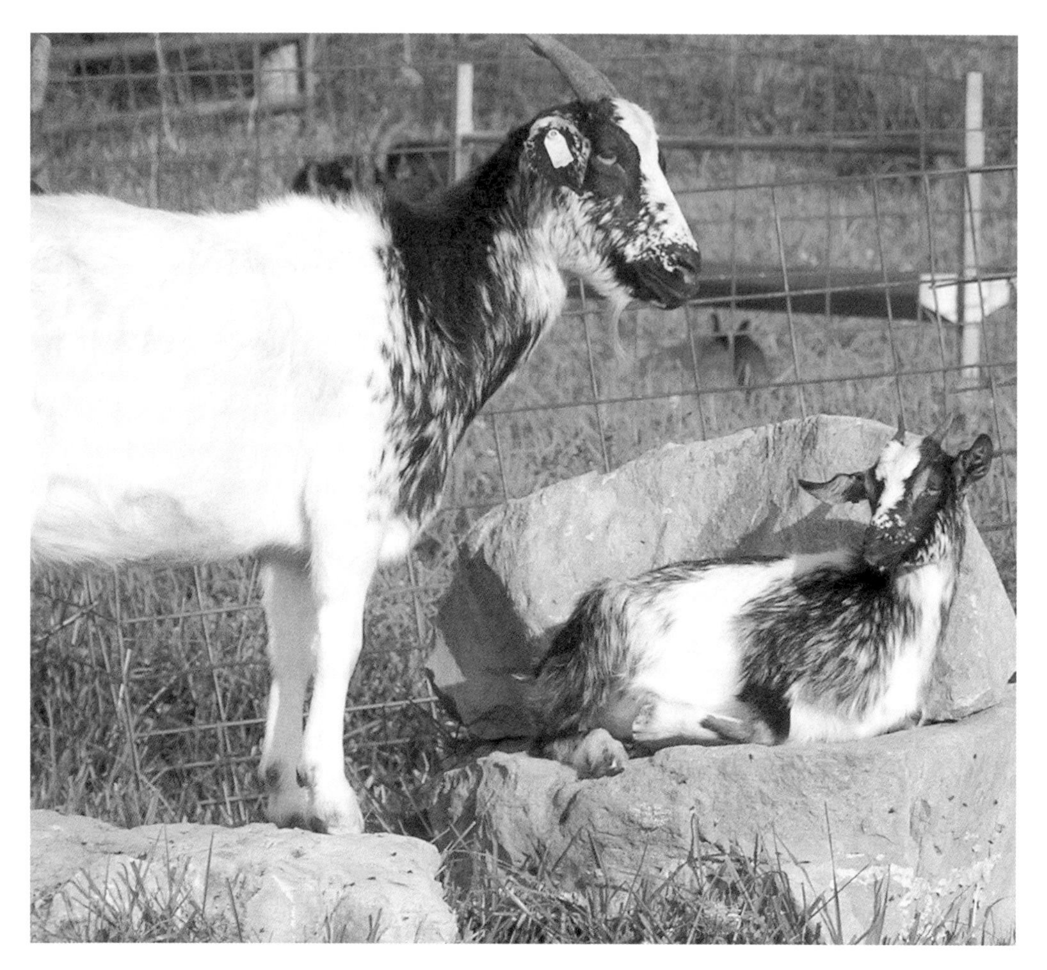

Figure 15.4 Accurate animal identification is essential if genetic rescues are to succeed. Ear tags are often used in cattle, sheep, and goats. Other species are marked by brands, detailed descriptions, or other tactics. Photo by DPS.

healthy population structure is the most reliable route to being able to select for increased production in the future. Therefore, in the early stages of a rescue operation, population structure needs to be the highest priority.

The results of population analyses (DNA or pedigree) can help drive some of these strategies. A low level of heterozygosity but a decently diverse array of alleles at the various loci in a population is an indication that there has been inbreeding across different herds or other subgroups. This situation can be corrected by deliberately mixing in animals from one subpopulation into another. In most situations this can be done by taking a male from each subpopulation and moving him on to another one. As long as all of the available herds are participating, nothing is likely to be lost in the process. This strategy makes sense in order to increase the relative number of heterozygotes in the population.

The contrasting situation is one of high heterozygosity across the population, which can indicate a past practice of more deliberate outbreeding. This situation can benefit from

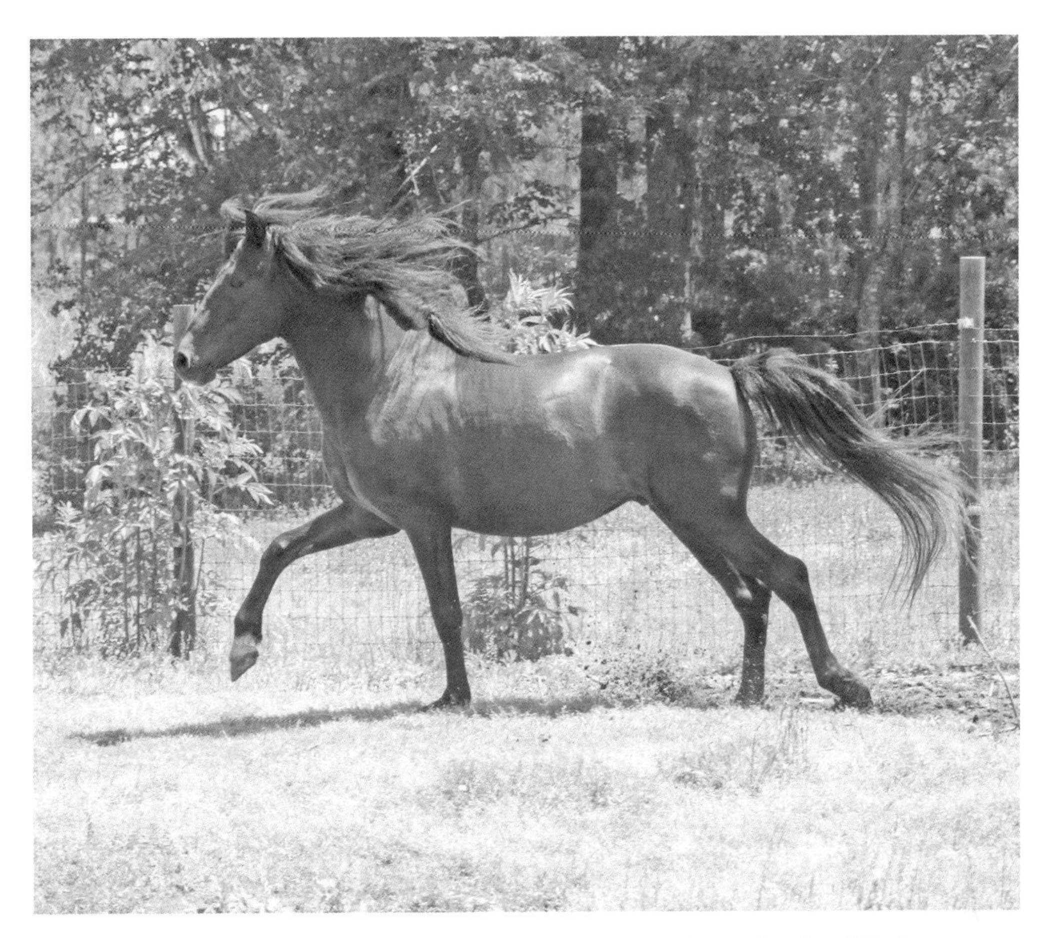

Figure 15.5 Animals from rare bloodlines or DNA types can only be used to their full advantage if they are identified and made available. This Marsh Tacky stallion was the last of his line, but has produced several foals that retain his genetic contribution to the breed. Photo by JB.

some subdivision of the population and at least limited isolation of the subdivisions from one another for a few generations. This situation is much rarer than those where inbreeding is the challenge.

The location and identification of specific individual animals with rare pedigrees or rare DNA variants makes it possible to use them more broadly for reproduction in order to balance out genetic influences in the breed (Figure 15.5). This can either be done by pedigree analysis or through the use of microsatellite or SNP analyses that can identify animals with rare genotypes. Regardless of the method used to identify rare individuals, it is wise to assure that they see broad enough use, either within a single or a few herds, that their genetic contribution is secure. The goal is to assure that rare individuals provide multiple offspring.

The details of how these rare individuals can influence a population can be subtle, and are important to consider. Each offspring of a rare animal gets 50% of the genome from that animal. Two offspring, however, get a total of only 75%, because the random 50%

of the second one overlaps with the 50% of the first one so that not all of what it receives from the parent is distinct from the first one. The result is that actually capturing the entire genome of any breeding animal is difficult. To get reasonably complete sampling of the genome it is necessary that multiple offspring be produced. Each of these must be used in reproduction because each has a unique 50% of the original genome, even though there is considerable overlap among them. To achieve over 90% coverage of an animal's genome, it must produce four offspring that see future use.

One option for enhancing the influence of a rare individual is to resort to some level of inbreeding. This can be done by repeated cycles of inbreeding the offspring of a rare animal back to the parental rare animal. The first offspring is 50% of the rare animal, while the offspring that result from mating progeny back to the rare animal go up to 75%. The influence of the target animal now predominates, and animals produced this way can be moved on to other herds to distribute this rare contribution more widely and to distribute it more evenly in the population without any further inbreeding. This tactic can distribute portions of the rare genome quickly and broadly. A different strategy is to use the first offspring of the rare animal that are only 50% its influence. These can be distributed widely throughout the breed by infusing them into other lines. This strategy works to conserve the individual genes of the rare animal, even if they never again predominate in any single individual animal. Forcing the genetic component of a rare animal to predominate in its descendants is only possible through inbreeding.

Salvaging the genetics of rare animals needs to be put into the overall context of an effective breed rescue that results in a sound population structure. The temptation might be to use the animal broadly over the entire population, but this strategy runs the risk of taking an underrepresented genome and making it overrepresented. While rare genomes do need a boost, that boost should only be used to assure a proportionate representation. The risk in overemphasizing rare bloodlines is that this comes at the expense of the more common bloodlines, which also have important and essential roles to play.

In some situations specific founders may have had minimal influence in descendants. At some point their contribution to genetic diversity becomes trivial, and any attempts to concentrate the influence cannot be all that successful. This is most likely to occur around the point where their influence is 10% or less. At this low level of founder influence, it is fairly safe to simply refrain from heroics to try to expand the influence, while at the same time trying at least moderately to assure that it does not become completely extinct.

Many breeders, especially of rare breeds, put great emphasis on tail male and tail female lineages (Figure 15.6). These are the influences that come through the generations all from males (sire, grandsire, great grandsire), and similarly for the female side. These are important, but it is very easy to overemphasize them. Over succeeding generations these influences become tiny when considered in the light of the entire genome. Where they do matter, though, is in the retention of specific variation of either mitochondrial DNA (from the tail female line) or the Y chromosome (from the tail male line). One solution to managing this influence is to simply assure that at least a few females are retained from each tail female line. Similarly, a few males from each tail male line can always be retained. This assures that the population retains the unique contributions of mitochondria and the Y chromosome from these lineages. It is unwise to allow either of these to go completely

sire	paternal grandsire	great grandsire	great great grandsire
			great great granddam
		great granddam	great great grandsire
			great great granddam
	paternal granddam	great grandsire	great great grandsire
			great great granddam
		great granddam	great great grandsire
			great great granddam
dam	maternal grandsire	great grandsire	great great grandsire
			great great granddam
		great granddam	great great grandsire
			great great granddam
	maternal granddam	great grandsire	great great grandsire
			great great granddam
		great granddam	great great grandsire
			great great granddam

Figure 15.6 Over several generations the "tail male" and "tail female" contribution of genetics becomes fairly small. In this four-generation pedigree, the light grey portion is coming from the original great-great grandsire, and similarly for the dark grey portion coming from the great-great granddam. The middle shade of grey comes from the ancestors that are not in these tail positions, yet over several generations these come to provide the majority of the genetic material in any individual animal. Figure by DPS.

extinct. It is also true, though, that these influences are small when considered in light of the entire balance of the genome. They are only a minor consideration among many others in trying to achieve a good balance of genetic diversity in a rescue population. In the breeder culture of some breeds, the tail male and tail female aspect of breeding takes on huge importance, and one that vastly overstates their relatively small role in maintaining genetic diversity over many generations.

15.2 *Subdivision of Populations*

Another general recommendation that is useful in nearly all rescue situations is to subdivide the population in order to reduce the risks of genetic drift as well as any threats from disaster or disease that come from concentration in a single geographic location. Subdivision redistributes the genetic variation of the breed and increases the chances that more of it will be successfully conserved (Figure 15.7).

Subdividing a population nearly always assures that each subgroup has a slightly different representation of the original genetic diversity within the population. Some subgroups miss out on certain variants, but others retain them. Usually this works out so that nothing is lost over the entire population, even though some variants may be lost in some of the subgroups. This contrasts with keeping everything together in one location, because then any loss due to genetic drift will be a loss to the entire breed.

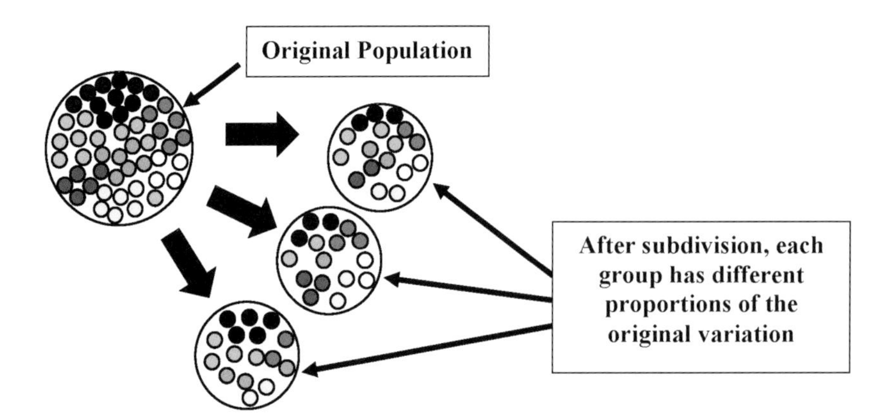

Figure 15.7 Subdividing populations helps save unique genetics in each subpopulation and reduces potential losses from genetic drift. Each subdivision loses some degree of variation, but the total overall loss of diversity is minimal. Figure by DPS.

15.3 Species-Specific Considerations

The theoretical aspects of a breed rescue hold true across the different species, but each has its own peculiar combination of characteristics that influence the practicality of what is done in a rescue situation. These boil down to differences in time to maturation and levels of prolificacy.

At one extreme are the larger species that mature slowly and generally produce only a single offspring at each birth. The most delayed of these are horses and donkeys, followed closely by cattle. Especially for these species, the assisted reproduction techniques can be helpful because they allow reproduction of individual animals at rates above the slow pace imposed by natural reproduction.

A second group of species has faster maturation as well as somewhat greater prolificacy. Goats and sheep fit in here. Nearly all breeds of sheep and goats mature more rapidly than horses, donkeys, and cattle. Most sheep and goat breeds, but not all, also tend to have twins or triplets (or more!) instead of only having singles. The quicker maturation and higher prolificacy work together to make the expansion of numbers faster and the management of genetic diversity easier than is the case with the larger species.

Swine and dogs fit into the next group, with fairly rapid maturation as well as the production of litters. While litter size does vary from breed to breed, it is nearly always above five or six, which provides ample opportunity for genetic management, selection, and expansion of numbers (Figure 15.8).

The most prolific species are also the fastest to mature: rabbits, chickens, ducks, and turkeys. These provide for a very rapid expansion of numbers that can easily be coupled with management of genetic structure of the population and selection for quality or production.

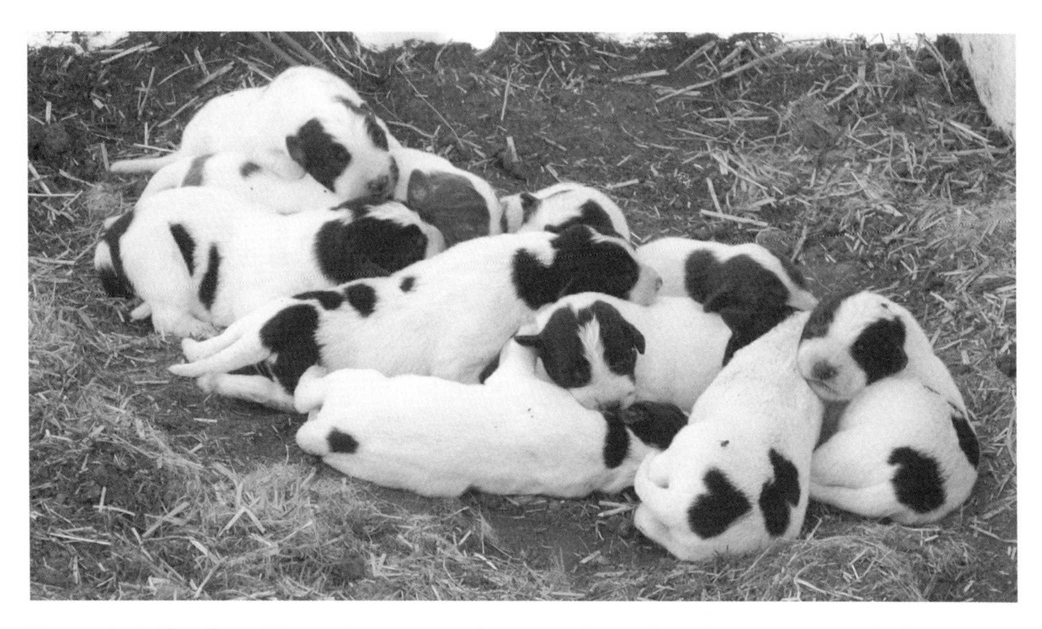

Figure 15.8 The sizes of litters that dogs produce provide numbers for expansion and selection. Photo by DPS.

CHAPTER 16

Specific Plans for Rescue Breeding

Strategies for success in population rescues will vary from one specific situation to the next. It is helpful to take a representative few of them to detail exactly how an effective rescue can proceed. Each rescue situation is unique, but several general patterns repeat often enough that they can serve as useful and practical templates. In this chapter, each individual rescue situation is discussed from its theoretical aspects and is then illustrated by a specific situation in which that sort of rescue proceeded. These examples highlight potential snags or aspects that can help guide other rescues. These rescue protocols have been successful with both breeds and bloodlines and can be adapted to either situation.

The basic idea within each of these examples is to expand the number of animals and to target saving as much as possible of the genetic diversity present and available in the original animals. Meeting these goals usually takes a few generations of careful attention and well-planned matings. Once these goals have been achieved, it is possible to transition to a sustained breed management strategy for the long term, as has been detailed in Chapters 13 and 14. An important overriding detail is to understand, in each situation, exactly in which animals most of the genetic variation resides. That allows breeding strategies to maximize retention of the variation.

In the specific strategies outlined below, reference is made to "generations" rather than "years." These strategies work equally well for different species, but in each species the generations take different amounts of time. Rabbits can squeeze in a few generations in a single year. Dogs require at least a year, as do goats, sheep, and hogs. In most situations getting one generation per year is only possible if the breeding animals are pushed a bit. Cattle go up to at least two years and more likely three as a minimum, while horses and donkeys require yet a few more years. Those species for which multiple years intervene between generations have the possibility of repeated matings of specific individual males and females beyond what is possible for those with shorter generation intervals. For example, a program that pushes sheep or goats pretty hard is unlikely to allow a specific female to be mated back to the same male more than one time if the males are cycled through the population as rapidly as possible. In contrast, a cow is very likely to have the opportunity to be mated to the same bull for at least two years, and maybe three because it takes that long for his sons to mature to breeding age. This delay is especially likely in the early stages of a rescue program. The opportunity for multiple pairings of two individual cattle, horses, or donkeys is simply for the reason that the gestation period and ensuing maturation of their offspring takes more years than does the production and maturation of a goat or a sheep.

The original animals in a rescue are called "founders." In some situations a great deal is known about these, while in others very little is known. More information is always better, but even in the absence of information it is still possible to proceed and to achieve success. Doing something is always better than doing nothing! In order to shorten some of the text, "G1" will refer to a "generation one" animal, which is the first generation produced after mating the founders. "G2" refers to a "generation two" animal that has one or two "G1" parents, and so on. Founders will still be referred to as "founders" because "F" alone can cause confusion with the nomenclature of "F1" as the "first filial generation" that many readers will be familiar with from courses on genetics.

Unfortunately, these protocols are inherently complicated, and they can be difficult to understand, even though every attempt has been made to keep them as straightforward as possible. It may help readers to grasp some of the more subtle aspects of how these protocols work if they chart them out. This approach might feel like a homework assignment, but that level of work should provide an appreciation of how the genetic material resides in different animals over time, over distance, and through the generations. This level of understanding enhances the grasp of how the principles play out within a population.

Each of these situations is defined by the initial founder animals that are available for the rescue protocol. They are the raw material that constrains the potential for success in each rescue situation.

16.1 One Male, Several Females

A reasonably common and somewhat dire situation for rescues is one in which only a single male is available along with several females. This situation often arises in a breed or bloodline where a long-term breeder has simply aged out or otherwise reduced a herd. At that point, all that remains are those animals the breeder chose to have around at the very end of what was usually a fairly long career. This situation raises the question of "how many animals are too few?" It is a question with no single correct answer. Each population has a different degree of inbreeding, and each is able to withstand inbreeding to varying degrees. A level of inbreeding that is easily tolerated by one family group can be crippling to another. In light of this, the initial goal is to expand numbers while also minimizing further inbreeding.

If every founder animal is completely outbred (which is very unlikely), then success could likely be had with a single male and five or so females. In most situations, though, it is a reasonable assumption that most of the founder animals are indeed related. In these situations it is difficult to ascertain just exactly how many animals will serve as a minimum because the level of inbreeding at the start is often unknown. Success is always more likely with more founder animals rather than fewer because more animals have potentially more genetic variation than is present in only a few.

During the early stages of the rescue, it is essential to document as much as possible about the founders. In most situations it is reasonable to assume (unless there is evidence to the contrary) that animals born within the same year are all sired by the same male. Depending on the species or specific situation, this might also be a logical assumption across years as well. For example, it is certain that cattle born in consecutive years are not a dam-daughter or dam-son pair. This sort of detective work can help, because even if it does not firmly establish relationships, it at least eliminates some relationships as possibilities. If there are three or more years separating the births of cattle, then parent-offspring relationships are possible. For hogs, sheep, and goats the assumption of dam-offspring relationship is a bit more tenuous due to the early maturation of those species.

For the founders to produce the first rescue generation, the only option is to mate the founder male back to the founder females. It is wise, early on, to freeze semen from the founder male. This serves as a backup if needed, and also creates the potential to use him long into the future. After that first round of mating, the first crop of rescue offspring (G1) will hit the ground. These will include both males and females, although this depends a bit on luck as well as on the number of founder females. It is rare to have a rescue with fewer than ten females in the founder group, so the assumption of both male and female offspring in this first crop is reasonable.

Among that first generation, the goal is to save all the female offspring, but also multiple male offspring. All of the G1 animals are half-siblings produced by that original male and the founder females. Young males for breeding should be retained from the oldest founder females whenever possible, because those females generally have the highest levels of genetic diversity and also have the fewest years of productive life remaining. How many of the young males to save depends on resources, but more is always better than fewer because they are insurance against losses due to accident or disease.

The population now includes the founder male, the founder females, and their G1 offspring. G1 animals are all half-siblings, and potentially some full siblings in those species that have litters. At this point it is ideal to subdivide the population. Groups should be based on any known relationships among the animals. The goal is to keep dams and their female offspring in the same group because this concentrates each founder genome into one specific group rather than spreading it around equally. Ideally each group should include a few of the oldest foundation females. They are joined with their daughters, and eventually their granddaughters. The G1 males should have semen frozen as insurance against loss.

To produce G2, each group of females should be mated to a G1 male that is a son of a founder female from a different breeding group. This strategy reduces the resulting inbreeding. The goal is to use the G1 males at the youngest age possible. Multiple G1 males are mated to the original foundation females as well as to their own paternal half-sisters, avoiding pairing them with full sisters. It is ideal to use at least three males. The females can be split into three groups or whatever number is realistic in a given situation. The G1 males that are destined for breeding should each be recruited from a different dam. Even in the case of litter-bearing species, multiple females need to contribute as the dams of future sires. While the founder male is an obvious potential source of a genetic bottleneck in the rescue, the founder females can serve equally as bottlenecks if only one or a few participate

Table 16.1 Rescue protocol with a single male and multiple females.

Matings in different generations	Female offspring to retain	Male offspring to retain
Founder male to all founder females	All G1, daughters stay with dams as herd is split into three	Three G1 from the oldest founder in each group
Three G1 males, each used on one of three groups of females that include founders (not dam) and their G1 daughters	All G2, each staying with dam	One G2 from each group, from oldest founder that has not previously provided a son for breeding
Three G2 males, each used on one of the three groups that does not include his dam	All G3, each staying with dam	One G3 from each group, from a founder female if possible.

in the production of breeding animals in succeeding generations. Broad and balanced participation of all founders is the goal. The general strategy is outlined in Table 16.1.

The second generation (G2) consists of a few different general sorts of animals. One is the product of the G1 males with the original foundation females. Their genetic background is 25% the founder male, 25% the founder female that is the dam of the G1 male, and 50% the G2 animal's own founder dam. This strategy has reduced the genetic influence of the founder male from his own 100% to a lower 25% in the G2 animals. Each of this type of G2 animal has a relatively low contribution from the founder male, but if that founder male has produced many offspring, then his total genome is still likely to have been passed along, even though it is not a majority contribution to any individual animal. Essentially nothing has been lost, but with the added benefit of the lowest chance of inbreeding in the future.

The second sort of G2 animal is produced by the mating of the G1 males to the G1 females. The genetic background of these animals is 50% the founder male, 25% one founder female, and 25% a different founder female. These animals are useful, but must be used cautiously to avoid the risk of having the founder male become a genetic bottleneck. This outcome is especially likely if the G2 males of this type are recruited for future breeding instead of the ones of the previous type produced by the founder females and therefore having only 25% the influence of the founder male.

The strategy of using young males back on the founder females is quite distinct from a more commonly encountered strategy that uses the founder male on his own daughters. In that situation the genetic influence in the G2 offspring from the daughters of the founder male would be 75% the founder male, and only 25% from one of the founder females. That strategy essentially erases the genetic diversity of the founder females, replacing it with the limited variation housed in the founder male's genome. This strategy should be avoided as it comes with considerable inbreeding and potential loss of vitality.

To produce G3, each breeding group provides one G2 male for use in one of the other groups. Depending on number of animals, infrastructure, and potential collaborators, the three groups could either be kept going or they could be expanded by splitting them into further subgroups. If the project remains based on three groups, each of these grows larger because of recruitment of the young females, although with the potential loss of some of the older foundation animals. Those older foundation animals are essential for as long as they are available, and every effort should be made to keep them productive for as long as possible.

The G3 group has animals of different basic genetic types. Founder females produce G3 offspring that are 12.5% founder male, 12.5% one founder female, 25% a second founder female, and 50% the third founder female that is their own dam. This demonstrates the wisdom of retaining males (and females) from these founder females, because the genetics of the founder females has now come to predominate over that of the founder male. This reduces the relationship of one G3 animal to the others, especially those from different subgroups. This strategy is the safest route to maximize the retention of the original genetic variation present in all of the founder animals while also partitioning it for maximum divergence in the different subgroups.

The G3 that is sired by G2 males and out of G1 females are fairly complicated: 37.5% founder male, 12.5% one founder female, 25% a second founder female, and 25% a third founder female. This has still reduced the influence of the founder male from the 50% in G1. The G3 offspring of a G2 male with a G2 female is variable, depending on whether the G2 female is from a founder dam or not. The genetic influence of the founder male in this type of G3 animal varies from 25% to 37.5%. The effects of sequentially saving back breeding males from foundation dams is outlined in Figure 16.1, and contrasts with that of using a founder male back on his daughters, as outlined in Figure 16.2.

The next cycle sees the use of G3 males recruited from each of the groups so that each was sired by a different G2 male. Each of these G3 males is used with a group of females that does not contain his dam, which also assures that it does not contain half-sisters if the females have always been retained in their own birth groups. In an ideal situation, the number of groups has been expanded beyond three by splitting each group further. If that is possible, then each subgroup will need its own unique G3 male. The genetic makeup of G4 is complicated because multiple generations of females are available as dams of the retained breeding males: founder females (0% founder male), G1 (50% founder male), G2 (25% to 37.5% founder male), and G3 (12.5% to 37.5% founder male). It is generally best to recruit breeding males from the original foundation females because they have the highest genetic diversity and least relationship to the founder male. If that is assumed, then G4 has some animals that have a genetic influence that is only 6.25% from the founder male, with the balance coming from a mixture of founder females. The relative influence of those founder females steadily increases, taking the population away from the genetic bottleneck of that original male. If different females contribute to different males in different groups, then the original genetic diversity has a maximum opportunity to be maintained.

A subtle and counterintuitive detail is that once the founder females are unavailable, it actually makes more sense to recruit the most recent generations as dams of males than it does those earlier generations. As an example, many of the G3 females have less influence from the founder male than the G1 females do. A detailed look at pedigrees can help breeders to make appropriate choices at this point.

The cycles of pairing young males with founder females can continue for as long as founder females are available. It is ideal that several of the founder females contribute offspring for as long as they are able. Eventually the project will have rescued the genetic material of the original founders and will also have expanded the numbers of animals. The

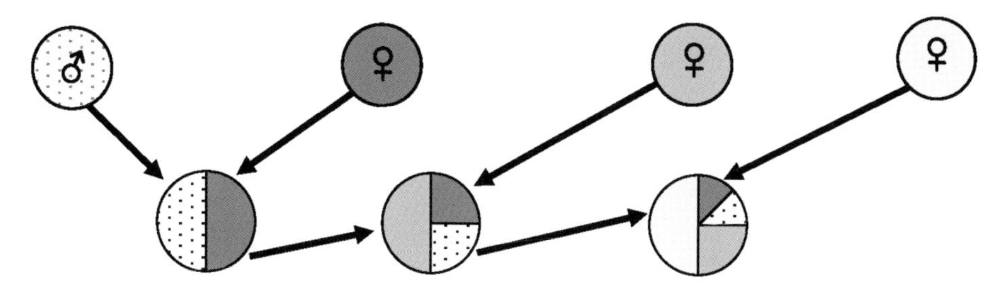

Figure 16.1 The strategy of saving sons from foundation dams and using those back on different foundation females sequentially reduces the influence of the founder male, preventing him from being a genetic bottleneck. Figure by DPS.

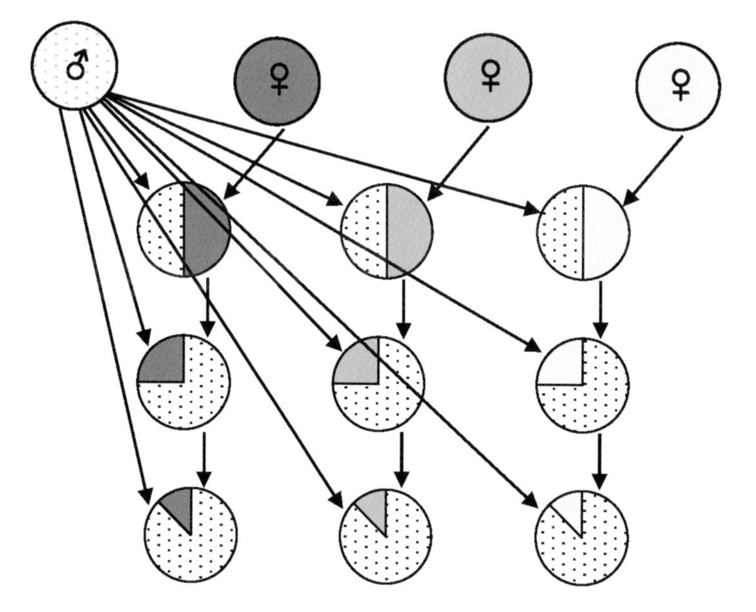

Figure 16.2 The opposite strategy of using a foundation male on his own daughters quickly replaces the genetic influence of the founder dams with the one founder male's genetic material, assuring that he is a bottleneck. Figure by DPS.

population can then be managed by the principles outlined in Chapter 14. That point is usually achieved by about G3.

16.1.1 *Jericho Goats*

Jericho goats are a strain of local Spanish goats from Alabama (Figure 16.3). These goats were stewarded over several decades by a breeder dedicated to conserving and selecting the goats local to her own family's landholdings. She developed these local goats into a productive bloodline, unique due to their origin as well as their environmental adaptation. The owner decided to stop breeding goats, and a portion of the herd was passed along to Shan and Courtney Norman, Spanish goat breeders dedicated to the breed and to conservation.

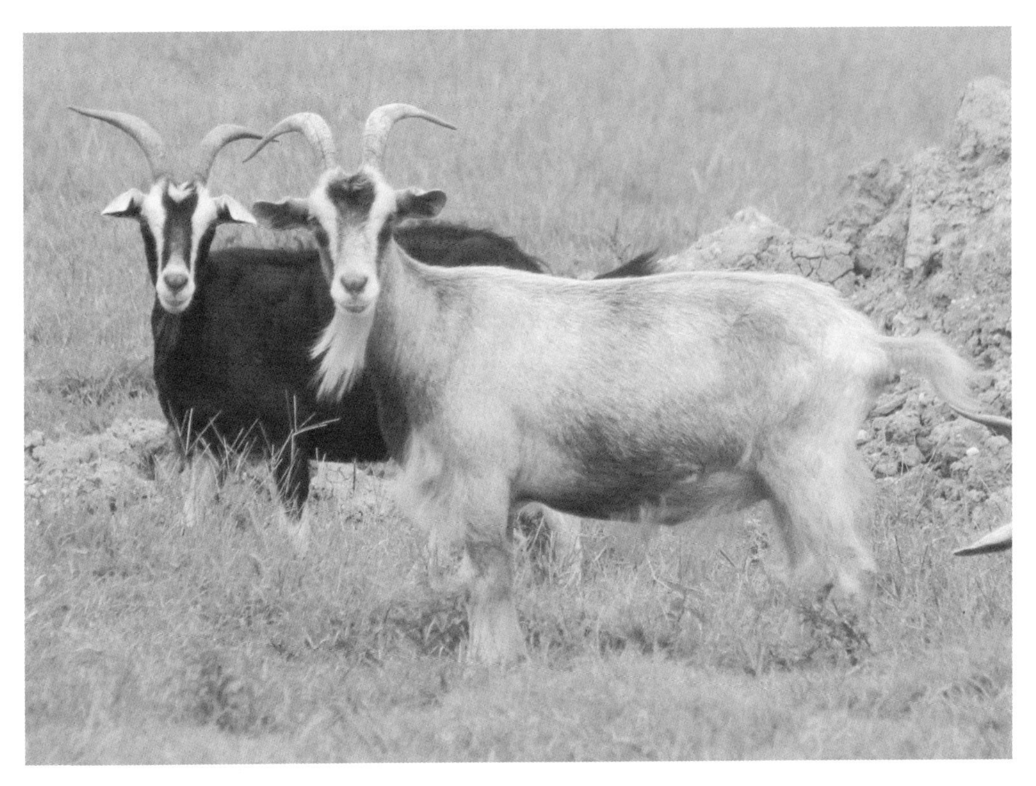

Figure 16.3 Jericho goats are a good example of the success possible with a planned rescue protocol that maximizes the influence of founder females. Photo by Courtney Norman.

The Normans were able to acquire a single buck and 15 original does. The general principles outlined above are achievable with this number of animals. The founder buck is mated to all of the does for the first one or two years. This provides for the birth of G1 kids. Each is 50% the original buck, 50% one of the does. G1 bucks are then used on the original does and their daughters.

As the G1 males mature, the herd is split into three; each group has five founder does along with their daughters. This can be somewhat difficult because the original founder animals have undocumented relationships one to another. In the case of goats, mothers and daughters often form long-term bonds and stick together closely. Paying attention to behavior can therefore help to sort the original founder does into groups of related animals. In the absence of behavioral clues, a second strategy is to rely on relative ages. Each group should include a few of the oldest females, and a somewhat equal representation of the younger ones year by year.

The G1 males selected for breeding should come from the oldest females to assure maximal genetic diversity. Once the G1 males have been used, the second generation is on the way. The G2 males are once again selected from the older founder females. At this point significant genetic distance begins to be present among the subgroups. Numbers have also increased, offering opportunities for selective retention of the best young animals instead of all of them.

After a few years of breeding the goats, the Normans were fortunate to have found another small herd of Jericho goats that had been started from the same original herd, but several years before they got their start. This offers great potential for conserving diversity. A few females from this other herd were introduced into the Norman's herd, and some buck kids were selectively retained from them in order to expand their influence. An alternative strategy would have been to use these females as one of the sublines which retains their influence and prevents its dilution.

The Jericho goats have a few single genes that offer glimpses of how these can be managed in a rescue. The founder buck has an impressive fringe of long hair down his back and on his legs. The Normans prefer smoother shorter hair on their goats. The temptation is to begin selection against the long hair immediately. Hair length in goats is controlled by very few genes, so it is easily corrected in the future. In contrast, inbreeding depression is not so easily rectified, so population structure is more important than hair length for early decisions. The original herd included four different colors. Color is a trivial characteristic, especially in Spanish goats, so it can be ignored in the early stages of rescue. Indeed, color variation is part of the heritage of the bloodline and should be maintained as a part of it.

16.2 One Male, Several Females, Some Inbreeding Depression

It is difficult to succeed in a rescue that is completely closed to outside influences when only a single male is available and significant inbreeding has occurred. In the case of a rare breed this might spell the end of the breed. In the case of a bloodline or strain within a breed, options exist for continuing on with at least a majority influence of that bloodline. While the principles outlined below will work with either situation (breed or bloodline), the assumption is that bloodline conservation is the issue at hand and that other bloodlines are available within the breed such that outcrosses are available that do not compromise the purebred status of the animals. Rescue situations under these conditions are complicated. Matings need to include two different strategies: bloodline-pure alongside introgression from another bloodline. These two demands pull in opposite directions and managing them simultaneously can be difficult to accomplish under real-world conditions due to limitations of space or pasture subdivisions.

The founder male and the founder females can all contribute to both the bloodline-pure and the bloodline-cross sides of this rescue. At the onset, two sorts of matings are accomplished.

1. The founder male is mated to half of the founder females as well as several females from other bloodlines within the same breed. The matings of founder male to founder female are all likely to be inbred and run the risk of some offspring being compromised.
2. A male from a different bloodline is mated to the other half of the founder females.

It is likely that a second round (or more) of matings is possible with the founder females. When this can be done, the specific founder females that were used for bloodline-pure and for bloodline-cross breeding should be swapped. This assures that each founder female has an opportunity to participate in each of the two strategies.

It is unlikely that all of the bloodline-pure matings will produce viable or hearty offspring, but any that do come along are especially important. They have proven that they are viable even in the presence of inbreeding. The bloodline outcrosses are very likely to be both vigorous and productive. The difference in vitality creates a real bias toward those bloodline outcrosses, and it is essential to remember that both types of offspring have important roles in the future of this rescue.

The G1 offspring consist of both bloodline-pure and bloodline-cross animals. Any bloodline-pure offspring that are full of vim and vigor are quite useful for future use and should be retained. The bloodline-cross offspring include two types: founder male x females from other bloodlines, and founder females x male from another bloodline.

G1 males should be saved from all three classes (bloodline-pure, bloodline-cross from founder male, bloodline-cross from founder female). The uses of these G1 animals vary. The bloodline-pure males are good candidates for the same strategy as the original founder male: both bloodline-pure and bloodline-cross matings. The bloodline-cross G1 males are used on bloodline-pure females (both foundation and G1) to yield a G2 that is 75% the rescue bloodline.

G1 bloodline-cross females from outside females are mated to bloodline-pure G1 males. Mating them back to the founder male is too close for comfort due to inbreeding. In contrast, the G1 bloodline-cross females that are sired by outside males can safely be mated back to the founder male for offspring that are 75% the original bloodline but 50% the founder male, or to a G1 bloodline-pure male for 75% the original bloodline but only 25% the founder male. G1 bloodline-pure females should not be mated back to their sire, nor to their half-brothers, because the results will have high levels of inbreeding. These can be mated back to G1 bloodline-cross males from the outside male, the results having a fairly low level of inbreeding and still having 75% of the influence of the original bloodline but only 25% the founder male.

G2 consists of a few bloodline-pure animals from the original founder females and the bloodline-pure G1 males (100% the original bloodline). It also includes bloodline-cross animals of two sorts. Those from the G1 descended from outside females are 25% founder male, 25% outcross female, 50% founder female (therefore 75% original bloodline). Those from the G1 descended from outside males are 25% outcross male, 25% founder female, 50% founder female. This is a different 75% representation of the original bloodline. The outcross (75%) G2 males can be saved for mating to some of the 100% founder females, and also to the 100% and 50% G1 females. The purebred G2 males (100%) are probably best taken back to the outcross 50% G1 females, but also to 100% founder females to which they are not related (not dam nor granddam). They can also be mated back to G2 bloodline-cross females that have different ancestors within the bloodline than those that account for that specific G2 male, as well as different ancestors from outside the bloodline. The goal is to maximize the genetic distance where possible, but to also maximize the influence of the original rescue bloodline.

This strategy quickly becomes complicated. And, unfortunately, the best advantage can be had from using multiple males from each of the various classes of offspring in order to maximize the diversity of the portion of breeding from outside the original bloodline. This can be impractical in many situations where a large number of small

Table 16.2 Rescue situations with a single male, multiple females, and inbreeding require close attention to detail.

Generation	Type of mating with resulting influences		
	Pure founders	Founder male outcross	Founder female outcross
G1	Founder male to founder females = G1 pure 100% (50% founder male) (50% founder female)	Founder male to outcross females = G1 50% (50% founder male) (50% cross dam)	Outcross male to founder females = G1 50% (50% founder female) (50% cross sire)
G2	G1 pure males to founder females = G2 pure 100% (25% founder male) (75% founder female)	G1 cross males to founder females = G2 75% (50% founder female) (25% founder male) (25% outcross female)	G1 cross males to founder females = G2 75% (50% founder female) (25% founder female) (25% outcross male)
		G1 pure males to G1 cross dam females = G2 75% (50% founder male) (25% founder female) (25% outcross female)	G1 pure males to G1 cross sire females = G2 75% (25% founder male) (50% founder female) (25% outcross male)
G3	G2 pure males to founder females = G3 pure 100% (12.5% founder male) (87.5% founder females)	G2 75% males to founder females = G3 87.5% (12.5% founder male) (75% founder females) (12.5% outcross female)	G2 75% males to founder females = G3 87.5% (87.5% founder females) (12.5% outcross male)
		G2 pure males to G2 75% females = G3 87.5% (depends on cross)	G2 pure males to G2 75% females = G3 87.5% (depends on cross)

breeding groups butts up against the constraints of infrastructure. The protocol is outlined in Table 16.2.

The result is a range of G3 offspring that are either 87.5% or 100% the original bloodline. At this point the job is essentially done, especially if the project is a bloodline rescue. An important point is that from this point on, matings should be planned to include the pairing of animals at all levels: 87.5% male to 87.5% female, for example, rather than constantly trying to decrease the outside bloodline's influence by consistently pairing the bloodline-cross animals with bloodline-pure animals. Only by including some degree of the outside breeding is it possible to avoid the reemergence of any inbreeding depression. Managing this cannot be accomplished if one side of every mating is 100% because that strategy slowly eliminates the introduced genetic material that is necessary for success in this situation. This strategy saves the essence of the bloodline and its favorable qualities while leaving behind the inbreeding depression. If a breed rescue (rather than a bloodline rescue) is the target, then a few more careful generations of matching influences are probably warranted, with selection for vitality at each generational step.

16.2.1 Palmer-Dunn Pineywoods Cattle

The Palmer-Dunn bloodline of Pineywoods cattle illustrates both the need for rescuing rare bloodlines and the challenges associated with such rescues (Figure 16.4). Palmer-Dunn cattle are the last remnant of a family bloodline owned by Muriel Dunn, who inherited the cattle and her love for them from her father, Elijah Palmer. The cattle were smooth and well conformed, and had the added benefit that many of them were polled in a breed that is usually horned.

After a few years of a rescue protocol it became obvious that at least some inbreeding depression was surfacing in this old family bloodline. While some of the animals that were produced were productive and thriving, others were flagging in production levels and vitality. The solution to this was to embark on a program that included outcrosses to other bloodlines of Pineywoods cattle. This solved the inbreeding problem while staying within the same pure breed. In addition to the bloodline-cross calves, calves were also produced that were pure Palmer-Dunn. Going down the two routes at the same time provided the opportunity to generate bloodline-pure calves, although with the risk that some may not be all that viable. Along with this strategy was the sort of "insurance policy" provided by the bloodline-cross calves, which are viable and healthy.

In this case the original bull was available along with eight cows and the bloodline-pure sons and daughters of these foundation animals. In order to maximize chances for success, semen was frozen from several of the bloodline-pure bulls produced from matings of the original bull and some of the founder cows. The semen can be used in the future with the bloodline-cross heifers to once again produce cattle that are productive and that have a majority of the influence of the original Palmer-Dunn genetics.

In this bloodline, the polled characteristic adds an interesting twist because it is a desired single gene that is not uniformly present in all animals. While some selection in favor of polledness is warranted, it also makes sense to fully include the horned animals that are produced in order to retain the other contributions they make to the bloodline.

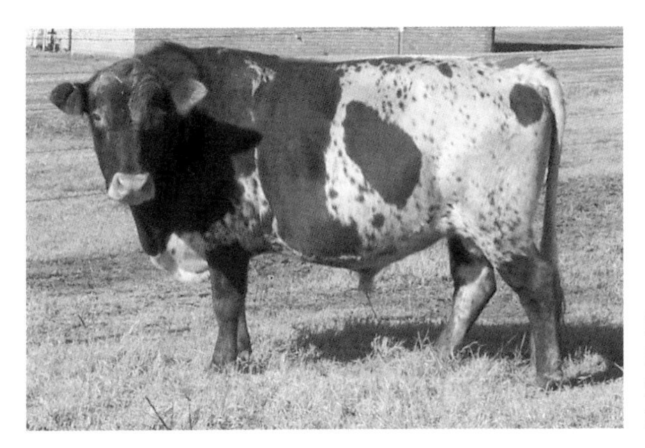

Figure 16.4 Palmer-Dunn Pineywoods cattle offer breeders important options within the breed. Photo by DPS.

16.3 Multiple Males, Multiple Females, All Variably Inbred

Sometimes a single herd of a rare breed remains, containing multiple males and multiple females. These surviving animals are all likely to be related to some degree or another due to the history of being the tail-end of a breed and in a single herd. The most common situation is a herd that has been closed for decades, with a breeding pattern of using a male for a few to several years, then replacing him with a son or two. Over several decades this breeding strategy drastically reduces genetic variation. Even in this situation it is possible to recover viability and productivity, along with building up numbers.

A first step in this case is to accomplish a complete inventory of animals along with their likely relationships. Animals born within the same year are all likely to have been sired by the same male, which helps establish year-groups as groups of half-siblings. Other hints as to relationships can be inferred from the behavior of the animals. Even if some of this information is not accurate it is still better than no information at all. The closest relationships are usually the ones easiest to document, and these are also the ones of most concern in planning out future mating strategies.

In this situation, the genetic diversity likely lies in both the females and in the multiple males. Semen should be frozen from the original males. This saves those individuals for future use. Saving eggs (oocytes) from the females is trickier, but it is possible to harvest embryos or oocytes if abundant financial resources are available.

A general strategy for this situation balances two opposing goals. One goal is to concentrate the influence of the individual founders through some level of inbreeding. Producing some offspring that are a relatively high percentage of each founder helps to avoid a short-term situation where the entire population is made up of animals with an even mix of each founder. While producing an even mixture of the founders sounds harmless, what this really ends up achieving is a situation with little distinction between the animals as well as little genetic distance between them. At that point nearly every mating is equally inbred.

A second goal is to maximize diversity across the breed by balancing founder contribution and minimizing inbreeding. This is nearly the opposite of the first goal, and in this case is done in order to make sure that all founders contribute to the succeeding generations without losing their genetic variations.

These two opposing goals can be accomplished by alternating the two strategies year to year with individual females. The founder females are linebred/inbred one year. This maximizes their genetic contribution to the resulting offspring. They are then outbred the next year, with the goal of achieving an even balance from the various founders. Males, in contrast, can be used every year in both strategies by assuring mating to an appropriate blend of females. This is illustrated in Figure 16.5.

A first step in rescuing this situation is to mate all of the available animals. For example, founder female D can be mated to a relatively unrelated male. If a son is produced, then at maturity he can be mated back to his dam. This is close inbreeding but provides for an opportunity to freeze semen from an animal that is 75% the influence of founder female D. This secures most of her genome for future use. While that son is maturing, founder female D can be mated to a different available male, and if a son is produced the process can be repeated because he will be 75% founder female D, but a different 75% than the

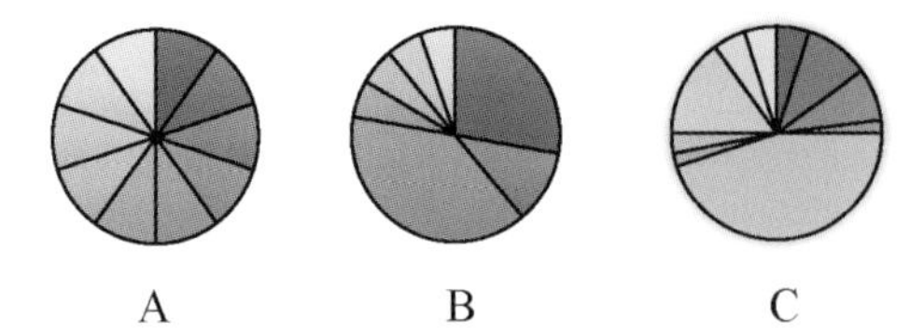

Figure 16.5 Managing founder influences so that some animals have a large contribution from specific individual founders can help to manage the population over time. Animal A has an equal representation of ten founders. Animal B concentrates the medium grey and dark grey founders, Animal C concentrates a different medium grey founder. This makes it possible to balance founders through the mating of animals of types B and C, while type A animals, if mated together, only contribute to the same even mixture. Figure by DPS.

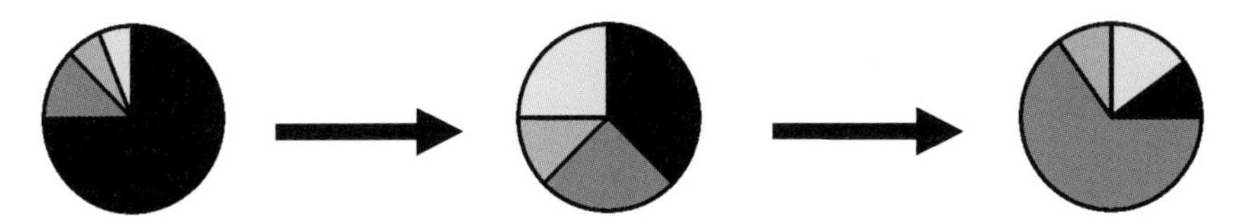

Figure 16.6 Alternating linebreeding and outcrossing can swing the genetic material back to concentration of specific founders in alternate generations, providing for genetic distance between animals. In this example the black influence goes from being dominant then to moderate and finally to minimal. The medium grey influence goes from moderate but then is increased to a majority. These swings are accomplished by alternating inbreeding and outbreeding from one generation to the next. Figure by DPS.

first one that was produced. The remaining 25% of the genetic material in each of these will be different, making it possible to access her unique genome without doubling up on any specific founder male. This strategy assures that any inbreeding is only to the one founder, and not simultaneously to several different ones. This is an extreme strategy, and success depends on the longevity and fertility of the founder females. It is, however, one strategy for assuring availability of their genetic material in the future.

This strategy is repeated across several females, and partitions the genetic variation so that relative genetic distance is developed between succeeding generations. These different strands can then be blended back together in the future. The danger of blending them completely at the outset is that once blended they cannot be separated from one another. Blending them fully reduces the genetic distance between animals and eventually every animal ends up fairly equally related to every other one. The key, as with most rescue strategies, is to try to assure maximum contribution from each founder. The consequences of this are illustrated in Figure 16.6.

This is a situation that can be helped along by superovulation and embryo transfer, although the cost of doing this is likely to vastly outpace the economic value of the first stages of the rescue. Embryo transfer helps to assure the production of both male and female offspring from each mating, with the additional advantage that the hardiest and most vigorous can be retained and used. A potential downside is that not all animals are equally successful in an embryo transfer program, so embarking on this strategy can lead to

Table 16.3 Mating plan for a rescue involving two males and multiple females, with a third male available in year 4. Males A and B along with females D, E, F, G, H, I, J are initially available, with male C being discovered only later. The goal is to both concentrate (inbreed) and distribute (outbreed) the founders over time.

Year	Line based on male A	Line based on male B	Line based on male C
1	Male A to D, E, F	Male B to G, H, I, J	
2	Male A to G, H, I, J	Male B to D, E, F	
3	Male AD to D, E, F, and B daughters from year 1	Male BG to G, H, I, J, and A daughters from year 1	
4	Male AH to mix of females	Male BE to mix of females	Male C to D, F, G, I, and some A and B daughters
5	Male AJ to mix of females	Male BF to mix of females	Male C to E, H, J
6	Male AF to mix of females	Male BJ to mix of females	Male CI to mix of females

over-selection for success in the system, while at the same time assuring that the animals that are less responsive can only contribute minimally. The outcome can therefore be counter to saving a majority of the genetic variation. The details of this mating strategy are outlined in Table 16.3.

16.3.1 Randall Lineback Cattle

Randall Lineback cattle are a landrace from New England with roots in Northern Atlantic cattle. Everett Randall managed his cattle for many decades by a strategy of using a single bull over the herd and then replacing him with a son. This provided for at least some knowledge of relationships among these founders by knowing birth years. The last of the cattle were rescued from slaughter by Cynthia Creech, who acquired seven cows and two bulls, but background information made it possible to add another founder bull and founder cow to the records even though they were not available for use in the rescue. A third bull was found a few years later, boosting the number of founders up to 12.

Fortunately, the three bulls were distant enough in age to be able to assume that they were not sired by the same bull. They also each had a different dam. This was helpful in avoiding a tighter genetic bottleneck than was already apparent from the low numbers and the historic breeding strategy of using single bulls and replacing them with sons.

The breeding strategy was to freeze semen from the original two bulls, along with the third bull that was found later. In retrospect this should have included more straws than were actually frozen. Two bulls were in Creech's herd and could be used alternately with the various cows. As bull calves were produced, these were mated back to their dams for calves that had a very high percentage influence of that founder female. In addition, several cows in every year were deliberately mated with a goal of producing calves that completely lacked any influence from some specific founders. This strategy avoided the herd becoming an even mixture of each founder. As long as some cattle were a high percentage of an individual founder while others were zero percentage, it was possible in the long run to minimize severe inbreeding in at least some matings well into the future. For most founders it was possible to produce animals that were 50% the influence of that specific founder, all

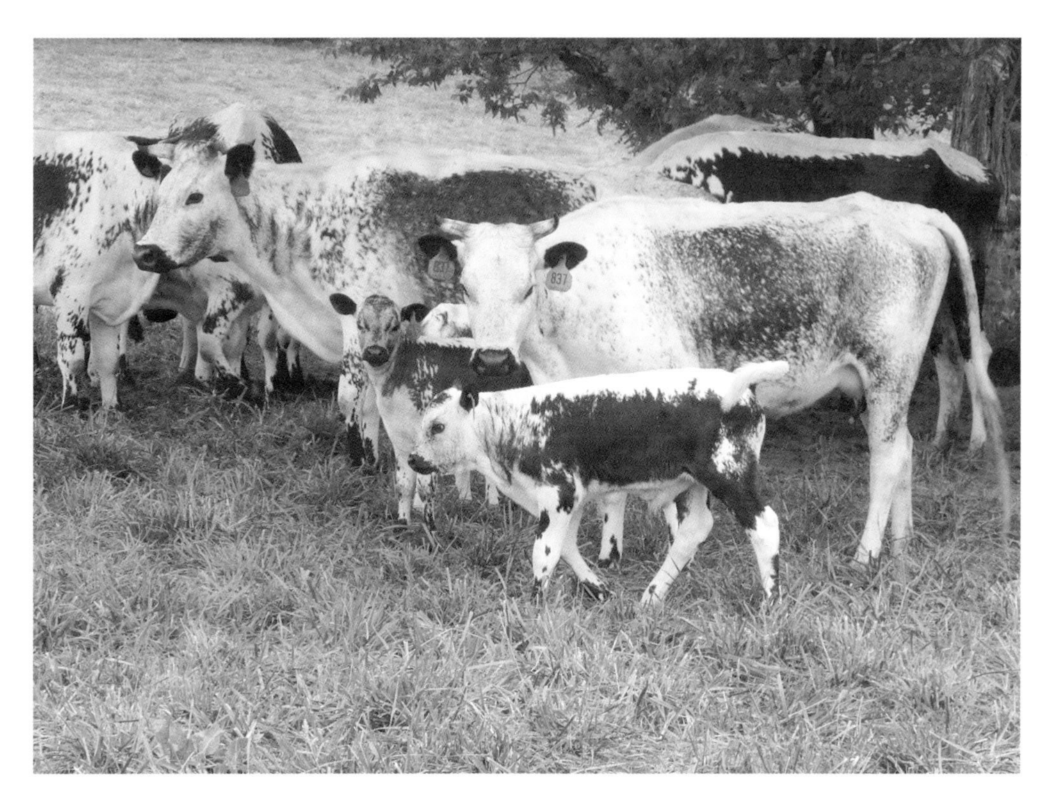

Figure 16.7 Randall Lineback cattle were brought back from the brink of extinction by a careful protocol of maximizing founders in some animals, and balancing founders in others. Photo by DPS.

the way down to 0% in other animals. These two extremes in the contribution of a specific founder could then be played off of one another in future matings. The relatively late inclusion of the third bull provided for his having a relatively low level of relationship to the other animals, allowing the production of animals that maximized the genetic distance he provided.

As the breed expanded it became possible to recruit other breeders to the cause, and having multiple herds minimized the risk inherent when all cattle resided in a single location. In addition, this provided for a variety of approaches and selection goals which also served to maintain diversity. Some breeders were more interested in beef production, while others emphasized the dairy side of this originally dual-purpose breed (Figure 16.7).

Another phenomenon that emerged in the breed was the birth of red linebacked calves. At the time of the rescue all animals were black linebacks, even though red linebacked animals were historically present in the breed. The red calves demonstrate that recessive genes can lurk even in the smallest populations, only to resurface in future generations. Retaining these red linebacked animals assures that the other genetic diversity that they offer to the breed rescue is not lost.

Some cows were discovered to be marginally fertile, which is a common problem in inbred populations. Various breeders took on this challenge by a combination of enhanced management and selection for fertility. The results of management and selection have seen fertility rates rise to 95% in some herds, demonstrating that conservation breeding protocols coupled with selection can indeed produce viable and productive populations of heritage breeds that were once near extinction. From a foundation of ten live animals, there are now well over 500 Randall Lineback cattle in the USA.

In the early days of the rescue, blood typing provided evidence of the uniqueness and validity of the breed and revealed that many Randall Lineback cattle had a variant that was very rare in all other cattle breeds. Later investigations based on DNA microsatellite techniques have similarly validated the breed's uniqueness and the need for rescuing this breed from extinction.

The breed, as expected, has relatively low levels of genetic variation as determined by microsatellites. This finding of low diversity actually helps breeders to safeguard the purity of the breed because any crossbreds are easily detected and can either be eliminated from the breeding program or used in an upgrading protocol. Importantly, the low variation means that animals with lapsed pedigrees due to non-registration can be typed for DNA, and can easily be included as purebreds when the results indicate that this conclusion is accurate. The results of the microsatellite study also illustrate the wisdom of subdividing populations as a guarantee against loss. Some microsatellite alleles are found in only certain herds and not in others. These rare alleles are especially prone to loss by genetic drift, and dividing populations is one way to minimize the chances of this loss across the entire breed.

16.4 One Male, Multiple Herds of Females

In rare cases an entire breed collapses across several different herds. This can result in remnant purebred females in a number of herds, but only a single or a few males. The most drastic is the situation with only one male. This situation usually arises when the females are being crossbred to other breeds, and therefore are not contributing to the recruitment of purebreds into their own breed. This specific situation can seem to be hopeless, but from the viewpoint of genetic rescue it actually can be reversed more easily and successfully than several other situations. The threat in this situation is that action will be too slow to be effective. Pure breeding must be instituted as quickly as possible.

One advantage of this situation is that it is very unlikely that severe inbreeding has occurred because the sudden collapse precludes long periods of close breeding within a small population. In addition, there is likely to be a robust level of genetic diversity contained in the different individual herds. The result is that the remaining females retain a great deal of the genetic variation of the breed. The challenge is to salvage the genetics in the females as completely and quickly as possible. The clock is ticking on those founder females, and it is ideal that each of them make multiple contributions to the next generations.

In this situation it is vital to freeze semen from the remaining male. He should then be used on all the herds, whether by natural service or by artificial insemination. The first crop of offspring (G1) is obviously a large group of half-siblings, and at first thought this would seem to be a very narrow bottleneck. However, when the G1 males are old enough, each herd should use a different one of these. Each of these will have been produced from a different founder female. The result is the G2, and the offspring produced from the founder females (rather than the G1 females) have reduced the founder male's influence down

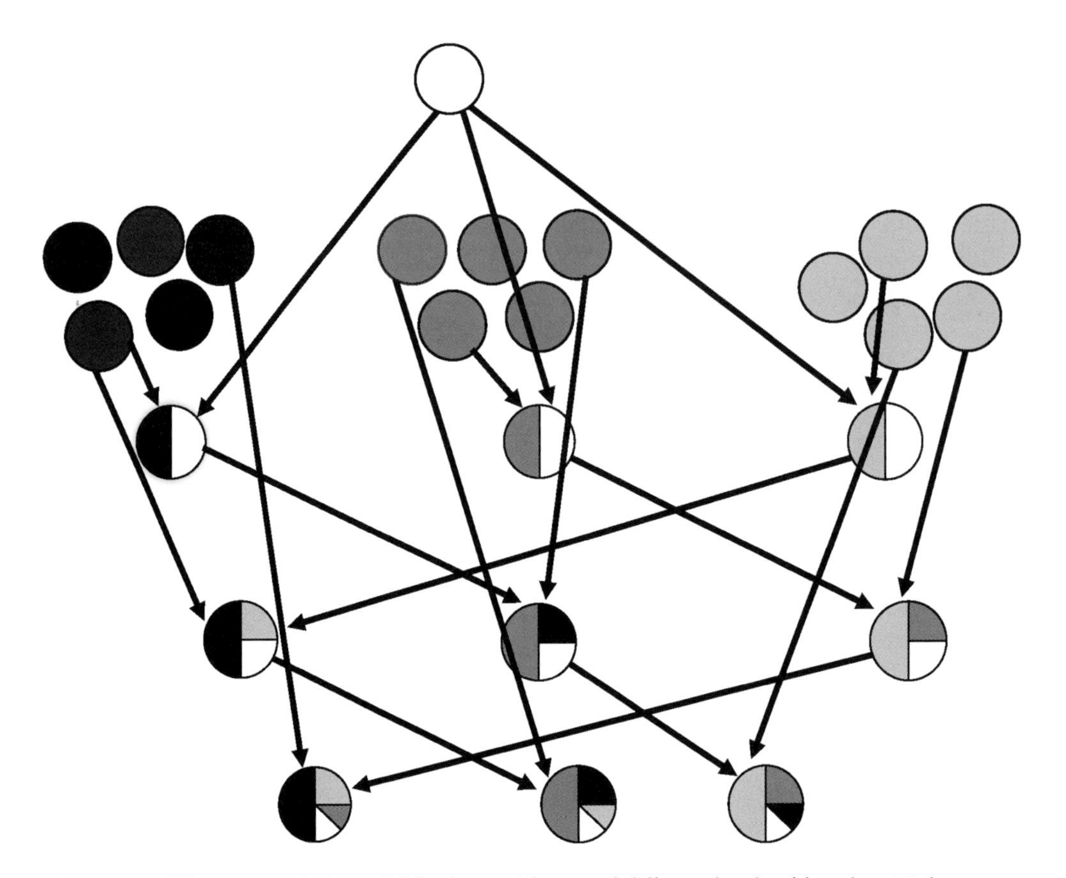

Figure 16.8 When one male is available along with several different herds of females, it is best to use that male in all herds. Sons from other founder females can then be saved after the next cycle. Over multiple cycles this saves the original genetic variation with no bottleneck. Figure by DPS.

from 50% to 25%. This is already progress, and if the cycle can be repeated again, the G3 animals will be down to 12.5% the influence of the founder male. With luck, one more cycle becomes G4 and is down to 6.25% which becomes negligible as the source of any genetic bottleneck (Figure 16.8).

A repeated strategy of selecting breeding males from the oldest unrelated founder females results in the retention of a maximum level of genetic diversity. While the founder male does influence all the animals, the portion in their genome that is not from him is quite different from animal to animal because they each descend from different founder females.

The peculiar aspect of this specific rescue is that by keeping the bottleneck as short as possible it is essentially possible to retain the entire range of biodiversity available in those original founders. Because they are unlikely to be inbred, they are likely to have considerable genetic variation. In contrast, longer bottlenecks lose more and more genetic variation at each generational step (Figure 16.9). Long bottlenecks cannot retain high levels of genetic variation. Short bottlenecks, in contrast, lead to minimal losses. Minimal loss is assured with quick and somewhat aggressive conservation rescue action. While this situation seems

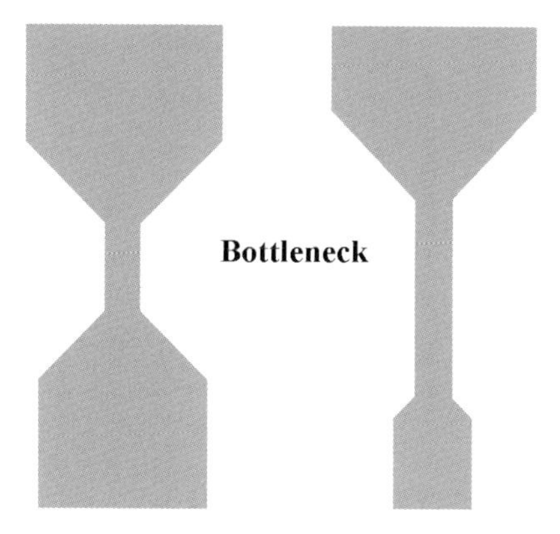

Figure 16.9 Genetic bottlenecks occur when population size declines. If populations quickly expand again, the loss of diversity can be minimized. Long bottlenecks result in more loss, so that eventual recovery is less than with a short bottleneck. Figure by DPS.

nearly hopeless at the outset, careful management can assure success that is beyond what can be expected from other starting points.

Aggressive conservation rescue action means maximizing the contributions of the founder females. They provide both sons and daughters to the program, which broadens the genetic differences among the animals. This is especially important on the male side of the population structure. For males, the "founder female" influence is manipulated to become predominant by the selective and sequential retention of sons from those old foundation females. Different males having different predominant influences from different founder females can be the key to success. These males can then be used to transition the breed from rescue to a very successful breed maintenance phase.

16.4.1 *Criollo Macabeo Cattle*

The Criollo Macabeo is an Iberian-derived breed of local cattle in the lowland tropical region of Ecuador (Figure 16.10). All Criollo breeds have a base in cattle introduced by the Spaniards centuries ago, and the breeds within this group have advantages of longevity, fertility, and adaptation to harsh environments. This, coupled with a moderate to small body size, has made them targets for crossbreeding with larger cattle. Crossbreeding has occurred to the point that many Criollo breeds have become endangered or extinct, a situation facing the Criollo Macabeo.

Fortunately, a single bull calf was born after the last purebred bull was taken for slaughter. About seven herds in the region still have purebred cows, most of which are in their teenage years with some in their twenties. Quick action is essential in this situation, because having the old cows contribute their genetic wealth is the key to long-term success.

Using this bull at the first opportunity, especially on the old cows, is the best strategy. Ideally, assisted reproductive techniques should be used. This is a good situation for

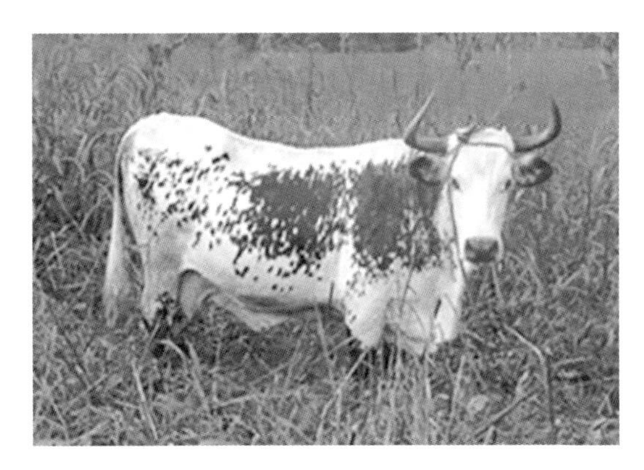

Figure 16.10 The Criollo Macabeo has many interesting traits of adaptation to the Amazonian tropics but was almost lost after bulls were taken to slaughter.
Photo by J.C. Moyano.

superovulation and embryo transfer, especially with the very oldest founder cows. It is an even stronger strategy in the second and third generations that use sons produced from the founder bull and a variety of founder cows, but is obviously only possible if those old original foundation cows are still alive and able to participate. The value in using assisted reproduction techniques to produce G2 and G3 is due to the subsequent calves having less influence from that original bottleneck male, and therefore having more potential advantage for wide use across the breed. Superovulation at the later stages assures that greater proportions of the cows' genomes make it into the succeeding generation. Multiple calves assure a broader rescue of genetic material.

As calves are produced that are low percentage influence of the founder bull, it is wise to begin rotating them between herds. That is, the G1, G2, and G3 bull calves of one herd should be used in another herd. An important caution is that it is ideal that all of the available herds should participate and contribute males to the effort. Relying on only one herd to provide all bull candidates must be avoided. This assures broad survival of the genetic diversity in the older females of each herd. If all the bulls come from only one herd, then eventually the genetic material from that one herd overtakes and swamps the genetic material in the other herds.

16.5 One Large Herd with Satellite Populations

One reasonably common situation with rare breeds is that one (or a handful) of breeders have kept the breed going in fairly reasonable numbers, but a few outlying stragglers are also available. This is a somewhat problematic situation because the genetic diversity ends up arranged such that the single herd contains a relatively large portion of the animals in the breed, but paradoxically only a small portion of the total genetic variation. In contrast the outlier herds contain few animals, but a large portion of the genetic variation needed to move forward. The irony of this situation is that the numerically stronger herd is important for the numerical future of the breed, while the outliers are disproportionately important for the genetic structure of the population. Balancing these contributions genetically, as well as politically, can be tricky.

Diligence and careful planning are required in order to balance the management of numbers as well as genetic variation. If all herds contribute, and if these contributions are

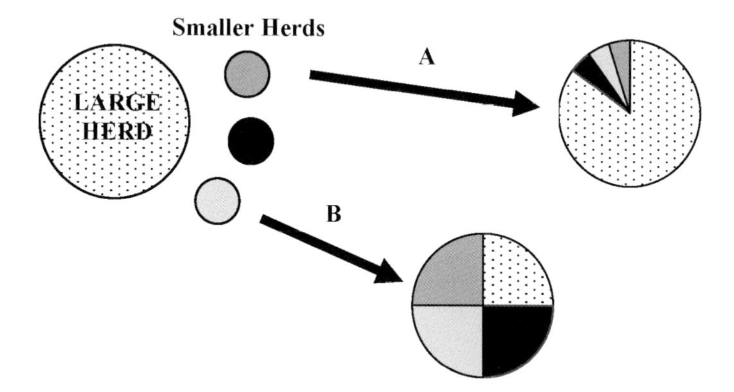

Figure 16.11 Carefully managed mating can balance the genetic contributions of one large herd along with outliers that are either individuals or small herds. If the large herd contributes most of the breeding animals (A), then the final genetic representation is unbalanced in its favor. If the outlier herds are used to balance their genetic contribution (B), then a more uniform contribution can be assured. Figure by DPS.

increasingly balanced across the population, then both numbers and genetic variation can be successfully saved. Drastically shrinking the influence of the large herd while drastically increasing the influence of the smaller ones leads to little net gain unless these changes are managed carefully.

The breed can be considered to be made up of mainstream animals from the large herd, and outlier animals in the small peripheral herds. It is important to use the outlier animals for reproduction and for the recruitment of offspring into the reproductive population. If outlier animals are available in both sexes, then it makes sense to mate some of them together. This takes their genetic uniqueness down to the next generation, along with their distance from the mainstream herd. The dangerous temptation is to rely on the mainstream herd as the main source for breeding males. In addition, the mainstream herd can end up being the majority source of females for any mating to outlier males. Relying too heavily on the mainstream herd for breeding animals over several generations results in replacing the unique genetic variation of the outlier herds with that of the mainstream herd. The strategy of mating outlier male to outlier female counteracts this to a great extent and assures continued production of animals that are distinct from the mainstream herd (Figure 16.11).

In contrast, it can be helpful for the mainstream herd to use animals from the outlier herds in order to balance out the genetic variation in the breed. In cases where outlier males are available, this is relatively easy to do because the males can be used for both sorts of matings (outlier male to outlier female and outlier male to mainstream female). In the case of females, decisions need to be made as to which strategy serves best, and this decision might change year to year as numbers build up. Ideally the pairing of outlier to outlier is accomplished sufficiently to result in expanded numbers such that these can serve as a ready source of genetic variation distinct from the mainstream herd.

16.5.1 Marsh Tacky Horses

Marsh Tacky horses are a traditional breed from coastal South Carolina (Figure 16.12). The breed survived as one large main herd in addition to several small scattered unrelated herds along with a very few unrelated individual animals. A first step in conserving this landrace was to identify animals and to try to document the origins of each animal as much as possible. In this case the origin was often traced back to a specific locality, if not always a specific pedigree. The different areas were isolated from one another, so it was logical to assume that horses from different areas were minimally related to one another.

Horses were mated so that various basic sorts of foals could be made available for future breeders. Many matings were "mainstream herd" where sire and dam both came from the one large herd. Other matings were between outlier animals where sires and dams from the various isolated herds were mated to one another. In most cases these outlier matings were between stallions and mares from different origins, with the important restriction that neither of the pair came from the mainstream herd. This strategy assures that genetic distance is maintained and can be used to balance out influences in the future.

In this situation many of the outlier animals were elderly. Every potential foal needed to be planned for maximal contribution to conservation breeding and population structure.

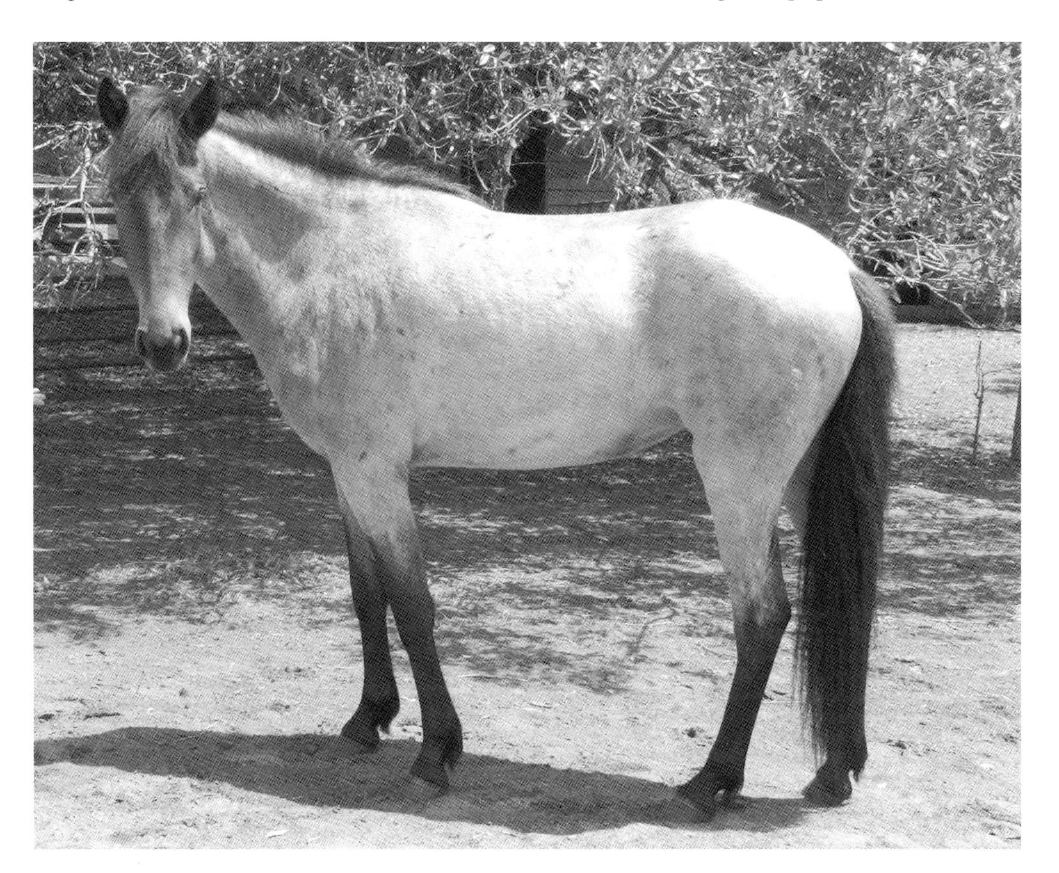

Figure 16.12 This Marsh Tacky mare is from a rare line but has now successfully produced foals from stallions of other rare lines. Photo by JB.

Each foal in this situation has the very real possibility of being the last one from that animal. This is distinct from the situation facing more common bloodlines where the redundancy of genetics among the animals makes it possible to be less restrictive in planning the pairing of elderly animals. A useful general rule is that aged animals (especially females) of rare bloodlines should always be mated to maximally emphasize their uniqueness and to avoid mating them to animals from other more common bloodlines. The mating of these outliers to more mainstream mates erodes their genetic uniqueness rather than building on it and maintaining it. At every opportunity these older females should be designated for producing bloodline-pure offspring. The younger generations produced by this strategy can see a broader range of use, simply because they have many more potential opportunities for contributions and these contributions can cover a broader range of options.

When the G1 and G2 younger outlier animals are available, it is possible and wise to accomplish matings that blend outlier and mainstream influences, although long-term success always should involve at least some matings that preserve these two sorts of original gene pools intact. This can be done handily by the preservation of frozen semen in most species.

16.6 Breeds with Multiple Rare Bloodlines

In many breeds a handful of rare bloodlines are available. In this situation it is possible to mate animals of one rare bloodline to those of another. The product of this is not a specific old foundation bloodline but is something more like a "rare bloodline composite." This strategy has the advantage of assuring that the animals of succeeding generations maintain genetic distinctions from other more common bloodlines. These animals can then be used in the future to balance out the influence of the more common bloodlines.

The strategy of mating animals of one rare bloodline to animals of another rare bloodline is much better than using the rare bloodline animals to mate to animals of common bloodlines. "Rare to rare" mating avoids the danger that the common bloodlines will simply absorb the rare bloodlines, resulting in their complete dilution. "Rare to common" mating performed over succeeding generations results in the original variation in the rare bloodline getting swamped by the genetics of the common bloodline (Figure 16.13).

16.6.1 Choctaw/Cherokee/Huasteca horses

One example of too few animals for stand-alone conservation includes the Huasteca and Cherokee horses that Gilbert Jones had during his horse-breeding career and that were passed along to Bryant Rickman (Figure 16.14). The Huasteca horses were only a single pair from the Yucatán in Mexico. The Huasteca horses were used with each other and also with Choctaw mates over the years. The resulting foals were varying influences of Huasteca and Choctaw breeding. An important detail was that the Choctaw horses used with the Huasteca mates tended to be from distinct families of Choctaw horses that were otherwise unrepresented among the bloodline-pure Choctaw horses used for the conservation project that specifically targeted Choctaw horses. As a result, not only was Huasteca influence common among many horses that were otherwise of Choctaw breeding, but the Choctaw breeding in these bloodline-cross horses was also unique and important for conservation

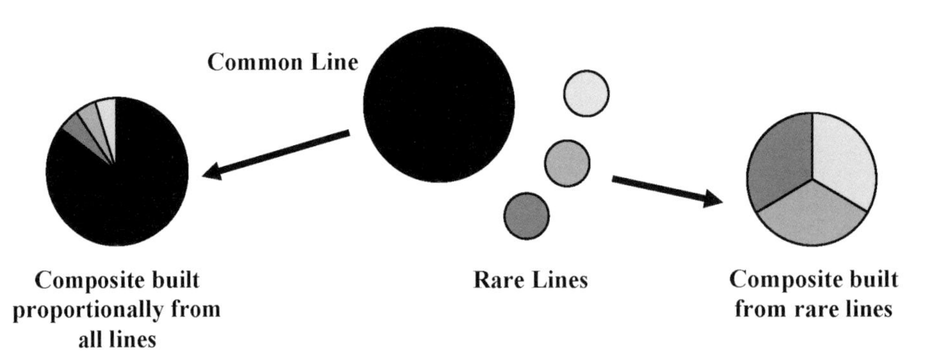

Figure 16.13 Animals of rare bloodlines should be mated together instead of back to a more common bloodline in order to create a "rare bloodline composite" that has a genetic identity unique from the more common bloodline. Figure by DPS.

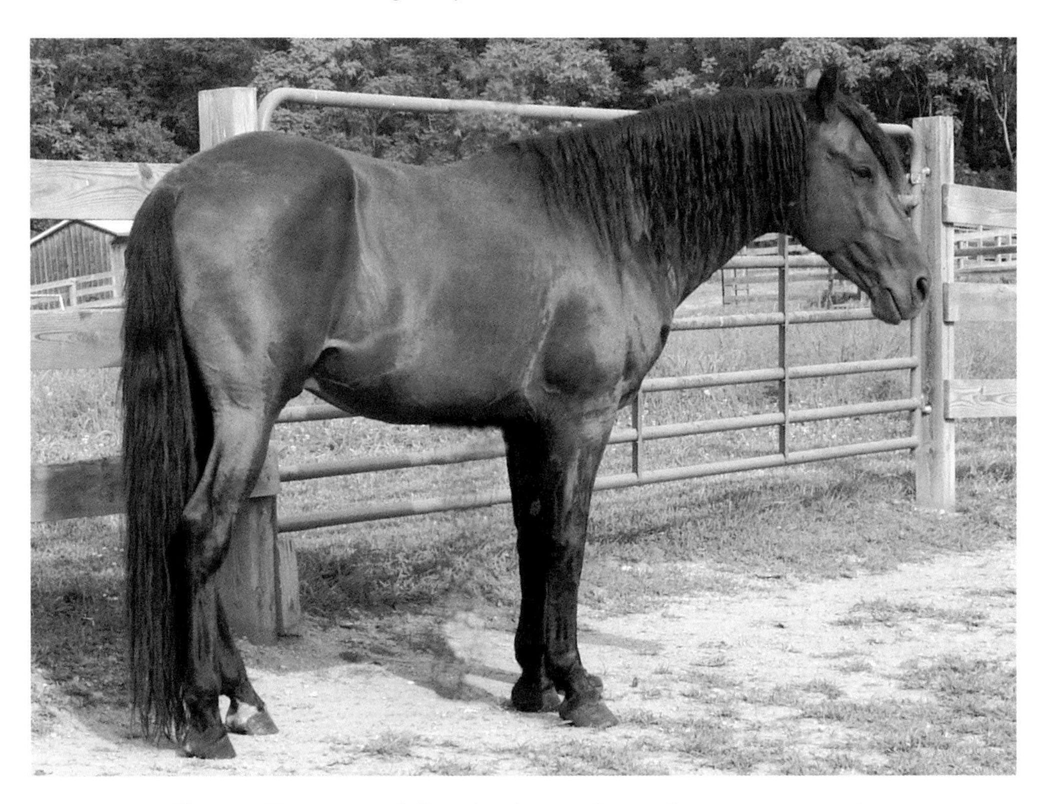

Figure 16.14 Choctaw, Huasteca, and Cherokee horses all contribute to a conservation program that blends these and also maintains genetic distances. Photo by DPS.

in its own right. A decision was made to include these "Choctaw/Huasteca" horses into the overall Choctaw horse conservation project, always keeping an eye on levels of the two sorts of foundation breeding in the horses so that the influences could be closely managed.

Due to the original low numbers of Huasteca horses, it is impossible to maintain a majority influence in very many horses because the only route to achieve that outcome involves considerable inbreeding. In the early days, a few parent-offspring matings were accomplished, so some horses were available that were 75% Huasteca. However, these few and the original Huasteca founders (100%) were all that were available from that bloodline. By careful attention to mating strategies, it is possible to produce a few breeding horses that have 50% of this Huasteca influence, or in a few cases even a bit more. If the Choctaw portion of these horses derives from different Choctaw families, then genetic diversity is adequate so that linebreeding to the Huasteca portion is of minimal threat. This strategy has indeed produced a consistent array of excellent horses over several generations.

Cherokee horses faced a similar fate to the Huasteca horses. Only a few horses remained, most of these with varying influences from older Cherokee, Choctaw, and occasional Mexican lines. These all came from the breeding program of the Corntassle family in Oklahoma. They were eventually brought under the umbrella of the overall Choctaw horse conservation project due to the fact that most horses had varying degrees of Choctaw breeding. Fortunately, there were more Cherokee horses remaining than was the case with Huasteca horses, providing for more options to produce horses with a majority of Cherokee breeding.

The result of previous decisions of breeders led to the situation of a final population that includes many Choctaw horses of 100% Choctaw breeding, along with somewhat fewer that are Choctaw-Huasteca, others that are Choctaw-Cherokee, and several that are blends of all three. The Huasteca and Cherokee influences bring unique strengths to the resulting horses, and therefore simply allowing them to drift to extinction or absorption through successive generations of mating to Choctaw horses is not all that logical. In this situation it is wise conservation to assure that many horses remain 100% Choctaw, and that others remain the various combinations. It is best to always produce some foals that have the maximum of Huasteca or Cherokee breeding that is possible. Over the years it has become impossible to have any Huasteca or Cherokee horses that are up to 100%. However, a strategy of alternating bloodline-pure mating with bloodline-cross mating allows the long-term production of majority-Huasteca and majority-Cherokee horses on into the future.

The recent discovery of a few Choctaw stallions in Mississippi, the last of an old local line, opens up opportunities for joining this line to the Oklahoma lines of the breed (Figure 16.15). In this case, the rare animals were a stallion and two sons from a now-deceased mare. One strategy is to mate each to Oklahoma Choctaw mares, generating foals that are 50% Mississippi breeding and 50% Oklahoma breeding. The females of one can then be mated to the males of the other, for 75% Mississippi Choctaw and 25% Oklahoma Choctaw foals. Ideally, with three animals, it might be possible to go one more cycle for a final result of 87.5% Mississippi breeding. At that point, the horses would include fillies as well as colts, and a viable line that is more than 50% Mississippi breeding would be available to breeders of Choctaw horses.

16.6.2 Rare Strain Pineywoods Cattle

Pineywoods cattle have a number of rare bloodlines that have dwindled down to very few animals. These stand in contrast to a few of the more populous foundation bloodlines such as Conway, Hickman, and Carter. In a few cases, the numbers within the rare bloodline are sufficient for survival after application of good conservation rescue protocols, as was

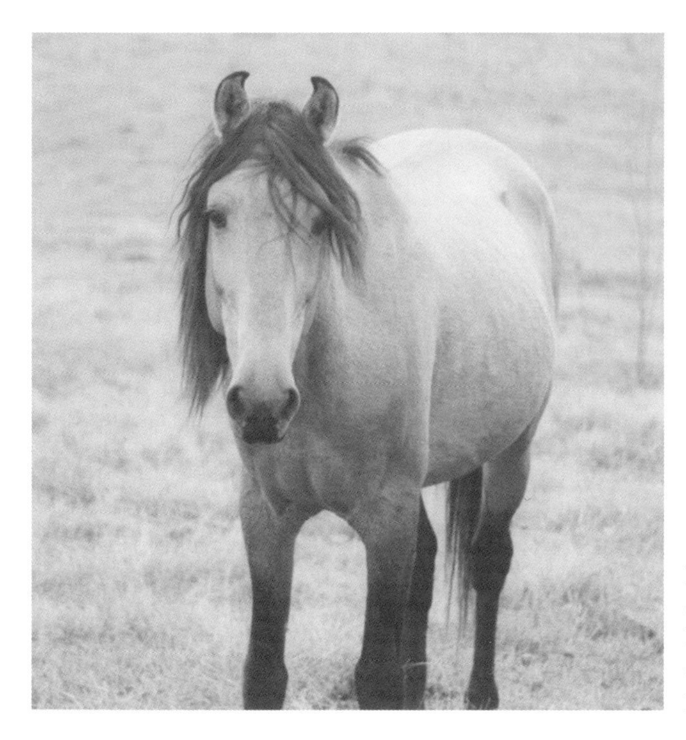

Figure 16.15 The recent discovery of old-line Choctaw horses in Mississippi opens new options for saving this rare breed. Photo by JB.

discussed above with the Palmer-Dunn line. In others the bloodlines are down to numbers that preclude any hope of survival without the inclusion of other genetic material.

Similar to the situation with other breeds that have rare bloodlines, the general recommendation is to mate the rare bloodline Pineywoods animals together. The result of this strategy is to produce a composite entirely based on rare bloodlines. These "rare bloodline composites" give the breed a genetic resource distinct from the more common bloodlines. Carefully managing the three basic sorts of animals (common bloodline, rare bloodline, and rare bloodline composite) provides genetic diversity for the breed's long-term success.

Fred Diamond has succeeded in building a "rare bloodline composite" based on a few individual animals from his old family line (Diamond) as well as those of the Seal, Garner, Ladnier, Bounds, and Griffin families (Figure 16.16). In most cases these influences came from single animals from the older herds that are no longer available. Blending them together maintains their unique contributions so that they can then be used either with one another, or in further composites with more common bloodlines.

16.6.3 *Java Chickens*

Javas are, by their standard, large and robust birds (Figure 16.17). Years of declining population size led to persistence of the breed in only a few pockets that were isolated from one another. As time went on, each pocket began to lose vigor and breed character. This decline was largely due to inbreeding depression, and further relegated this breed to be a trivial relic from the past. Fortunately, Peter Malmberg, of the Garfield Farm Museum, was able to assemble birds from the remaining few strains and cross them with one another.

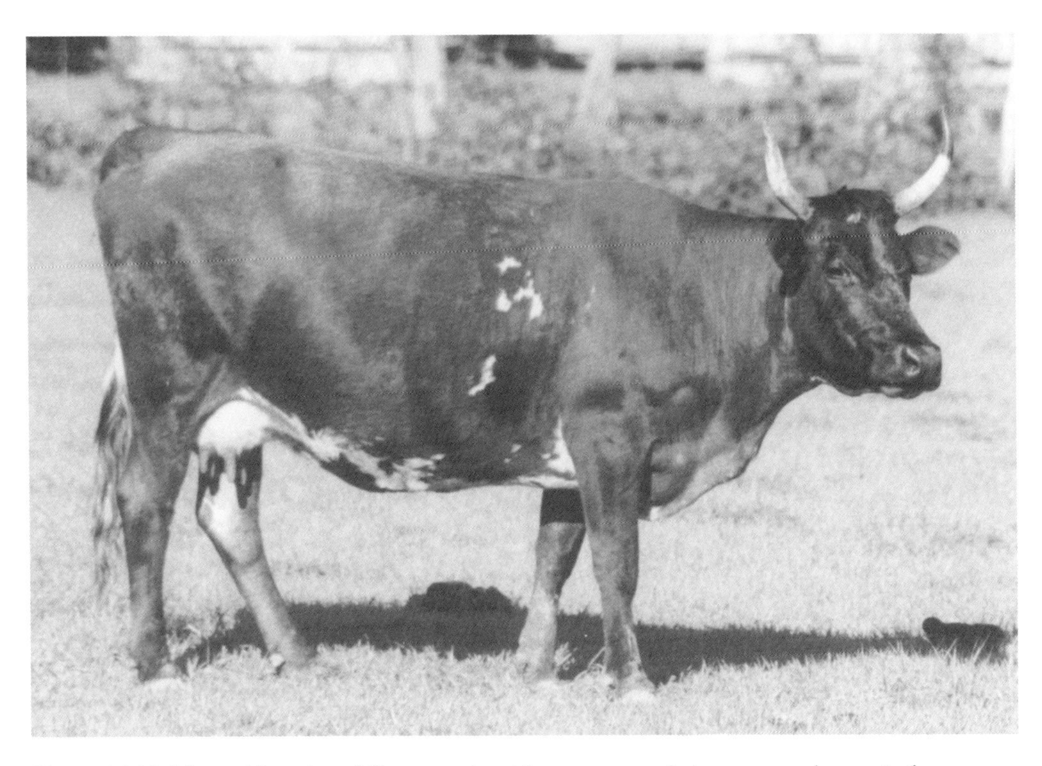

Figure 16.16 Many old strains of Pineywoods cattle can now only be conserved as part of a rare bloodline composite. Photo by DPS.

The resulting birds benefitted from the hybrid vigor of the cross, and regained both vigor and breed character.

At this point it is important to consider next steps for the Java and other breeds like it, as outlined in Figure 16.18. One strategy is to continue to work with the composite population that resulted from the cross. A single composite is likely to again undergo decline as the interrelatedness of birds increases over time with no possible outcrosses. A second strategy is to closely monitor the original, subpar strains and maintain them as reservoirs of genetic variability for the future. This strategy, unfortunately, requires a few breeders to maintain birds of compromised vigor and production. A third option is to carefully manage the original strains by adding in about one quarter or one eighth breeding of the other foundation strain in order to hopefully improve overall viability and breed character while still maintaining important genetic differences in the strains. This is likely the best choice because it is practical for the breeders, and is also not likely to fail genetically. A fourth choice could succeed as well as the third strategy. Combine the strains, then quickly subdivide the resultant crossed population into several different locations and breeding populations to allow new strain differences to emerge. The transfer of breeding animals among such populations needs to be carefully monitored to assure that the entire population does not go in a single direction, with one genetic strain influencing all others. The challenge is to maintain breed type, breed character, vitality, and genetic strength. All of these are greatly influenced by the existence of relatively unrelated bloodlines within a breed.

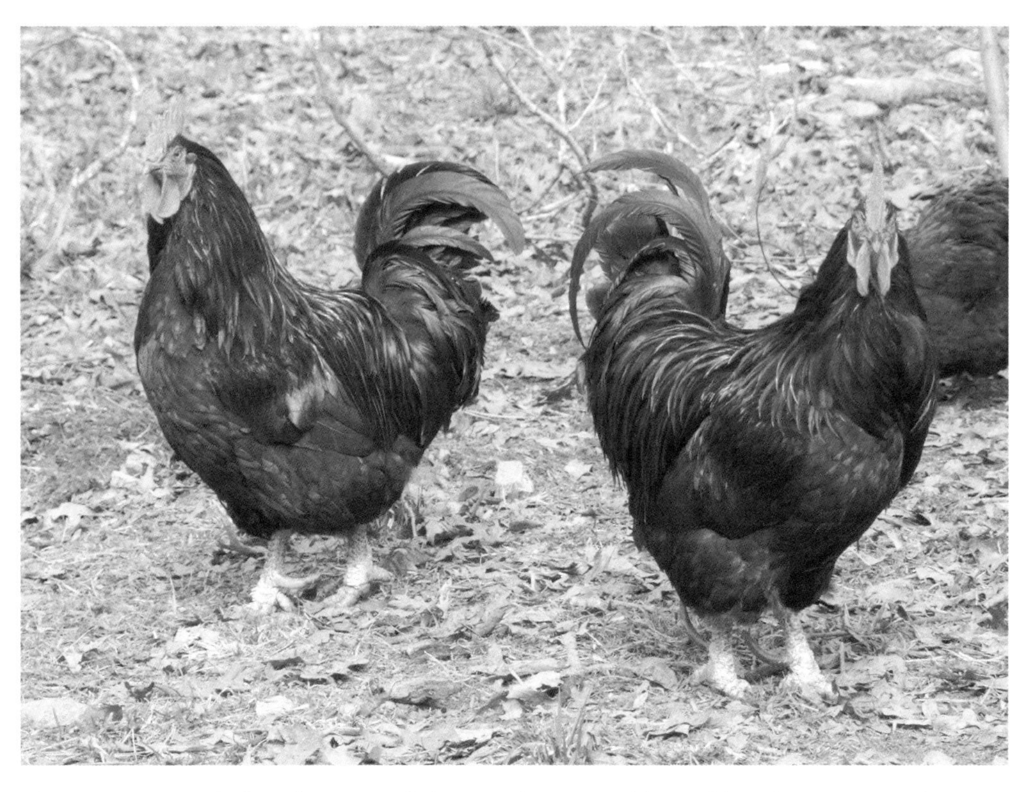

Figure 16.17 Java chickens have recently become the target of focused breeding programs that are bringing back the vitality, productivity, and original breed type that once characterized the breed. Photo by JB.

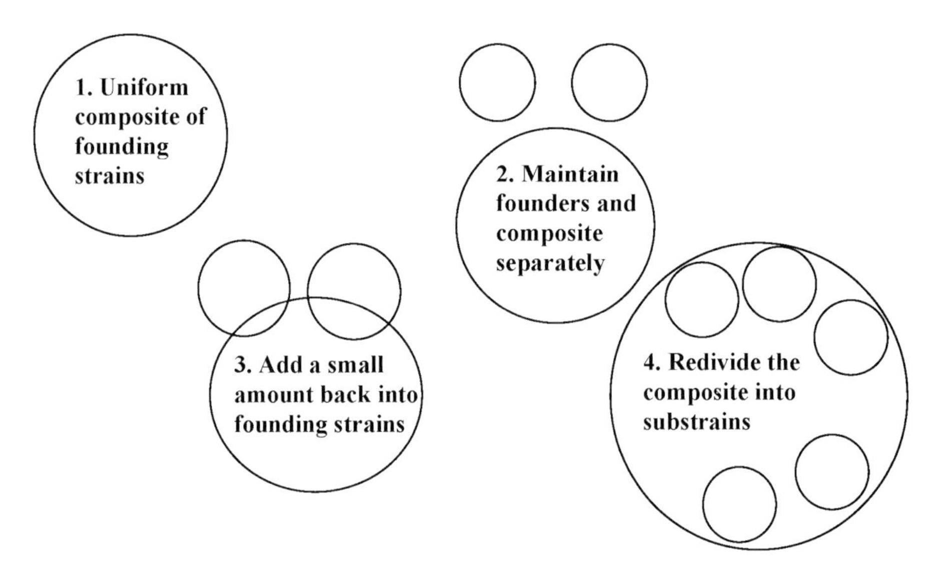

Figure 16.18 Different strategies for managing the genetic diversity in Java chicken populations after an initial cross of unrelated strains has boosted vigor and productivity. Figure by DPS.

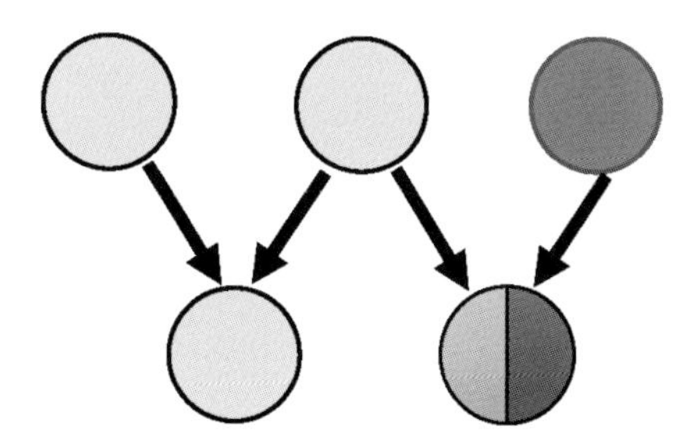

Figure 16.19 Mating an older female (light grey) to her own bloodline provides for a younger generation of that bloodline that has more potential longevity and numbers for breeding. Mating her to a different bloodline (dark grey) removes that opportunity, perhaps forever. Figure by DPS.

16.7 Too Few Animals for Stand-Alone Conservation

Occasionally the numbers of animals in a breed or bloodline fall below what is realistically needed to maintain the line in isolation. In the case of a breed, this spells the end of the breed. In the case of a bloodline or strain within a breed, some good options are available. This is similar to the situation described above with rare bloodlines that show evidence of inbreeding depression, although a few distinctions can be made in planning out strategies for conservation in this situation.

Animals of the rare bloodlines can be used for maximum benefit to achieve the long-term goal of maximizing genetic diversity. In the case of older animals, and especially older females, their reproductive potential is often limited, and every offspring is important. In this case, mating should be limited to within the bloodline in order to maximize retention of the bloodline's genetic material (Figure 16.19). Younger animals that are produced can be used more broadly, and mated both within the bloodline and outside of the bloodline, because they can potentially contribute genetic material for many more years than the older animals can.

Upgrading back to the rare bloodline is a good alternative to genetic erosion because it concentrates rather than dilutes the original strain. The process begins with an outside male mated to the original females. Two or three male offspring are then saved (Figure 16.20). These males are then used, at the youngest possible age, back on the original females. The resulting offspring are then 75% the original strain, and ideally the tactic of using new young males as soon as possible is repeated to yield a crop of offspring that are 87.5% the original strain. This works especially well if the males are recruited from different founding females, rather than the same one repeatedly.

Success depends on the number of the original females, their kinships to one another, their ages, and their longevity. In many cases it is possible to generate a population that is largely the original genetic material of the old strain. This can be useful for overall breed diversity and genetic health. While the general outline of upgrading to enhance a rare strain is presented here, each case is unique and specific plans must be tailored to each specific situation.

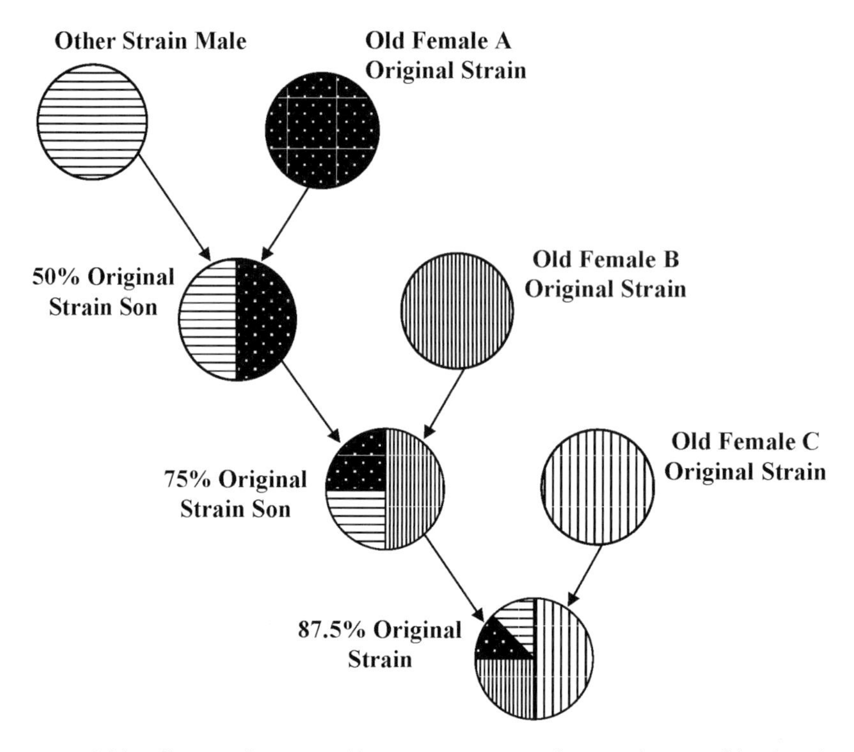

Figure 16.20 A bloodline can be rescued by using a strategy that wisely uses older females of the line as well as their sons. This is a variation of more common upgrading schemes. Figure by DPS.

16.7.1 Eggerton Myotonic Goats

One bloodline of Tennessee Myotonic goat was developed by Sarah Eggerton of Texas (Figure 16.21). The bloodline was reduced down to three females after lightning killed the only remaining buck. A son of one of the does was produced by another bloodline of buck, resulting in a buck that was 50% Eggerton. While this initial buck was growing, a second buck of yet another line produced some 50% Eggerton kids. These bucks were used back on the Eggerton does, resulting in bucks and does that were 75% Eggerton breeding. One of these was used back on the sole surviving doe, providing a buck that was 87.5% Eggerton, and he could then be used on some of the daughters of the other does, providing for a group of animals that had between 50% and 75% the influence of the old Eggerton line. With an earlier start and more initial females, this rescue could have generated a group with even higher proportions of Eggerton breeding, but considerations of eventual inbreeding limited the final percent of Eggerton breeding that was possible.

16.8 Single Animal of Conservation Interest

In some situations, only a single animal remains from a bloodline or is otherwise of special conservation interest for reasons such as possessing some unique characteristic. An entire rescue based on a single animal is impossible, but a few strategies can work to assure the broad genetic contribution of a single animal back into its breed. If the animal is the

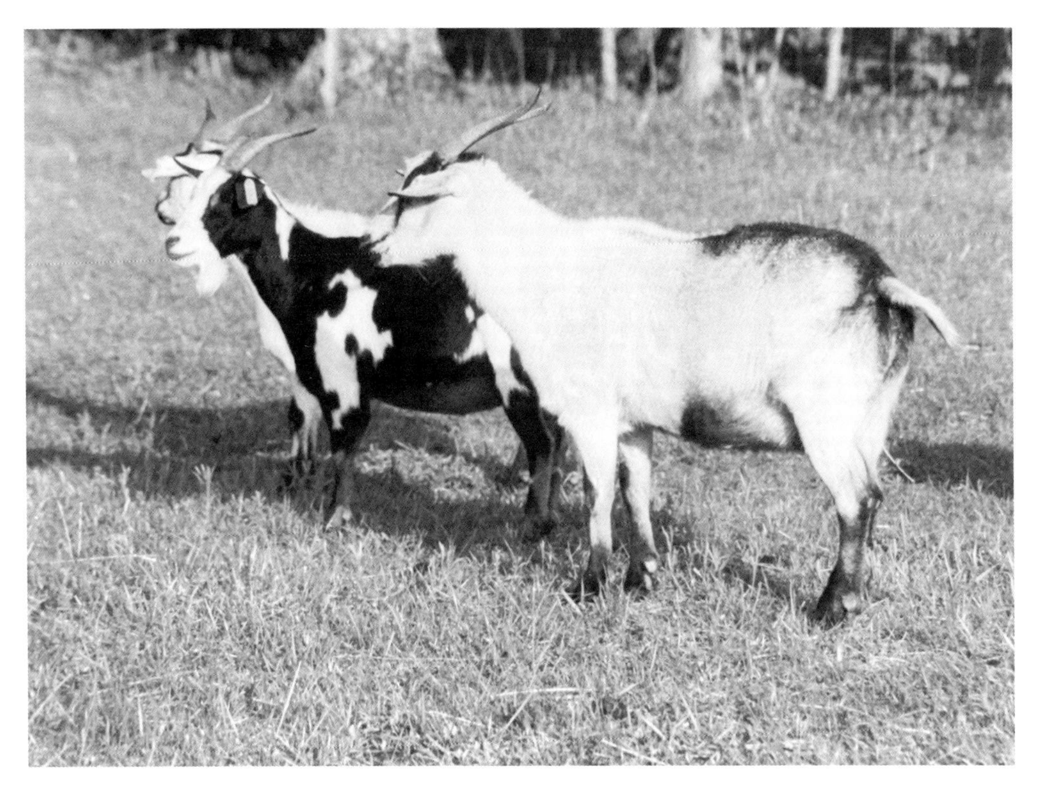

Figure 16.21 Eggerton Myotonic goats were a distinctive bloodline that went down to three surviving females. Careful attention to rescue conservation breeding produced upgraded bucks. Photo by DPS.

last survivor of a distinct breed, then obviously conservation in a pure-breeding sense is unrealistic.

One strategy that has been successful when the situation involves a remnant of a bloodline is the mating of a rare animal to an animal from another bloodline within the same breed. This produces a G1 offspring that is 50% the influence of that one rare animal. If luck holds and the G1 offspring is of the opposite sex, then it can be mated back to its parent, the result being a G2 that is 75% the influence of the original animal. The number of generations for which this is successful depends entirely on the individual animal involved. There is no really good predictor of when repeated backcrosses to the one individual will begin to fail due to inbreeding depression. It is therefore generally safest to stop at the 75% level, although some animals have gone up to one more generation (87.5%) with no ill effects (Figure 16.22).

This strategy of successive back-mating to a foundation animal works out slightly differently for males than it does for females. Males can easily produce several different G1 offspring from different mates, and the female offspring can then be mated back to their sire. In the case of an initial female, progress will be slower unless financial resources for embryo transfer are available. An additional note is that litter-bearing species have the advantage of multiple offspring following a single mating, which usually opens up a

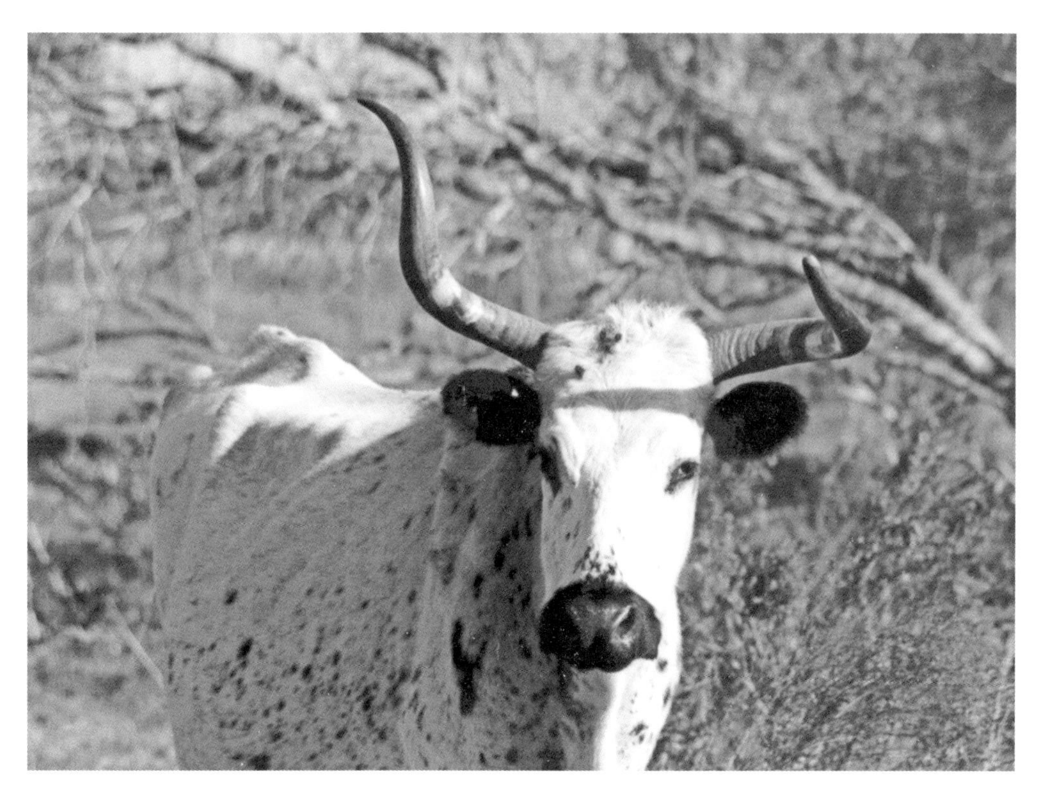

Figure 16.22 This Texas Longhorn cow is the result of three generations of cows mated back to the same original sire, so she is 87.5% his genetic influence. She was productive and hearty, but that result cannot be guaranteed for every instance of such close inbreeding. Photo by DPS.

variety of options much earlier than with species that produce only a single offspring per birth.

It may be possible to use this strategy repeatedly, depending on species and lifespan. This example assumes that the initial animal of interest is a female of the targeted bloodline A. The initial bloodline cross is to bloodline B. This produces a G1 animal that is 50% A, 50% B. This animal is mated back to the parent for a G2 offspring that is 75% A, 25% B. The founder animal from bloodline A is next mated to a different bloodline (C) using a similar two-generation approach. The resulting G2 is then 75% A, 25% C. The final result is that the 25% of the two different sorts of G2 animals is from different bloodlines (B for one, C for the other). This maximizes the diversity of the portion of the genome that is not coming from the bloodline A, which provides genetic distance so that these can either be used by pairing them together or pairing them sequentially with other outside animals (Figure 16.23).

16.8.1 Glendhu Leicester Longwool Sheep

The strategy of repeated outcrossing to different bloodlines followed by inbreeding back to a vanishing bloodline was used successfully with Flora Glendhu, a Leicester Longwool ewe from the original Tasmanian importation by Colonial Williamsburg that reintroduced this breed into the USA. Flora Glendhu was the only animal imported from one of the source

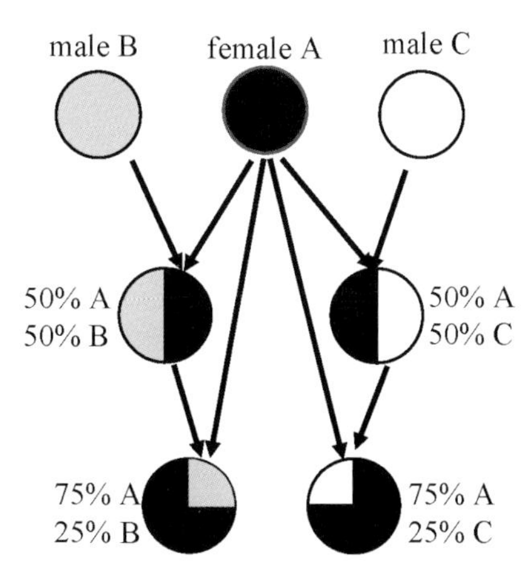

Figure 16.23 Targeted inbreeding can produce breeding animals that are 75%, or even 87.5%, the influence of specific rare or otherwise genetically valuable animals. If this is done from different mates over time, the "non-rare" piece of the genome is different for each animal, providing for inbreeding that is only targeted on that one rare or desirable animal. Figure by DPS.

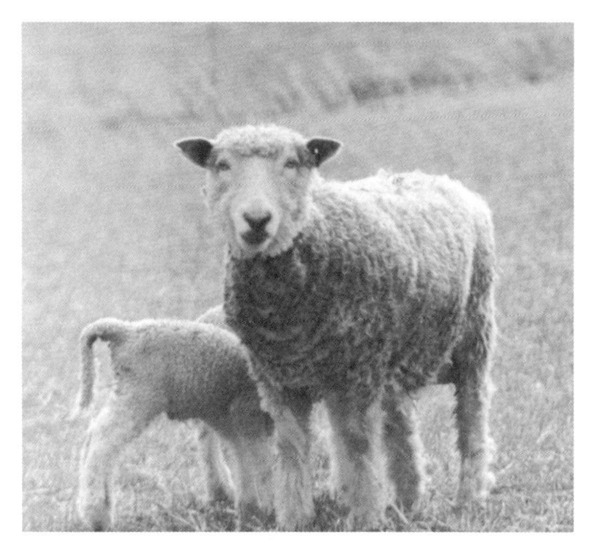

Figure 16.24 Flora Glendhu was able to make a lasting genetic contribution to the Leicester Longwool breed in the USA despite her being the only animal imported from one of the original Tasmanian foundation flocks. Photo by DPS.

herds. She represented unique founder genetics, and was stout, hardy, prolific, and a good mother (Figure 16.24). She was not only rare, but was also a highly desirable example of the breed.

It was possible to mate her to a ram of another bloodline. Fortunately, she produced twin lambs: a ram and a ewe. The ram lamb was then mated back to her, with the final result of lambs (fortunately, a ram and ewe) that were 75% her influence. Rather than using that 75% ram lamb back on her, it was decided to mate her to a ram of a different bloodline to produce another set of twins. The ram lamb of that set then repeated the entire process to produce lambs that were 75% her influence, the balance being 25% that was different from the first cycle.

This strategy succeeded in producing two rams and two ewes, each 75% the old Glendhu breeding with the other 25% having no overlap in the two sets of twins. The result is that 94% of her genetic material was made available from the two rams, boosted up to 99% by including their twin sisters. The two rams were then used widely in different flocks. Her daughters also were included in breeding programs. Through her sons and daughters that had 75% her genetics, her influence in the breed was assured. The genetic material that once had limited availability in a single ewe was thereby used broadly to strengthen the breed with her genetic diversity but also her phenotypic excellence.

16.9 Frozen Semen Available from Historic Stores

Rare breeds include many that were once popular but have subsequently dwindled to rarity. Many of these once-popular breeds have stores of frozen semen available from males long dead. This is especially the case for cattle. Conservation breeders can use this to their advantage because it is possible to use the older semen stores in contemporary programs. The use of the semen can follow the same strategy as that outlined above for using outlier or rare bloodline animals in live breeding.

In situations where multiple sires of multiple bloodlines are available it is possible to come close to resurrecting the traditional breed by the use of frozen semen for several sequential generations. This strategy essentially replaces contemporary genomes with those from the past. Care must be taken to not completely eradicate the contemporary genomes, but in most cases, this is not a realistic fear in most breeds due to the ease and availability of contemporary animals used for live breeding.

This situation is different from the more usual rescue situations that involve populations where the majority of the genetic variation resides in females. The majority of the genetic variation in this situation is in the semen that was frozen long ago and the bulls providing this semen are the founder animals, in contrast to the contemporary females.

One strategy for maximizing the genetic contribution of the older frozen founder bulls' semen is to mate the females produced at each generational step back to other sires using their semen that was frozen long ago. While this would be unwise across an entire breed, it can make sense to accomplish this tactic for several generations in at least some portions of most breeds. The result is animals that have increasingly strong representations of long-gone genomes. Using frozen semen from sires long dead offers an opportunity to dip into a breed's genetic storehouse back before any genetic bottleneck existed. The use of older frozen semen is an opportunity to recapture some of those earlier phenotypes in breeds that have seen dramatic changes in breed type over the years. In many cases these old types are still quite useful. Some breeds have seen varying degrees of sanctioned introgression from outside breeds over the years. This is usually fairly recent, and in this situation the opportunity to take remaining purebred females back to long-dead sires can rejuvenate purebred lines that are free from introgression.

16.9.1 Shorthorn Cattle

The historic fates of Shorthorn cattle have interesting twists with important lessons for breed conservation (Figure 16.25). The Shorthorn was once popular in its own right and

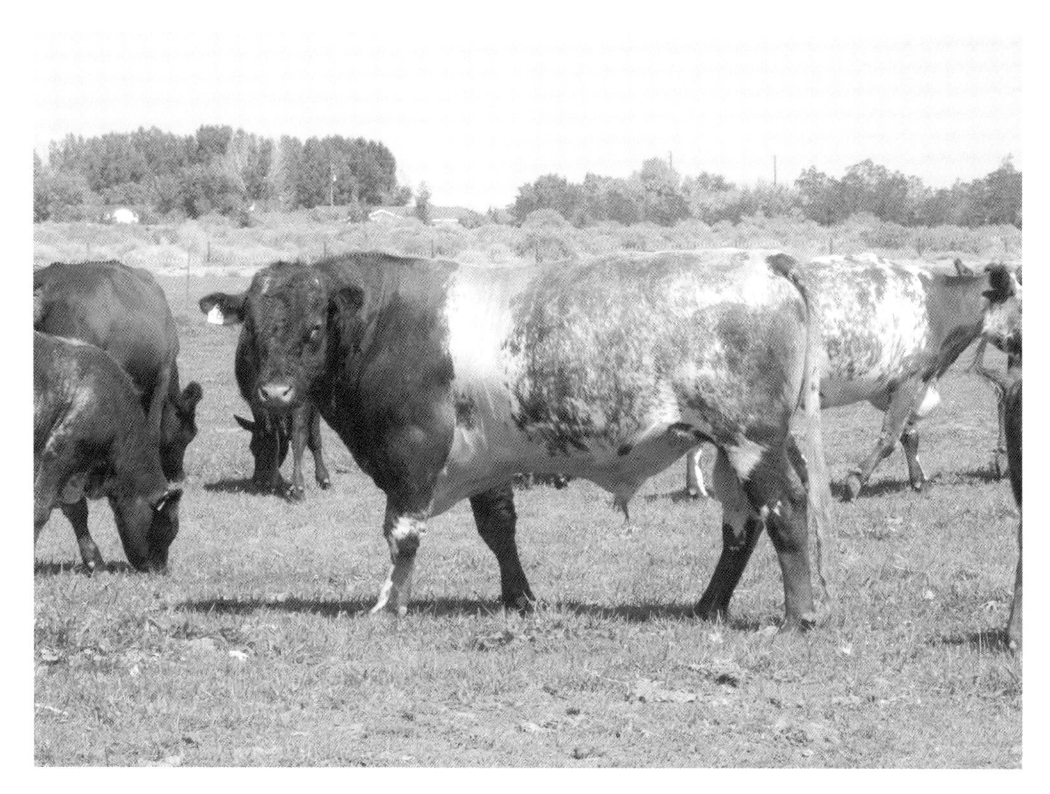

Figure 16.25 Shorthorn cattle are a breed that can greatly benefit from a large store of historically important purebred sires. Photo by JB.

was broadly used across the world to influence many other breeds. The Shorthorn's popularity began to decline, and it became relatively common practice to include influences from other breeds to modify the breed's phenotype according to the then-prevailing fashions and changing demands. Shorthorn populations throughout the world underwent considerable introgression either to increase meat production or to increase milk production depending on producer goals for this originally dual-purpose breed.

As is common in many breeds, conservation-minded breeders have always appreciated the original type of the breed and have therefore stuck with the purebred populations. The USA now has more of this purebred remnant of the breed than any other country, making the purebred American Shorthorns an international conservation priority. This remnant purebred group are identified as "Heritage Shorthorn" or "Native." "Native" might be a bit confusing, but in this context, it refers to being "native to Yorkshire and other regions original to the breed." This group of cattle has several real advantages that can lead to successful conservation. One advantage is that the breed associations accept such animals into the registry, and identify them as the unique resource they are. This gives the cattle a distinct identity within the breed and cleanly separates them from cattle that have introgression from other breeds. A second significant advantage is that a number of bloodlines within this elite group are available to breeders. Frozen semen stores from past decades add considerably to this diversity and bring forward traditional types that are increasingly in demand as the market once again emphasizes efficient cattle that can fatten on grass alone.

Cattle breeders also benefit from the many advanced assisted reproduction techniques that are more readily available for cattle than for many other species. Frozen semen, even if only available in limited amounts for some bulls, can be used with cows that are superovulated with subsequent embryo transfer in order to produce more than a single calf. The heifers produced by matings of contemporary cows with historic semen can then be put back to historic bulls, increasing the relative influence of the historic genetic material. The males produced by such a strategy can also be grown out, and their semen frozen to increase the availability of these historic genetics.

16.10 Managing a Genetic Defect

Some rare breed populations bring along with their advantages a few disadvantages in the form of specific undesirable genes. These genes must be dealt with carefully. Especially in a rescue situation, an approach involving drastic culling is likely to lead to extinction rather than success. This is complicated by the fact that modern technology often brings the rapid development of tests for genetic diseases or other undesirable genes. This opens up the possibility of widespread testing of breeding stock. The cascade of decisions that follows any testing is important. Rather than the culling of all carriers, in most breeds it is usually more logical to simply avoid mating them together. This is especially true in rare bloodlines and in rare breeds.

Avoiding the mating of carriers together instantly eliminates the production of affected offspring for those defects that are due to recessive genes. Fortunately, this includes most defects in most species. This single strategy is sufficient to assure good animal welfare while also maintaining the genetic diversity that is housed in the carrier animals. The offending gene can then be tracked through the generations, assuring that carriers are never mated together. This also ensures that the frequency of the gene in the population is decreased while not simultaneously removing so many animals that genetic variation for other traits is lost.

16.10.1 Akhal-Teke Naked Foal Syndrome

Akhal-Teke horses represent an important foundational root for all horse breeds (Figure 16.26). The breed rarely produces naked foals that are due to a recessive gene. When two copies of the gene are present, the result is the birth of a hairless foal that dies soon after birth. Breeders are understandably eager to avoid the birth of affected foals and a genetic test is now available that reliably identifies carriers as well as horses that are free from the allele. In this rare breed, a detailed herd book analysis can be coupled with widespread genetic testing for the gene in order to identify carriers as well as categorize them as being from common or rare bloodlines.

Different decisions may well be appropriate for carriers from common bloodlines in contrast to those from rare bloodlines. In the case of the common bloodlines, it is likely that non-carrier animals are available. In this situation, it is no loss to the breed to remove the carriers from reproduction, provided that such an action is not removing animals that

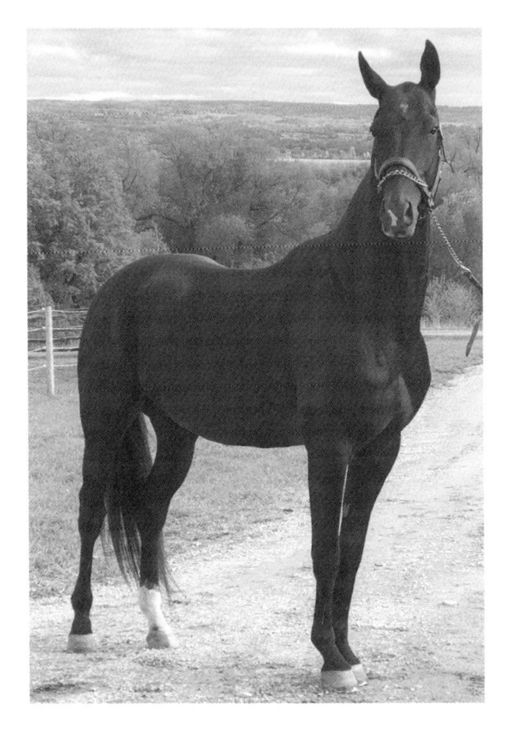

Figure 16.26 Akhal-Teke horses can benefit from the wise management of the rare recessive lethal gene the breed has. It is possible to manage the gene while also assuring good genetic variation. Photo by JB.

are truly excellent in traits other than this single gene. In the case of rare bloodlines, the breed can clearly lose a great deal from culling all of the carriers. It makes sense to use carriers from rare bloodlines, but only as mates to horses that test negative for the gene. This assures that their genetic variation that is so essential for breed survival is passed along to the next generation, but without the birth of affected foals. A few generations of this approach should reduce the frequency of carriers by selectively retaining non-carriers. Even if breeders decide not to reduce the frequency of the gene, the practice of not mating those carriers to one another still eliminates the production of affected foals regardless of the frequency of the gene.

In this case both the breeders and the breed association have important roles. The breed association needs to educate breeders carefully and fully as to the issues surrounding the genetic disease and its control. At the same time, the association needs to wisely formulate rules and strategies that control the mating of carriers to one another, while also avoiding the trap of devaluing the carriers. One potential solution among several is the institution of a rule that insists on the genetic testing of all stallions. The stipulation can then be made that only mares that are tested as negative for the gene can be mated to carrier stallions. This is essentially requiring that stallions all be tested, and that mares mated to carrier stallions be tested with negative results. Mares mated to non-carrier stallions would not need to be tested, but certainly could be.

It may be necessary to somehow boost the economic reward for using a carrier stallion to counter any inherent bias against carrier stallions. This could be done by reducing or eliminating registration or other fees, especially if the testing of foals from carrier stallions is required as a further step in tracking the gene.

CHAPTER 17

Putting the Lessons Together: Dexter Cattle

The dynamics of Dexter cattle include a host of issues that usefully illustrate many of the important details in breed management and conservation. These details relate back to wide ranging aspects of breed biology including breed definition, breed type, managing gene pools, selection, use of assisted reproductive techniques, breed analysis, breed maintenance, and the rescue of small populations. None of these aspects are unique to Dexter cattle, but the breed serves as a handy reference point for nearly all of them and how they can all be considered together to strengthen and maintain a breed for long-term success.

Irish cattle breeds have varying histories, and were first standardized during the 1800s although that process continued until fairly recently (Table 17.1). The earlier Irish cattle population was more variable than any of today's descendant breeds, which is a common trajectory as a landrace becomes standardized.

Both Dexter and Kerry cattle were registered in the same herd book in the early days of the breed association. Some early observers considered Kerry and Dexter cattle to be a single breed, with the difference being that Dexters have the single gene that confers dwarfism. Genetic evidence is now available to show that this simplified version was in fact not the case. Breeders always considered the two breeds to be different from each other despite their both having black color and horns. It appears that minimal crossing between the two gene pools took place so that genetic differences between them persist to this day. This goes back to the importance of a breed's definition. One definition of these two populations yields one gene pool with two varieties separated by a single gene. The second definition, the accurate one, reflects the fact that the two populations are indeed different breeds with complex underlying distinctions that warrant maintenance in isolation from each other.

The other Irish cattle breeds have other interesting details. A Droimeann cow named Big Bertha is the oldest recorded cow. She lived three months shy of 50 years, having produced 39 calves. Droimeann and Irish Moiled cattle are both dairy breeds, and both have the distinctive lineback pattern that ranges from nearly all colored with a white stripe down the back, to intermediates with speckled sides, to nearly all white with colored ears, eye rings, muzzles, and feet (Figure 17.1). This pattern also occurs in several Scandinavian breeds, and

Table 17.1 Irish cattle breeds are now standardized, but the range of colors, horn status, and body sizes reflects an earlier more variable population.

	Dexter	Kerry	Droimeann	Irish Moiled	Bó Riabhach
Organized	Pre-1900	Pre-1900	2016	Pre-1900	Not yet
Color	Black, dun, red	Black	Black lineback Red lineback	Red lineback	Brindle
Horns	Horned	Horned	Horned	Polled	Either
Size	Dwarf	Normal	Normal	Normal	Normal
Use	Dual-purpose	Dairy	Dairy	Dairy	Dual-purpose
Origin	Southwest	Southwest	Southwest	North	North central

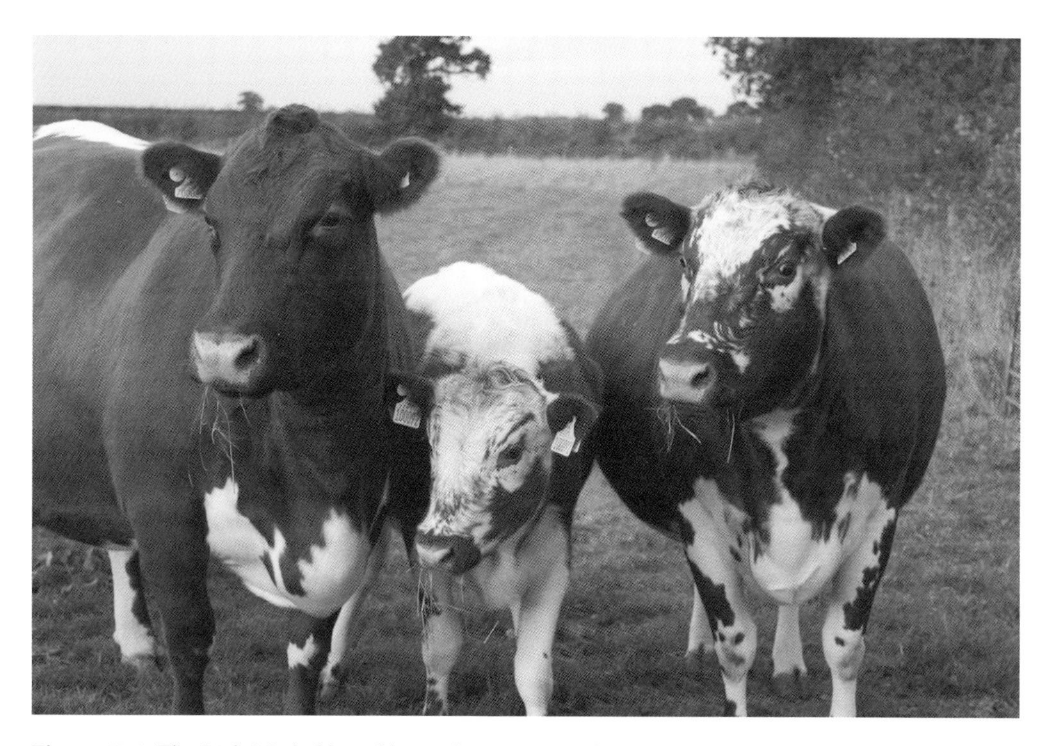

Figure 17.1 The Irish Moiled breed has a distinct origin from the southwestern Irish breeds. Photo by JB.

one theory is that it arrived in Norway and Sweden with cattle plundered by the Vikings. The Bó Riabhach breed is brindle, and is still fairly early in the process of being defined as a breed. The Irish breeds reflect the definition of breeds by an interaction of geography, breeder selection, and external characters such as color, horns, and dwarfism.

The fate of the Dexter breed follows that of many other breeds. In the early 1900s the breed was relatively common, and was exported to various countries such as the USA, South Africa, and England. In the mid-1900s the breed fell out of favor. Low numbers interacted with the privations during World War II to threaten the breed's existence. Many herds were lost to record keeping. In the late 1900s the breed's fate once again changed.

An enthusiastic new generation of breeders has now expanded numbers, so that the breed is no longer considered at risk of decline and extinction. The relatively short bottleneck has assured retention of a great deal of the breed's genetic variability.

Distinct groups of Dexter breeders have chosen a few different pathways for going forward within the breed. Some of these differences have generated a great deal of emotion, with a few breeders insisting that their approach is the only single valid approach for the entire breed. However, no single specific breeding philosophy can be validated as the only correct way forward to the exclusion of all the others. They each can serve as useful points to discuss the practicality of realizing goals and the long-term consequences of the different approaches. Constructively managing divergent goals is one of the great challenges on the political and cultural side of breed conservation. Any strategy that allows different philosophies to peacefully coexist benefits the breed involved. A closer look at the biology involved can inform breeders as they make these important decisions.

Dexters come in two basic types, both of which are small. The dwarfism of the short-legged type is due to a single gene. Cattle with one copy of the gene are achondroplastic dwarves. Cattle with two copies are aborted late in gestation with severe developmental abnormalities. This presents the breeders with a challenge because mating two short-legged dwarves together comes with a 25% chance of this negative outcome. It is tempting to suggest that an easy solution is to eliminate the gene. However, breeders with long experience insist that the traditional short-legged dwarves have very real advantages in adaptation and production, and even in temperament. They should not be discarded lightly.

The availability of a test for this gene has led to two responses. Many breeders simply avoid the gene altogether, which then runs the risk of the gene going to extinction. Other breeders have adopted the strategy of avoiding the mating of two carriers. Both strategies succeed in assuring that no abnormal calves are produced. Importantly, the strategy of continuing to use carriers with non-carrier mates provides for the continuation of a trait that is recognized as useful by several breeders. This trait is also traditional for the breed, even if not uniformly present in all animals of the breed.

Demand for breeding stock changed somewhat as a consequence of a test being available for dwarfism. Carriers of the gene now have a somewhat lower monetary value than those that do not carry it, although this varies from situation to situation. Semen from carriers likewise meets with less demand than semen from non-carriers. However, it is important for non-carriers to be mated to carriers. Breeders therefore need to assure that carriers of both sexes are broadly available in the breed.

Most Dexters a century ago were black, horned, dual-purpose, achondroplastic dwarves (Figure 17.2). Dun, red, and non-dwarf calves always popped up from time to time and were fully included as purebreds. Due to the consequences of the dwarfism in the breed, and to the horns, many current breeders have opted to select for animals that are not dwarf, not horned, and not black. Many breeders target red, polled, non-dwarf cattle, a type that is distinct from the original cattle a century ago. This selection has changed the overall style of the breed away from its original form. While this change of average breed type is true of the Dexter and is an easy target for some level of condemnation, such changes are also true of most other breeds if contemporary types are contrasted to historic types.

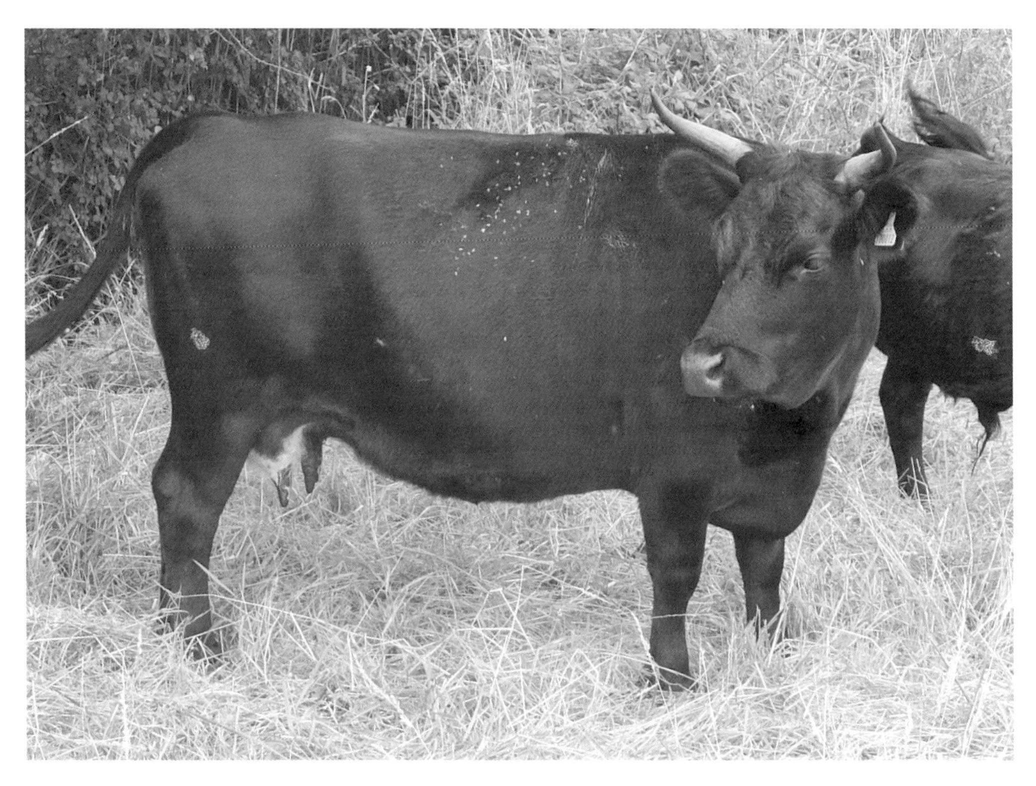

Figure 17.2 The traditional type of the Dexter breed is important to maintain. Photo by DPS.

The history of genetic influences in the breed can be superimposed over the variation that is provided by the single genes affecting color, dwarfism, and horns. These genetic influences help to flesh out an understanding of the breed that can guide breeders with different goals. The influences that go into the current Dexter breed in the USA and the UK include the following.

1. Irish. These are founders imported up to 1920. The breed was originally Irish, although all modern Irish animals now come from recent reimportations from the UK.
2. Early English. These are founders imported up to 1920.
3. American. These are founders that were registered without traceback to Ireland or England up to 1920.
4. Later English. Imports from England after about 1920. These importations generally occurred during the 1950s.
5. Colorado. These are animals from a herd with a known foundation that goes back to the first three influences (Irish, Early English, and American). This herd continued purebred breeding, but pedigrees and registrations lapsed in the final days of the herd. Only later was the herd recovered as a purebred resource, but the lapses raise doubts for some breeders.
6. "Other" are a handful of registered animals from the mid-1900s that lack registered parents. This was when the breed's popularity was at its lowest in the USA. These are

very low in number and not much is known about them. This designation needs to be included for completeness.

7. Parndon Bullfinch. This influence comes from a bull imported from the UK. His pedigree includes a single female ancestor with an untraced lineage. She was born in the early 1940s during the chaos of WWII. Most people accept this animal as a purebred. She originated in a purebred herd that had many other cattle with carefully documented pedigrees.
8. Woodmagic. These are from the Woodmagic herd in England, which was maintained for decades in isolation from other herds. The owner heavily selected cattle for a specifically small but non-dwarf type that some breeders find objectionable, but others consider to be very desirable.
9. Grade animals. These are only from some limited English lines, and rarely or never appear in the USA herd book. During and after WWII, the UK carefully tracked upgraded animals. The breed association in the USA has never allowed upgrading.
10. Saltaire Platinum. This imported influence introduced the polled gene into the breed from his granddam born in 1984. Different breeders hold different opinions on the origin of this bull and the polledness he brings to the breed. Tracking the influence of his controversial polled ancestor allows breeders to make their own decisions with complete information.
11. Lucifer of Knotting, born 1985, is an imported bull. His influence is controversial among breeders because of his type and temperament. The controversy mostly centers on one of his ancestors, and it is this influence that is tracked under this heading.

The exact breakdown of these foundation influences is politically charged, with individual breeders accepting or rejecting certain ones. The final combination of what is acceptable varies considerably, so this is not a neat pattern of concentric circles each with its next layer of inclusion. Many breeders accept all of these various influences as typical of the breed. Other breeders reject many of them. In between these extremes are several breeders that accept certain combinations of them, although the specific ones that are acceptable vary considerably. The important detail is that knowing the breakdown of these foundation influences in individual animals makes it possible for breeders to make informed decisions that are congruent with their own breeding philosophy. This process is greatly helped by a detailed herd book analysis that traces these various influences in all cattle. Such an analysis does not assess the relative value of each of these, it only lays out that they exist and makes the information available to breeders.

One unique portion of the American breed is based on Irish, Early English, and American influences. None of these persists solely on their own, although currently about 100 cattle descend from these three origins and no others. This core, for breeders in the USA, is the most restrictive portion of the breed. This part of the breed has minimal connections to other international herds of the breed, and as a result is a high priority for conservation. Due to its low numbers it would benefit from targeted breeding based on enhancing numbers and avoiding further loss of the genetic variability available in these animals.

The most restrictive approach taken in the UK involves a slightly different array of the early influences. The cattle currently in the UK have moderate to minimal overlap with

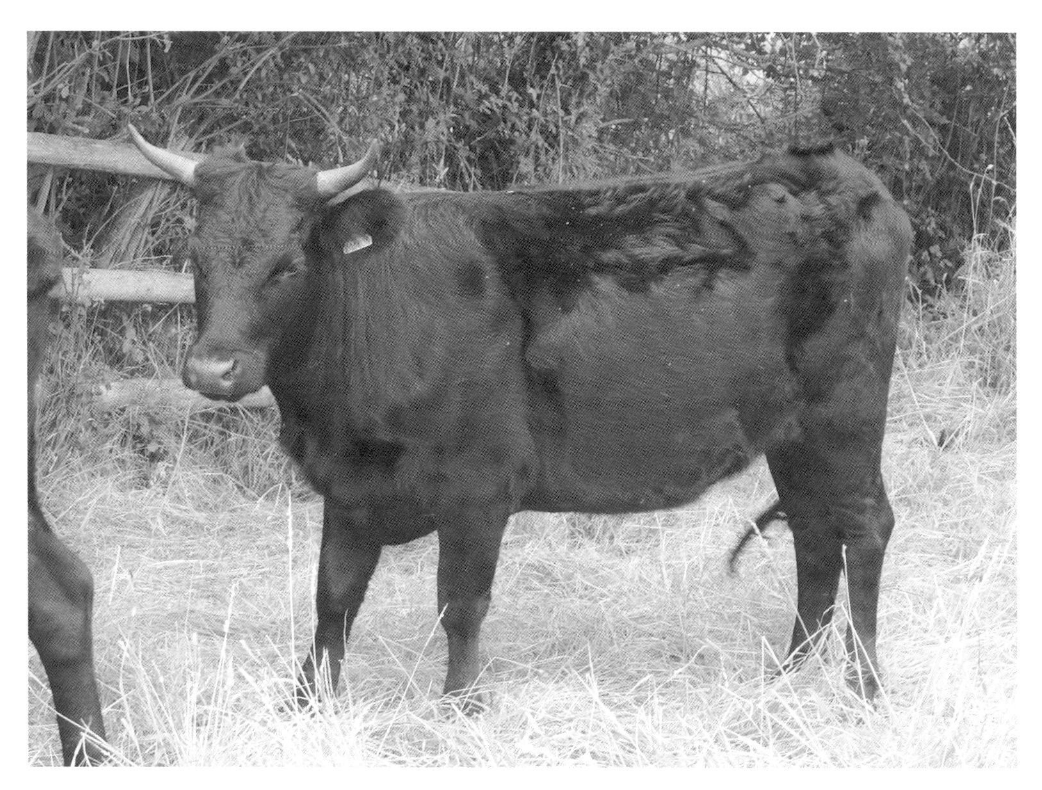

Figure 17.3 This Dexter heifer is one of few remaining in the UK that traces back to only the earliest threads of the breed. Photo by DPS.

Later English cattle in the USA. The result is that this most restrictive UK group stands alone as a unique genetic resource. This group is only about ten living cattle (Figure 17.3). Fortunately, it is possible to boost numbers and genetic variability by using semen frozen decades ago from several bulls that qualify as members of this group. This is an important difference between the restrictive British group and the restrictive American group, because the American group has minimal access to semen frozen decades ago. The frozen semen provides British breeders with the possibility of a successful rescue of these older bloodlines despite the low number of living representatives.

The most restrictive USA group and the most restrictive UK group are mutually acceptable to one another. They dip into the foundation of the breed in different ways, so it is wisest and best to assure that the breeding protocols in both countries keep their unique bloodlines intact while also assuring that reciprocal exchanges occur. As bulls are produced from the USA and UK lines, and crosses occur between the lines, it is especially important to freeze semen so that it is available long into the future. Expanding the numbers of these rare foundation threads in the Dexter can be important in the overall population structure of the breed in both the USA and the UK, and opens up several options for breeders. Whether or not they use these options is a personal decision but having them available makes sense for wise conservation. It is especially important for semen to be frozen to standards that will allow it to be imported from one country to the other.

Most American breeders would add the Colorado animals to the restrictive core that is available in the USA. Some breeders would object to this due to the lack of exact pedigree information on these animals. Accepting these into the herd books is an example of recovery of purebreds. The decision in this case is based on the history of a known foundation of specific registered animals, and breeding in isolation since that foundation. To that can be added the phenotype of the animals, which is typical for the breed. They are therefore "native on appearance" in addition to the evidence based on history. A final step could easily include DNA profiling, comparing these cattle to others from the restrictive early foundations of the breed in America. Colorado animals should be the target of a rescue that emphasizes expansion of numbers. It is logical to include influences from the "Irish, Early English, American" group because of the similar foundation of the two groups. The result is a useful composite of these rare influences that can stand on its own due to sufficient genetic variability.

Breeder opinions begin to diverge as one steps out of these most restrictive groups. The influence of Parndon Bullfinch is accepted by all except the most restrictive breeders. It is easy to trace his influence, though, and because it is a point of concern for some it is wise to do so. The reason for tracking this is that it is then possible for the most restrictive breeders to assure that this influence does not completely swamp all other bloodlines within the most restrictive group. The influence of this line is more completely accepted in the USA than in the UK.

The Woodmagic influence has broad acceptance by all except a few UK breeders. The Woodmagic influence pervades many cattle in both the USA and the UK, although animals that have only this influence are now rare. Given the origin in a single herd and the low numbers of cattle that are solely of this bloodline, it is likely unrealistic to think that a rescue program based on absolute bloodline purity would be possible. The objections to the Woodmagic herd are based on distinctions in the DNA profile when compared to other bloodlines of Dexter cattle in the UK. This is assumed by many to be the result of introgression from other breeds, but the studies that indicated these results did not include other breeds that were available in the locality of the Woodmagic herd and that would have been the most likely source of any introgression. The results, therefore, could simply be due to foundation effect, isolation, genetic drift, and selection. This underscores the need for DNA sampling to be very complete at the outset of defining a breed, and for any breeds suspected as sources of introgression to also be sampled. When sampling is incomplete, the results can be used to exclude animals that should have been included.

A few influences are very minor and probably inconsequential. They can still be traced for completeness. The "other" cattle that are untraced from the mid-1900s are very few in number, and do not raise significant questions for anyone. They offer only a little breed vitality or heritage, and do not need to be the target of any heroic rescue effort. Grade cattle are only an issue in the UK, and not in the USA. This situation could change, depending on the level of any ongoing importation of genetic material or cattle from the UK into the USA.

The two more recent influences of Saltaire Platinum and Lucifer of Knotting are the most controversial, with some breeders shunning any inclusion of these. Due to the popularity of polled cattle, Saltaire Platinum now occurs in the pedigrees of about 75% of the breed in the USA. The polled character comes only from it and from no other source. This is an example of the power of selection to change a breed, especially when a single gene of large effect is the cause of a desired phenotype. Some breeders reject this influence, even though it might be well below 1% of the breeding of an animal. This hearkens back to issues of upgrading, selection for breed type, and the question as to the level of genetic influence required for an animal to be considered purebred. The controversy over Lucifer of Knotting is similar and his influence likewise occurs at a low level in some animals. In this case both his temperament and his type are suspect, and are the reasons that some breeders shun his influence in their cattle. These influences from these two bulls are common in the modern breed, despite their controversy among some breeders.

It is important to understand how the different threads interact. The most restrictive portions of the breed can only be replenished from those same portions, while the least restrictive portions are more open to influences from across the breed. This phenomenon has the practical outcome that targeted conservation attention needs to be devoted to the portions of the breed with the most restricted definitions. Animals from the most restricted groups can easily be used back into the other groups without a loss of identity. The opposite is not true: using the most inclusive groups back into the most restricted groups will lead to their extinction and their unavailability to future breeders. Saving the most restrictive groups is therefore effective in conserving the overall genetic diversity of the breed for future generations of breeders. This can sound like a preference for the restrictive groups over the others, when in fact it is simply a strategy to assure that all of the various threads are kept intact for future breeders.

The potential fate of these different threads is an interesting final tapestry. How to make these actually work together for all involved is the conservation challenge. Today's Dexter breed descends from these 11 different foundations. It is currently increasing in popularity to the point that the breed could be considered to no longer be a conservation target as a rare breed. However, within the larger breed are these smaller groups of uniquely bred animals that are now vanishingly rare and could be lost. They could well be important for a genetically secure future for the breed. Dexters therefore are a good example of a breed within which rescue protocols can still find good use, even if that is at the level of bloodlines rather than the entire breed.

It is valid to acknowledge that different breeders have different goals (Figure 17.4). The

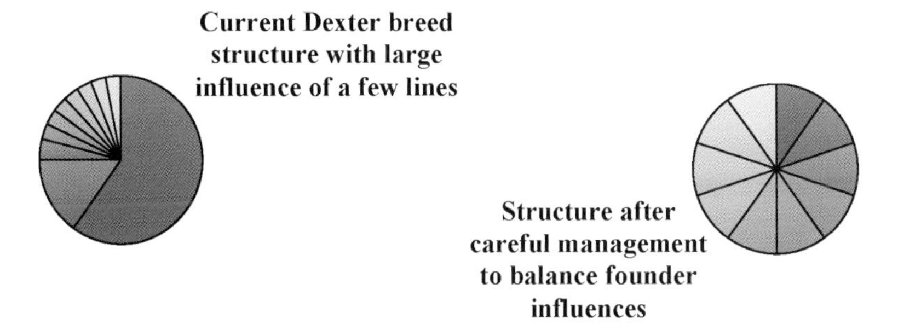

Figure 17.4 A secure future for the Dexter breed is best served by broad cooperation among breeders in the USA and UK to assure that the rarest influences do not vanish by absorption into more common influences. Figure by DPS.

goals of no single group should be allowed to nullify the desires of the others. The breeders will then be able to select out what they desire from among these various threads. This emphasis will strike some as odd, but it is the strategy that works to conserve the maximum diversity possible for use by the broadest range of breeder philosophies.

CHAPTER 18

External Factors Affecting Breeds

Forces that are external to breeds and their breeders have important influences on breed survival. These influences can be either positive or negative, and they must be recognized and managed for breeds to succeed. Breeds must survive and serve in an environment dictated by external factors that include cultural use, market demand, and governmental regulation. Otherwise, they quickly become trivial and only of interest to a handful of dedicated breeders who are keeping the breed as a hobby. Although the hobby approach can and does succeed in saving breeds from extinction, conservation is most secure and effective when breeds serve some demand from the outside world (Figure 18.1). Breeds that are useful have a much better chance of long-term survival than those that find no appropriate practical use, provided that narrow, single-purpose uses are not the only yardstick used in making the determination of the usefulness of a breed.

18.1 Market Demand

One essential aspect of breed survival is the demand for the breed. Market demand for breeds can have a huge impact on breed numbers, but must be carefully weighed against other motivations for stewards of rare breeds. The whole array of motivations for keeping and breeding rare breeds varies dramatically. At one end of the continuum are people who are motivated by a sincere concern for the biodiversity of a particular breed, as well as safeguarding and expanding a genetic resource to fit into a production niche. At the other end are those who are more self-serving and have motives that stem from a desire to cash in on the demand for rarity or to enhance their own sense of importance. In between these two extremes lie most breeders, who are interested in breed survival but also have concern for a reasonable and justified economic payback from the breed. Secure market demand can bring security to a breed by providing positive outcomes for the entire spectrum of breeders.

It is fortunate for the long-term survival of many breeds that rarity itself is appealing, so that in the present era the truly rare breeds are unlikely to undergo complete extinction. Nearly every breed can indeed survive if it is stewarded by breeders that are motivated to avoid breed extinction. The downside of this approach is that such breeds can quickly

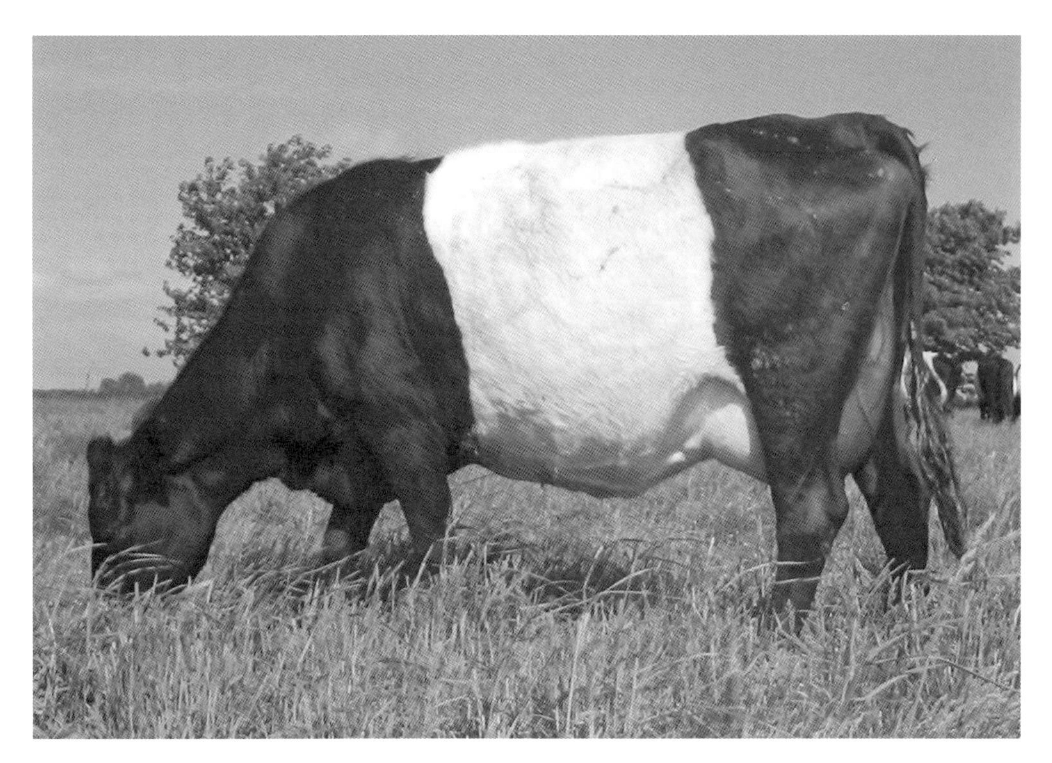

Figure 18.1 Dutch Belted cattle offer traits such as forage efficiency, longevity, walking ability, and milk production that assure them a secure future with dairy farmers who need this combination in their herds. Photo by Winifred Hoffman.

become viewed as oddities with no real purpose other than their rarity. Most rare breeds deserve better than that because they are useful and productive in an appropriate habitat and for an appropriate purpose. They should ideally remain part of a functioning and productive agricultural landscape.

Demand for a breed has a few subtle but important aspects. Breeds for which demand is high seldom become rare. In contrast, breeds for which demand is chronically low will always find survival to be challenging. While politics and breed culture can both play a role in effectively managing demand, other more direct external factors are usually more important and can lead in the direction of either success or failure.

Breeds are most sustainable when the demand for the breed comes directly from its products or services. Brisk demand assures the continuity of a breed when its products and services are distinctive and highly desired. Healthy commodity-based demand assures that breeders will reap monetary rewards for their efforts in producing the breed. The result for such breeds is a secure niche in agriculture. Dog breeds, while not usually considered commodities, likewise face various demands, and fluctuate in popularity according to the interplay of various external factors. Shaping a breed to meet those demands can be essential to breed survival.

Breed demand falls into several categories. A very healthy situation for a breed would be for it to fit market channels that already exist. Products most obviously include meat, fiber,

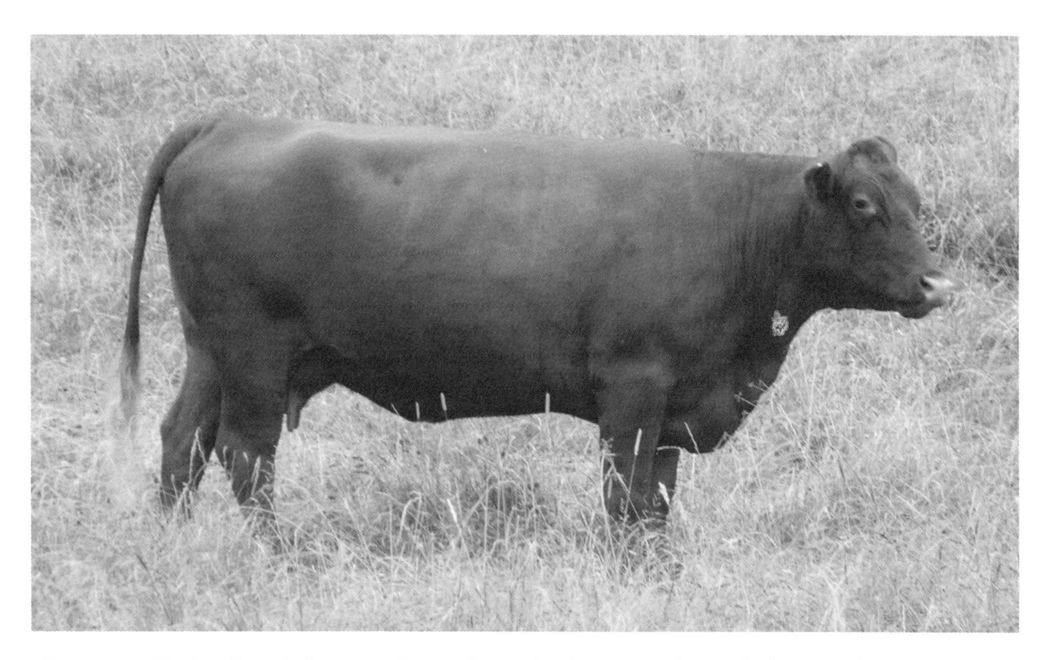

Figure 18.2 Red Poll cattle have attributes that make them a ready-made fit to modern production needs. Photo by DPS.

eggs, or milk, but services such as draft, grassland management, pest control, and wildfire fuel abatement can also be desired. Rare breeds with "ready-made" markets are the rarest of the rare, largely because if a breed had already fit mainstream market demand, then it would have never suffered rarity in the first place. A few such breeds do indeed exist and their reasons for rarity usually rest in some factor other than production. For breeds such as Red Poll cattle, for example, the fit is already there with mainstream agricultural demand. The challenge is to make that connection more obvious to candidate breeders in order to enhance demand for this productive breed that consistently excels in pounds of calf weaned per cow exposed to a bull (Figure 18.2).

Rarity is another category of demand, but a market based solely on rarity has potential problems. A few breeders have tried to assure or prolong breed rarity, usually by overly restrictive registry procedures. This is a strategy used to preserve their own market advantage by virtue of already being involved in the breed rather than having to buy-in anew. Self-serving breeders also occasionally target a specific rare breed, but then quickly get out of the breed as numbers increase and prices fall from the initially high levels provided by the novelty or exotic market. Breed rarity, as an end in itself, invites a departure from the healthy linkage of breed demand to commodity and production concerns. At that point, the market is likely to serve conservation poorly, if at all. Rare dog breeds are especially susceptible to becoming the target of fads. Dog breeds are more adequately served when demand rests on their ability to perform various tasks, including their important service as companion animals that offer a specific package of desirable traits to their owners. Rare and newly imported chicken breeds are rapidly going down the road that values rarity on its own instead of a link between specific production traits and demand for them.

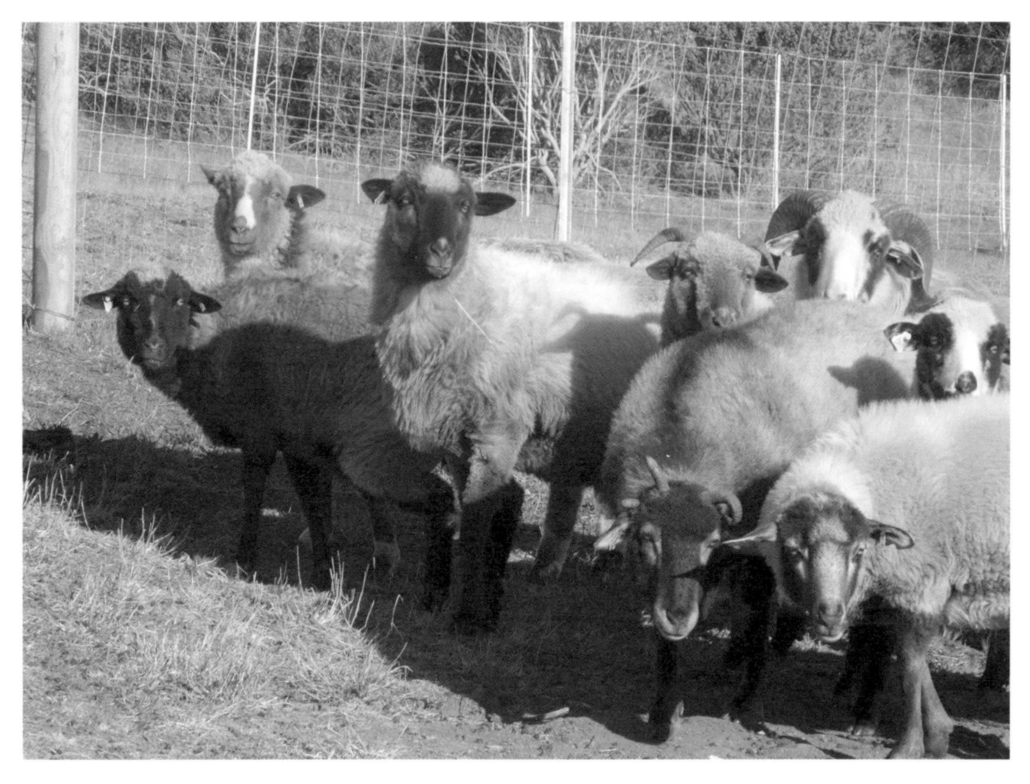

Figure 18.3 Navajo-Churro sheep were long penalized in mainstream markets because of their small carcasses. This trend has now reversed, assuring a stronger market for breeds with a small body size. Photo by DPS.

Many rare breed products fall outside of the norm for agricultural commodities, which is indeed one common reason for breed rarity. In many cases they still fit well into alternative markets. One example is the relatively small lamb carcasses produced by many rare sheep breeds. Large carcasses have long been desired by meat packers that control most of the mainstream commerce in lamb meat in the USA (Figure 18.3). In such situations, it can be necessary to develop and serve alternative markets that create increased demand for specialized products that are outside the mainstream. Fortunately, in the case of smaller sheep, demand has grown in favor of smaller sheep that are a better fit for the desires of many ethnic minorities. This example of changing targets for market demand is one powerful argument for saving rare and unusual breeds. Some breeds are likely to be a good fit for future demands and they are ready-to-go as a complete genetic package to meet those demands.

The development of alternative markets can easily include breed-specific or breed-labeled products where the uniqueness of the product becomes an asset instead of a liability. A recent phenomenon has changed what have been minor specialty markets (small lambs, for example) into a broader demand, to the extent that the market now readily accepts more variable products than a few decades ago and a wider variety of breeds find a production niche more easily. Some early success with fattening hogs on acorns to produce specialty

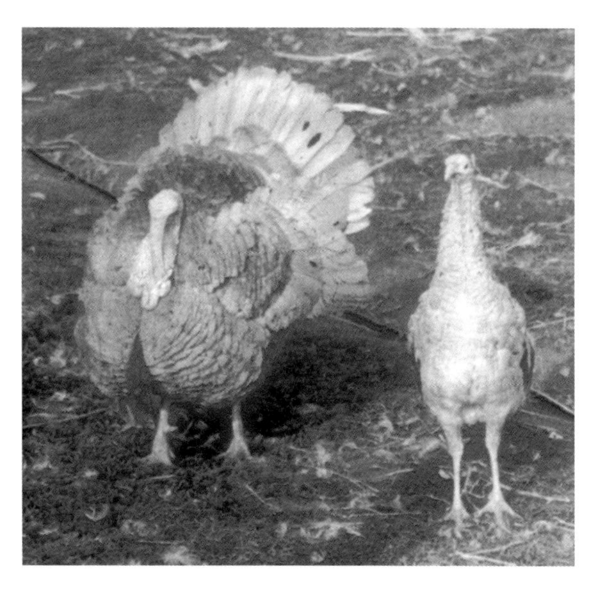

Figure 18.4 Demand for heritage turkey varieties has increased the hatchery demand for poults, resulting in increasingly secure breed resources. Photo by DPS.

hams further illustrates how the match of the right breed, right process, and right market can dramatically change the fate of a breed. Likewise, fat-rumped sheep such as the Karakul are an awkward fit for mainstream markets but are highly desired and gain a premium when producers can connect to the minority groups that favor this type of sheep.

The amazing turnaround in the fate of standard turkey varieties testifies to the potential benefits of product-specific promotion to foster breed conservation and expansion (Figure 18.4). Populations of nearly all varieties of heritage and standard turkeys had collapsed by the late 1990s. A targeted program coordinated by The Livestock Conservancy and Slow Food USA increased the demand for these birds as holiday fare. The numbers of breeder birds furnishing poults then steadily increased year by year. This provided these historic varieties with a more secure place in the agricultural landscape. While still vanishingly small when compared to the total national demand for turkeys, the resulting ten-fold increase has assured a much more secure population structure for many heritage turkey strains.

Promotional programs for rare breed products have been very effective across several breeds, such as the "Save the Sheep" contest run by *Spinoff* magazine in the late 1990s, and the current "Shave 'Em to Save 'Em" program run by The Livestock Conservancy. These promotional efforts link users of wool with rare breed producers. The result is an increased awareness of the wonderfully wide array of fibers produced by rare breeds. This has increased the demand for fibers produced by pure breeds and has boosted income to producers. These efforts successfully target an audience that is uniquely and powerfully situated to help conservation efforts by linking fiber purchases to rare breed conservation programs. These efforts have ushered in an awareness among fiber artists to the plight of rare sheep breeds and the uniqueness of their wools. The result is an increased appreciation and demand for breed-specific wools, all through connecting a large community of end-users with those that are committed to producing these fibers from purebred animals.

18.2 Crossbreeding

Several rare breeds are rare for the peculiar reason that their crossbred offspring have high value. For some of these breeds, it makes more economic sense in the short term to use purebred females for crossbreeding rather than for the production of purebred offspring. The result of such a market imbalance is that the production of purebred daughters and sons can become dangerously low as high numbers of purebred dams are crossed rather than bred pure. The next generation of purebreds is simply not being produced, and breed numbers dwindle.

Excellence in crossbreeding has endangered several breeds. Spanish cattle in the Americas (loosely termed "Criollos") are a good example, and include the Florida Cracker (Figure 18.5) and Texas Longhorn cattle in the USA. These cattle survive and produce well in compromised environments. They are genetically distinct from other breeds of cattle and are therefore a high conservation priority. Their unique genome provides for vigorous and productive crossbred offspring with both Brahman cattle as well as Northern European cattle. The excellent survival and production ability of half Criollo calves has led to purebred Criollo cows being mated with bulls of different breeds, with the subsequent retention of the crossbred heifers. What has been lacking in many locations is enough pure breeding to assure that the pure Criollo cows are available for crossbreeding in the future. Several countries have come to mourn the loss of the purebred Criollos as overall cattle productivity has

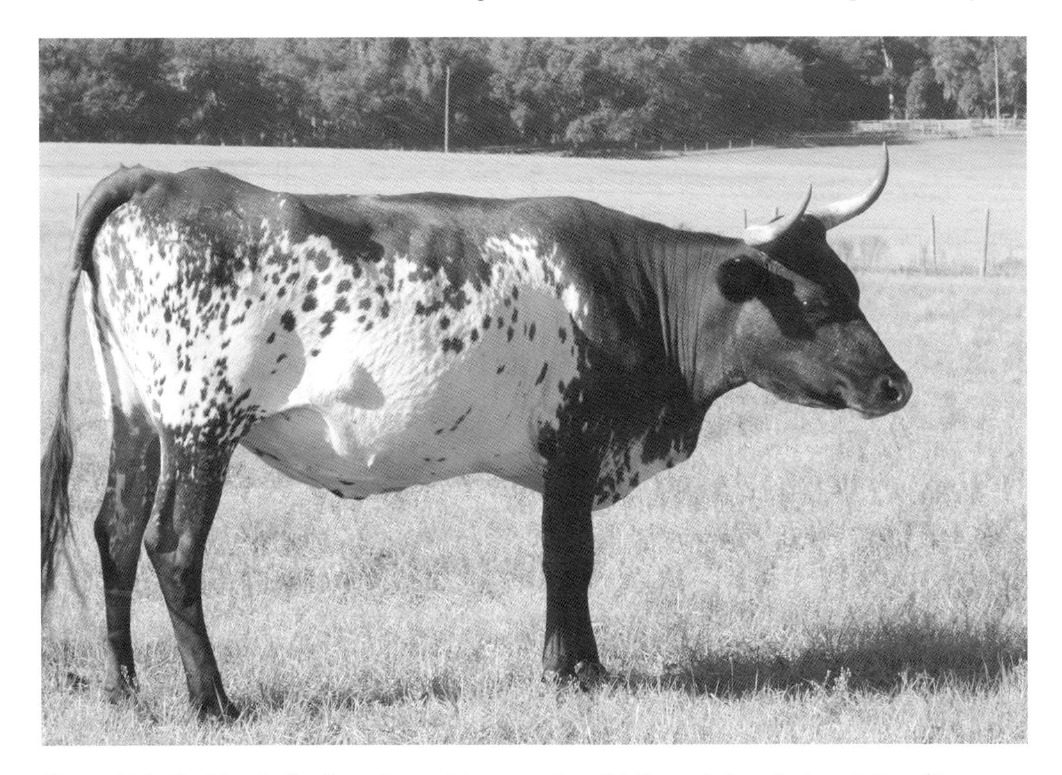

Figure 18.5 The Florida Cracker, along with most other Criollo cattle breeds, is a victim of its own success in providing cows for crossbreeding programs. Photo by DPS.

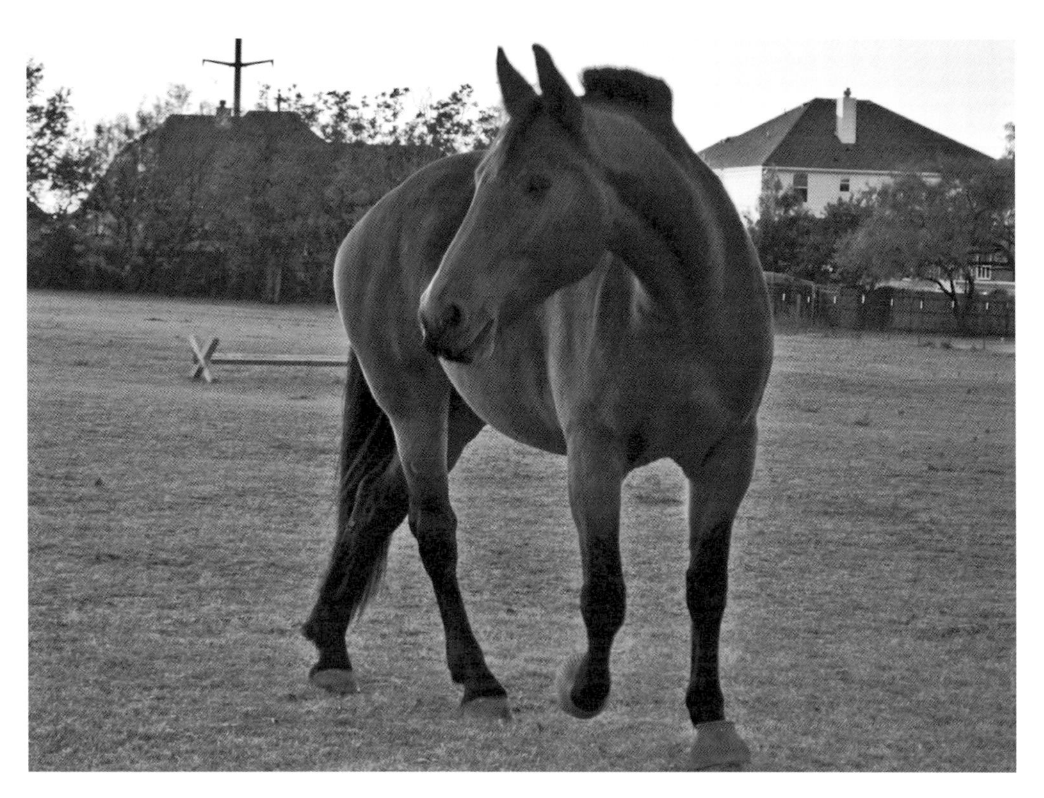

Figure 18.6 Partbred Cleveland Bay foals can be more valuable than purebreds, which can be detrimental to purebred recruitment. Photo by JB.

fallen when the Criollo influence has dropped below 25%. This pattern has been repeated with local types of Criollo cattle in most countries of Latin America. Fortunately, the adaptation of the Criollo is increasingly sought so that many of the Criollo breeds are experiencing numerical growth. Unfortunately, many local strains of the Criollo slipped to extinction before producers realized their true value.

Other examples of crossbreeding leading to purebred decline include several horse breeds. These include some Warmbloods, such as the Cleveland Bay (Figure 18.6) and Irish Draught, as well as a number of pony breeds such as the Connemara. Losses in these breeds come from an inadequate recruitment of the traditional heavier utility type that produces wonderful sport horses when paired with Thoroughbred mates. In some breeds the resulting crossbreds are simply lost to the breed. In others a more insidious loss occurs because these crossbred sport horses have been included in the herd book. The result is that the older, heavier, utility type is mixed in with the lighter, athletic, modern sport type under the same breed name. As breeders select breeding stock, they tend to favor the modern athletic type with no regard to its mixed pedigree. By this process the original heavier type becomes rare or lost despite the continuity of the breed name. This ignores the fact that in many instances the modern sport horse is a hybrid (and a good one, at that) springing from the traditional heavier utility type mated to light horse breeds. Very few horse breeds have been able to counter this trend.

One strategy to avoid losing the heavier original type in horse breeds is the use of a "part-bred" herd book which lists the crossbreds and recognizes the parent breed's influence on them, but does not allow them to replace the traditional type as breeding stock. Such a strategy very effectively recognizes the excellence of these crossbreds (athletic performance) while protecting the traits that the pure breed has (reproducing athletic excellence through crossbreeding).

Excellence in crossbreeding is especially perplexing as a cause for breed rarity because it is the breed's excellence that is endangering it. In a few situations breeders have been able to capitalize on crossbreeding excellence while conserving the pure breed. Blanco Orejinegro cattle, a Criollo breed of Colombia, are prized for their resistance to certain parasites. Breeders of these cattle are providing purebred bulls for use on commercial dairy cattle to impart this resistance to the commercial crossbreds. This strategy serves the breed much better than using Holstein semen on the Blanco Orejinegro cows. The path these breeders have followed has saved the breed from extinction so that the breed can serve future generations with its useful characteristics.

Some breeds used for crossbreeding have never been all that common, for the simple reason that not many were ever required to fill the need for the crossbreeding sires. This is especially true for those breeds whose males are the ones used in crossbreeding. For most of its history, the American Mammoth Jackstock has had only one purpose: to provide jacks for mating to mares to produce mule foals. This role is satisfied by relatively low breed numbers, which has had implications for breed survival. Fortunately, the increasing use of the breed for riding donkeys has increased demand as well as numbers, although at some risk of changing breed type.

18.3 Regulations

In some situations, external regulations, usually governmental, can profoundly affect rare breed conservation. Recent moves in several European countries to insist upon scrapie-resistant genotypes in breeding rams have certainly changed breeding choices in several breeds. To some extent this trend is being mimicked by breed associations in the USA, as well as by some individual states. This can rapidly change breeds by limiting choices of breeding stock. When a ram fails to be used solely because of his scrapie-resistance genotype it is not only the single gene that fails to be passed along, but also his entire genome that has been culled. This specific example becomes very complicated as regulations, biology, and breed dynamics all interact in unexpected ways that can have profound consequences for breed survival.

The approach to scrapie control diverges strongly from country to country. Some countries rely on resistant genotypes, despite at least some evidence that the resistance is actually a prolonged incubation period for the disease. This period may be longer than the lifespan of most sheep so that clinical cases do not develop. In contrast, other countries insist that any imported sheep be of susceptible genotypes, but free of scrapie. This approach assures that regardless of the biology of resistance (long incubation versus true freedom from the disease agent), these countries are very unlikely to be importing any problems along with select carrier sheep. The Icelanders have long experience in eradicating scrapie and insist on

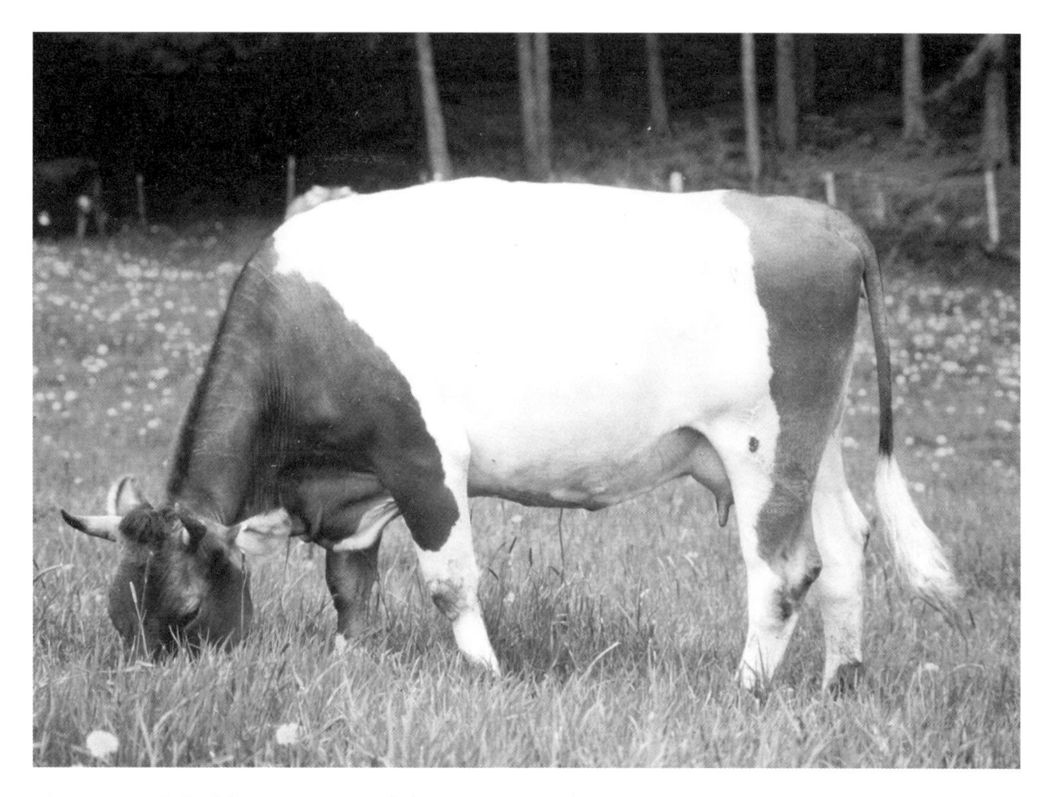

Figure 18.7 Belted Swiss cows nearly became extinct due to bull licensing laws in Switzerland. Photo © Evelyn Simak.

an approach that does not involve elimination of "susceptible" genotypes. Their record of success is impressive, with the progressive elimination of this disease over time so that the few cases in Iceland have only occurred in a few isolated geographic pockets.

The USA is somewhat different than most other countries in having very little governmental oversight of animal breeding. In several European countries, for example, only licensed, registered bulls and stallions are allowed to reproduce (Figure 18.7). This can and does have a profound impact on the status and type of breeds. In some situations, this is good because the officials have a traditional and conservative eye for breed type. In other situations, contemporary fads can drastically change a breed and the government's participation assures that little can be done to counter this. Such a pattern occurs commonly with Warmblood horse breeding throughout most of Europe. Another example is the bull licensing regulations that have been one reason for the near-extinction of Dutch Belted cattle in the Netherlands, and have also been the reason behind the near-loss of linebacked and colorsided cattle breeds in a number of countries.

Selection goals can be fickle, changing over time. When these changing selection goals are combined with governmental sanctions the result can be dramatic. Haflinger horses have gone from a lighter riding type to a heavier light draft type, and now back to the original lighter riding type. Changes back and forth like this can easily damage the genetic structure of a breed.

Regardless of specific regulations, a key issue in any situation is whether effective conservation is taking place or not. The specific practices that are in place in purebred selection programs have a large influence on this. Conservation can thrive under a variety of specific rules, as long as a sound philosophy which guards breed type and breed purity is appreciated.

18.4 Imports

Rare breed imports present a complicated array of issues for breed conservation. Some importations of rare breeds are a benefit to conservation while others are a threat both in the country of destination and in the country of origin. While some imported breeds are likely to be involved in constructive conservation endeavors, others are likely to detract from serious livestock breed conservation. Imported animals are almost always highly selected stock that come into their destination with good documentation and at great expense. This gives the imports an instant advantage in credibility and publicity over numerous local breeds that are in peril. This is especially true of local breeds that are raised in extensive or traditional situations because the breeders in those systems have rarely participated in breed organization or promotion.

Rare breed importation into the USA encompasses two main issues, each of which can have different influences on conservation. The first is the importation of a breed that is new to the USA. The second is the importation of new breeding stock into a breed that is already present in the USA. Imports can help to broaden the range of breeds available. They can provide a needed boost to breeds already in a country. Imports can also pose a variety of risks.

One fairly basic consideration for imports relates back to the fact that these breeds then become international, rather than national, resources. This outcome is potentially good because it vastly reduces the risk of loss due to natural disaster or political upheaval. A core concern, though, is whether the different countries that host the breed have reciprocal recognition of purebred animals. In many examples, this recognition is not reciprocal. This makes the country receiving the importations a sort of "dead end" because those animals cannot participate in the breed in the opposite direction. This is the unfortunate pattern for many international breeds, and it largely precludes the potential advantages open to a truly international breed. Few breeds manage effective reciprocity all that well. This can stem from registry regulation, breeder culture, or governmental regulations. The goal should always be easy reciprocity to assure that the international breed remains a single gene pool.

The Clydesdale horse stands out as a very good example of a breed that has managed full international reciprocity. This is true not only at a theoretical level through registry rules, but also at a very practical level because the breeders in various countries (most notably the UK, USA, Australia, and New Zealand) send horses in various directions (Figure 18.8). This is distinct from the breeder culture in many breeds in which animals only move in one direction.

The effects of imported breeds and bloodlines vary, and any summary is bound to be at least somewhat incomplete by not reflecting a host of finer details. With that disclaimer, it is possible to put imported breeds into four general categories.

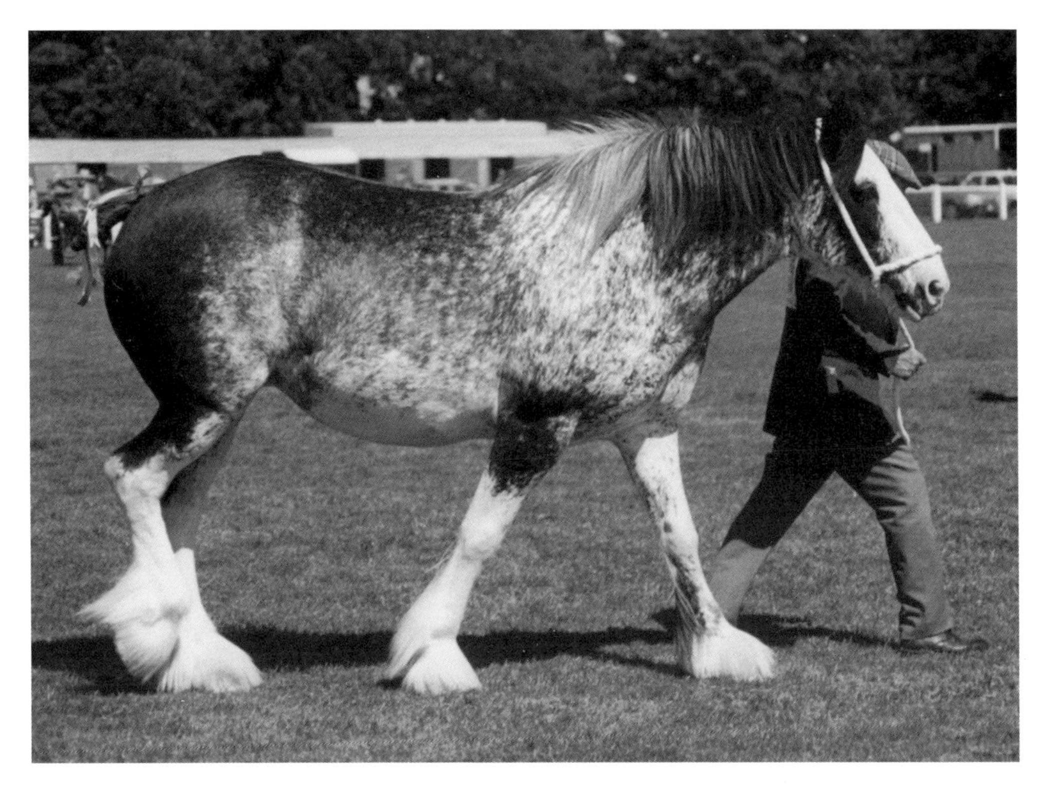

Figure 18.8 Clydesdale horses are a truly international breed, with breeding animals exchanged among all of the countries hosting this attractive draft horse. Photo by DPS.

- Imports that contribute substantially to conservation efforts.
- Imports that enhance American bloodlines.
- Imports that hamper conservation in their country of origin.
- Imports that endanger American bloodlines or breeds.

18.4.1 Imports That Contribute Substantially to Conservation Efforts

Imports that contribute to conservation are success stories and are a real boon to the conservation of the breed. Breeds that fit into this category include those that are endangered in their homelands, usually by political or geographic threats. The Meishan hog breed is a good example of a breed with a very extreme phenotype that is important for conservation (Figure 18.9). This is one of the highly prolific Chinese hog breeds. In a strange twist of fate, the populations in China are now greatly endangered, while the descendants of imports to the USA are much more secure and are carefully managed in conservation breeding programs.

The Caspian horse has long been endangered in its Iranian homeland (Figure 18.10). The danger was once from political upheaval, followed by a period during which the breed lacked a targeted conservation program in Iran. Fortunately, the breed's situation in Iran is now changing in a very positive direction. For several years, though, imports from Iran were more likely to be used for conservation in the UK or the USA than they were in Iran. The

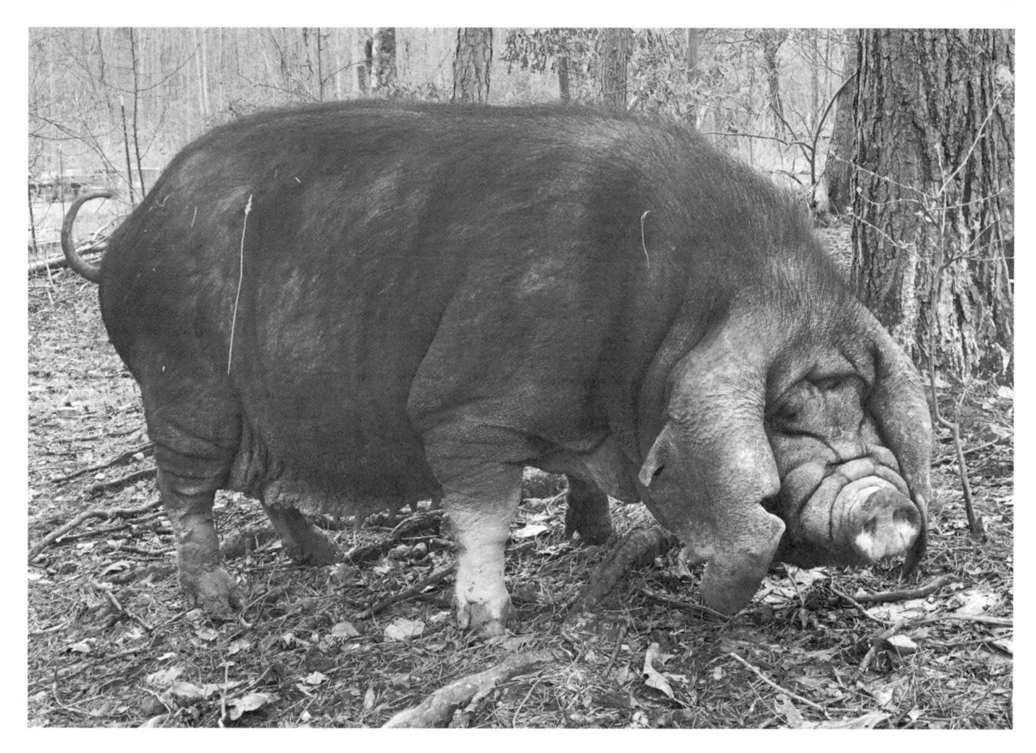

Figure 18.9 The Meishan hog breed is much more secure in the USA than it currently is in China. Photo by JB.

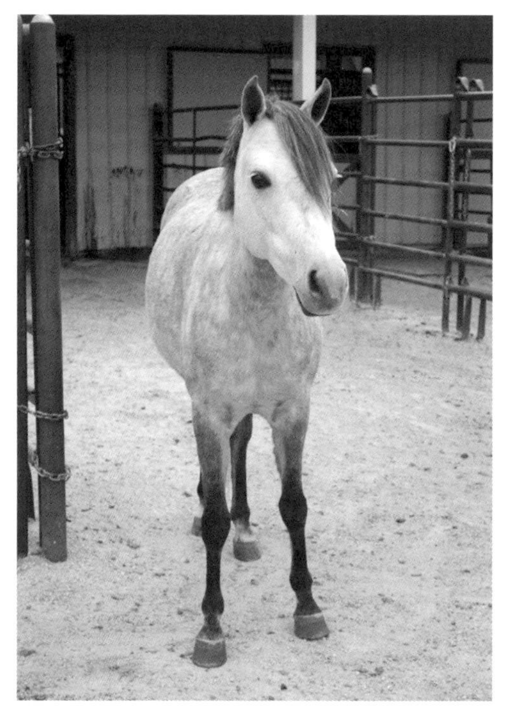

Figure 18.10 Caspian horses are more secure for having been imported to several countries around the world. Current efforts to enhance communication and breeding across international boundaries are working to secure this unique breed's place. Photo by JB.

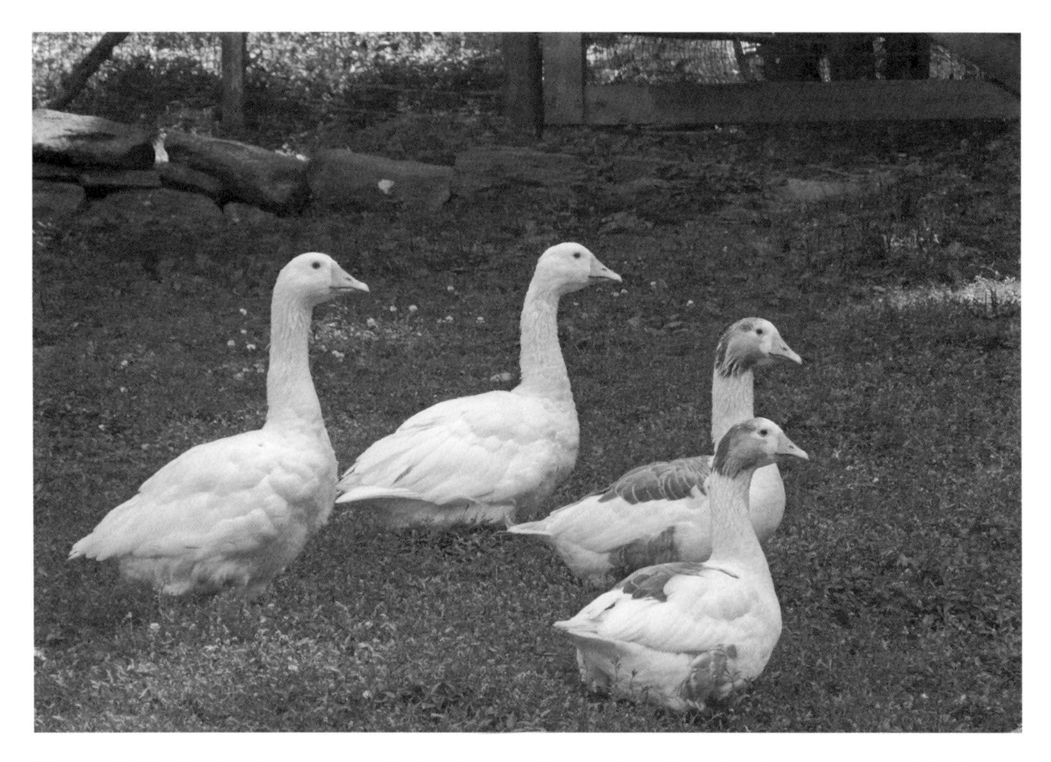

Figure 18.11 Shetland geese are a distinctive, small goose breed that has become more globally secure through its American population. Photo by DPS.

goal with this breed and others in a similar situation should always be to foster meaningful conservation in the country of origin. In the absence of such programs, conservation is best served by the representatives of the breed that have been exported to other countries. Those imports need to be stewarded with this in mind.

Ankole cattle are another example. They are few in number in the USA, and historically numerous in their central African homeland. However, the situation in Africa is rapidly changing, with rampant crossbreeding of the breed to enhance milk production. While it is impossible to know the exact situation, the fact remains that members of the breed in the USA are very likely to remain purebred and act as a genetic reservoir of this breed for the future. They need to be managed well in light of the possibility of rapid and unforeseen changes in breed numbers in Africa.

Other importations that contribute substantially to conservation are somewhat surprising. One is the Shetland goose, a small and distinctive goose breed imported by Nancy Kohlberg of Cabbage Hill Farm in New York (Figure 18.11). The geese in the American population have increased their numbers beyond those in Britain, and in the process have significantly contributed to the array of divergent goose breeds available in the USA. The efforts of Cabbage Hill Farm in New York and Holderread Waterfowl Farm in Oregon have assured that this goose breed is now more globally secure, both genetically and numerically. Happily, the conservation efforts in the UK are now also increasing the breed's numbers there, including the important discovery of previously overlooked bloodlines.

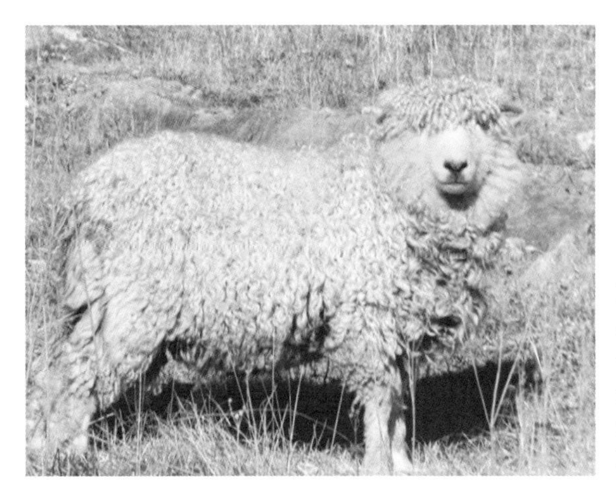

Figure 18.12 The American populations of the Leicester Longwool are able to receive influences from all the international populations of the breed, in contrast to those in other countries. Photo by DPS.

Poitou donkeys are another imported rare breed success story, largely through the efforts of Debbie Hamilton of Vermont. Her assurance that the breed in the USA is reciprocal with the breed in France is the result of hard work over a long time. This specific effort has made it possible for the small American representation of this breed to have an important impact on the breed's survival both in France and in the USA. A genetically significant portion of the breed is in the USA, and Debbie's diligence assured that the international breed can benefit from it. Debbie is unfortunately now deceased, but her efforts serve as a reminder that careful attention to both conservation breeding and the external factors of breed survival can outlive the people involved.

Some importations could not have been predicted to lead to significant contributions to global breed conservation but have ended up doing just that. Leicester Longwool sheep were imported by the Colonial Williamsburg Foundation as an appropriate breed for their historical interpretation program (Figure 18.12). At the time of importation, the breed in the UK, Australia, and New Zealand was thriving and was at least somewhat commercially relevant. It was difficult to foresee that the USA's contribution would be significant for this breed. Fifteen years after the importation, the numbers of this breed in the USA have risen while those in Australia and New Zealand have plummeted. The USA population, based on a blend of Australian, New Zealand, and English breeding, has therefore emerged as an important genetic pool based on the various international strains of this old and unique breed. In addition, the USA population is the only one that is open to influences from all other sources due to the intricacies of import-export regulations in the various countries holding this historically pivotal standardized breed. The ongoing importation of semen from New Zealand, Australia, and England to bolster Leicester Longwool sheep in this country is an example of enhancing American bloodlines through importation. This breed serves as an example of unique opportunities for American breeders to help manage an international breed in a way that no other country is able to, due to import restrictions.

A common thread for most of these importation success stories, as well as for others, is that the imported animals of several of these breeds are more likely to contribute to conservation following importation to the USA than they were to make contributions in their home country. This is unfortunate, as breeds are always best conserved in the region from which they originated. For breed conservation to be successful with these imported animals, it is essential that a broad genetic base be imported. It is also important to assure that the imported animals are managed for maximum genetic viability with good representation of all founders. A casual, non-deliberate breeding program is much easier in the short term but is very unlikely to succeed in accomplishing long-term conservation goals.

18.4.2 Imports That Enhance American Bloodlines

Imported additions to existing breed populations in the USA offer potential conservation benefits. These must be used carefully, or they risk diluting the uniqueness of American populations instead of invigorating and broadening them. This sort of import is especially useful for breeds with small American populations that are all interrelated.

Several breeds in the USA can benefit from the occasional introduction of new genetic material from other populations of the same breed that have been isolated for long periods of time. This functions to even out the genetic variation in the breed, and also counteracts any tendency for genetic drift or inbreeding that can compromise a breed. Dexter and Shorthorn cattle stand out as breeds long present in the USA that could benefit from infusions of new genetic material. Large Black hogs have recently benefitted from the infusion of new boar lines from the UK. Shetland geese are a more recent import, and could benefit from imports derived from populations that were not present in the original importations.

18.4.3 Imports That Hamper Conservation in the Country of Origin

Imports damage the breed in the country of origin when irreplaceable bloodlines or animals are removed from conservation programs in their country of origin. Fortunately, examples of these are relatively few. In the last few decades, the export of many Galloway and Highland cattle from the UK into Germany has resulted in some drain on those breeds. These imports were less likely to remain documented or to contribute to purebred breeding programs in their countries of destination, and therefore many were lost to their breeds. The Highland and Galloway breeds are numerous enough to sustain the loss, but the underlying principle is troubling if rare breeds become involved.

A similar phenomenon can and does occur in horse breeds when high-performing and select breeding stock is exported. This can result in a slow and steady drain of the top of the breed from the country of origin. The breed in its country of origin thereby suffers an erosion of quality and potential and can become relegated to second-class status among countries holding the breed. The consistent export of Narragansett Pacer horses from the USA to the Caribbean islands in the 1800s was a major reason for the eventual extinction of the breed. The exported horses were not used for pure breeding in their destinations, and eventually the breed collapsed in the USA due to inadequate numbers. This sort of exportation is never in the best interests of breed conservation, although in rare cases such exports are the only hope that some animals will be used for breed conservation. This is true if they are unlikely to be used in their home country for purebred breeding.

18.4.4 Imports That Endanger American Bloodlines and Breeds

Imports can easily endanger unique American breeds as well as unique American bloodlines within international breeds. The negative effect of imports is usually accomplished

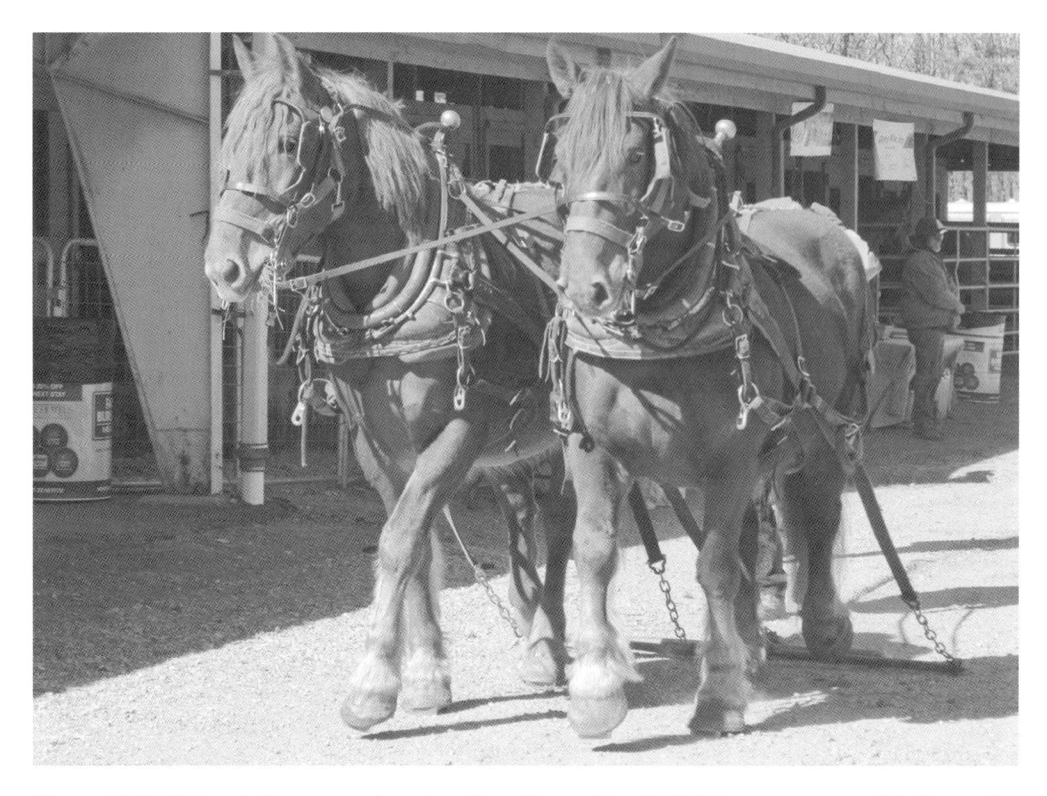

Figure 18.13 Uniquely long-term American bloodlines of the Suffolk horse are now all influenced by more recent imports from the UK. Photo by JB.

by direct competition for space on farms. The competition disadvantages local genetic resources, with the common result that the imports supplant either local breeds or local bloodlines that are impossible to replace. This group of imports demands close attention.

Imports of new bloodlines into breeds already present in the USA can be a great benefit, but they must be managed wisely. A strong tendency is for newly imported animals to be very widely used, and through this they can end up replacing existing local bloodlines. This defeats the purpose of strengthening existing lines, and instead simply replaces them with something new. An example is the Suffolk horse, which has a long presence in the USA as a valued farm work horse (Figure 18.13). The breed is English, and breeders in the USA tend to add in English horses from time to time. This has resulted in the situation where no Suffolk horse in the USA now has only the long-term American bloodlines. These unique portions of the breed are now no longer accessible as intact identifiable resources. It is important to be sure that the imported influences do not entirely replace the older, original American stock, which plays an important role in maintaining the diversity of international breeds.

The threat from imports varies greatly from breed to breed. Devon cattle in many countries, notably excluding the USA, allow at least some crossbreds or grades to be included as purebreds. Thus Devon cattle in the USA have largely avoided inclusion of Salers breeding, and as such serve as a reservoir of a more original genetic resource for this internationally distributed breed.

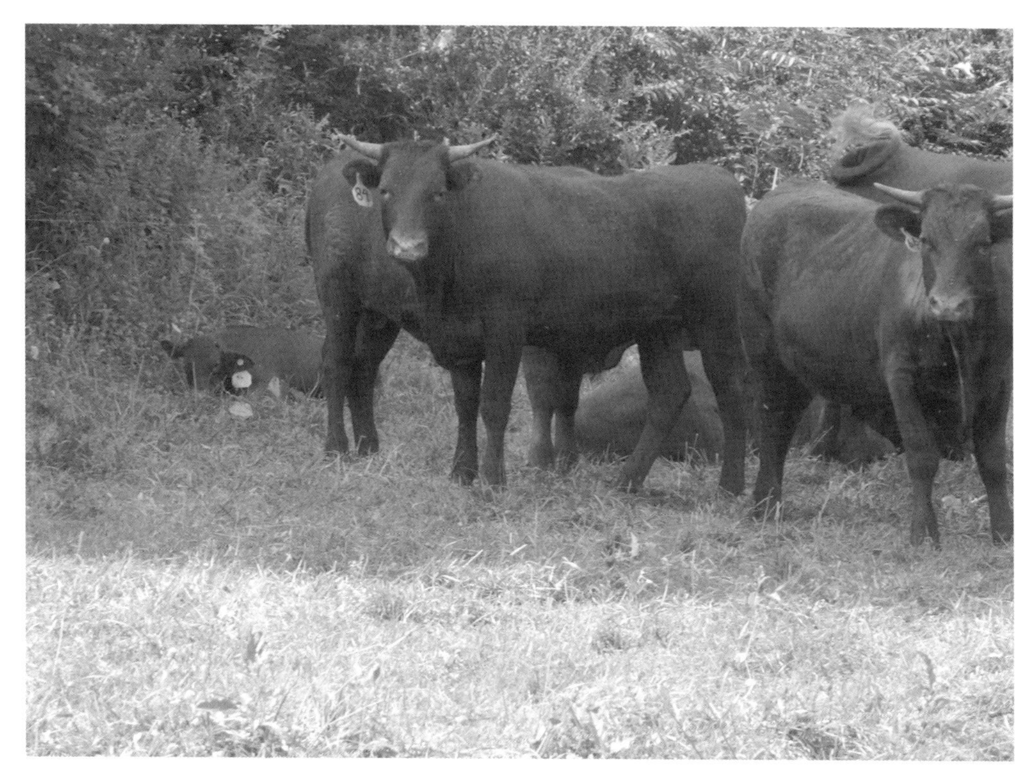

Figure 18.14 The emerging popularity of imported lines of Devon cattle has imperiled old, uniquely American bloodlines. Photo by DPS.

A new and paradoxical threat has also emerged for Devon cattle in the USA (Figure 18.14). As the Devon has become valued for its excellence in grass-fed beef production, demand for the breed has grown. Several breeders have promoted the use of semen from New Zealand Devon bulls in an effort to enhance the grass-fed potential of the breed. The result has been a steady decline in purely American bloodlines, and the American portion of the breed is indeed in danger of disappearing through what is essentially upgrading with New Zealand sires. This is ironic as the full potential of the American lines could well be lost before it is even documented.

A similar situation has developed with the Dexter cattle breed over the last century (Figure 18.15). While never all that numerous, the American population has the distinction of including animals that descend entirely from imports from Ireland and England in the early 1900s. The majority of this breed in the USA has been influenced by later imports from England that included many "appendix" cattle that have influences from a number of other breeds. While the Dexter influence still predominates, the paradox has arisen that the USA is now the main reservoir of the original Irish lines, these having now entirely disappeared in Ireland as well as in other countries.

The same potential threat also faces Jacob, Karakul, and Tunis sheep. The American type of each of these breeds is distinctive, and in some instances is closer to the original than what could now be imported. In addition, the long isolation of the American lines of these

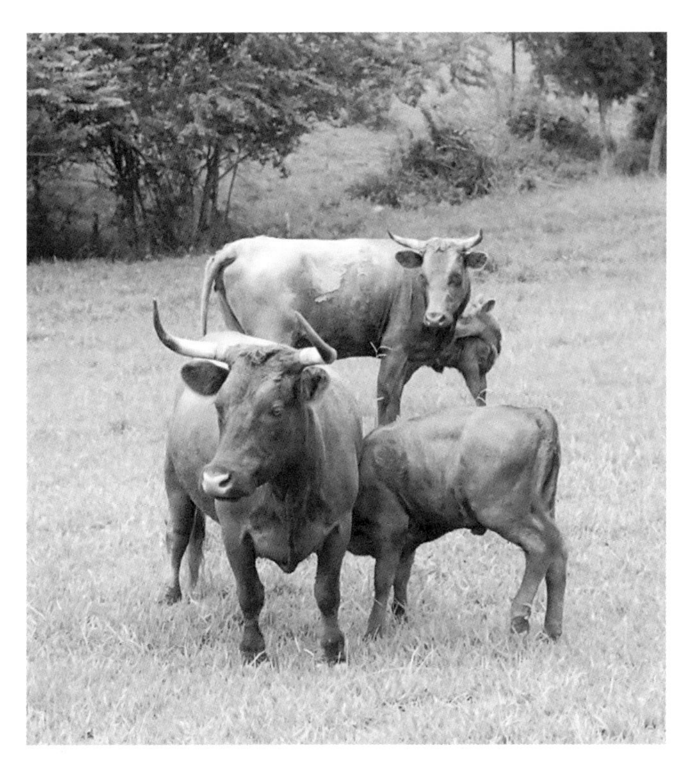

Figure 18.15 Bloodlines of American Dexter cattle now include more cattle of traditional bloodlines than herds in any other country. Photo by JB.

breeds from other international sources has led to these lines being very distinct, to the extent that the American version of all three of these breeds is recognized as a unique breed independent from other national populations. Breeding stock being imported to America results in the erosion of the unique American bloodlines, which then lose their status as being distinct from the international breed.

Another example of a breed that could be damaged by importation is the Dutch Belted dairy cattle breed, because America has long served as the major reserve of genetic material. The breed in the USA has a long history of uninterrupted purebred breeding, while the breed in the Netherlands experienced several decades of decline enforced by bull licensing laws. The populations in the two countries are now fairly distinct, and while some reciprocal exchange is appropriate, it is also true that imports from the Netherlands could eventually swamp the uniquely American population if they are used extensively.

The threat to American bloodlines is more subtle in some other examples. Ancient White Park cattle in the USA are the result of importation in the mid-1900s, and occurred before the latest genetic bottlenecks in Britain. American bloodlines were then augmented by a recent importation of semen that was so widely used that fully pre-bottleneck animals are now rare or nonexistent. Any pre-bottleneck cattle that remain are valuable because they can have the potential to contribute greatly to the long-term survival of this ancient and pivotal cattle breed.

In another example, a Sorraia stallion was imported from Portugal with plans to use him on Colonial Spanish mares within the USA. While superficially similar in type, the mares come from a variety of origins. Crossbreeding between branches of a family that have been

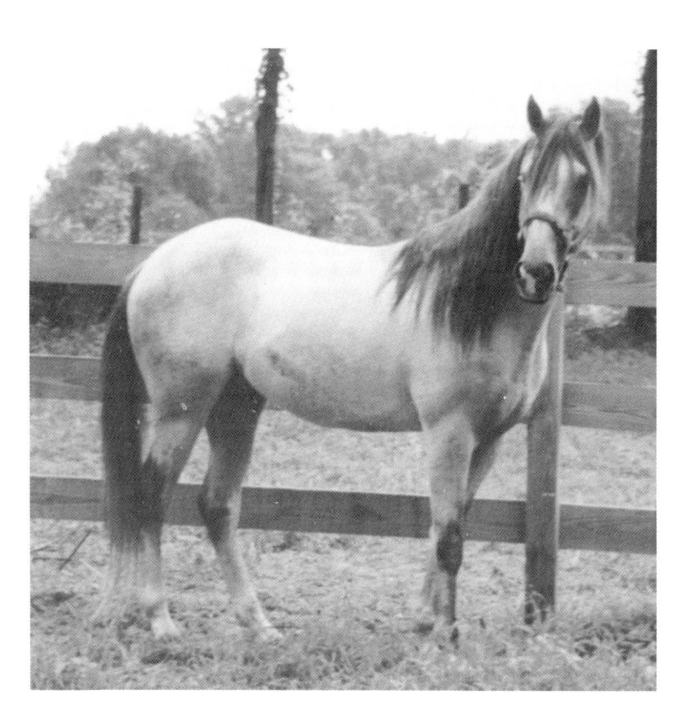

Figure 18.16 The Iberian-derived horse breeds such as the Florida Cracker occur throughout the Americas and have strong phenotypic and genetic similarities. Despite this, imported horses nearly always have a greater economic value than locally produced animals. Photo by DPS.

separated for several centuries could well end up displacing some of the unique attributes and genome of the Colonial Spanish horse in the USA. This is not likely to occur to a very damaging degree, but the level of interest in an imported horse is greater than that in locally produced ones. Because of this attraction, imports can displace locally produced animals of similar quality and higher conservation value.

The phenomenon of imported animals having better name recognition and higher cost than local animals can have a surprising result on popularity in some cases. The various branches of the Colonial Spanish horses in North and South America closely resemble one another (Figure 18.16). The local branches of this family are all rare, with some in peril of extinction. In spite of this, the imported Peruvian Paso, Mangalarga, and horses of other related breeds enjoy great popularity and command a high dollar value even though similar North American horses could be had for a fraction of the price. This phenomenon does great damage to local breed resources because it focuses attention on the imports, each of which takes up a stall that could be housing a locally produced horse. These imports divert attention away from uniquely American genetic resources that are closely similar to the imported resource.

Some imports do more than simply displace bloodlines; they instead displace entire rare American breeds, usually by occupying barns, stalls, and pastures that would otherwise be devoted to raising rare breeds that are already in the country. These imports include some breeds that have become real threats to the maintenance and survival of our unique breed resources. Some of these are relatively common breeds that have been recently imported, such as the Boer and Kiko goats, whose impact is felt by Spanish and Tennessee Myotonic goats. Another example is the Dorper hair sheep which is displacing Katahdin, St. Croix, and Barbados Blackbelly sheep (Figure 18.17).

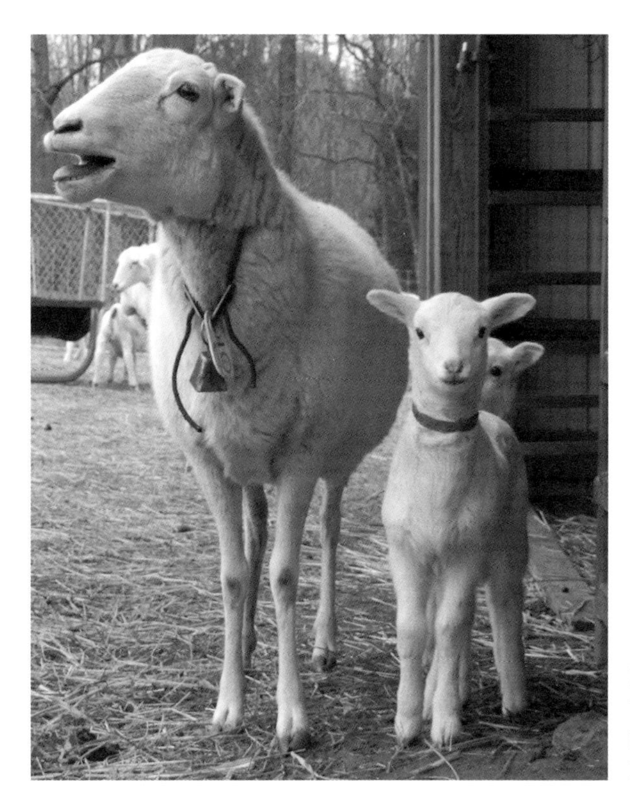

Figure 18.17 The recently imported Dorper endangers local hair sheep breeds, such as these St. Croix ewes. Photo by JB.

Similarly, in an effort to document the potential of Iberian-based cattle breeds for beef production in the South, the United States Department of Agriculture (USDA) imported the Colombian and Venezuelan Romosinuano breed. This is a useful and productive breed and is being used in breed comparison studies in Florida. The local Florida Cracker, a cousin breed to the imported Romosinuano, is in dire straits and is not included in these studies, even though it is available right down the road from where the research is being accomplished. Private endeavors as well as public ones often repeat the illogic of ignoring the local resource by documenting an imported relative, which then displaces the local resource and further contributes to its extinction. This happens at great expense and effort while similar local genetic resources are relegated to second-class status.

The importation of Wensleydale and Teeswater sheep semen has posed a direct short-term threat to other luster longwool breeds in this country, such as Cotswold, Lincoln, and Leicester Longwool. The USA breed associations for Teeswater and Wensleydale sheep designate ewes of these three longwool breeds as the only recognized recipients of this semen to establish a base for the upgrading to high-grade sheep of these two breeds. The irony of this situation is that the breeds from which these ewes come are rare in their own right, and in some cases rarer than the imported resource. These breeds providing the ewes for crossbreeding are US representatives of internationally recognized breed populations that contribute to international conservation. The Wensleydales and Teeswaters in the USA, however, will be the result of upgrading. In the case of the Teeswaters, the upgrades will be eventually recognized as full members of the breed back in the UK, but currently this is not to be allowed for the Wensleydale. Hopefully, this will change. Upgraded sheep only make sense for conservation if they are able to contribute to international breed numbers or conservation efforts for Wensleydales and Teeswaters. The result of this complicated situation is that these two rare breeds directly threaten others (even if temporarily), with no significant long-term contribution to global security of any of the five breeds involved.

A further conservation implication in the luster longwools (Leicester Longwool, Lincoln, Cotswold, Wensleydale, Teeswater) is that these breeds tend to compete directly with one another for space on farms. As a general trend the overall numbers of longwool sheep remain fairly constant, but within that number the relative numbers of the individual breeds fluctuate. This means that a space taken by a Wensleydale or Teeswater upgraded sheep is very likely to have been filled by a purebred Cotswold, Lincoln, or Leicester Longwool, rather than by a crossbred or non-longwool sheep. This becomes a zero-sum game in many instances, with the import displacing and preventing meaningful conservation of another breed in danger and already long-established in this country.

In a somewhat similar vein, Shetland sheep have surged in popularity. When first imported to the USA, this breed was on both the British Rare Breed Survival Trust and The Livestock Conservancy rare sheep breed list, although only for the peculiar reason that the large populations on the Shetland Islands were not considered in the UK numbers. The breed is now a conservation success story and has become much more secure numerically. A large part of the success is not only the many advantages these sheep have for smallholders, but also the fascination with a breed from a remote corner of the globe. Many sheep enthusiasts now keep Shetlands, while the multicolored and finer-fleeced Romeldale remains an American breed in very real danger of extinction.

Several horse breeds are similarly problematic, at least potentially. Each horse occupies a slot that then becomes unavailable for other horses. Endangered American breeds must compete with several imported breeds for attention. The imports include many British pony breeds, for which the breed dynamics can sometimes result in America being a dead end because imports arrive to the USA, but no reciprocal exports are ever undertaken. This is in contrast to the healthier situation, now increasingly realized and appreciated, that all countries with a breed need to be key participants in the breed's international survival strategy. Imports with little hope of reciprocity usually contribute little to conservation of their own breed, and at the same time also take up spaces that horses of uniquely American origin could have occupied. This is an especially strong threat to local breeds such as the Newfoundland Pony that descend from foundation influences introduced well before the process of breed standardization occurred (Figure 18.18).

Other imports are more difficult to classify as to their net effect on global conservation. Effective conservation of the primitive and feral breeds is problematic outside of their original habitat. Soay sheep, Arapawa goats, and Exmoor ponies belong in this group. It is important to question whether any of these breeds that is so closely associated with a specific distinctive environment can be effectively conserved outside of that environment. These questions have no easy answers.

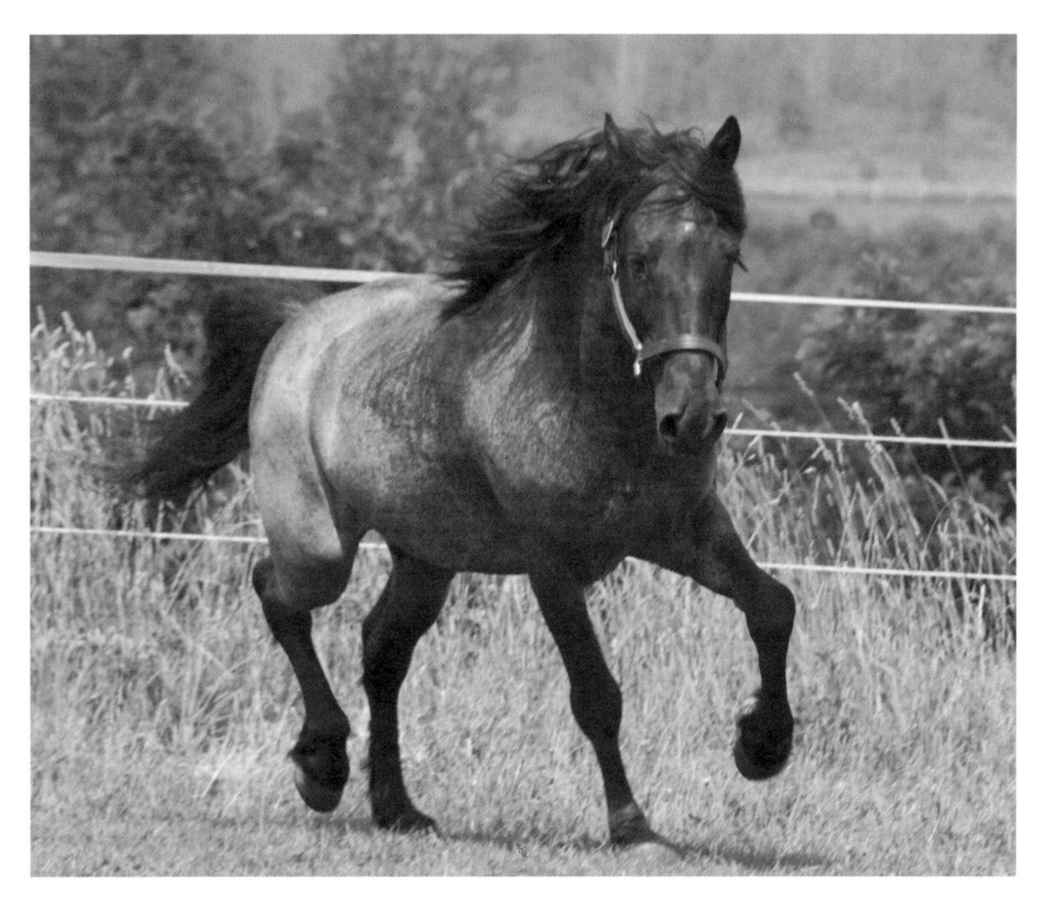

Figure 18.18 The Newfoundland Pony is a distinctive Canadian breed with a long history. Its foundation includes ponies from the UK that arrived well before breed standardization was underway. Photo by Judith Johnson.

18.4.5 Assessment of Importations

Imports of rare breeds or new bloodlines of existing breeds are frequently problematic for conservation. The reason for this is that imports tend to be cared for by dedicated individuals with great enthusiasm, loyalty, and economic resources. These are the very sorts of advocates that are needed for the rare breeds already endangered in the country receiving the imports. Their energy and talents would have greater effect focused on the high priorities that are already present rather than importing new priorities. Exceptions do exist where imports do not hamper conservation priorities and do indeed accomplish significant conservation work. These few cases are worthy of celebration as valuable conservation successes, although it remains a fact that imported breeds generally have little positive effect for conservation of rare breeds. Imports can do a great deal of damage to conservation efforts for local breeds. Any program with imported breeds, especially those that are recently or newly imported, needs to be very carefully evaluated as to its consequences, both for the breed in question as well as for other endangered breeds.

CHAPTER 19

General Principles for Breed Associations

Consideration of the cultural and political aspects affecting breeds is essential for long-term successful breed maintenance. These aspects are often the source of the most daunting challenges facing breeds. Other than recommending that everyone play nicely together, not much more can be added. "Play nicely together" is easy in theory but notoriously difficult in practice because it often means people working together despite having very different underlying philosophies and goals, all of which are legitimate. However, breeds are doomed in the long term without some level of broad and inclusive action by breeders and other advocates. As a result, "playing nicely together" is the key to success.

The history and fate of the American Quarter Horse illustrates well the importance of cooperation (Figure 19.1). In the middle of the 1900s there were several different registries for American Quarter Horses, and none of them were all that successful. Breeders then got together, and decided that it was possible to respect one another and respect one another's stallion without the need to mate their mares to that stallion. This was a turning point. The breeders joined forces and today the American Quarter Horse is the most numerous of any registered horse breed on the planet. Working together despite legitimate differences remains a basic component of successful breed security. This level of cooperation is especially essential for managing the rarest of the rare and for assuring good outcomes for breed rescue situations.

Successful breed management demands an effective collaboration between several different stakeholders. Breeders have an essential role, as do associations and registries. Associations and registries for many breeds are one and the same thing, although some breeds separate out the two roles so that associations delve more into promotion and showing while registries only track and validate animals.

Breed associations are groups of people with a shared interest in a specific breed. While this may seem obvious, the fine details can become complicated and can splinter rather than unite people. Issues involved in breed associations are vitally important to the maintenance and conservation of pure breeds of livestock. Some of the issues are procedural, and others are political, but all must be addressed for breed associations to do their job successfully. Breeds are biological entities, but in the modern era they cannot realistically

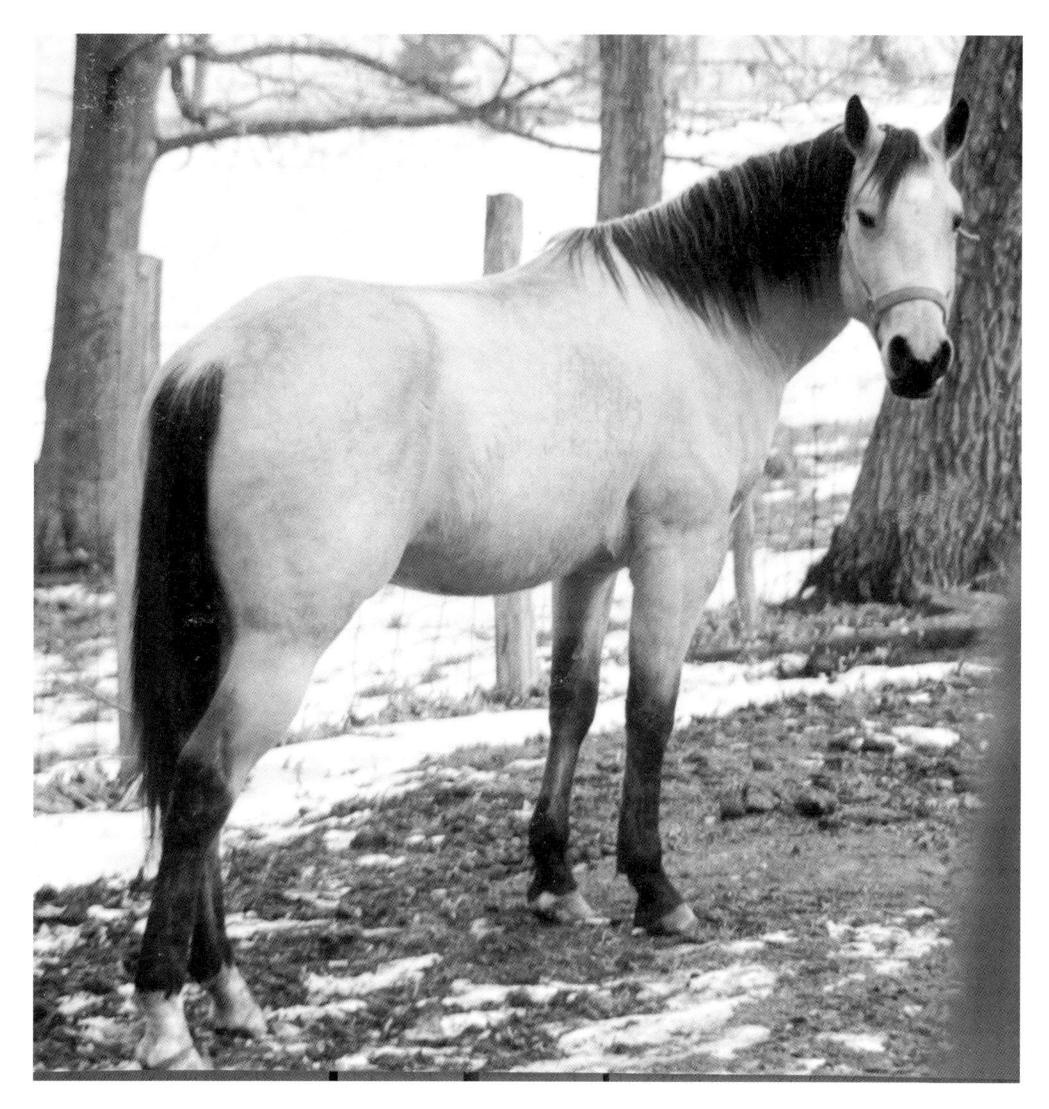

Figure 19.1 The Quarter Horse benefitted from breeders creating a culture of actively working together to promote the breed. Photo by DPS.

survive without the support and wise stewardship that come from a well-functioning breed association.

Many breeds are rare because of political and organizational failure on the part of breed associations. Success for all breed associations has a similar array of characteristics: timely communication, inclusiveness, frank discussion without rancor, and efficient processing of registrations. Failure in any one of these can lead to a weak and ineffective breed association that does the breed more damage than good. Breeds must not only survive the physical environment; they must also survive the political environment of their own breeders! Sometimes the internal political threats to a breed's existence are the most significant ones and overshadow any biological or market issues challenging the breed.

Understanding the philosophies and characteristics of breed associations can help them to work more smoothly. Some associations are driven almost completely by market forces. These include some very large and powerful associations that govern popular and numerous breeds and for which economic forces predominate. Some breed associations tightly focus their activities on issues of breed maintenance and genetic identity, while others are most concerned with social interaction among the breeders of the breed.

People join associations in order to belong to a group of people with shared interests. It is important for all breed associations to reflect on group identity and goals so that the activities of the group can serve the breed effectively. Successful associations, especially for rare breeds, serve a host of important functions including marketing, conservation, genetic management, and discussion among breeders. They also educate breeders, members, and the general public about the breed.

Each association member brings certain strengths, needs, and perspectives. All of these must be managed effectively to assure that individual member needs are met, while also meeting the shared goals of the group. Each member likely has a slightly different priority for the different issues confronting the breed and the association, but all must work together for the common good of the breed and the association. Deciding which of these individual agendas fit within the association's job description is difficult and may sometimes be rancorous, but setting priorities is essential if associations are to avoid diluting their efforts by attempting to be all things to all people.

19.1 Purposes of Associations

Two important purposes for nearly all associations are communication and education. Most associations also operate a breed registry as a third important purpose. Some breeds split the registry from the association and use the association more for management of shows, educational programs, and documentation of animal performance. Both approaches have merit and either can succeed. Management and promotion of the breed are at the core of every association's purpose. These can be accomplished in a variety of ways that best suit the association and the breed.

Associations, networks, and even individual breeders all benefit from deciding on a purpose for the association. This is commonly called a mission statement. A mission statement should be a conscious effort to decide the reason for the existence of the organization. Mission statements define goals and direct the actions of associations. Short, pithy mission statements are always best, as these are easy to keep before the members. They are also easy to use as yardsticks against which to measure decisions as they affect the breed. Mission statements should not become some irrelevant detail gathering dust on a shelf. They should be constantly before the members, and especially the leadership. In this way the mission statement is the touchstone against which actions and programs are evaluated. Good mission statements help to avoid drift in attitudes and actions. Avoiding drift away from the central mission can greatly help in avoiding dissension and conflict among members. Having all participants engaged in a single mission goes a long way to ensuring united and effective action.

A very telling passage from *Alice in Wonderland* comes to mind:

"Would you tell me, please, which way I ought to go from here?"
"That depends a good deal on where you want to go," said the Cat.
"I don't much care where," said Alice.
"Then it doesn't much matter which way you go," said the Cat.

A lack of conscious direction nearly always assures little to no progress in getting to a destination. This is just as true of associations as it is of individual breeding programs. Legitimate goals for associations, networks, and individual breeders are numerous and include breed conservation, management of populations for long-term viability, commercial success in marketing products and breeding stock, increase in breed numbers, show ring wins, production of breed products, and production of breeding stock. The list is nearly limitless, and unfortunately some of these goals are mutually exclusive. Having a specified mission statement and goals helps to direct actions toward a successful outcome.

Associations and networks can work only if breeders are truly engaged and involved in the best interests of their breed. Association, network, and breeder should all be working together to achieve common goals. The success of any one of these should contribute to the success of all three.

19.2 Membership

Breed associations usually have different levels of formal membership. Many associations limit full membership, with voting privileges, to active breeders that register animals. This is logical, because these are the individuals with the greatest stake in the decisions and activities affecting the breed. Other associations open full membership to all owners, whether breeders or not. This last point is trivial to several breeds but is of great importance to horse breeds in which many owners are not breeders and never will be. These non-breeder members do have an important stake in many decisions concerning the breed, especially details of showing and performance.

Associate members usually are adults who do not own animals of the breed, while junior members are youths (Figure 19.2). Both associate and junior members have some interest in the breed, but usually do not have voting privileges. Such members are indeed part of the association and can contribute to the discussion that goes into decision-making even if they lack a vote.

Family memberships are also a part of many breed associations, and usually involve a financial saving over multiple individual memberships. Some associations limit voting rights to one vote per family membership, some allow two. A significant reason for family memberships is that the individuals covered by the membership can each conduct official business (registrations, transfers) with the breed association. This can greatly simplify registry and association function as delays are avoided when one family member is unavailable for signature on breed association documents.

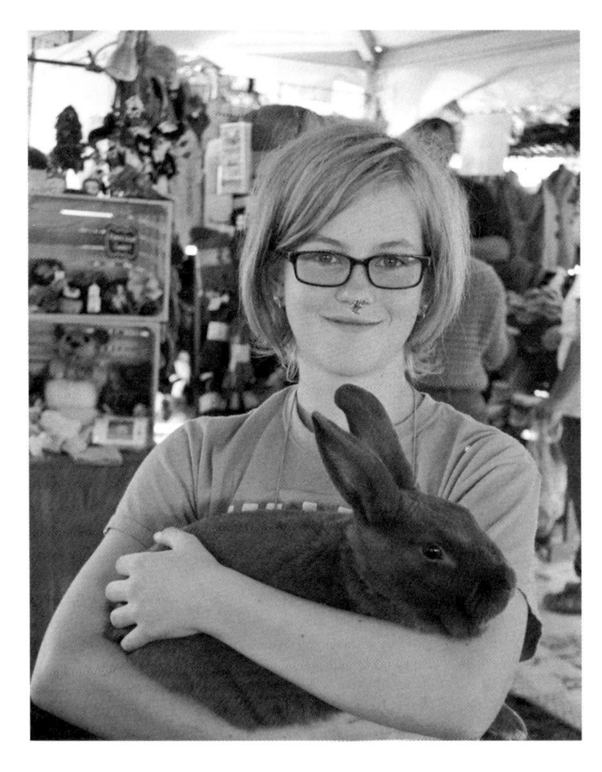

Figure 19.2 Youth are the breeders of tomorrow, and are an essential part of breed associations. Photo by JB.

19.3 Breed Associations for Endangered Breeds

Endangered and rare breeds bring with them a host of issues that are less important for common breeds. One important goal of associations that serve rare breeds is to try to locate and include all breeders of purebred animals into the association. It is also important to try to include all purebred animals into the registry, while excluding all non-purebred animals. This is much easier to state than it is to accomplish, but this goal is critical for effective breed conservation. Associations benefit from having this as a stated goal that is kept before the members. Appropriate inclusion and exclusion of animals can be fraught with difficulty, and each association handles the challenge differently.

Details of the genetic management of breeds are especially relevant to rare breed associations. While associations for common breeds tend to focus more on the genetic improvement of production, associations for rare breeds must also pay close attention to genetic aspects of breed population viability and management.

19.4 Communication

Communication is one of the vital functions of a breed association. It is probably even more important than registry functions for the long-term survival of most breeds. For rare and endangered breeds, the communication network brought together by the association can be critically important to the survival of the breed and its expansion. Communication involves just about every aspect of breed business: news about breeders and animals, shows, successful promotion efforts, marketing, husbandry, and management. Communication is especially important concerning the dispersal of animals from herds that are being discontinued for whatever reason. Communication also involves education of all members as to any genetic and political issues that face the association and the breed. The importance of communication can hardly be overstated.

Effective communication embraces a variety of mechanisms. Newsletters have long been a common method used by breed associations to communicate with members and interested members of the public. Newsletters are nearly always assumed to be part of an association's service to its membership. The advantage of newsletters is that they stand as a reasonably permanent record of association activity. Small associations usually encounter problems in getting timely submissions of sufficient material for newsletters. This can be a major headache for an editor who is generally an unpaid volunteer. For many large associations, the newsletter has evolved into a magazine format with a fully paid staff.

As the digital age advances, more and more associations dispense with a printed newsletter or magazine, and resort to a web-based system of communication. This can both cut costs and speed up communication. A potential downside is that significant numbers of rare-breed enthusiasts live in situations where access to the internet is limited or nonexistent. Associations must be careful to have strategies that facilitate member participation as fully as possible, with no hint of relegating those with limited computer access to second-class status. Offering a printed as well as a web-based alternative for association communications can do this fairly effectively. Email or internet-based chat lists are becoming increasingly common as either official or unofficial forums for communication on topics of interest to breeders. These electronic formats have the advantage of being quicker than print media, so that time-sensitive information is more likely to reach its desired audience than it is through more sporadic newsletters.

One disadvantage of communication based on email or other messaging modalities is that it is written rather than verbal. It is fairly common for unintended inferences to be read from hastily composed messages. Another disadvantage is the more casual tone that often accompanies the use of email. This can result in significant misinformation or miscommunication unless wisely monitored and moderated. Misunderstandings must be rapidly defused before they escalate into nasty disputes. These are all too commonly encountered in electronic forums. Having a significant subgroup that is dedicated to maintaining a positive and open discussion forum within the chat group can assure that the group remains very successful for everyone. For electronic forums to serve as conduits for official breed association business, they must be closely monitored and may need to be open only to members of the association in order for sensitive internal issues to be discussed and managed as constructively as possible.

In addition to formal associations, breeders also organize and communicate in many informal ways. These form what is loosely called "the network" and provide a significant way of connecting breeders to one another to share information and ideas as well as news of current interest. One very powerful asset that networks bring to breeders is alerting them to emergency dispersals so that important portions of breeds are not lost (Figure 19.3). Networks have been essential in rescuing some specific strains of various breeds. They are an important part of the community that develops around a breed. This aspect is only likely

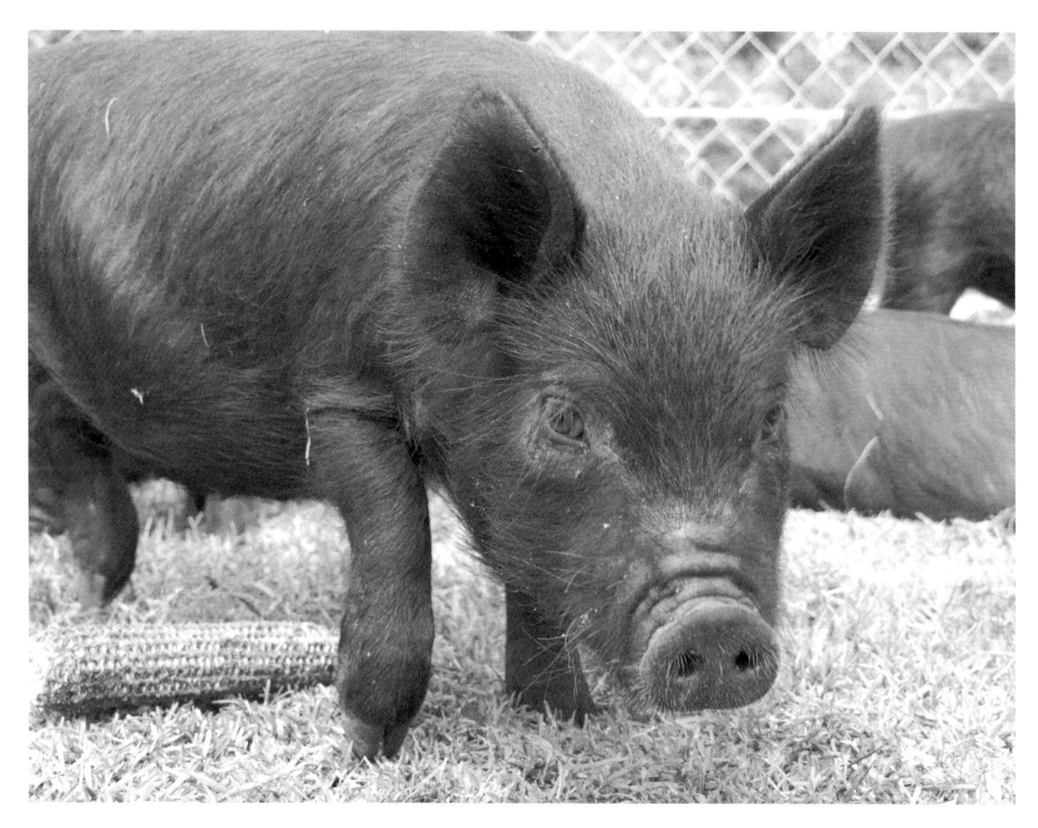

Figure 19.3 Communication networks can be indispensable in placing animals. Some endangered lines of Guinea Hogs have benefitted from networks that were able to rescue them after owner situations changed and endangered their survival. Photo by JB.

to increase in importance and degree in the future as electronic communication becomes more widespread.

Unfortunately, gossip is also rapidly shared through informal networks and if not managed properly and promptly it can be disastrous to a breed and its breeders. Unsubstantiated allegations, or even accurate ones, can do irreparable damage not only to individual breeders but also to group integrity and loyalty. Public electronic forums are extremely poor avenues for addressing conflicts and rivalries.

19.5 Multiple Breed Associations

Breeding of purebred livestock is generally undertaken by people that are passionate about the breed and its future. Breeders with an enhanced sense of this passion characterize many of those involved in the conservation of rare breeds. This passion can be a positive attribute or a hindrance to conservation depending on how it is managed. It is all too common for breeders of rare breeds of livestock to disagree on various points, and for those disagreements to result in splits of associations so that multiple associations end up serving single breeds. Splits within an association also split a small breed into yet smaller populations.

Each of those populations is then more endangered than it once was as part of the previous larger whole. This is because small populations face biological risks from inbreeding and physical risks from disasters such as fire or storms. There is also the very important fact that small groups simply have fewer resources for outreach, promotion, and education than larger groups. Larger groups are much more likely to grow than small groups.

Some of the disagreements that result in splits are significant because they originate back in the very concept of a specific pure breed and what it should entail. Most splits indeed take this form, and are usually the result of two conflicting philosophies. Generally, one camp is more inclusive than another. No single answer fits this dilemma. Situations do arise in which the more inclusive breeders are failing to adequately conserve the breed as a purebred resource. Equally, the more exclusive breeders can easily be eliminating animals that rightly belong in the pure breed. These issues have been dealt with in previous chapters of this book, and an important part of the solution is for associations to develop a philosophy that helps them make these important decisions consistently rather than haphazardly. Moderating the extremes of opinion on this and other issues is a vital role for breed association leadership. Careful and attentive management of an association can blend these varying extremes of breeder philosophy into an endeavor that allows both extremes to maintain their identities, while pursuing common goals related to the breed.

Much of the work of an association takes real effort. All those efforts are duplicated when multiple associations exist. This includes registries, newsletters, legal corporate responsibilities, breeder recruitment, and a host of other issues. This aspect alone suggests that fewer associations are a better choice for most breeds. The duplication of effort drains energy and resources, and also detracts from other vitally important tasks such as breed promotion and broader communication among all of the breeders.

The advantages of multiple associations coming together to form a single breed association are alluded to above with the American Quarter Horse. Once the breeders decided to coexist under a single umbrella, the stage was set for the breed to become the most populous horse breed in the world. The association has taken this breed to a position that is enviable in modern horse breeds. The foundation breeders who are most stringent in favoring the traditional look and breeding are able to thrive and function within the overall framework of a breed association that also includes factions devoted to halter conformation shows, rodeo competition, reining competitions, and racing with horses heavily influenced by Thoroughbred breeding. Each segment of the breed benefits from the resources of the larger breed and is thereby able to achieve its own goals, even those that are not all that widely shared throughout the entire breeder community.

A contrasting situation currently exists among Colonial Spanish horse breeders (Figure 19.4). Splits among breeders of this breed have resulted in several names for the breed, including Spanish Mustang, Spanish Barb, Barb, Tacky, Florida Cracker, and others. This is a numerically small breed regardless of which horses are included in the count, yet it currently has some 16 associations for fewer than 3000 horses! Some of these associations are built around a single geographically defined population (Florida Cracker, Pryor Mountain). Others are broader and more inclusive (Spanish Mustang Registry, Southwest Spanish Mustang Association, Horse of the Americas). Unfortunately, many of the splits

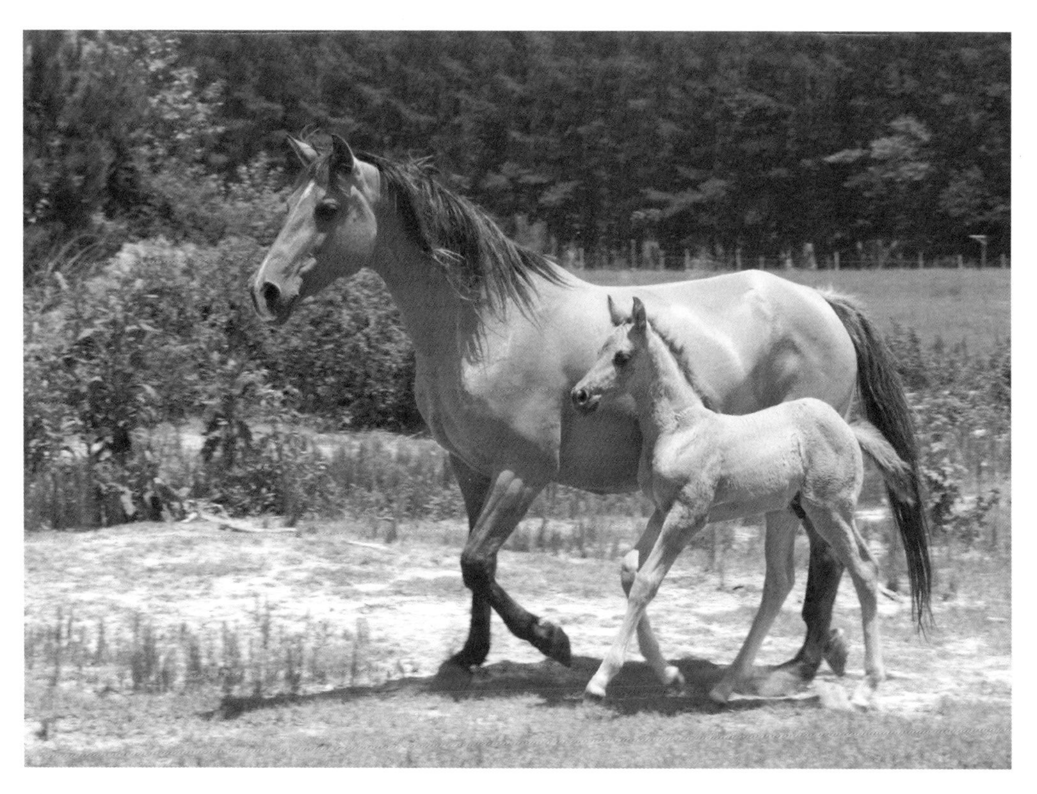

Figure 19.4 At one point, the Colonial Spanish horses were served by as many as 22 different associations. The Marsh Tacky is one of those distinctive local strains that is served by an independent breed association. Photo by JB.

occurred between strong personalities that were passionate about the breed, and those are the splits most difficult to heal. Each has good reasons for deciding what should be excluded and what should be included. However, when the whole group of horses is examined, they generally resemble one another more than they resemble any other breed resource. In that situation, grouping these under a single association would help to foster conservation. It would also contribute to broader promotion efforts to increase demand for this unique American breed, while still providing space for those with a more restrictive outlook to pursue their own goals.

Unique in association history was a very inclusive effort in the establishment of the Jersey-Duroc Record Association in 1883. This association absorbed associations that targeted red swine breeds including Victoria, Kentucky Red Berkshire, Red Guinea, Red Spanish, and others. The result of combining these was the composite Jersey-Duroc breed, now simply known as the Duroc. The success of the association could be considered to have come at the cost of extinction to these founder breeds. However, they were all fairly closely related and shared a common foundation. Combining them resulted in a remarkably successful breed based on all of the components. The Duroc is noted to this day for its hardiness and productivity and is currently one of the most internationally popular hog breeds. The success of the Duroc springs in large part from an effective and inclusive association.

19.6 Codes of Ethics

A code of ethics is a common way for an association to convey to its breeders their responsibilities to the breed as well as to the association. The usual minimum requirement from most associations and registries is that the breeder or other applicant for registration of animals accurately represents pedigree and registration information. The existence of various breeds and various breeders will add a variety of other issues to this short version. Ethics can easily be called into question, even when all parties are well meaning. The trick is to avoid penalizing the well-meaning honest mistake, while penalizing intentionally dishonest actions. This is not always easy, and as codes of ethics become more and more complex it becomes increasingly difficult to bring the corporate wisdom of the association to bear in any given situation.

Some few associations are more active in the area of ethics and insist that business dealings by breeders and members meet certain standards of disclosure and honesty. Most of these guidelines and rules are an attempt to avoid customers dissatisfied by the misrepresentation of animals. The identity and preparation of animals for competitive showing can be a frequent subject of codes of ethics, including the masking of birth defects or color markings in certain breeds.

Codes of ethics are sadly necessary, if for no other reason than when many people are involved in associations (which is good), disagreements are sure to arise (which is bad). Expectations of breeders and members must be clearly specified. Penalties can include fines, limitations on registration or showing privileges, limitations on other association-related benefits, or outright expulsion. Penalties must be articulated to correspond to the varying degrees of severity of breaches of ethics that can be encountered. Sanctions must be fairly and wisely applied. Penalties are certainly appropriate in some situations, but it is important to understand the effect of such punishments because they can quickly undermine any economic stability for affected breeders. Nasty disputes that end up in sanctions run a very real risk of alienating bystanders as well as the parties that are directly involved. This can severely damage a breeder community and ultimately the breed.

19.7 Educational Programs

Breed associations are all ideally involved in education. This aspect of associations is a key component for the long-term success of the breed and the association. One aspect of education for a breed association is the education of its own members and leaders. This is frequently overlooked. Lack of effort on this front can result in unfocused and unsuccessful breed associations. Exactly how to educate members is a tough question. All members, and especially new members, ought to have reasonably detailed knowledge of the breed, its unique traits, its history, and its historic and present function. This is asking a lot of anyone, but if all members have knowledge of these key points, then discussions and activities can gain a great deal of consensus and support from the membership. Promotional pamphlets and breed standards can serve as educational tools to establish a shared understanding of these topics.

It is especially important to educate members about the husbandry and management needs of the breed. This must consider the historic role that the breed has played, its current role in agriculture, and appropriate management techniques to assure breeder success. This is important not only for the survival of the breed, but also for continued selection for historic type and performance. Much of this knowledge is being lost as older breeders pass away and new breeders join the ranks who have little or no connection to the breed, its heritage, and the culture in which it existed. At the very least, a resource list of publications should be available. If at all possible, interviews of older breeders and their children should document the culture and husbandry of the breed. Efforts like this can do a great deal to support future conservation of both type and function of breeds. Breeder members must also be educated about the basics of animal breeding and breed maintenance. Assuring an educated group of breeders can avoid common pitfalls that detract from the survival of breeds.

Equally important are educational efforts aimed at those outside the breed association, including the education and enlisting of new members and new breeders. This aspect is crucial to sustaining and expanding a support base for the breed. Failure here can easily lead to a diminishing base of breeders and enthusiasts for any breed. Promotional pamphlets, internet websites, strategically placed advertisements for the breed and association, and participation in appropriate public events are all useful ways to accomplish this.

Education of the general public about the breed and its products is also useful to help create a sound and consistent market. Assuring a secure place for breeds within production agriculture assures their future as genetic resources. Examples include The Livestock Conservancy's successful effort to educate the public about the desirability of traditionally raised standard and heritage varieties of turkeys, along with the "Shave 'Em to Save 'Em" program promoting rare breed wools. The target is to link a genetic resource with public demand through education.

19.8 Research

Forward-looking associations are interested and involved in research. The level of research varies from investigations into breed history to the analysis of the molecular genetics of the breed. All levels are useful. At one extreme, the studies are very inexpensive and at the other they are tremendously expensive due to the technology, equipment, and personnel needed to succeed.

Historical research can help to direct conservation programs by putting a breed in its appropriate context. Landraces that are adapted to harsh local conditions, for example, can be and should continue to be used and tested in similar environments. Breeds with certain unique uses (mule-producing jacks, for example) should continue in that niche in order to maintain selection pressures that developed the breed in the first place. History can also help to identify the different bloodlines in a breed and aid in their conservation management so that none becomes extinct, and the breed remains genetically healthy.

Many breeds also have a need for research on the inheritance of specific unique traits, such as functional characteristics or more cosmetic details such as color. Research on the characteristics of the breed can greatly help efforts to conserve and expand breeds with attention to traditional types and roles of the breed. Research is also especially useful when deleterious traits surface in breeds. This research makes it possible to pinpoint the causes of

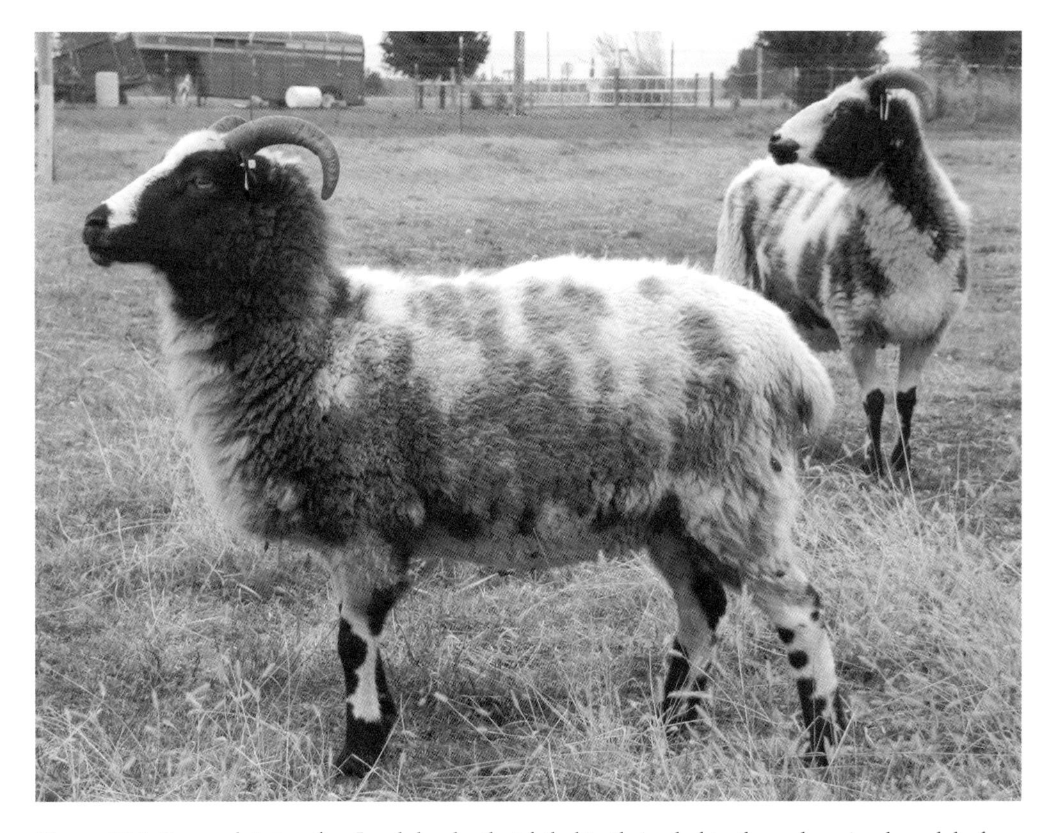

Figure 19.5 Research into a few Jacob lambs that failed to thrive led to the only animal model of human Tay-Sachs disease. Photo by JB.

these negative traits and develop appropriate strategies for their management or elimination without endangering the genetic health of the breed.

The importance of some research findings goes way beyond the individual breed involved. Breeders of American Jacob sheep pursued the diagnosis of rare lambs that failed to thrive (Figure 19.5). The result was finding a mutation similar to the one responsible for Tay-Sachs disease in people. This is the only animal model of this devastating human neurologic disease and helps medical advances. The trait only affects a small portion of the breed, so documenting it in no way damaged the breed but has resulted in great benefits to humans.

19.9 Recruiting and Training New Breeders

Breed associations need to assure that new breeders are entering the breed. New breeders are the only mechanism for providing continuity of the breed, but their recruitment is frequently overlooked as a deliberate and necessary activity by breed associations. Not only must new breeders be recruited, but they must also be welcomed and then trained to be able to make critical selection decisions that conserve breed type, heritage, and utility. Failing to do this is to fail in effective breed conservation.

Dissension can easily arise between older, traditional breeders and newly recruited breeders that bring with them new cultural and husbandry perspectives. Breeds need both types of breeders to succeed. Without the older breeders, the breeds would not exist in the first place. Without the new breeders, the breed will cease to exist very quickly. Moderating the differences that can arise between older and newer breeders is essential to securing the future of breeds. A culture of respect and appreciation between these two types of breeders should be deliberately fostered. Breeds need both a history and a future, and both old and new breeders are essential to this.

In order for a breed to remain viable, it is ideal that all breeders be seed stock producers. This means that all breeders should be producing animals that will be useful in purebred breeding programs. This broad base of contribution to the pure breed assures that no single breeding program, and therefore no single bloodline, dominates the others and narrows the genetic base. For this ideal situation to occur, new breeders need to easily and openly be able to receive the fruits of the experience of more experienced breeders. Secret techniques for breeding superior animals all too easily pass into oblivion with the deaths of breeders that zealously guarded them. Such secrets are notoriously slow to be rediscovered. Breeders need to set aside extremes of the competitive spirit, and instead take pride in watching the next generation grow in knowledge and competence. Effective mentoring of new breeders is not only satisfying, but also invaluable for a breed's survival.

Developing the next generation of breeders has several important facets. One of these is conveying the cultural heritage of the breed, and this is where a rich history of stories about the breed and its breeders becomes useful. Stories such as a boyhood spent chasing deer in the South Carolina swamps on the backs of Marsh Tacky horses enrich and inform the continuing use and selection of the horses. The preferential use of four-horned Navajo-Churro rams in certain Navajo healing ceremonies similarly puts the maintenance of this variant in an important cultural context. All breeds have a heritage and culture that needs to be collected, safeguarded, valued, and preserved in order to maintain the cultural relevance of the breed.

In addition to historical lore, the fine points of selecting breeding stock need to be taught (Figure 19.6). The details of what to select, and why, are extremely important to convey to the next generation. For standard turkeys, the selection of birds that are both large as well as sound and functional is a tough call, and the knowledge of how to do this is carried in the heads of poultry breeders such as Glenn Drowns and Frank Reese who have long and effective experience in selecting birds for function in modern turkey production. The rarity of the system means that only a few breeders survive with the knowledge to make that system work. Only by having older, experienced, successful breeders eagerly and generously convey the subtleties of points of selection is it possible to assure that this rich knowledge is not lost. Transfer of this sort of knowledge usually takes personal interaction because much of the detail is difficult to condense down to a written format. Breeder training short courses and field days can be very helpful in transmitting important details of breed selection to the next generation.

A great deal of knowledge and observation goes into successful breeding programs. It is difficult to articulate and share some aspects of these. Breed type, for example, is more easily appreciated visually with live animals than by a written presentation. An appreciation

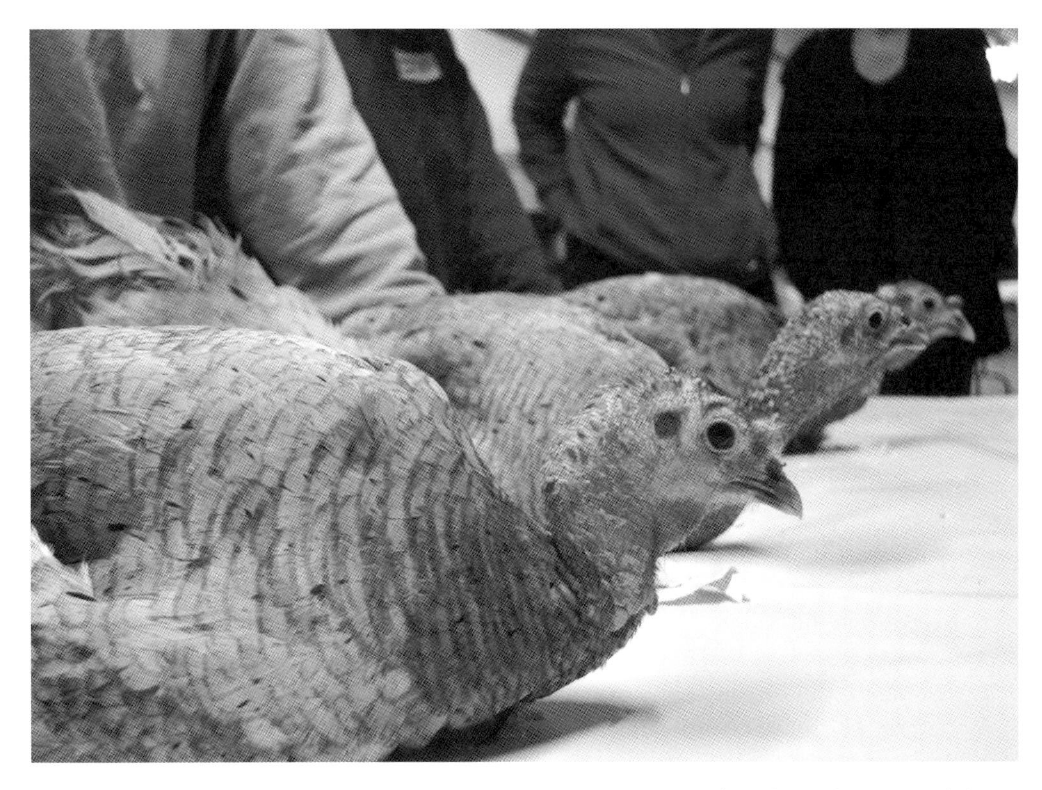

Figure 19.6 Workshops such as The Livestock Conservancy's poultry breeding selection workshops are a great way to encourage and train up the next generation of breeders. Photo by JB.

for the interaction of breed type and breed function is also important. This needs to be conveyed to younger breeders so that the conservation of type has an appropriate and logical context rather than becoming a triviality of purebred breeding that appeals only to fanciers.

19.10 Breed Promotion

Breed promotion is multifaceted but is a key component of every successful breed association. It involves educating breeders, as well as the general public, about the breed's products and potential. The goal is to encourage and promote demand for the breed. This is made easier when a breed has unique products. Many breeds do offer unique products, and it is important to promote these. In addition to products are the valuable services or functions of breeds such as the crossbreeding potential of Florida Cracker or Pineywoods cows or the remarkable brush clearing abilities of Tennessee Myotonic goats. Each time the purebred product finds a market, purebred breeders benefit and so do the breeds they steward.

It is not enough for a breed to excel in some special niche; the word must also get out so that those interested in the product or service will know where to get it. The goal of promotion is to accurately portray the breed's excellence so that a loyal and satisfied following is established. Breed promotion is only successful if it is based on facts that reflect the breed's uniqueness and superiority.

Promotion must also reflect the breed and its identity. For this to be successful the association must have clear knowledge of the breed and its history. By being firmly rooted in this knowledge it is possible for the breeders and the association to value the character and function of the breed, and to promote these attributes in the marketplace.

19.11 Breed Sale Events

Many breed associations host annual sale events. These sales serve as a promotional tool that brings breeders, buyers, and other interested folks together in a setting where animals are available for viewing and purchase. Most of these breed sales are auctions. They are an opportunity for new enthusiasts to get started with the breed (Figure 19.7).

Breed sale events work best when old, established breeders support them by consigning select animals so that the sale reflects the top end of the breed. This is one situation where it is vitally important for breeders to realize that the good of the entire breed takes precedence over the short-term benefit to individual breeders. Especially in the early years of such sales, it may well be that the prices are somewhat below those possible by private treaty sales. A multi-year commitment to assuring high quality lots for the breed sale can help to assure that the long-term fate of these sales is good and strong. Sales which become a dumping

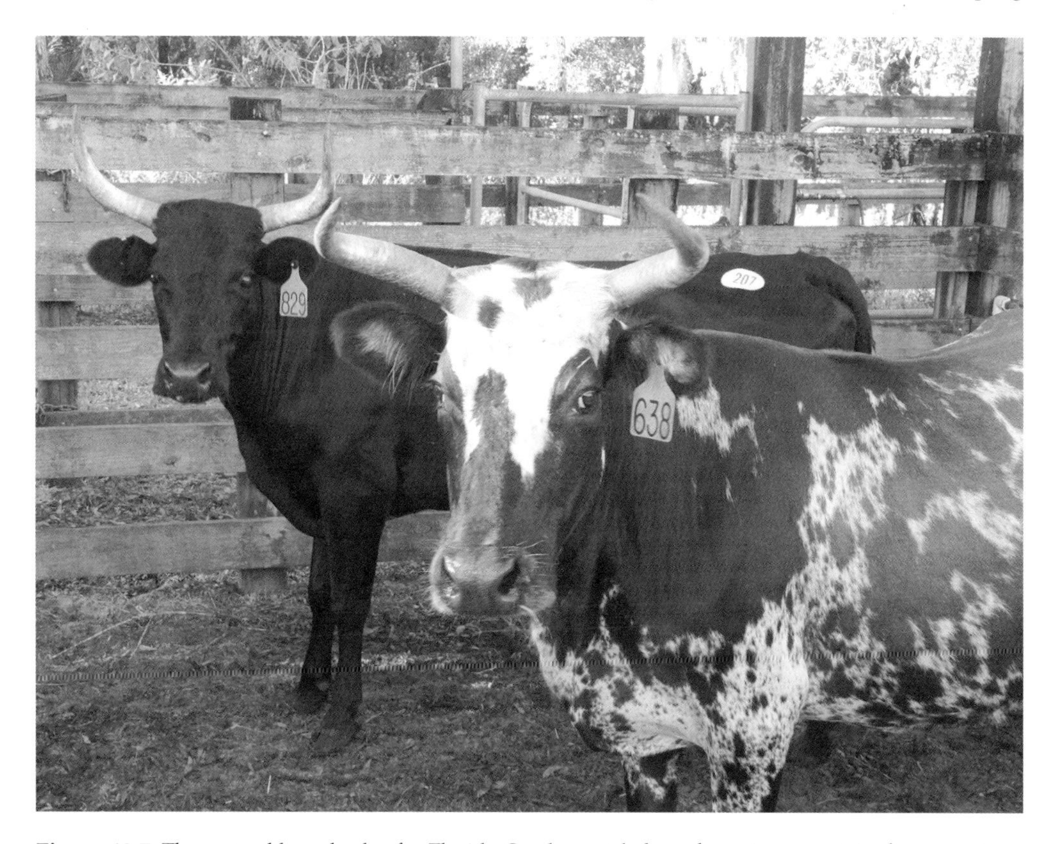

Figure 19.7 The annual breed sales for Florida Cracker cattle have been important in disseminating breeding stock and recruiting new members. Photo by DPS.

ground for second-rate stock will damage the breed and will not encourage newcomers to join those working with the breed.

Sales committees must be visionary, hardworking, and neutral in order to assure that the sale is run fairly and is successful. For many breeds it may be necessary to constrain consignments of breeders. For example, large numbers of breeding males at a sale can easily result in an overall weak sale, with numbers of animals going for slaughter instead of for breeding. This reduces the prices to commercial levels, which is not in the best long-term interest of a breed sale event. A strategy to circumvent this problem is to only allow breeders to consign males if they also consign three or more females to the sale. Specific invitations or requests to larger and established breeders for consignments of select females will generally assure a successful sale.

19.12 Assuring Continuity

Breed associations also have to assure continuity of the association as leaders age out and are lost to the association (Figure 19.8). This is especially the case for association founders. Assuring continuity has inherent difficulties, especially in smaller associations. Founders of associations tend to be energetic, knowledgeable, and opinionated. This is an ideal

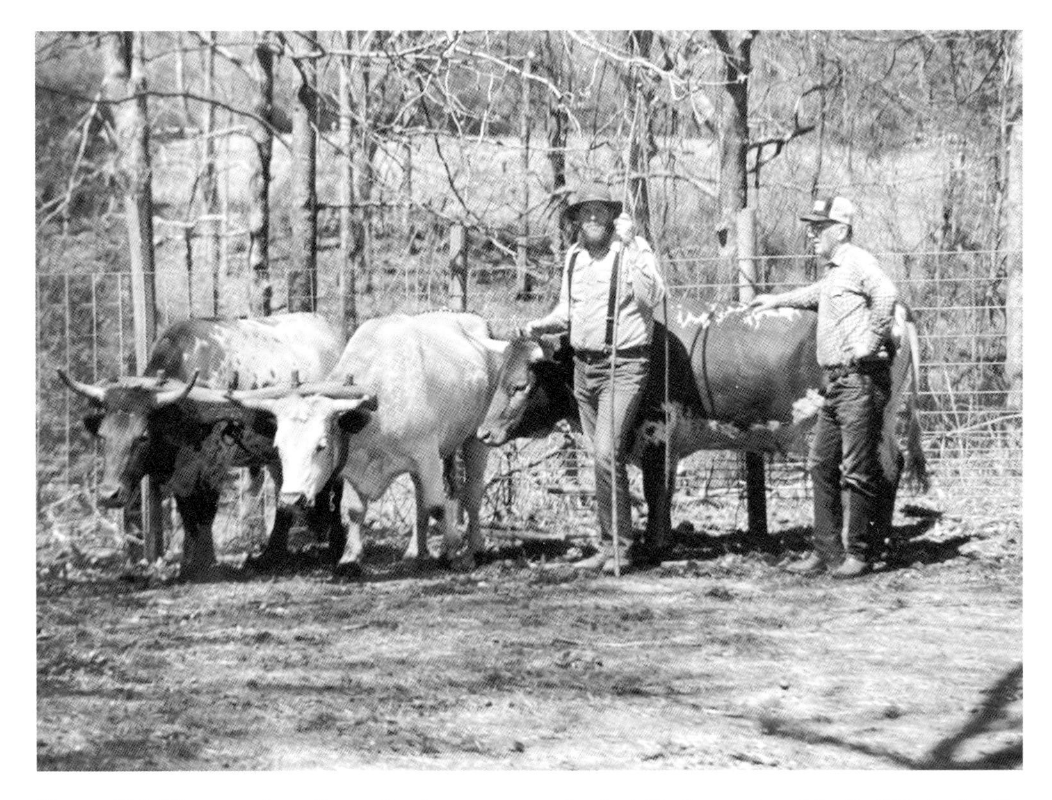

Figure 19.8 Pineywoods cattle continuity was assured as Jack Baylis mentored Justin Pitts in details of training and using oxen and managing cattle. Justin, in his turn, is currently mentoring the next generation. Photo by DPS.

combination of traits to establish an association, but the "opinionated" part can become a real roadblock to recruiting and empowering the next generation of leaders.

Unfortunately, failure to recruit and train that next generation of leaders eventually leads to the collapse of an association. This is an all-too-common fate for associations that are built around a few charismatic individuals. This can happen directly from selfish retention of control by those founders, but also happens more subtly by the founders simply not stepping back a bit and providing vacant spaces for others to fill. Those others generally have a different way of accomplishing their tasks, and this can be off-putting to those that first established procedures and cultural norms. In the long run, though, an association benefits from a variety of approaches, nearly in the same way that a breed benefits from genetic variation. While too much variation can be damaging, too little will invariably cause collapse. Between these extremes lie the associations that have talented senior leadership that encourages and facilitates capable junior leadership to step up and guide the association.

CHAPTER 20

Practical Details of Breed Associations

20.1 Forms of Association

Breed associations rely on some level of organization. Organizational details usually follow only a few different forms, but the development and organization of each breed association is individual. The various forms of organization have both practical and legal ramifications that affect how they succeed in their various functions. The legal aspect of associations is usually not considered to be terribly important among small groups. However, as associations become larger and interactions become less personal, it is vital for associations to function well as legal entities. This prevents an association's legal issues from spilling over and becoming personal legal issues for the members and leaders involved.

20.1.1 Private Associations

One mode of organization that is rarely used among breed associations is private ownership. This mode can work very well, although by the very nature of this organizational form it is less participatory than other forms because the owner is the final authority for all decisions and financial responsibilities (Figure 20.1). This can have advantages as long as the owner is dedicated to the advancement and persistence of the breed. This is always the case in the early days of a private association, and the few private breed associations that exist generally have indeed functioned well for the advancement of the breeds involved, especially in their early days.

A significant weakness of private ownership is the difficulty of assuring continuity of services and philosophy when ownership eventually changes as the original owner either ages, unfortunately dies, or simply loses the level of interest that was present when the breed association was started. The transfer of the association from one owner to the next must be carefully considered. Few rules exist to guide this process because it is a private rather than a public transaction. During a transfer it is especially important to assure that the records of the association do not become lost due to inattention. Transitions of registry ownership prove contentious for some registries that are privately held, and it is best for the breed if orderly plans for succession are in place.

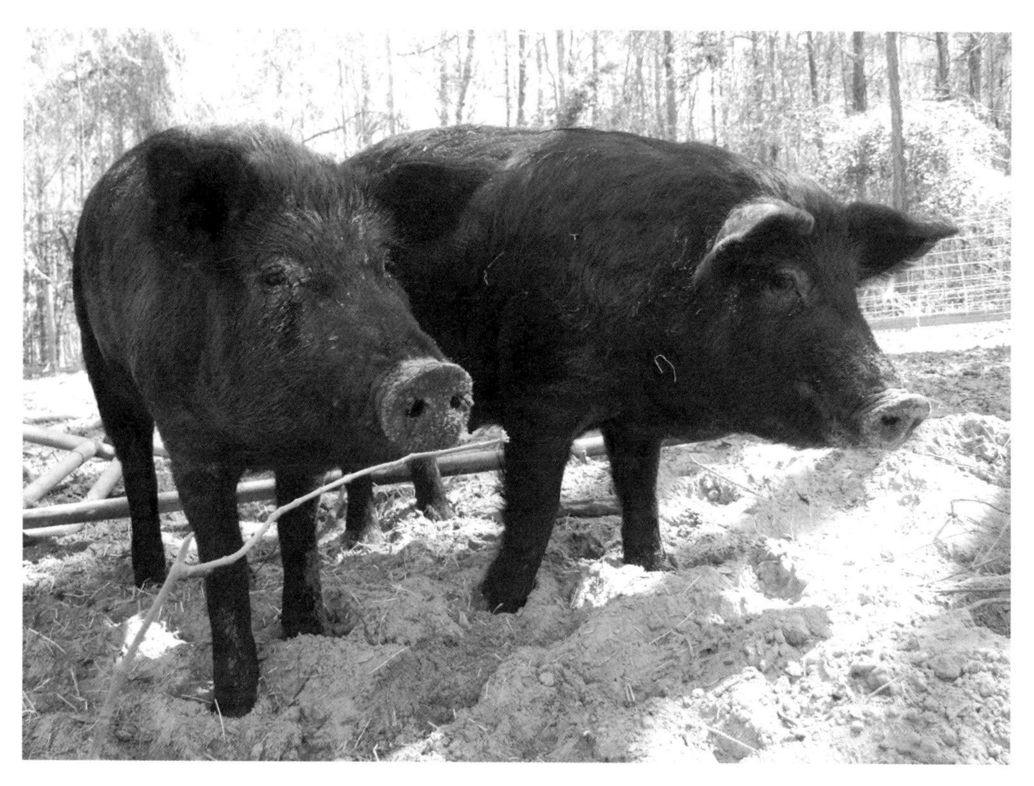

Figure 20.1 Mulefoot hogs have long had a privately held registry. Photo by JB.

A few examples of privately held associations illustrate some of the issues with this form of organization. The American Indian Horse Registry has functioned for several decades as one of the registries for the Colonial Spanish horse. Sole ownership passed decades ago to a new owner through outright purchase, providing for continuity albeit with a subtle shift in emphasis toward more traditional bloodlines within the breed. This is a boon to conservation. Another registry for Colonial Spanish horses is the Horse of the Americas. It was also passed to new owners through purchase, and a participatory form of governance is in place through the use of directors, each representing one of the strains of this important landrace. Directors have a high personal stake in the breed and its future, and are engaged and active in breed activities.

The organizational model of privately held associations does not inherently require the association to be responsive to the breeders and others they serve. Sometimes this has served breeds poorly because breeder concerns have not been addressed and difficult issues are not effectively managed. This can be especially true when income is registration-based because the incentive of the owner is then to relax registry rules to allow the overeager recruitment of breeding animals. This is a common risk in dog and pig breeds, where litters are born but not every member of a litter should go on to a breeding career.

Changes in owner attitude with time or with age also threaten breeds managed by privately held associations. There are multiple examples of owners becoming elderly, with a decreasing ability or interest in serving the breeders of the breed. Owners can also become resistant to sharing registration or pedigree information, resulting in a loss of information which is essential to breed survival. Strategies for avoiding this are ideally in place before they are needed. Succession for privately held breed associations has proven to be problematic for many breeds.

20.1.2 Unincorporated Associations

Sometimes a group of breeders begins as a loose network. This level of casual association can be very effective in breed conservation, especially in the early days of organizing a breed and its breeders. Spanish goat breeders have very successfully discovered many old lines of these traditional goats, despite only recently moving from a loose network to a more defined organization (Figure 20.2). In the interests of long-term breed survival, it is usually best for these networks to eventually adopt a formal structure in order to assure continued success. Following the general guidelines for an incorporated association is a good plan from the earliest days of group activity because this makes future change less challenging.

The advantage of an unincorporated association is the freedom from reporting duties, legal responsibilities, and formal rules. The disadvantage is that a lack of these can result in a level of organization that is not high enough to effectively monitor the breed and its fortunes.

Landraces are especially likely to lack formal associations, and this can place them in peril of loss by the attrition of elderly owners and breeders. Gulf Coast sheep breeders have historically gone down two different paths of organization (Figure 20.3). One involves the formal Gulf Coast Sheep Breeders Association, which functions like most other breed associations with registries and bylaws. This group has long had a formal registry. The second organizational model is a looser organization, undertaken by the Coastal South Native

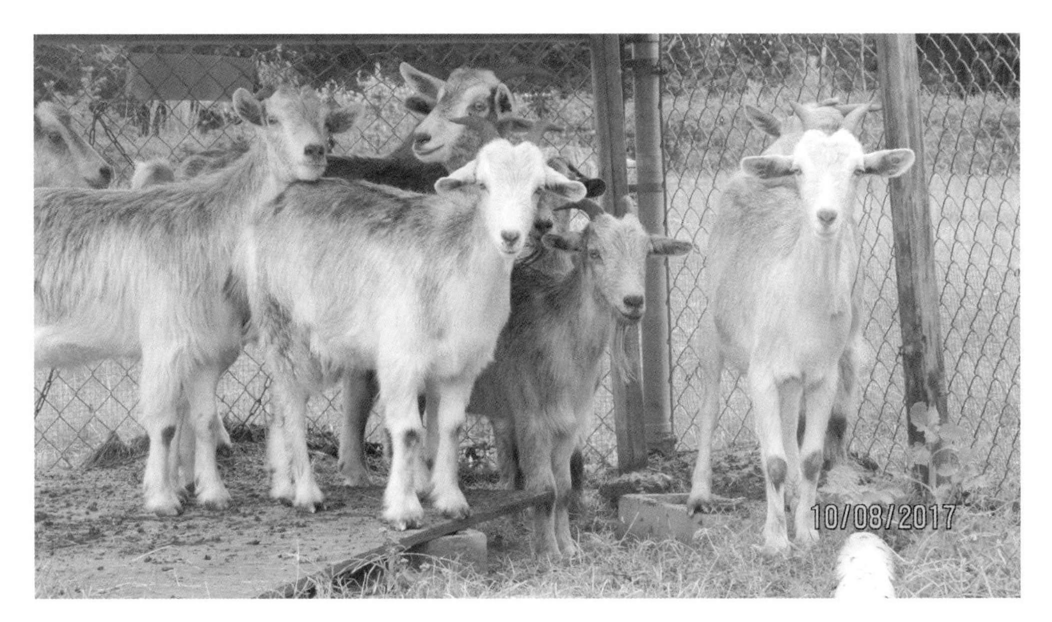

Figure 20.2 The organization of Spanish goat breeders began as a very informal network that was highly successful in finding old foundation herds of pure stock. Photo by Courtney Norman.

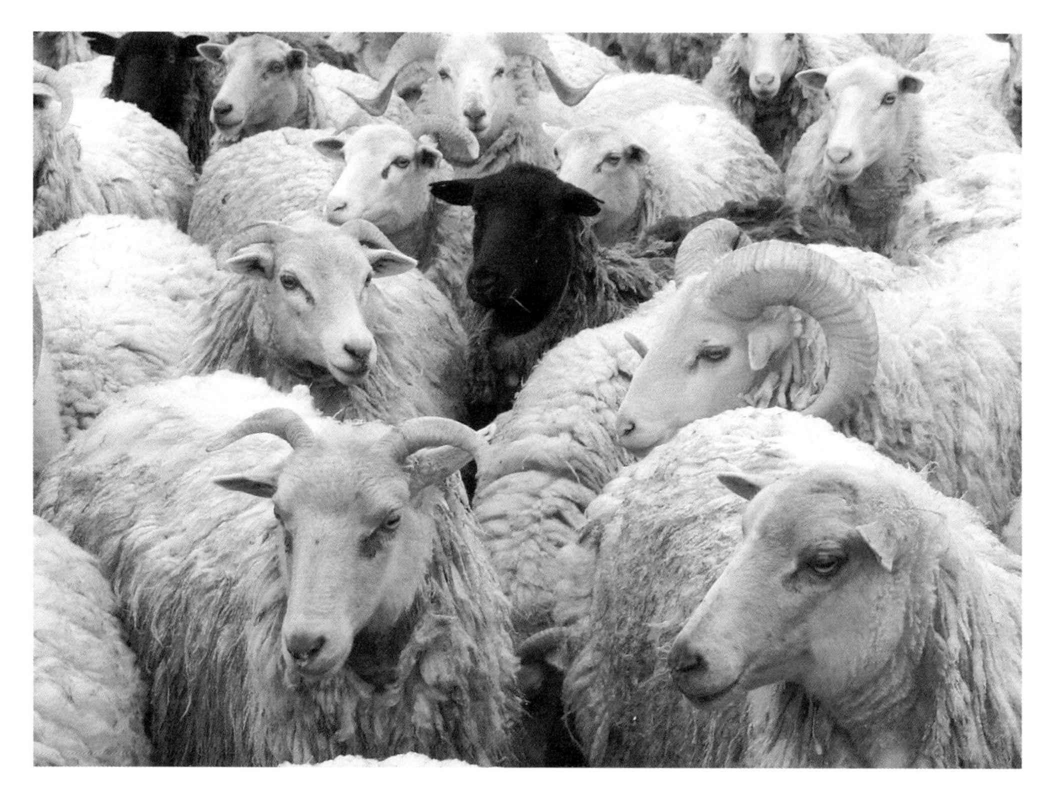

Figure 20.3 Gulf Coast sheep breeders have organized in different ways to serve the breed. Photo by JB.

Sheep Flock Alliance. This group recognizes certain flocks of traditional sheep, encourages their pure breeding, and manages exchanges between flocks. Each of these two types of organizational structure serves the breed and the breeders in different and constructive ways. Fortunately, the Gulf Coast Sheep Breeders Association has begun to explore creative ways to expand beyond the usual framework of a restrictive registry to document and better serve traditional flocks raised in extensive systems by long-term owners. If this succeeds it will serve as a useful example of effective landrace conservation that encompasses traditional systems as well as serving newcomers from outside that original community.

20.1.3 *Incorporated Associations*

Members of most breed associations eventually organize themselves as corporations that are managed democratically and are controlled by member votes. This organizational style clearly clarifies the tax status and legal obligations of an association. It also formally addresses the issues of personal versus corporate liability for the board and officers. Corporations in the USA are chartered at the state level, and as a result the specific laws vary as to requirements and costs. It is nearly always necessary to have local legal assistance when incorporating a breed association.

Breed associations can choose between non-profit or for-profit status for their corporation. The distinctions have tax and legal ramifications. The non-profit status does have some advantages, but also has complicated reporting requirements that may make this choice a poor one for many smaller associations. One advantage of non-profit status is the ability to obtain grants from various sources, as well as the ability to receive tax-deductible contributions. The for-profit associations circumvent some of the reporting procedures but have disadvantages such as ineligibility for certain sources of funding such as the grants and tax-deductible contributions available to the non-profit associations. It is rare for associations to be making enough money to truly be considered profitable, especially for rare breeds, so non-profit status usually makes good sense for most of them if the requirements for reporting can be met.

20.2 Bylaws

Bylaws dictate the organizational structure of the association, and must be tailored to meet legal requirements for associations, especially if the association is incorporated. These requirements vary from state to state and complying with them must be done on a case-by-case basis. Bylaws of associations must be carefully developed because they govern the legal aspects of the association and dictate the management of the association in terms of leadership, selection of leadership, terms of office, and financial responsibilities, as well as the management of any association business such as shows, registrations, meetings, or other activities. Bylaws are generally accepted by vote of the membership and contain procedures for their amendment.

Bylaws need to be stringent enough to provide for continuity and consistency within the association, but also flexible enough to allow changes when necessary. Procedures for changes need to be practical and not overly cumbersome. Members should have easy access to the bylaws so that the association is sure to always operate within their guidelines. Guidelines on developing and revising bylaws are readily available in various books, and example bylaws are provided in Appendix 4. Discussion with other breed associations can often provide useful guidance as bylaws are developed.

Procedures for amending bylaws are extremely important and need to be explained and codified in the bylaws themselves. As associations change over the years, and especially as membership either grows or shrinks dramatically, it usually becomes necessary to amend bylaws to assure that association functions can continue in an efficient manner. For changes to be legitimate, the process by which they are made needs to be clearly explained and accurately followed. In most associations, changes can be put forward by either the membership or the board, and then usually must be approved by a vote of the entire membership. This can be done either at an annual meeting or by ballot from the entire membership. Annual meetings have the disadvantage that only a portion of the membership is likely to attend. Busy people (especially people with young families or active businesses) are the least likely to be able to attend, and are among the most important people to engage in association work. Ballots from the entire membership are more inclusive and offer fewer opportunities for accusations of a deal done behind closed doors. In the case of a non-profit association, changes in bylaws need to be recorded with the state granting the non-profit status.

Bylaws can be quite detailed or can more broadly lay out the procedures of the association. Fine details, including specific amounts for fees and dues, are best left out of the bylaws because any changes to these will need to be accomplished through the cumbersome procedures required for formal changes. Including too many details in the bylaws can make management difficult over long spans of time.

20.3 Board of Directors

Incorporated associations are required to have a board of directors. Commonly the board of directors is elected from the membership. Voting for the board of directors is frequently restricted to breeder members, and usually excludes associate members who are either youths, non-breeders (for most species), or non-owners. Some horse breeds allow non-breeder owners to vote because they constitute a significant portion of membership and have a direct interest in decisions that affect showing and competition. A few common variations include a division of the board into regions or districts so that relatively uniform representation is assured to all members across the nation. Each district or region usually has a designated number of positions on the board and is able to fill those by direct election.

The directors are usually elected from the membership at a time interval that is established in the bylaws. A common strategy is to have an odd number of directors to avoid tie votes, and for the directors to serve terms of multiple years. Three-year terms are routine across many associations. In most associations these terms are staggered so that roughly one third of the board members are elected in any given year. For new boards this would mean one third of the directors serve a one-year term, one third a two-year term, and one third a three-year term. Each director that is elected in succeeding years serves a three-year term. The result of staggered three-year terms is the continuity of leadership for the association that is greater than would be the case if all director terms started and ended at the same time. In addition, the recurring inclusion of new board members also assures that new ideas and approaches are made available to the board. Term limits are typical in most associations, and the most common is a limit of two consecutive terms. This assures not only continuity but also periodic infusions of new leadership.

Changing board membership brings new dynamics that serve to avoid stagnation. A potential downside to these periodic changes, especially with small boards, is that a large and sudden shift in leadership can be disruptive to the continuity of services and association culture. In some situations, board takeovers have been instigated and successfully accomplished by replacing several board members simultaneously through the normal election cycle. This is indeed democratic and can bring desired and much-needed change in some situations. However, the change can be so rapid and acrimonious that the association suffers loss of members and breeders, as well as some loss of loyalty from those who remain. Any sudden change in direction or philosophy needs to be carefully considered and also carefully accomplished in order to avoid doing more damage than good.

Boards of directors vary in their activities and responsibilities. Some of this variation is due to differences in bylaws, while other variation is simply due to differences in association culture. For most associations, the directors provide leadership and are especially crucial in developing and maintaining policy. In larger associations it is generally the board of directors that establishes policy and oversees the executive director, who is basically their employee. The executive director is responsible for establishing, maintaining, and changing procedures, which essentially implement the policy decisions that are made by the board. The executive director also oversees the rest of the paid staff.

Meetings of the board of directors always have legal requirements for a record of the proceedings in the form of minutes. Board procedures must be spelled out so that orderly meetings are possible, usually following *Robert's Rules of Order* which are readily available in book form. Fortunately, these rules are the norm for many livestock organizations, and most people have at least some familiarity with them.

20.3.1 Directors and Officers

Members of the board of directors are ultimately responsible for the fate of the association, and in most states that also includes the fiscal fate of the association. Beyond their legal responsibilities, members of the board usually have important informal responsibilities by setting the tone for the entire breed association. The association benefits when board business is accomplished in a businesslike and open manner. The association is diminished when board members are self-serving and manipulate the association through secret deals. Setting the tone of the overall association and its activities is a crucial responsibility for board members.

The board of directors is responsible for a great deal of what works well in an association. This includes factors beyond the more formal responsibilities and activities that it has by virtue of the bylaws. The board must set an example to the general membership by eager participation in the association and its activities. Some boards function strictly as a governance body whereas others are involved in the day-to-day functions of the organization. The former is more typical of a mature organization, while the latter typifies many small or young organizations. Ideally members of the board volunteer for a variety of responsibilities, such as planning and preparing for meetings, sharing their knowledge and experience with members through newsletters and other communications, and contributing key abilities to the association such as specialized training (legal, veterinary, fiscal, writing, design).

Directors and officers set the tone for the entire breed association, and a few general recommendations are wise to assure that this works for the positive benefit of the breed. Contentious issues will emerge from time to time, and how the directors handle these is important. Suggestions to aid resolution include the following.

- Table a decision for a future meeting if there has been contention, conflict, or any intimidation.
- Consult with outside experts to get outside perspectives.
- Review the mission statement and the bylaws to check for congruence with previously stated goals and to see if a similar situation has been addressed earlier.
- Think long term rather than short term about the future of the breed.

20.4 Networks of Breed Associations

A few organizations are available that provide resources that help to consolidate and inform the individual associations. One of these is The Livestock Conservancy, which is especially helpful in organizing and providing information for rare breeds and the associations

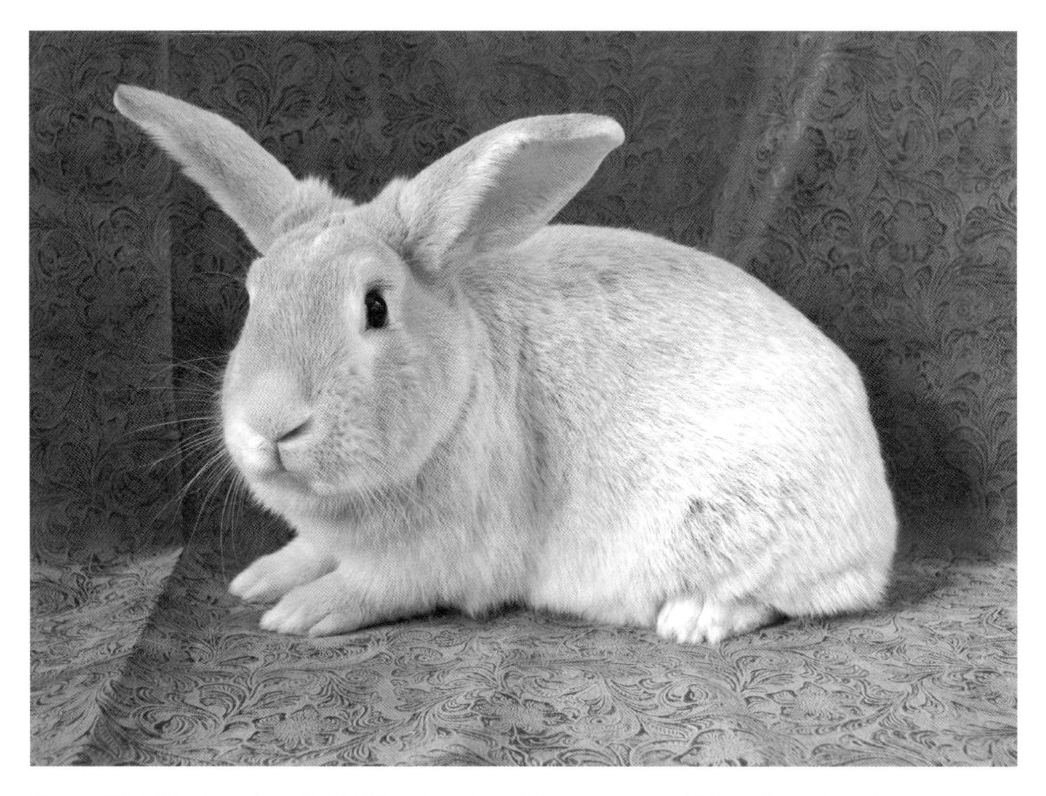

Figure 20.4 The American Rabbit Breeders Association serves rabbit breeds, such as the Crème d'Argent. Photo by JB.

serving them. Other consortia of herd book associations exist, such as the National Pedigreed Livestock Association. Most of these umbrella entities, other than The Livestock Conservancy, target larger breed associations. These larger consortia frequently engage in political lobbying and other large-scale functions.

A few associations work across an entire species with a full range of association functions including animal registration. These include groups such as the American Rabbit Breeders Association (ARBA) (Figure 20.4), the American Kennel Club (AKC), the United Kennel Club (UKC), the American Dairy Goat Association (ADGA), and the American Goat Society (AGS). The breeds served by these associations benefit from sharing expenses for registry functions as well as for organizing shows. This is a boon to the numerically smaller breeds, as they are able to maintain timely support for registry functions and to participate in shows without bearing the responsibility of organizing them single-handedly. A possible negative, however, is that underlying philosophies for breeding and breed maintenance can easily become shared broadly across breeds rather than being tailored to each individual breed. The result is that some blurring of breed distinctions has occurred over years of selection under a single guiding philosophy.

A few organizations, such as the American Poultry Association (APA) and the Society for the Preservation of Poultry Antiquities (SPPA), function in nearly the same manner as the multi-breed organizations. These two serve multiple species and their various breeds but lack the registry function that is associated with the umbrella organizations that serve the mammalian species. The breeders of many of the more populous poultry, rabbit, and dog breeds have stand-alone breed clubs to help organize various programs, but still depend greatly on the umbrella organizations for organizing and disseminating information and activities of interest to the breeders. This accomplishes breed-specific issues efficiently because many of the more mechanical details are still managed by the umbrella organizations.

Other cross-species organizations have somewhat different goals and purposes. Cattle breeders are served by the Dairy and Beef Councils, as well as state and regional cattlemen's associations. These organizations are much more involved with the economic dynamics of these industries than they are the issues of purebred breeding and breed maintenance. The same is true of the National Pork Producers Council (NPPC), the American Sheep Industry (ASI), and the National Turkey Federation (NTF).

20.5 Promoting the Association

Promotion is very important if the association is to secure its rightful place as the hub of breed activity. Active promotion is best if built upon a base of association integrity and competence, but these two in the absence of active promotion are insufficient to ensure the success of an association.

The reputation of the association is based on many different aspects that reflect the complexity of an association's work and responsibility. One aspect of an association that is critical to its reputation is commitment to the breed and bylaws. Only a sincere and clear-headed dedication to the breed and its management can enable an association to convey the message of the breed to the public. Bylaws must serve this mission, and the association must adhere to them in an honest effort to secure the status and future of the breed.

The reputation of the association is also earned by its service to members. This is not always an easy job description. Associations must serve as central sources of information and services and must be available to offer these to members. Large associations that have centrally paid staff accomplish this relatively easily. It is much more difficult for smaller associations that are staffed by volunteers, because these volunteers will be the recipients of many requests for information and services on behalf of the members as well as the public. While some members can be unrealistic in their demands on even the largest and most well-staffed association, it remains true that reasonable requests must be acknowledged and met efficiently and pleasantly if the association is to attract and retain members. The cost in time, effort, and financial resources is significant, especially for small associations. All of these need to be understood and considered by volunteers and by the board as it develops budgets.

20.6 Association Responsibilities

Associations have various responsibilities to breeders as well as to the breed. These are usually congruent, but occasionally it is possible for the breeders' interests to be at variance with those of the breed. It takes dedication and neutrality for the association to assure

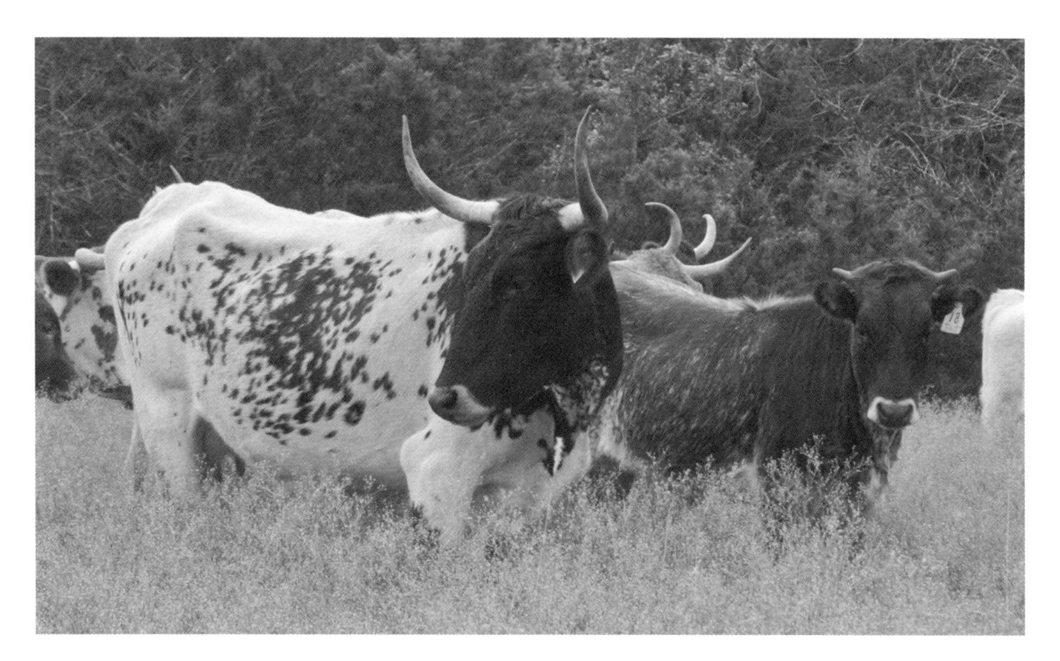

Figure 20.5 The Cattlemen's Texas Longhorn Registry has managed to preserve the original type of the breed despite pressures to yield to fads for certain colors or extreme horn length.
Photo by DPS.

that the needs of the breed are met while not damaging the situation for the breeders. Difficulties arise when short-term commercial interests conflict with the long-term survival and integrity of the breed. Examples are changing fads in type or purpose of the breed, where a new or off-type may be in temporary high demand (Figure 20.5). These can result in significant economic benefit to some breeders but can also irrevocably change the breed type.

20.6.1 Conservation Responsibilities

One obvious responsibility of breed associations is to provide education about purebred breeding and breed characteristics to current and potential breeders. This needs to be a very active role of the association. To neglect this is to assure that less organized or less informed sources will flow into the vacuum left by association inactivity. Without a well-thought and articulated stance on conservation and purebred breeding, the association and the breed are both likely to drift from fad to fad.

Attention to the conservation needs of the breed also helps to set the culture of the breeders to attend to the long-term needs of the breed. This is a subtle but important role for associations. The association should be the leader in assuring effective conservation management of the breed according to sound genetic and organizational principles.

20.6.2 Reporting Pedigree Information

Associations generally maintain complete pedigree records for their breed. This is important information to breeders as well as to others interested in the breed. Pedigree information

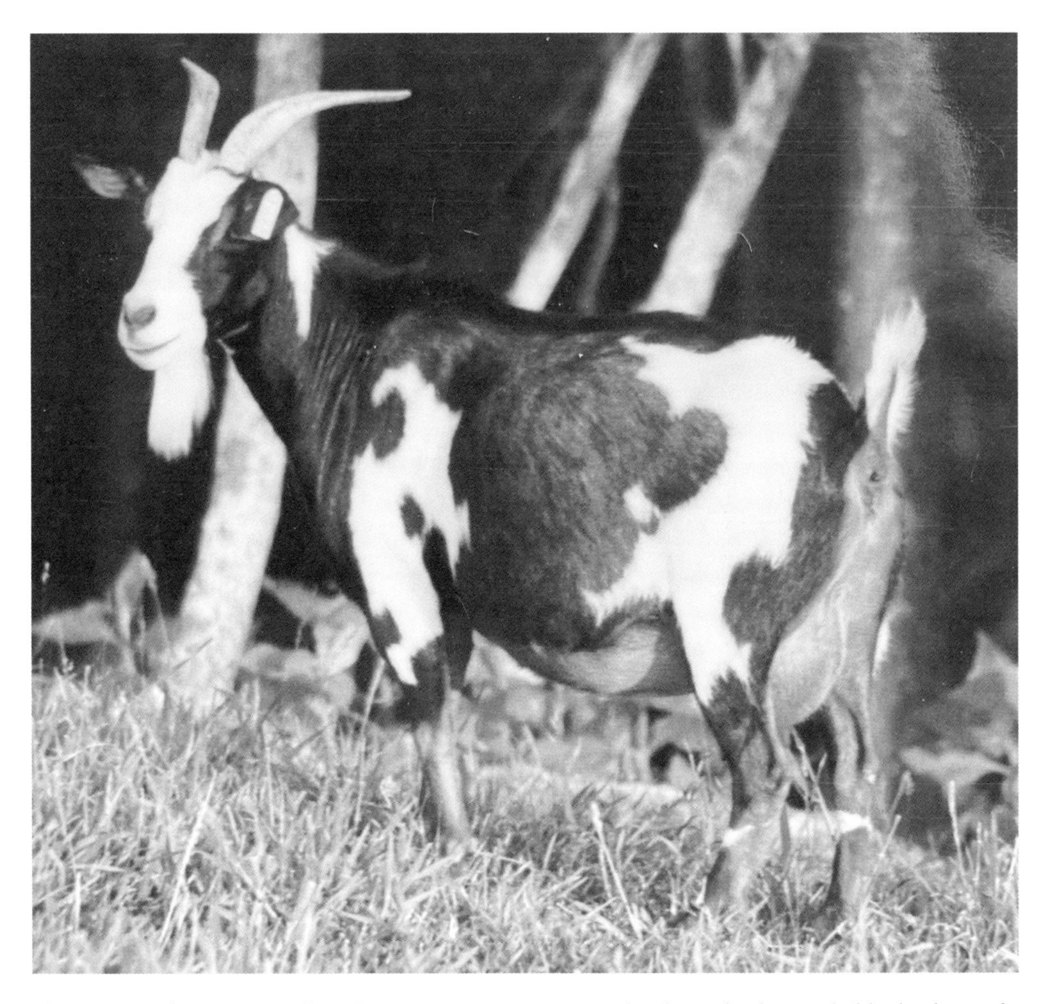

Figure 20.6 The Myotonic Goat Registry is one association that has a freely searchable database of pedigrees for all registered goats. Photo by DPS.

is valuable, and it is worthwhile for each association to actively decide to whom pedigree information should be made available and under what conditions. Some breeders may feel that pedigree information on animals in their ownership should be privileged. Others will have no disagreement with free, open, and total sharing of such information with any and all who request it. Breed associations need to decide which of these approaches to follow.

It is generally in the breed's best interest for pedigree information to be widely shared and available. This sets the tone for open and complete communication within the association and can be very helpful in establishing a constructive and mutually supportive culture within the breeder community. Several breed associations have websites with searchable pedigree databases (Figure 20.6). These serve well to allow breeders and buyers to locate stock of most interest to them in an easy and affordable manner. In some associations, a nominal fee is charged for pedigree information, but an increasing number of associations find that the benefits of freely sharing this information vastly outweigh any disadvantages.

20.6.3 Reporting Breed Health Status

Associations should be aware of the general health issues confronting the breed and should communicate these to breeders and members. An important aspect of genetic health is the occurrence and incidence of genetic defects within the breed. Reporting of specific genetic diseases can become politically heated. It is best if the information is stripped of any identity linking it to specific breeders or animals. Anonymity comes closer to assuring full disclosure than any other strategy does. This suggestion is targeted for the association, but it is also true that individual breeders should be encouraged to fully share the details on animals they have produced to anyone interested in them. The final call rests with the individual breeder.

Although anonymity of health reporting does have the drawback of limiting the actions that interested people can take to select against specific defects, it does assure that breeders are not carelessly nor needlessly smeared. It is highly likely that misinformation will occasionally be conveyed, so procedures should be in place to minimize the damage that can occur. When an anonymous reporting scheme is actively pursued it generally develops that owners and breeders step up to the challenge of disclosing information more publicly. This is especially true of defects for which testing is available. The list of genetic defects is constantly increasing in number. In a situation where animals can be DNA tested either as carriers or as free of the variant, it is becoming increasingly common for that information to be made public by breeders so that customers can make informed choices.

Any health or genetic information disclosure should come with education about how to use the information. For example, in many rare breeds the draconian measure of culling all animals that carry certain recessive traits or structural defects is likely to assure the constriction of the gene pool and the eventual demise of the breed. In this case the breeders need to be educated as to the wise and necessary use of carriers, and how to do this with minimal risk of expressing the undesired traits or defects.

20.6.4 Reporting Measures of Genetic Diversity

The genetic status of a breed is one dimension of its overall genetic health. Association actions in this regard should include periodic reports on the status of bloodlines within the breed, overall population levels, popularity trends within the breed, and other trends that are important to maintaining the breed as a viable population. Incidence of specific genetic variants (rare variants such as polledness or dwarfism in some breeds, and color or gaitedness in some horse breeds) should also be evaluated and communicated to the breeders on a periodic basis. Reporting these characteristics assures that breeders are alert to variants that could otherwise slip to extinction.

20.6.5 Programs to Save Herds in Peril

The development of action plans for rescuing herds that are in peril of being disbanded through commercial channels (this generally means slaughter) are a necessary responsibility of the association. Programs to fend off sudden loss of genetic material need to be articulated in advance of their need, because the need generally occurs after a catastrophe such as a natural disaster or the sudden disability or death of a breeder. In such situations, quick and

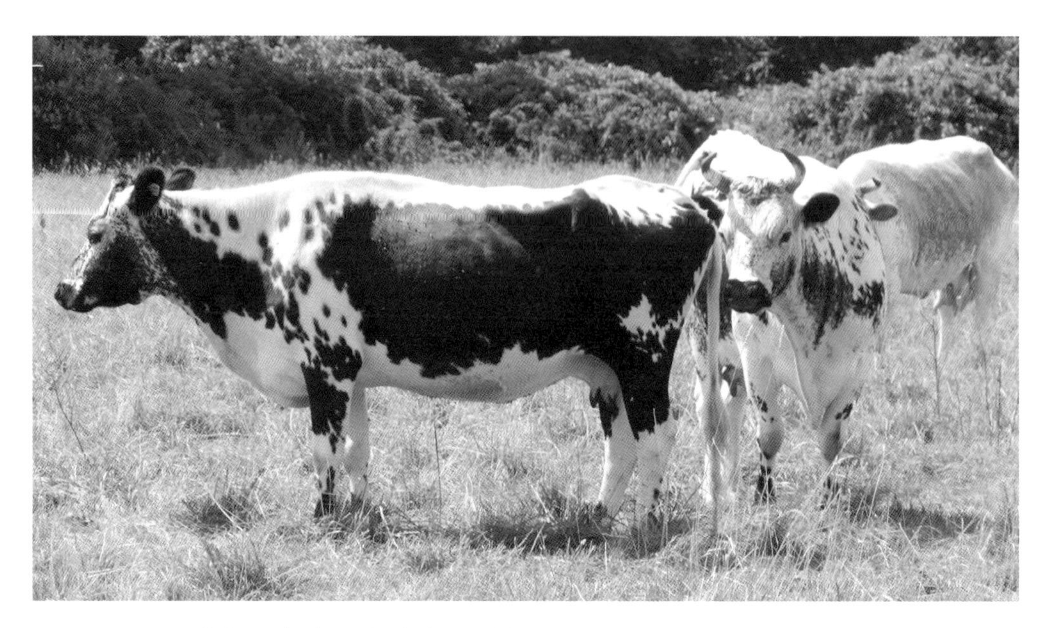

Figure 20.7 Randall Lineback cattle all descend from founders that were rescued from slaughter. Rescues do not have to be this dramatic (and perilous) if breeders and associations plan ahead for finding and placing herds or animals at risk of being lost to the breed. Photo by JB.

informed action is needed without the luxury of time to develop effective strategies on the spur of the moment (Figure 20.7).

Associations can help to build a breed culture of informed awareness concerning dispersals. This should ideally result in each breeder having a plan for the dispersal of his or her herd in case of accident or other disaster. Association plans should very much be only a last resort to use when individual breeder plans fail.

20.6.6 Development of Long-Range Conservation Plans

Associations are critically important stewards for a breed. They should actively develop mechanisms for the long-term maintenance of a breed that involve all factors affecting breed survival. Included are economic parameters such as products, marketing, and helping to sustain a brisk demand for the purebred product. "Certified Angus Beef" is a very good example of a breed association undertaking effective breed product marketing and reaping a huge reward from increased demand for the breed. The marketing of heritage turkeys for Thanksgiving is a similar success story, and one that needs to be repeated for every breed.

Also included are long-range breed maintenance plans that detail the association's actions to maintain the breed as a genetically viable and useful entity. Conservation plans should be based on the accurate assessment of the status of bloodlines within the breed. Plans can be formulated for assuring that different bloodlines survive throughout the breed. Plans to cryopreserve appropriate genetic materials for long-term storage should be implemented and should involve targeted sampling to assure the broadest possible representation of the breed. Special attention should be paid to the inclusion of an adequate sample of all distinct bloodlines within the breed. This can be accomplished by individual breeders, but will be more effective if coordinated by the breed association. Participation in the National Animal Germplasm Program (NAGP) can provide technical support and other resources for this endeavor. The Livestock Conservancy is a partner in this program and can help coordinate breeder activities with it.

20.6.7 Dispelling False Rumors Quickly

Associations, by their very nature, are groups of people. Groups of people always involve politics, as well as other social dynamics. Rumors tend to be part of the whole package of a breed association, but ideally the board and other leaders within the breed can dispel false rumors quickly and effectively. More effective yet is for associations to build an open, accurate, and effective communication style that prevents any need for a rumor mill. It is especially the responsibility of breed leaders, such as the board of directors, major breeders, and the staff, to avoid very deliberately contributing to false rumors and negative behavior. This sets a positive tone for communication among the breeders and is of great benefit to the entire breed and its community of breeders and consumers.

20.7 Conflict of Interest

Certain conflicts of interest are nearly inevitable in a breed association, and it is wise to deal with these before problems develop. One source of conflicted interest occurs when the registrar or secretary is also a breeder. This is a very common state of affairs in small breed associations, where funds are not available to outsource the registry function.

Most breed inquiries are directed through the secretary or registrar, which is why a breeder in such a role can have an inherent conflict of interest. It would be easy to skim off purchase inquiries for oneself, or for close associates, friends, or partners. To prevent even the appearance of this, it is wise for a specific packet of information, including members' and breeders' names and addresses, to be forwarded to all inquiries. This strategy allows the inquirer to then take the next step of contacting breeders in a specific area or breeders with specific animals of interest. In the interest of fairness to all, it is always wisest to forward complete information to any inquiry. Some larger associations limit the information they send out to only include that from the same region as the inquiry. It is always safest to forward reasonably complete information so that any impression of favoritism is prevented. The recent tendency for much information to be web-based diminishes the control-point of the registrar or secretary, which usually serves everyone well.

Another source of conflict can occur with boards of directors or other officers that are responsible for making breed and registry rules. Such rules can degenerate into protecting self-interest unless association members are careful to establish an association culture in which breed interest supersedes all other interests. Specific examples of shortsighted rule-making include changing the exclusion of cryptorchidism as a disqualifying defect in the stallions of some breeds. The self-interest of breeders with such stallions could easily overrule long-term breed welfare.

A similar conflict of interest in some landrace populations has resulted in early and complete closure of herd books, thereby eliminating many purebred animals from the registered breed. On the other hand, at least one landrace herd book included a few known crossbred animals because prominent individuals had already heavily invested in those animals before their crossbred character had been realized. These are both examples of short-term self-interest overriding the breed's long-term welfare. All breed associations should be diligent to create an association environment that engenders a high regard for the long-term integrity of the breed and the association itself.

20.8 Local and Regional Groups

Some breed associations have regional or local subdivisions, especially if the association is large. These regional and local groups may have formal status but most often are groups that arise to allow for greater local communication and activities, such as shows and meetings, field days, and other get togethers. Developing a formal status for these groups can assure that all breeders are speaking and acting in accordance with the philosophy and general procedures of the association (Figure 20.8).

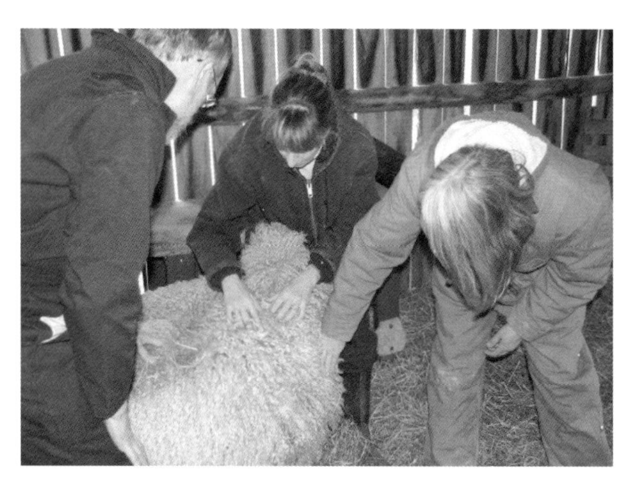

Figure 20.8 Local groups of breeders can host educational field days and other outreach efforts to advance their breed, promote its products, and build strong communities of breeders. Photo by Gail Groot.

CHAPTER 21

Registry

The functions of a breed registry are subtly different to those of a breed association, although most breed associations usually take on registry functions as one of their activities. Registry functions include many things that help the genetic management of a breed such as documenting, managing, and monitoring the mating and genetic contribution of individual animals, as well as the dynamics of the breed as a whole. These functions are especially important for rare breeds.

21.1 Registration

The most basic function of a registry is to validate animals as being of a specific breed. This is usually based on recorded pedigrees. Registration function is essential if a breed is to persist into the future, as it assures breeders, regardless of where they are, that animals with the validation of registration are truly members of the breed. That knowledge allows breeders to confidently include such animals in purebred breeding programs.

Validation of animals as representatives of a specific breed is usually done by the registration of individual animals rather than groups of them. Registration links an individual animal by some sort of unique identification (description, tattoo, ear tag, microchip, brand, or photograph) to a registration certificate. Individual validation is the most common approach for large animals of relatively high individual monetary value such as horses, cattle, donkeys, llamas, and alpacas. This strategy is also used for dogs.

At the other extreme, a different strategy has been used for poultry breeds. In general, poultry have no form of identity validation aside from external phenotype (Figure 21.1). Traditional breeds of poultry are gaining market acceptance as a premium product, and a move toward flock validation is gaining momentum. Such validations have been accomplished in the past by breed clubs and by the APA, whose programs are seeing a resurgence in interest. The goal is to validate populations of purebred poultry as members of their breed in order to aid breeders in marketing efforts. This serves some of the same functions as individual registration in the larger mammalian species, while at the same time avoiding

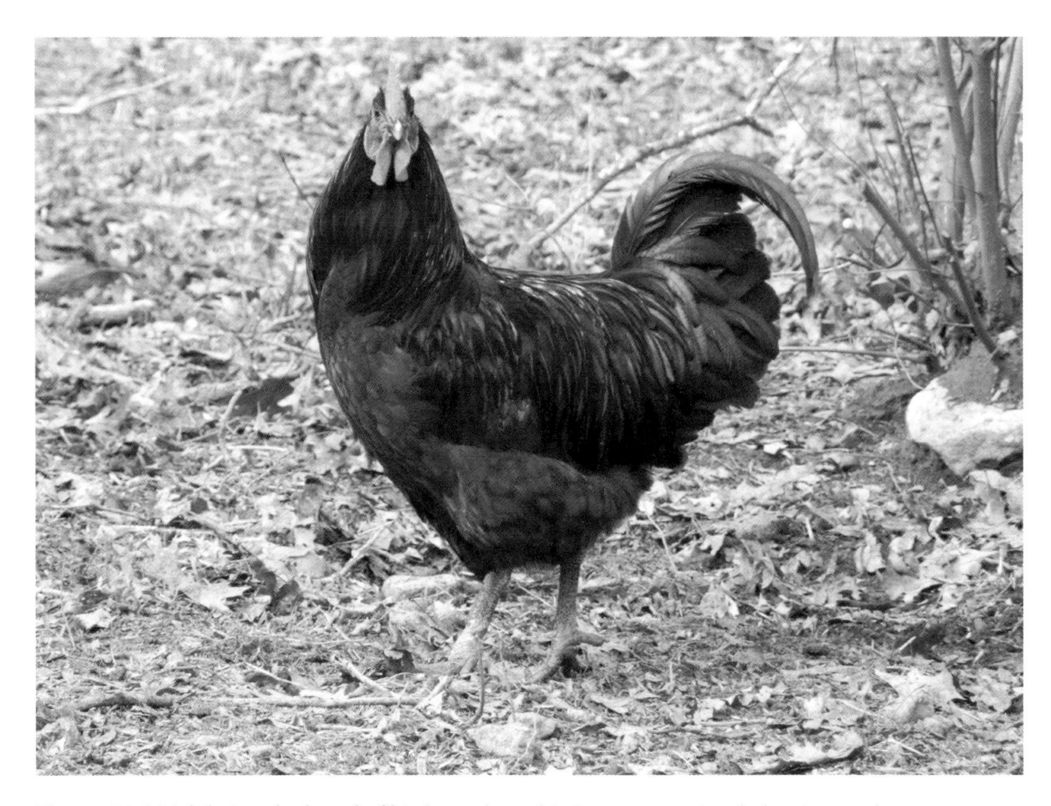

Figure 21.1 Validating the breed of birds, such as this Java rooster, is a balancing act between expense and effort on the one hand, and the economic value of the validation on the other hand. Photo by JB.

the individual identification of birds that is costly and cumbersome relative to the economic value of individual birds.

In between the extremes of poultry and large stock lie swine, sheep, and goats. Nearly all breeds of these species do have individual registration and validation. Most swine breeds require litter registration, followed by the individual registration of select older or adult animals intended for breeding. For some breeds of sheep and goats, especially the adapted landraces, the approach based on individual animals may need to be reconsidered. Herd-based approaches may be more practical for many breeders, especially the traditional breeders so important to the maintenance of these breeds in their original settings. The challenge with a herd-based system is knowing how to develop an evaluation process that will assure breed integrity by only including purebred animals, while also avoiding the labor, effort, and expense that individual registration entails.

21.2 Pedigrees

Pedigrees are records of animal ancestry. Recording pedigrees is a function of most breed registries. The recording of pedigrees accomplishes distinct goals. Pedigrees validate an individual animal's ancestry within the breed. The validation of pedigree adds to the

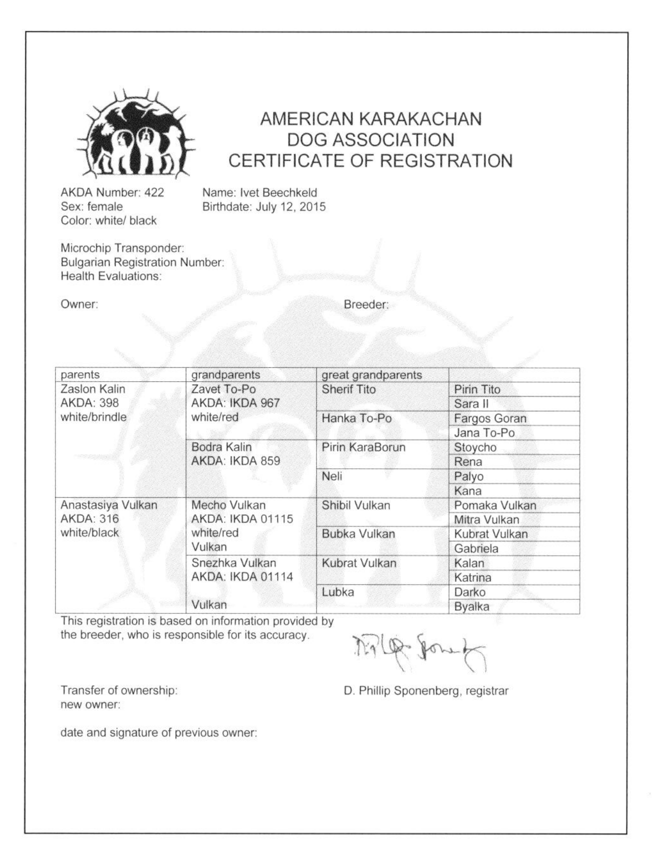

AMERICAN KARAKACHAN
DOG ASSOCIATION
CERTIFICATE OF REGISTRATION

AKDA Number: 422 Name: Ivet Beechkeld
Sex: female Birthdate: July 12, 2015
Color: white/ black

Microchip Transponder:
Bulgarian Registration Number:
Health Evaluations:

Owner: Breeder:

parents	grandparents	great grandparents	
Zaslon Kalin	Zavet To-Po	Sherif Tito	Pirin Tito
AKDA: 398	AKDA: IKDA 967		Sara II
white/brindle	white/red	Hanka To-Po	Fargos Goran
			Jana To-Po
	Bodra Kalin	Pirin KaraBorun	Stoycho
	AKDA: IKDA 859		Rena
		Neli	Palyo
			Kana
Anastasiya Vulkan	Mecho Vulkan	Shibil Vulkan	Pomaka Vulkan
AKDA: 316	AKDA: IKDA 01115		Mitra Vulkan
white/black	white/red	Bubka Vulkan	Kubrat Vulkan
	Vulkan		Gabriela
	Snezhka Vulkan	Kubrat Vulkan	Kalan
	AKDA: IKDA 01114		Katrina
		Lubka	Darko
	Vulkan		Byalka

This registration is based on information provided by the breeder, who is responsible for its accuracy.

Transfer of ownership: D. Phillip Sponenberg, registrar
new owner:

date and signature of previous owner:

Figure 21.2 Registration certificates usually indicate the pedigree of the animal, along with any details of identification. This links the certificate to a specific individual animal. Figure by DPS.

individual identity of an animal and can help to guide breeding choices. Pedigree information for some breeds goes beyond ancestor identification and includes detailed information about ancestors such as color, size, production characteristics, show ring wins, or other performance. Pedigree information is useful in making breeding decisions, and is especially useful to buyers selecting animals to complement their own existing bloodlines. While not all breeders in all breeds track pedigrees, for rare breeds the pedigree can become an essential part of managing the population for long-term survival. Pedigrees should be available for animals of all rare breeds.

It is important to separate the concept of registration from that of pedigree records as each serves a distinct role.

Registration specifically validates individual animals as being of a designated breed, while pedigree records specifically validate ancestry. Most registration certificates include an individual number that serves to track a specific animal and identify it and its pedigree, and most also include a printed pedigree, with the result that many people equate registrations with pedigrees even though they are two different things (Figure 21.2). The registration is critical to the survival of pure breeds of livestock, while the pedigree is valuable for the genetic management of the breed.

Registration without pedigree information is appropriate for some breeds. This is especially true of landraces that experience multi-sire mating. Detailed pedigree information for individual animals tends to be less and less available as animal size and individual value diminish. Individual pedigrees (and indeed registrations) are rare for poultry who are at the small end of the size range, but are routine for cattle and horses at the larger end. Sheep and goats vary from breed to breed as to their requirements for registration and pedigree records, although the general trend is for pedigrees to be complete for these species.

Within all classes of livestock, including poultry, individual breeders of elite stock do indeed document and rely on pedigree information. For poultry breeders the validation of pedigrees usually never goes beyond the individual breeder, while for most other species registry involvement takes this activity to a higher level. For these non-poultry species the independent validation of pedigree information is helpful as animals move from breeder to breeder or owner to owner. Registration serves to make the information more publicly available and also certifies the accuracy of the information by a neutral party (registrar) rather than one with a direct interest in the animal (breeder).

The validity of pedigrees varies immensely from breed to breed and species to species. Pedigree accuracy can very much become a sort of holy grail to breeders, but its usefulness must be put into a practical context, or the pursuit of accuracy can easily overwhelm scant resources. For species with high individual value (horses, cattle, alpacas) it is not too unusual for each animal presented for registration to be DNA typed. This provides for parentage verification, which validates the pedigree stated on the registration application. The cost of such verification is a relatively small fraction of the value of the animal, and it makes sense in such situations to pursue this avenue of accuracy. For breeds raised in more extensive settings (range cattle, range horses) the practicality of this strategy begins to diminish because obtaining the required blood, tissues, or hair can be expensive and logistically challenging due to the fact that animals need to be gathered, restrained, identified, and sampled (Figure 21.3). In many situations the validation only minimally enhances the value of the animal, and is therefore unwarranted as a practical management tool.

Species with relatively low individual commercial value, such as sheep, goats, and poultry, are almost never validated by checking the DNA of offspring and parents. The registries of these species rely on the honesty of the breeder about the parentage of the animals presented for registration. Some mistakes are inevitable and can creep in from intentional fraud or even just from honest mistakes that are a part of everyday life. The significance of the mistakes depends on their extent. A few of the larger registries for these species undertake spot checks in which occasional animals are pedigree-validated by a DNA test of the animal and its parents. This serves as a check to assure that misidentification is rare, while also signaling to the potentially fraudulent breeder that they risk detection.

Pedigrees serve as the raw material for an overall assessment of the genetic diversity within a breed. This can become critically important to the survival of the breed, because when genetic diversity becomes too restricted the overall vitality can begin to fail. Pedigree analysis can quickly document the extent to which this is occurring and can also lead to breeding strategies to help alleviate the problem by targeting the increased use of under-represented lines.

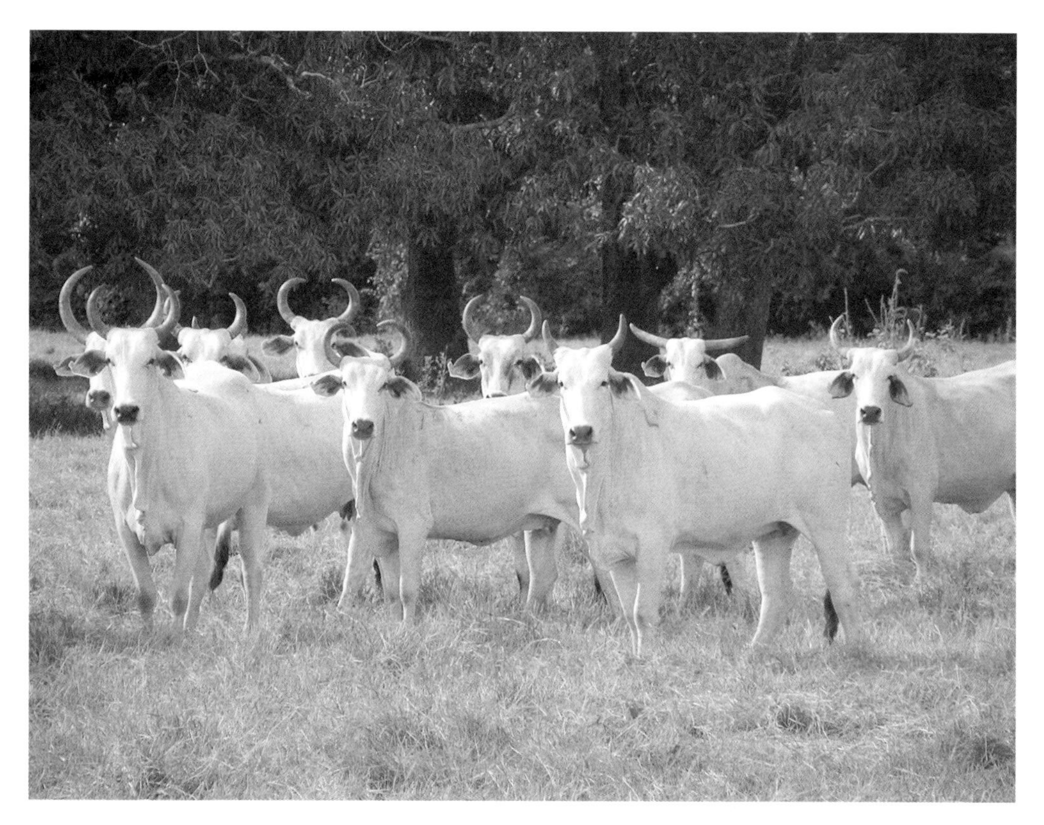

Figure 21.3 Cattle on extensive ranges can be difficult to gather, and in many situations, this precludes sampling for DNA verification of parentage. Photo by DPS.

The generation back to which pedigree information is useful is controversial. Information back to parents is likely to be insufficient for many breeding management decisions. Information on grandparents is truly useful in most decisions, but further back it becomes much less of a practical issue. This is because the contribution of a great grandparent is small enough to be negligible for most purposes. Some breeders make pedigree research a passion, and trace animals back through tens of generations. This is interesting historically, and is truly useful in a few cases, even though it has little biological impact in most situations. The effective management of some breed populations very much depends on pedigrees that are extensive and cover many generations. In those situations, a pedigree that covers many more than two generations is nearly always essential.

21.3 Pedigree Recording Systems

Pedigree information is usually considered to be of utmost concern to breed associations and is one of the main reasons for interest in associations. Pedigrees have become synonymous with purebred livestock, and while their importance to certain breeds is less than others (landraces and poultry, for example), details of pedigrees can be essential in managing the genetic status of a breed.

Older methods to track pedigrees nearly all involved either hand-written or typed lists. These served well for years but have the drawback that their preparation can be very tedious for the registrar. Pedigrees are generally full of numbers (such as registration numbers) and also generally unique names, including farm names and individual animal names. The character of the information is such that transcription errors are likely. Most errors do not result in any major disruption of the breed, but they can greatly limit the ability to accurately probe into the genetic heritage and history of a breed.

New systems of tracking pedigrees include several computerized database systems. These are important tools in population management and are used by nearly all large registries and umbrella organizations that serve several breeds. Systems have been developed by different organizations that are very specific for individual breeds. Other more generic options are also available that will work with a wide variety of breeds. Database systems generally provide for entry of individual animal data such as registration number, sex, date of birth, color, parentage, owner, breeder, and other important details. The program then automatically fills in the pedigree portion of the record from the sire and dam information. This approach reduces the chance of transcription errors because the same data do not require repeated manual entry into the system. The value of the database systems is that they can be used to generate other important information, such as inbreeding coefficients, the offspring of a specific sire or dam, animals under specific ownership, geographic distribution, or numbers of registrations per breeder.

An example of a widely used database program is *Breed Society Record and Ped eView* by Grassroots Systems LTD (sales@grassroots.co.uk). Another very widely used database program is *Breeders Assistant* (http://www.tenset.co.uk/). The International Species Identification System (ISIS) is a non-profit organization that works with, but is not exclusively for, zoological institutions worldwide. ISIS provides software and technical support for animal information databases, studbooks, and population management tools that are used to accomplish the long-term conservation management goals of their members. They developed the program *Single Population Analysis & Records Keeping System* (SPARKS). SPARKS offers the option to manage populations by groups if individual identification of animals is not possible, as is the case with much of the poultry and some landrace breeds kept in the USA.

21.4 Litter Recording

Swine, dog, and rabbit breeders are likely to use litter recording systems because these serve well to track the multiple offspring born to these species (Figure 21.4). Specific protocols for litter registration vary, but generally the breeder of a purebred litter notifies the association of the birth of the litter, with information about the parentage of the litter, as well as the numbers and sexes of the offspring. The litter registration makes the members of the litter eligible for later individual registration, which is frequently completed at a later date for selected animals in the litter. This recording method serves as an important check on the accuracy of registration information for litter-producing species.

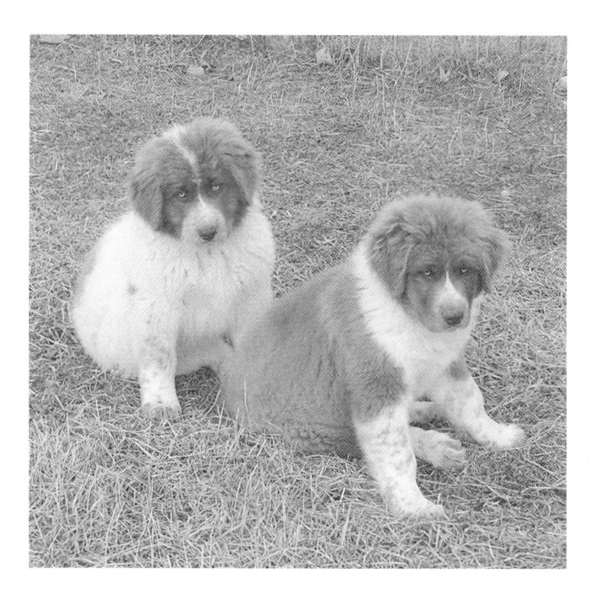

Figure 21.4 Enrolling litters for later individual registration is a strategy used by some dog and swine breeds.
Photo by DPS.

21.5 Stud Reports

Stud reports are used by some breed associations, usually for horse breeds, to track the level of breeding activity that is accomplished within the breed. These are usually annual reports that are filed by breeders after the breeding season. They generally include identification and registration information on the male, and similar information for all females to which he was mated during the year's activity. These reports can then be used to anticipate the production of the following year. It is common for breed associations that use stud reports to restrict subsequent registration only to those animals whose parents have been included. The reports are used to monitor breeding activity, and check the accuracy of the identity information of animals presented for registration.

21.6 Selective Recording Systems

Some breed associations have restrictions on registration, so that decisions regarding which specific animals to register are imposed by the association and not by the individual breeders. Few such associations exist in the USA, but Warmblood horse breeding in most of Europe is characterized by this system. Breeding stock, especially males, must be evaluated by a committee for conformation and performance before being allowed to stand as a registered breeding animal. These tightly controlled systems can enhance and improve a breed, and in some situations are essential to conserving the breed as a traditional genetic resource. Selective registration, however, can succumb to fads or current fashions, resulting in a change within the breed from a traditional to a more modern and uniform type. This is especially the case with Warmblood horse breeding where the blending of bloodlines and the selection to a single ideal has resulted in the homogenization of these once unique breeds.

Clun Forest sheep breeders use a different and useful strategy for the selective registration of lamb crops. In this breed, it is only permissible for breeders to register a percentage of each lamb crop. The specific animals included in the registration are left to a breeder's discretion, but the rule that only a percentage of lambs born can be registered forces each breeder to exercise selection in the lamb crop. This approach does not constrain the specific strategy or philosophy for keep-or-cull decisions but does insist that these decisions must be occurring in every flock. A potential drawback is that this, and all registration systems, ultimately depends on the honesty of the breeder in filling out total lamb production so that the correct number can be registered.

21.7 Registrations Are Important

Although registration figures are not entirely accurate for all breeds, they do provide a good estimate of the purebred breeding within a breed, and do so much more quickly than other measures such as a complete census of live animals. As an example, any breed that is commonly used for crossbreeding (such as Finnsheep or American Brahman cattle) may have a much higher census than would be reflected in the registration figures (Figure 21.5). As a result, any assessment based on total census would significantly overestimate the level of purebred breeding that is occurring.

Registrations allow for the tracking of individuals within a breed. Regardless of how many times a specific animal changes hands, the registration certificate can follow in order to maintain that animal's individual identity within the breed (Figure 21.6). By documenting the identity of any individual animal, it becomes less likely that these animals will be lost to the breed, especially in cases such as death of owner or other disruptive catastrophes.

Registrations help breed associations to monitor the status of breed populations and dynamics of the different lines and strains within the breed. Much of this monitoring is only possible if a reasonably high percentage of the breed is registered. It is nearly impossible to gain an accurate idea of breed populations or trends in the absence of a high registration percentage.

Registrations are the easiest and most expedient way to validate animals as being purebred examples of the breed. All conservation breeders should strive to keep registrations up to date and complete. For most breeds, this is the only way to ensure that animals and breeding programs can make their appropriate contributions to the breed.

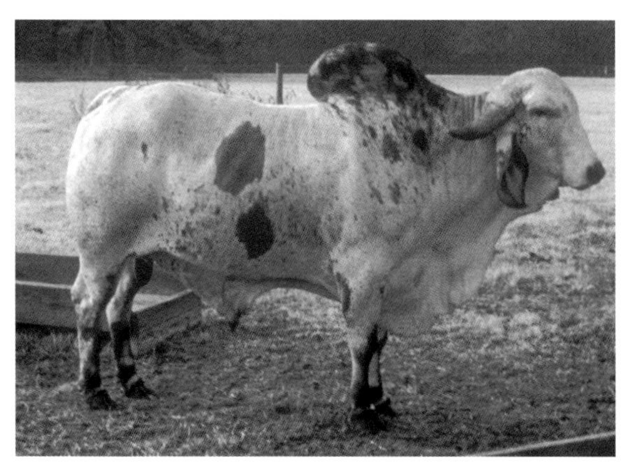

Figure 21.5 Some breeds, such as American Brahman cattle, are widely used for crossbreeding. For many of these the registration figures underestimate the actual population, while still reflecting the level of pure-breeding activity. Photo by DPS.

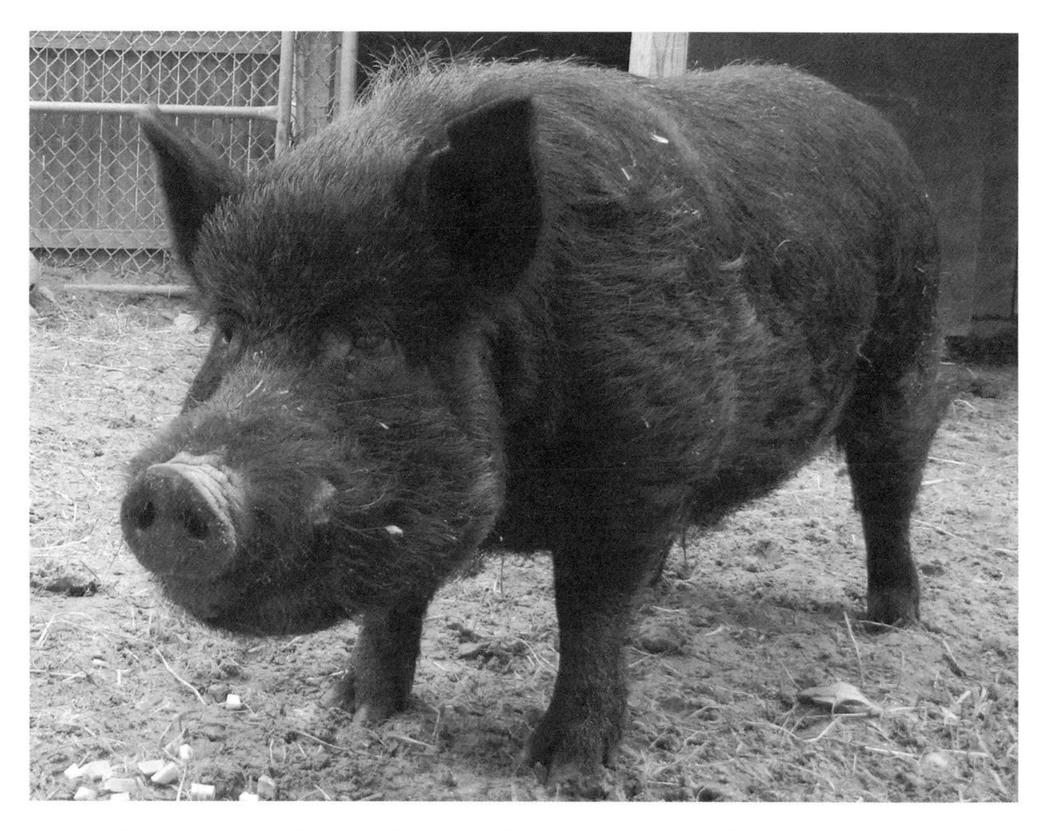

Figure 21.6 Registration of animals from rare bloodlines, such as this Guinea Hog boar, allows their identity to follow them throughout their careers, even as they move from herd to herd. Photo by JB.

21.8 Closed Herd Book Registries

Most breed associations have closed registry herd books. This refers to a requirement that only animals with a registered sire and dam are themselves eligible for registration. No progeny originating from unregistered stock are considered for registration. This requirement serves to make the population completely closed to outside genetics. This is the most common strategy for standardized breeds and is especially true of international breeds of British origin (Figure 21.7). This practice of complete genetic isolation of breeds arose in the 1700s and 1800s from English work with the Shorthorn cattle and Thoroughbred horse herd books, both of which were organized around this principle. By the late 1800s and early 1900s this strategy had become synonymous with the term "purebred livestock," so that even landrace breed associations, such as that for Texas Longhorn cattle, eventually adopted this same defining principle.

Closed populations do serve to isolate breeds, and as a consequence consolidate them as repeatable, predictable genetic packages. This is particularly useful in the early history of breeds, as long as the initial stage of inclusion of foundation animals was broad enough to involve most or all of the breed. In well-defined breeds that have long histories of pure breeding, the strategy of a closed herd book can be very constrictive because the genetic

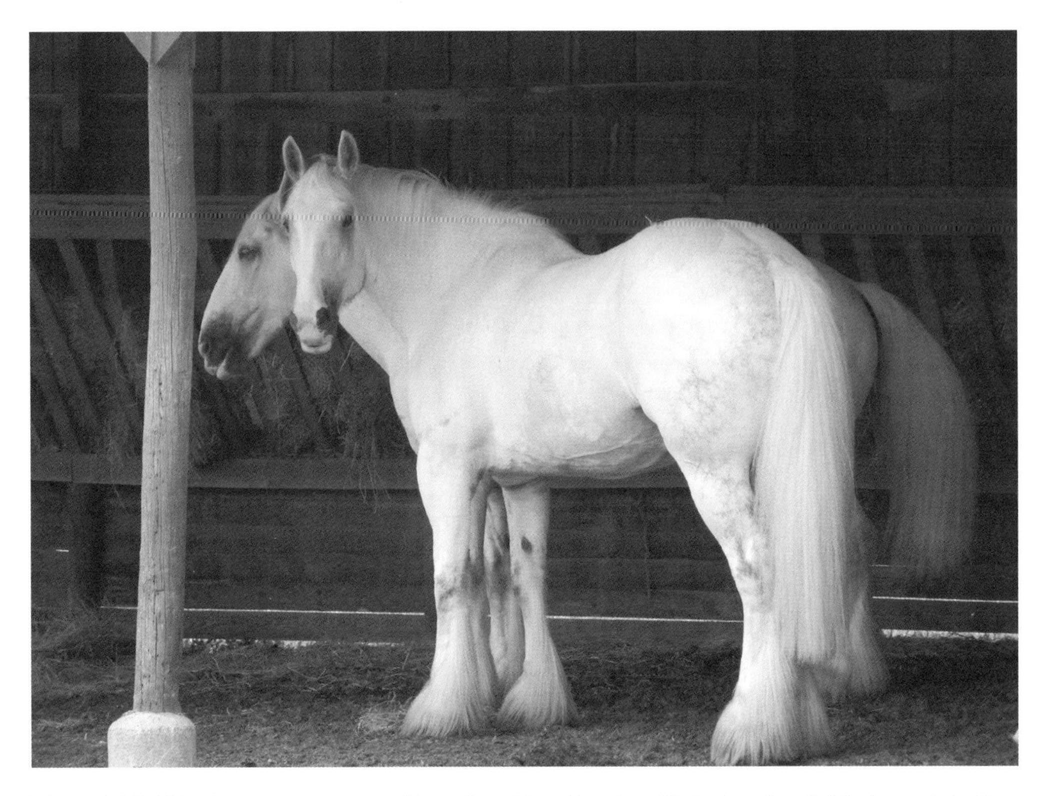

Figure 21.7 Shire horses are managed in a closed herd book, with foals only eligible for registration if they come from two registered parents. Photo by JB.

variability that is essential for vitality tends to diminish in each succeeding generation of breeding.

Some of the downsides to the complete closure of herd books are now being seen in a few different situations: older breeds (Thoroughbred horses), breeds with breeding practices that lead to genetic erosion (Holstein cattle), or breeds in species that have short generation intervals (dogs) because the consequences of tight genetic isolation play out in fewer years than they do in those with longer generation intervals. Some of the earliest closed breeds are now in their second or third century of this management strategy. Future strategies for managing pure breeds as repeatable genetic packages that retain enough variability for vitality promise to become increasingly important in the coming years, and may require modifications of strictly closed gene pools imposed by closed registries.

For a closed herd book to be valid in a genetic sense, it must include the vast majority of the breed. It is all too common for recently structured landrace herd books to close before a reasonably high proportion of the animals that are actually members of the landrace have been included. Closing the books restricts the numbers of breeders and animals within the population recognized as valid by the registry. As a result, the breeders of herds that have been included benefit from the restricted supply. This is shortsighted when considering the importance of the fate of breeds as genetic resources. With few exceptions, tightly closed herd books are inappropriate for landrace or local breeds.

In addition, herd books of even the oldest and most closed breeds should be open to the inclusion of animals that can be documented as purebred but that have been lost to the breed through a variety of situations. In this case the candidate animals should be rigorously validated as indeed purebred. Following success in that investigation, they should be included as full members of the breed. Multiple examples of situations where this can greatly help breeds with closed herd books can be cited, including Leicester Longwool sheep, Dexter cattle, and a few others.

21.9 Open Herd Book Registries

Few purebred breed associations follow an open herd book principle for organizing the breed population. This strategy is most common among landrace populations for which it is likely that good and typical representatives of the population remain outside the registered population for many decades after a herd book is organized. That is, the registered populations of these breeds tend to represent only a portion, and frequently a small portion, of the entire breed. In such breeds it is wisest to keep the herd book open to allow for inclusion of these purebred animals as they come to the attention of the association.

The key to operating an open herd book as an effective tool for genetic resource conservation is to assure that only representative animals are brought in. The goal should be to include every legitimate representative of the breed, and to exclude all non-representative animals. This is a tough line to draw and will vary from situation to situation and breed to breed. A few examples may help.

A group of traditionally minded Texas Longhorn cattle breeders banded together after the main portion of the association began going down a path selecting for big, smooth, long-horned, speckled cattle that diverged dramatically from the original type of the breed. The original association has a closed herd book, but the closure occurred after the inclusion of a few cattle with Hereford and presumed African blood types. The cattle with the foreign introgression are fully included in the breed and have become among the more popular bloodlines. In response to this situation, a group of breeders decided to develop an association that would continue to accept cattle after a visual inspection. Following success at that step, blood typing (later replaced by DNA technology) was used to assure that the cattle had Criollo blood types of the traditional Texas Longhorns. Female offspring of registered cattle could then be registered without further inspection, although all bull calves were DNA typed regardless of parentage. Newly accepted foundation animals (those with no background in the herd book) were still accepted. They did need to go through the inspection and genetic documentation step, but once they succeeded, they were included as full members of the breed (Figure 21.8). The result has been that the new association (Cattlemen's Texas Longhorn Registry), though maintaining an open herd book, has been able to guard the pure genetic resource more closely than the older associations with their prematurely closed herd books that had started with lax initial inclusion procedures as well as ongoing selection away from rather than toward traditional breed type.

In contrast, the Navajo-Churro sheep breeders have chosen a system that inspects each and every animal presented for registration, even if it comes from a long line of registered sheep. The goal is to assure that the traditional phenotype is recognized and perpetuated.

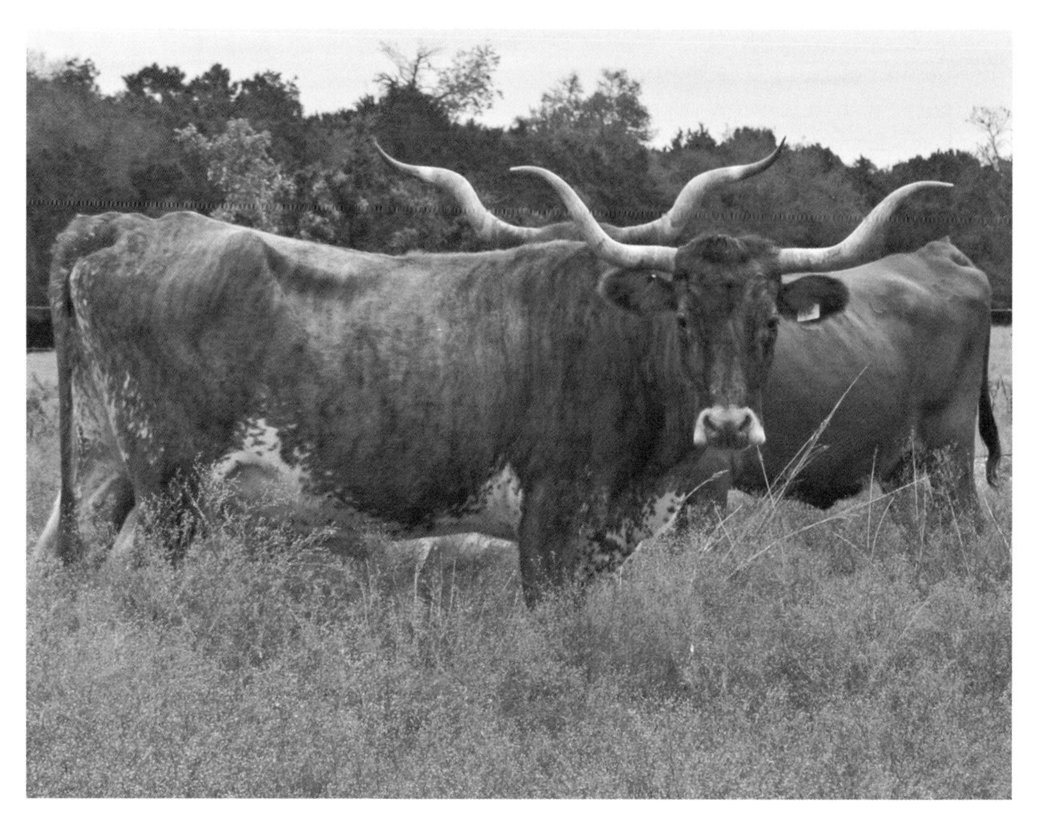

Figure 21.8 The Cattlemen's Texas Longhorn Registry uses an open herd book with strict evaluation of candidate animals to assure breed purity and conservation success. Photo by JB.

Inspection includes fleece type and structure, which is all-important to this breed. This more restrictive approach assures that the desired phenotype and its underlying genotype does not drift out of existence. This is an excellent example of selection for traditional type that is assured by the requirements of the association. This relates back to the function of a breed association to successfully manage a breed as a genetic resource. Inspection procedures can be resource-intensive but can be managed in such a way as to be practical. Breeders of Navajo-Churro sheep in areas where the sheep are numerous can get their sheep inspected on-site, with qualified English-, Spanish-, and Navajo-speaking inspectors. In addition, it is possible to submit photos and fleece samples, a strategy that allows more far-flung isolated breeders to participate in the breed. Broad participation is assured and facilitated, while still safeguarding the genetic resource.

Several American landrace populations use open herd books to good advantage. Among these is the large group of Colonial Spanish horse registries. Many of these will accept new horses following a visual inspection and an evaluation of the horse's history and population of origin. The associations vary in the extent to which the herd books function as open books. Some add horses relatively easily, while others are much more restrictive. Either philosophy presents both positive and negative aspects, depending on the overall goal for conservation purposes.

Florida Cracker and Pineywoods cattle breed associations both use open herd books. This works well when old lines of these breeds are newly discovered. As time proceeds, fewer and fewer of these are discovered, but they do still come to light occasionally. Any such discoveries are genetically important to these breeds and need to be fully included in the breed.

The Tennessee Myotonic (Fainting) goat registries are also open. One of the associations requires photographic documentation of the stiffness of the goats presented for registry, which is the main criterion for inclusion. This presents a subtle problem in that not all myotonic (stiff) goats are of traditional Tennessee breeding, so that the breed has become confused with this single genetic trait. As a result, it is likely that nontraditional goats are registered along with traditional goats, and this poses a threat to the original genetic resource. This situation has no easy solution, especially because many traditional Tennessee Myotonic goats remain unregistered and to close the books would be to forever deny them their legitimate role in the breed's future. Recent developments in other registries are attempting to surmount these problems by addressing foundation sources as well as breed type. As a response to the risks of the purity of newly encountered Myotonic goats, one registry has now limited the "open" option to females, so that bucks may no longer be brought in unless they have registered parents. This still leaves the herd book open, but a bit more cautiously than before.

The breeders of Damara sheep in Southern Africa follow yet another protocol. Some of these sheep are maintained in large, multi-sire, extensive flocks. Others are maintained in single-sire pedigreed flocks. Both systems have advantages for the breed. In this case the pedigreed flocks participate in a flock book, but entry is still available for sheep in the extensively raised flocks after individual inspection for congruence to breed type (Figure 21.9).

Open herd books are entirely appropriate for many breeds, especially for those with local origins. Such a strategy for breed maintenance brings with it great responsibility for the association to be clear-headed about the character and importance of breeds. As breeds go in and out of favor it can easily happen that during periods of popularity many non-representative animals are presented for registration. And, in periods of less interest, it is easily possible for good, representative animals to slip from the registered population and potentially be lost from the breed. Either situation is bad for the breed, but no easy solution solves both problems.

21.10 *Registration of Crossbreds and Partbreds*

The registration or recording of crossbred animals into separate sections of purebred registries has been a very contentious issue for a number of breeds. On one side of the issue are people who are adamant that no crossbreeding should ever occur with the breed, and that to do so is to assure the demise of the breed. On the other side are breeders who hold that any and every animal with a drop of purebred blood should be registered.

Recording or registration of crossbreds goes back to the genetic definition of breeds, and the need to maintain them as genetic pools. In addition, it validates the role that several breeds have to play in crossbreeding for commercial excellence. Maintaining the consistency of the entire package should be of the utmost interest to purebred breeders. To lose the package is to lose the breed.

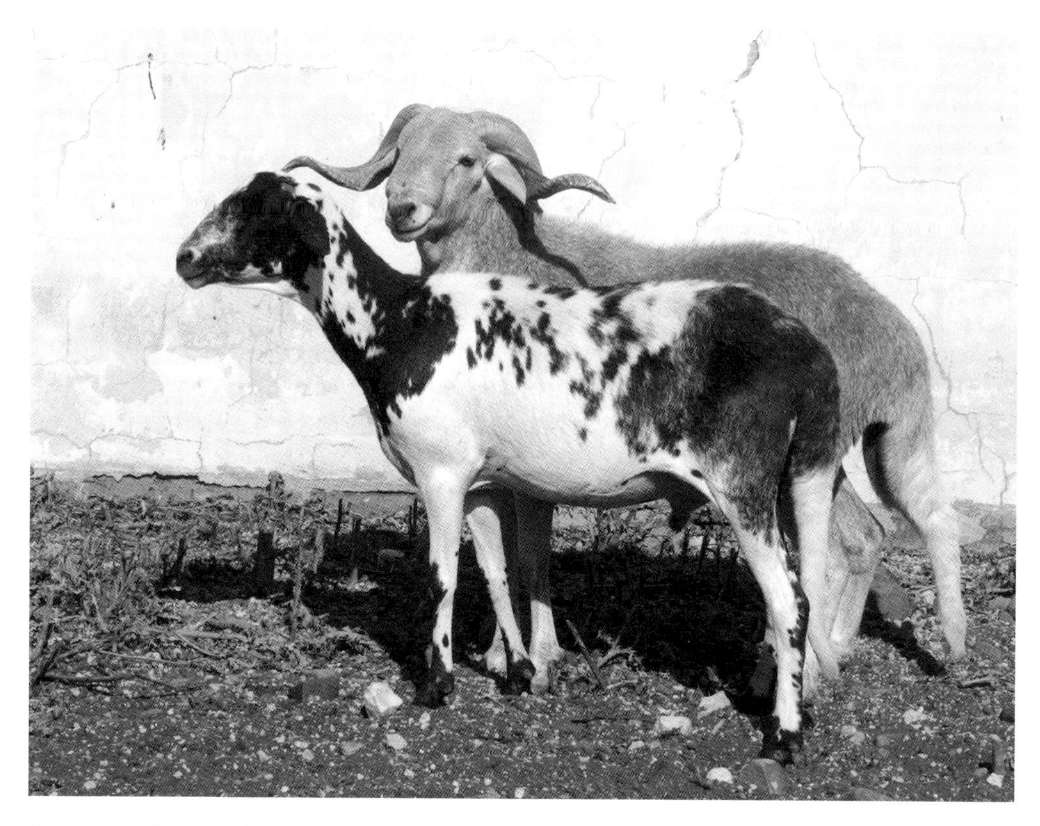

Figure 21.9 Damara sheep are managed both in registered single-sire herds as well as multi-sire extensive herds. Both systems contribute to the viability of the breed. Photo by DPS.

In order to protect the genetic integrity of several breeds it is prudent to identify and register known crossbreds. This allows breeders to "grade up" to purebred status, by clearly identifying animals that are known to be partly of outside breeding. By this strategy, even if a 75% purebred animal looked purebred it would be unlikely to be misidentified and misregistered as a purebred animal. Registering the crossbreds or upgrades in herds of serious breeders gives these animals a specific identity. This greatly reduces the chance that they, or their offspring, will be presented to the registry as purebreds, whether deliberately or accidentally. In order to prevent the registration of crossbreds as purebreds, it may be wise to provide a specific strategy for the registration of crossbreds and upgraded animals, such as those developed by several registries.

In addition, the registration of crossbreds can eliminate any temptation to register them as purebreds based on performance or phenotype. For example, some pony breeds have a modern "sport" pony type in addition to the more traditional cart pony or general farm use type. The traditional type has been essential in providing certain characteristics to the crossbred sport type, but is in danger of disappearing if the modern, crossbred type is allowed to be registered into the purebred herd book. Registration of crossbreds in an appropriate section of the herd book would allow them to reflect the excellence of the pure breed in producing the sport-horse type.

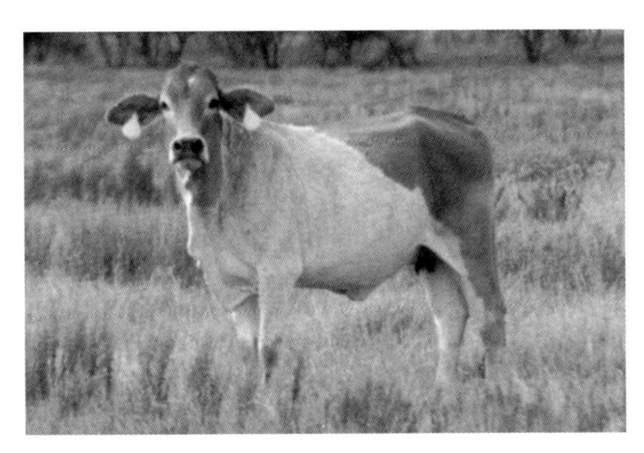

Figure 21.10 First-cross cows with a Brahman parent can be certified, providing them an identity that helps assure demand for pure Brahma cattle to use in crossbreeding systems. Photo by DPS.

Some breeds, such as the American Brahman, have also capitalized on the recording of crossbreds as a specific strategy to emphasize the ability of the breed to contribute to crossbred excellence. Their certification program identifies Brahman-crossbreds, which helps to increase the demand for purebreds used to generate those crossbreds (Figure 21.10).

21.11 Registration for Extensively Raised Landraces

Registration, or certification, of purebred status for landraces is problematic, especially when these breeds are raised in their traditional extensive, multi-sire herds. Attention to purebred identity and adherence to good breed management practices can become very real issues in such situations. One solution is the original formal, if loose, association of breeders developed by Spanish goat breeders. Spanish goat breeders could be listed with a loosely defined association. This facilitated communication among breeders, devotion to purebred breeding, and increased demand. As time goes on, though, this somewhat loose structure is almost invariably tightened. That phase is underway among Spanish goat breeders, and their association will eventually more closely resemble other more formal systems with fully functional registries.

Another potentially useful strategy was developed by traditionally minded Gulf Coast sheep breeders (Figure 21.11). They formed a loose association called Coastal South Native Sheep Flock Alliance and designed a series of accepted practices to assist in breed maintenance.

- No other breeds of sheep are to be kept on the same property as the Native flock. This is because crossbreeding is too likely when multiple breeds are kept, and recognition is by flock rather than by individual sheep. Sheep recognized as "Native" by the Alliance include those registered as Gulf Coast Natives by the association (Gulf Coast Sheep Breeders Association), which is more formally organized, as well as those sheep coming from a Native flock as described and accepted by the Alliance.
- A brief history of the flock is written and kept on record by the Alliance. This includes sources of sheep, their origin, and approximate dates.
- Any later additions to the flock are noted as to the source flock, sex, and year of addition. Ideally additions will only come from flocks recognized by the Alliance or individual sheep registered by the Gulf Coast Native Sheep Association.

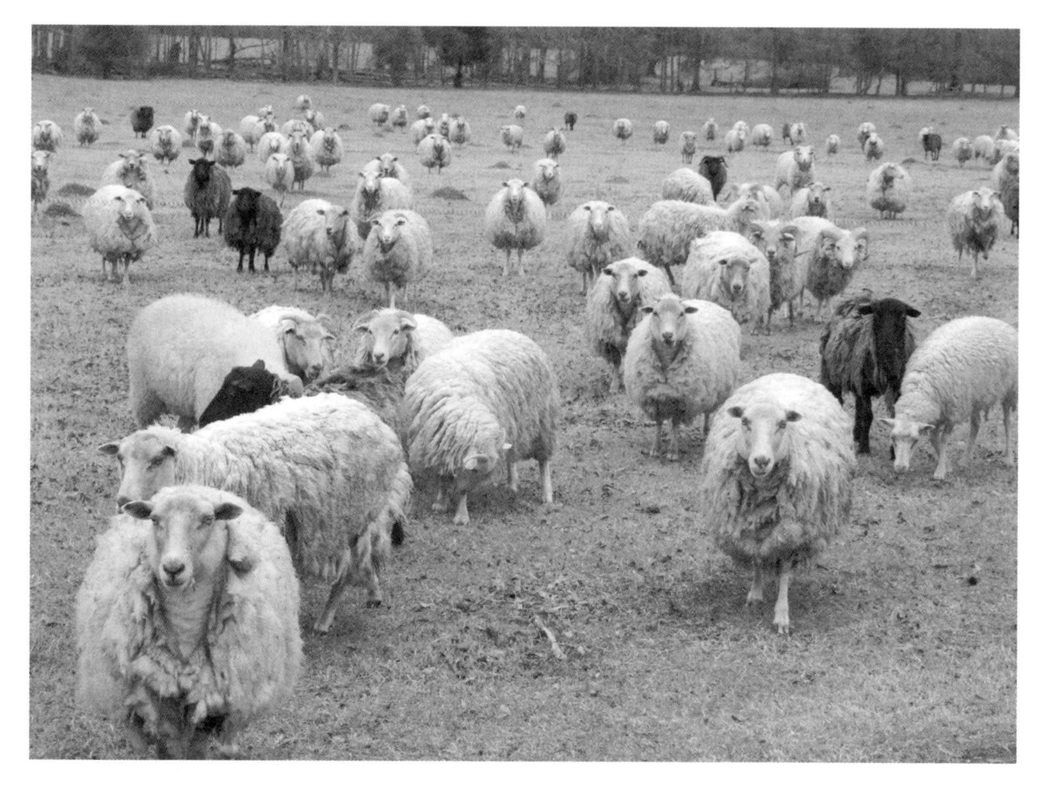

Figure 21.11 Gulf Coast sheep, along with other American landraces, benefit from an open registry that is committed to inclusion of purebred members of the breed. Photo by JB.

- Each flock participant gives an annual update on approximate numbers of sheep and sources of any additions to the flock.
- In cases where breeders have divided their sheep into separate flocks for breeding to maintain different lines, these are noted and tracked.

Sheep sold from participating flocks can be certified as "Native." Sheep in newly formed flocks can be individually registered by the Gulf Coast Sheep Breeders Association following adherence to their rules. Alternatively, the flock can be certified by providing the information shown above and meeting the requirements listed there. Fortunately, the two general approaches to breed management (individual registrations versus extensively raised flocks) are being considered as essential options for this local landrace and are likely to emerge as options within a single association.

21.12 Starting a Registry

The initial steps in starting a registry have profound effects on the later efficiency and completeness of registry function. Careful action at the outset usually results in a better final outcome down the road. This is especially true for landraces or for other breeds that have not previously had registries.

As much information as possible should be captured about the founding population. When background pedigree information is known, the ancestors of the animals should be registered first. This is true even if these animals are deceased. Following the registration of these founders, the descendants that are actually alive can be enrolled in the registry. Every effort should be made to individually register any animal that does indeed have an individual identity, even if only in a breeder's memory. While each age cohort should ideally be registered in sequence, as a practical matter for landraces it is often only possible to register ancestors before descendants and not within an entire age cohort. This strategy may seem sloppy, but it still allows computerized systems to work effectively.

It is also ideal to link each founder to a specific bloodline. This can help greatly in monitoring and managing genetic diversity into the future. In the case of larger animals (horses, cattle) most or all of the animals will have individual pedigrees and identified ancestors. Even in those species it can be helpful to also include the bloodline identity. In the case of smaller livestock (sheep, goats, and certainly poultry) the bloodline is often the only level of identity that is possible. Many registry software programs do not do a good job of tracking bloodline information, but it is possible to track this using spreadsheets or database systems. Bloodline affiliation can be a very useful tool in managing many breeds.

CHAPTER 22

Breeder Responsibilities

Breeders have a great many responsibilities to the breeds that they manage. Breeders gave us the breeds we cherish, and breeders are certainly capable of managing them so they can be passed on to future generations. Without engaged and dedicated breeders, breeds lose their relevance and risk being relegated to the status of trivial artifacts or becoming extinct. Breeders are essential for breeds!

Breeders have responsibilities that go well beyond themselves. These include responsibilities to the breed and its genetic health, as well as to the breeder community. Responsible breeders leave the breed in better shape than they found it, and also leave the community stronger than when they entered it. In contrast, irresponsible individuals can do real and lasting damage to both the breed and its community of breeders.

One important obligation of breeders is assuring that the registration of animals is kept current. Failing to do this leads to purebreds that are not registered, and the recovery of unregistered but purebred animals back into a breed is often difficult or impossible. Failing to keep up with registrations means that a breeder has not fulfilled all of the duties that the responsible breeding of purebred animals entails.

The usual point where many animals are lost to conservation is at herd dispersal upon a breeder's death (Figure 22.1). While this is never an easy situation, wise breeders assure that their wishes are clearly spelled out for dispersal of herds upon their death. In many cases animals have been lost because details of animal identification and registration have not been available. When these details are locked in a breeder's head, they become lost as soon as that mind is unavailable for whatever reason. Keeping animals identified and ensuring that registrations are up to date are essential to avoid losing all of a breeder's hard work.

An effective way to avoid loss of genetic material is through sales to other breeders over time. This can make dispersals less of a crisis. If breeders assure ongoing sales or transfers of purebred, registered stock to other breeders over several years, then upon a breeder's retirement or death most of the work has already been done. Effective breeders with consistent sales and transfers to others assure an ongoing contribution to the breed. Even if one breeder's herds do become lost through some disaster, the contribution of those animals

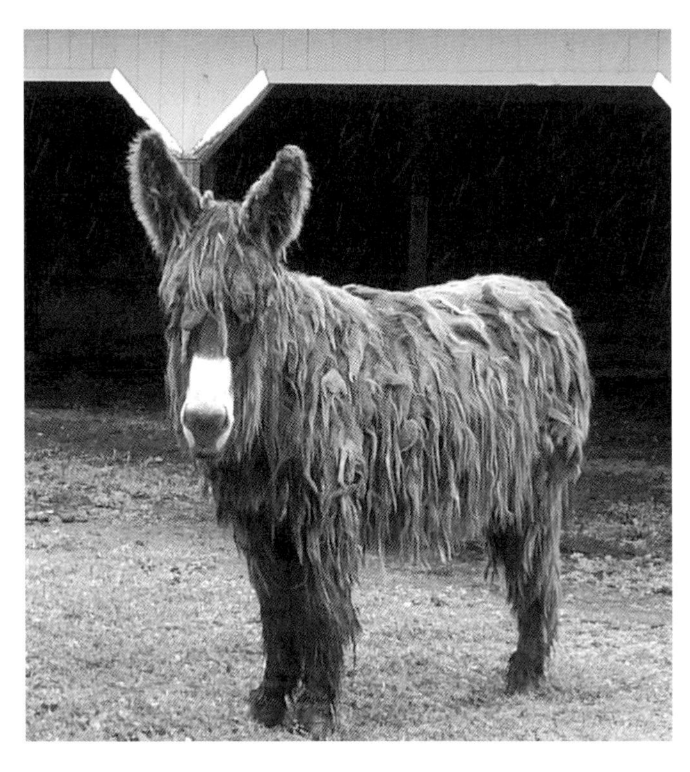

Figure 22.1 Debbie Hamilton's careful planning assured that her conservation work with Poitou donkeys outlived her to continue making a positive contribution to the breed. Photo by DPS.

to the breed does indeed continue because they have been shared with others all along. The ideal situation is for breeders to consistently sell top-quality stock to other committed producers. This strategy guarantees that no disastrous situation in the home herd can result in the complete loss of any benefits brought to the population by a good individual breeding program.

Another responsibility of breeders is to manage the breed type in such a way that it falls within the range for the breed. This implies that both management and selection will be appropriate to the specific genetic resource that is being managed. This can be a subtle and powerful concept yet is likely to be overlooked by many breeders. While many breeds will thrive under ideal management and abundant resources, some breeds will only maintain their traditional genetic heritage by being placed in environments that challenge them to retain their adaptive traits and remain productive. It is the breeders that must provide for that environment, and for the selection of the animals that are best adapted to it.

Breeds of livestock and poultry are an important part of food security. Breeds of dogs have important roles in modern society that range from effective companionship to the more obvious tasks that working dogs accomplish. The loss of genomes, whether through breed extinction or through changes within breed type, reduces the options for meeting future needs. Industrial strains present an interesting challenge to breed variability. They are exquisitely productive and are increasingly used for production. This results in their replacing other breeds that once had productive roles in various settings. However, the industrial stocks have very reduced biological fitness. They do not adapt well outside of their narrow setting, and therefore cannot meet future needs if these depend on a variety of environments. Widely divergent breed choices must be available, intact, and viable in order for the demands of changing agricultural systems to be met. Breeders are essential for this task!

Breeders also have important responsibilities to their associations and registries. Among these are providing accurate and timely information. This can include notification of births, deaths, and ownership transfers, all of which help the registry to maintain accurate and current records. More contentious, but equally important, is alerting the association to the production of any defects or known genetic diseases within pure or crossbred examples of the breed. Only by having this information can associations take early and effective measures to assure that the breed remains healthy and viable. Additionally, breeders can contribute to a positive and constructive culture within an association that facilitates the entry of newcomers and enables them to become long-term contributors to the breed and its future.

22.1 Master Breeders

Master breeders are those individuals that constructively breed their animals and make them available to others. They are uniquely able to assure animals that are true to type, as well as productive. They are often able to do this by an almost instinctive feel for animal breeding that relies on intuition as much as conscious thought (Figure 22.2). These established breeders have responsibilities in training new breeders, but new breeders also have a set of equally important responsibilities.

New breeders that aspire to become master breeders need to cultivate a combination of attitudes and abilities. To successfully acquire the knowledge that is required to progress toward being a successful breeder it is ideal to have:

- passion for the breed
- commitment to the long-term success of the breed
- adequate financial resources to manage and maintain a breeding population
- a clear-headed commercial or utilitarian outlook that does not sacrifice breed type or heritage
- personal integrity
- an "eye" for good stock and for type
- pride without arrogance
- an ability to listen to and learn from diverse resources
- reasonable freedom from assumptions.

This list is a tall order but one which continues to be fulfilled by many talented people working with a wide range of breeds.

Passion for the breed is critical for long-term success in the breed. Certain breeds resonate strongly with certain people, and these are the combinations that work best. When new breeders select breeds, or strains within breeds, it is important that they find a project that inherently appeals to them. Passion is difficult to force into a situation where it is not already present, and passion about a breeding program is a key component for the

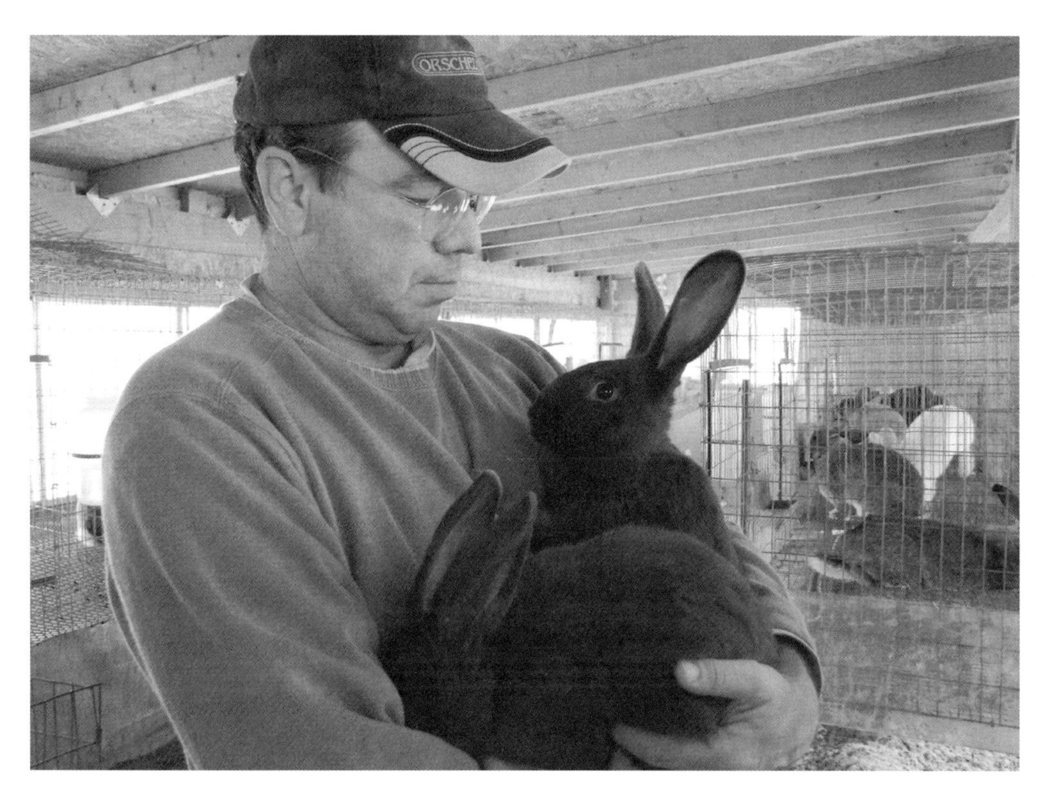

Figure 22.2 Master breeders like Eric Rapp are consistently able to evaluate stock and to produce high-quality animals from generation to generation. Photo by JB.

long-term dedication that is necessary for success. Passion allows breeders to overcome temporary setbacks that are inevitable in any breeding program.

Commitment is important because breeds benefit much more from long-term programs than they do from short-term endeavors. It is almost invariably damaging for breeders to acquire stock and then disperse it all after only a few generations of breeding. While dispersals occur for a variety of reasons, a committed breeder will work diligently to place key breeding stock in the hands of committed breeders rather than dispersing animals indiscriminately or sending them to slaughter. Similarly, informing family and friends of wishes for a herd's dispersal may be a final gift to the breed in which a breeder has invested a great deal of effort, time, and resources. Breeding programs can only really contribute to breed maintenance if they take a long view rather than a short one, and commitment is key to this.

Finances must be adequate in order to maintain breeding stock. In most cases the products of the breeding program should cover the cost of maintaining breeding stock. Some people, however, find it difficult to deal with the outright commercial aspects of most breeds of livestock. When it becomes emotionally impossible to send excess animals to other breeders or to slaughter, animal numbers build up and become greatly in excess of what is needed for breeding programs. These excess animals do not contribute to effective breeding programs, nor do they contribute to the positive cash flow needed to maintain breeding stock. This can have a decidedly negative effect on a breeding program. The presence of excess animals also increases the animal load on the environment, which can be directly detrimental to any top-notch stock in the same location. Adequate financial support and management of numbers are very important aspects and must be carefully considered before embarking on a breeding program for any breed.

Most breeds benefit from a practical commercial approach that also acknowledges breed type and heritage. An extreme commercial approach can ignore breed type, and this results in changing breeds away from traditional breed type. A better but more subtle approach links selection for commercial utility to stay within the constraints of traditional breed type. Morgan horses, for example, have a number of bloodlines that are a park horse type rather than the earlier, traditional multipurpose farm horse type. This change was largely driven by market forces and breeders willing to sacrifice breed type for commercial gain. This eroded the uniqueness of the breed, and the result has not been an effective strategy for breed maintenance.

Moral integrity of all breeders is necessary to safeguard the reputation of the individuals, the association, and ultimately the animals themselves. Records must be honest, and animals must be honestly represented to both registries and customers. Breeders that resort to anything less than an honest presentation of animals eventually do damage to their own reputations as well as to the breed. Breeders that sell stock should not only consider the one immediate sale but should also endeavor to generate customers that are so pleased with the animals and their performance that they come back for future sales. This requires an honest and accurate presentation of the animals as well as honest and fair business dealings.

Developing an "eye" for breed type and good stock is a subtle but important ability that master breeders possess. For many people this is almost instinctive and therefore difficult to describe. It is even more difficult to train other people in how to achieve "eye." Eager young breeders can go a long way by seeking out older breeders and not only talking to them, but also trying to see through that older breeder's eyes when inspecting animals. It is especially helpful to inspect and evaluate animals alongside an old established breeder, because this activity brings many subtle but powerful details to bear. Livestock judges can help greatly in this by inviting young breeders to evaluate livestock alongside them, asking the young breeders "what do you see?" rather than telling them up front what the experienced breeder sees. Forcing younger breeders to actively inspect and evaluate stock is an essential component of developing an eye for type and evaluation.

Having an eye for livestock helps master breeders to predict production potential from external clues. There is a fundamental importance in developing this ability. By linking external type to underlying performance potential, the breeder is able to select those animals most likely to succeed. Modern, statistical methods can certainly facilitate the selection of animals. It is important to remember that our current productive breeds were all developed over years by master breeders that used only their eyes and their brains. Eyes and brains therefore form a powerful tool set that should never be undervalued.

At a very basic level, master breeders have usually honed their skills in evaluating animals by closely observing them over many years. Certain levels of performance tend to go hand-in-hand with certain conformational traits. It is tempting to say that "form follows function." The reality is more along the lines that "form and function go together." Being

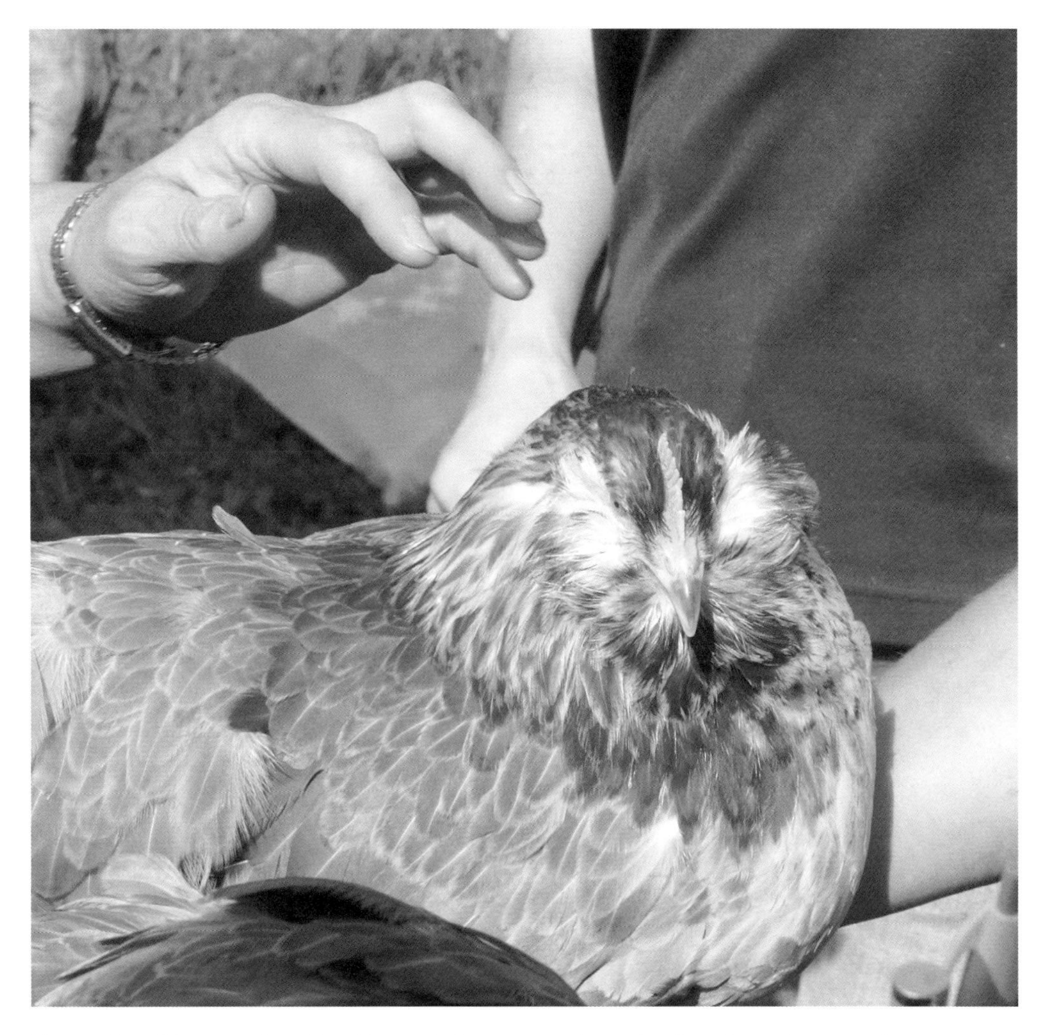

Figure 22.3 Clinics such as The Livestock Conservancy's poultry breeder training sessions can transmit the knowledge and techniques of master breeders to a new generation of breed stewards. Photo by JB.

able to recognize the relationship of these two is an important trait of master breeders (Figure 22.3).

Good breeders are constantly evaluating the performance of their animals and noting which conformational traits are typical of high producers and which are typical of low producers. This linkage is especially important when considering longevity of production because most animals that remain sound and productive over long lifespans have conformation that contributes to that success. In general, they have smooth, stout conformation that contributes to skeletal soundness over years. They also have good deep body capacity that contributes to efficient use of feedstuffs.

In addition to the evaluation of individual animals, master breeders are also able to place each of these animals in a context within the population, whether this is within the herd or the entire breed. This attention to the genetic structure of the entire group is vital to long-term success. Once again, this can be nearly instinctive for some breeders who have an uncanny ability to pair animals in order to produce a truly exceptional next generation.

Taking pride in the fruits of a breeding program without being arrogant is also important for master breeders. Most successful breeders are reasonably unassuming and listen effectively to others. They can sort through what is said and can learn something from just about anyone. They can also put this stored knowledge to good use. Arrogance precludes the receipt of information and defeats many breeders because they are missing important bits of information or technique. Most master breeders can easily be missed as the geniuses they are simply because they engage in minimal self-promotion.

The greatest master breeders have all of these attributes, and such people are very rare. Becoming a master breeder is slow, complicated work. Identifying and nurturing young breeders along the path to achieving these skills is an important responsibility for older breeders and breed associations.

22.2 Breeds, Breeders, Associations, and the Future

The future has always seemed dark and mysterious, and doomsayers have pointed to a downward spiral of culture and life throughout all eras of history. Without being unnecessarily pessimistic, it is possible to point to some very real threats to the future of breeds, breed integrity, and the function of agricultural systems. Fortunately, it is also possible to point to some bright spots on the horizon. These bright spots are presently increasing in brilliance as well as size.

Several threats that are unique to this time in history confront breeds and their integrity and use. Some threats are subtle and internal. Among these is the philosophy of absolute breed purity that keeps breeds completely isolated from any and all outside influences. This model for breeds and their maintenance is rather recent, having developed only in the last couple of centuries. This model differs from the traditional course of breed development, which insisted on utility and predictability but only as they served functional ends. Anything that contributed to the predictable package was considered fair game, and the concept of complete genetic isolation was not in force. It remains to be seen whether complete genetic isolation will eventually result in a gradual, ever tightening constraint of inbreeding depression for many breeds. Of all the threats facing breeds, this may be the most insidious and dangerous, because it is imposed by breed advocates that are in no way trying to diminish breeds and their utility. This is not to denigrate breed purity as a useful and wise concept. Instead, it is to insist that breed purity be kept in its original and useful context as it relates to utility.

Communication and transportation advances in the last century have also posed a threat to breeds and their integrity. This threat has usually arrived from a gradual homogenization of regional and international cultures, with the result that unique products and the animals that provide them are much less recognized and valued than they once were. Communication and transportation have resulted in ever-increasing consolidation of the production and marketing of agricultural products so that point-of-origin producers must follow the dictates of this consolidation to be successful. Globalization is the final stage of this process, and if unchecked can result in a very severe diminishment of genomes worldwide that produce unique, satisfying, healthy, and interesting local products. Against this trend is a fortunate reemergence of interest in more local resources, approaches, and knowledge that can all contribute to a secure place for breeds.

The cultural environment for breeds and breed maintenance is also increasingly changed. Breeds that were once valued as essential ingredients to local and regional agricultural production and cultural identity have become somewhat trivialized as "lifestyle endeavors" for those wealthy enough to indulge themselves in this activity. These breeds, while saved, have moved from essential partners in survival to a nonessential pet or hobby status. This switch in cultural environment changes the selection environment in which the breeds survive and persist and can only result in genetic changes as well. This moment in history provides the last access that many cultures will have to the previous generations of traditional, local ways of life. It is critical to access that deep well of knowledge and wisdom before it disappears forever.

The very basic endeavor of animal use and ownership is also increasingly under attack from a wide variety of angles. Some of these involve concerns over animal welfare. These need to be countered by producers assuring that animals are managed humanely and well. Other attacks are related to environmental concerns. These tend to lump all animal production into a single category based on the industrial model. This ignores the real and significant environmental benefits that come from many non-industrial production systems.

Not all is doom and gloom. An increasing number of people, both producers and consumers, are realizing that a sustainable and local agricultural system has great advantages for people, animals, and the environment. The growth of this view of agriculture will help to provide rare and traditional breeds with a secure future as the connection of breed, place, and production system becomes recognized and appreciated by larger numbers of people.

Finally, it is important to remember that generations of breeders have given us the breeds that we enjoy and use today. The future hope of breeds and their conservation lies with breeders as stewards. With a few tools and some encouragement, they are very much equal to accomplishing this important task and accomplishing it successfully (Figure 22.4).

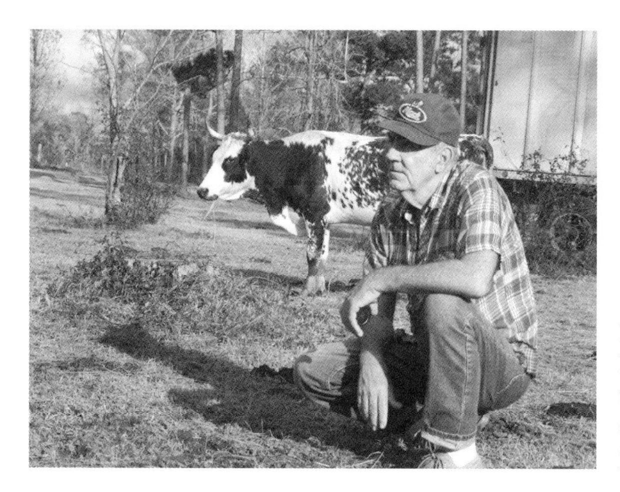

Figure 22.4 Breeders like Fred Diamond gave us the breeds we have today, and breeders will be essential stewards on into the future. Photo by JB.

APPENDIX 1

Phenotypic Matrix for Colonial Spanish Horses

This Colonial Spanish horse matrix score sheet was developed by D.P. Sponenberg and Chuck Reed. Horses are scored on various aspects of conformation and type. The final decision is not a simple average of scores, but rather a closer look at the number of non-typical (high) versus most typical (low) scores. The head character weighs heavily in the final determination, especially if the body scores well. A horse with a body that is very typical but with a head that is very nontypical is still rejected because such a horse is unlikely to be Colonial Spanish.

most typical score 1	fairly typical score 2	intermediate score 3	fairly nontypical score 4	least typical score 5
		HEAD PROFILE		
Concave/flat on forehead and convex from top of nasal area to top of upper lip (subconvex). Uniformly slightly convex from poll to muzzle. Straight.			Dished, as in Arabian. Markedly convex.	
		HEAD FROM FRONT VIEW		
Wide between eyes but tapering and "chiseled" in nasal/facial portion. Wide between eyes with sculpted taper to a fine muzzle is very typical.			Wide and fleshy throughout head from cranial portion to muzzle.	
		NOSTRILS		
Small, thin, and crescent-shaped. Flare larger when excited or exerting.			Large, round, and open at rest.	
		EARS		
Small to medium length, with distinctive notch or inward point at tips.			Long, straight, with no inward point at tip. Thick, wide, or boxy.	

<table>
<tr><th>most typical
score 1</th><th>fairly typical
score 2</th><th>intermediate
score 3</th><th>fairly nontypical
score 4</th><th>least typical
score 5</th></tr>
<tr><td colspan="5">EYES</td></tr>
<tr><td colspan="2">Vary from large to small (pig eyes).
Usually fairly high on head.</td><td></td><td colspan="2">Large and bold.
Low on head.</td></tr>
<tr><td colspan="5">MUZZLE PROFILE</td></tr>
<tr><td colspan="2">Refined with top lip longer than the bottom lip.</td><td></td><td colspan="2">Coarse and thick with lower lip loose, large, and projecting beyond upper lip.</td></tr>
<tr><td colspan="5">MUZZLE FRONTVIEW</td></tr>
<tr><td colspan="2">Fine taper to nostrils, slight outward flare, then inward delicate curve to small, fine muzzle that is narrower than the region between nostrils.</td><td></td><td colspan="2">Coarse and rounded or heavy and square.
Minimal tapering curve.</td></tr>
<tr><td colspan="5">NECK</td></tr>
<tr><td colspan="2">Wide from side.
Sometimes ewe-necked.
Attached low on chest.</td><td></td><td colspan="2">Thin.
Long.
Set high on chest.</td></tr>
<tr><td colspan="5">HEIGHT</td></tr>
<tr><td colspan="2">13.2 to 14.2 hands high.
Over 15 hands atypical.</td><td></td><td colspan="2">Under 13 hands.
Over 15 hands.</td></tr>
<tr><td colspan="5">WITHERS</td></tr>
<tr><td colspan="2">Pronounced and obvious.
"Sharp."</td><td></td><td colspan="2">Low.
Thick and meaty.</td></tr>
<tr><td colspan="5">BACK</td></tr>
<tr><td colspan="2">Short and strong.</td><td></td><td colspan="2">Long, weak, and plain.</td></tr>
<tr><td colspan="5">CROUP PROFILE</td></tr>
<tr><td colspan="2">Angled from top to tail, usually at 30°.</td><td></td><td colspan="2">Flat or high.</td></tr>
<tr><td colspan="5">TAIL SET</td></tr>
<tr><td colspan="2">Low, tailhead follows croup angle, "falls off" croup.</td><td></td><td colspan="2">High, tailhead up above the angle of the croup.</td></tr>
<tr><td colspan="5">SHOULDER</td></tr>
<tr><td colspan="2">Should be long, and at an angle of 45–55°.</td><td></td><td colspan="2">Short, and steeper than 55°.</td></tr>
<tr><td colspan="5">CHEST SIDEVIEW</td></tr>
<tr><td colspan="2">Deep, usually accounting for half of height.</td><td></td><td colspan="2">Shallow, less than half of height.</td></tr>
<tr><td colspan="5">CHEST FRONTVIEW</td></tr>
<tr><td colspan="2">Narrow, with an "A" shape.</td><td></td><td colspan="2">Broad, with chest flat across.</td></tr>
</table>

<table>
<tr><th>most typical
score 1</th><th>fairly typical
score 2</th><th>intermediate
score 3</th><th>fairly nontypical
score 4</th><th>least typical
score 5</th></tr>
<tr><td colspan="5">CHESTNUTS</td></tr>
<tr><td colspan="2">Small, often absent on rear.
Flat rather than thick.</td><td></td><td colspan="2">Large, and thick.</td></tr>
<tr><td colspan="5">COLOR</td></tr>
<tr><td colspan="2">Any color.
Black-based colors common.
No bonus or penalty for any color.</td><td></td><td colspan="2">No color is penalized.</td></tr>
<tr><td colspan="5">REAR LIMBS FROM REAR VIEW</td></tr>
<tr><td colspan="2">Straight along whole length, or inward with close hocks and then straight to ground ("close hocks"), or slightly turned out from hocks to ground ("cow hocks") but not extreme.
Legs very flexible.
At trot, the hind track often lands past the front track.</td><td></td><td colspan="2">Excessive "cow hocks."
Heavy, bunchy gaskin muscle, tight tendons.</td></tr>
<tr><td colspan="5">FEATHERING ON LEGS</td></tr>
<tr><td colspan="2">Absent to light fetlock feathering, though some have long silky hair above ergot and a "comb" of curled hair up back of cannon.
Some horses from mountain areas have more feathering than typical of others, and lose this after moving to other environments.</td><td></td><td colspan="2">Coarse, abundant feathering as is seen in some draft horse breeds.</td></tr>
<tr><td colspan="5">REAR</td></tr>
<tr><td colspan="2">Contour from top of croup to gaskin has a "break" in line at the point of the butt.</td><td></td><td colspan="2">Contour from top of croup to gaskin is full and round "apple butt" with no break at the point of the butt.</td></tr>
<tr><td colspan="5">HIP FROM REAR</td></tr>
<tr><td colspan="2">Spine higher than hip, resulting in "rafter" hip.
Usually no crease from heavy muscling.</td><td></td><td colspan="2">Thickly muscled with a distinct crease down the rear.</td></tr>
<tr><td colspan="5">HIP FROM SIDE</td></tr>
<tr><td colspan="2">Long and sloping, well angled, and not heavy.</td><td></td><td colspan="2">Short, poorly angled.</td></tr>
<tr><td colspan="5">MUSCLING</td></tr>
<tr><td colspan="2">Long and tapered.</td><td></td><td colspan="2">Short and thick "bunchy."</td></tr>
<tr><td colspan="5">FRONT CANNON BONES</td></tr>
<tr><td colspan="2">Cross-section is round.
Palpate below splints.</td><td></td><td colspan="2">Cross-section is flat across rear of bone.</td></tr>
</table>

APPENDIX 2

A Protocol for Bloodline Analysis

A protocol for conducting bloodline analysis is useful. This analysis is rarely accomplished by the software packages that will readily handle DNA results. As a result, investigators need to figure out the goals of the analysis, as well as the steps to accomplish it. This is only one of several options.

The database can be arranged in columns with the following headings.

- Identification number of individual animal (registration number in most examples).
- Year of birth (needed later so that potential live breeding animals can be located).
- Name.
- Sire's identification number.
- Dam's identification number.

These five data points usually need to be manually entered, and then the following can be computed automatically from information entered for founders.

- Sire's name.
- Dam's name.
- Percentage of founder or bloodline 1.
- Percentage of founder or bloodline 2.
- Percentage of founder or bloodline 3.
  (And so on up to however many founders or bloodlines are present in the population.)
- Inbreeding coefficient five generations.
- Inbreeding coefficient ten generations (the inbreeding coefficients are computed from another source and merged, and can be derived from pedigree analysis or ROH from DNA techniques).

Once complete, the database can be copied or exported as "values only" which leaves the formulas behind. Only the calculated values remain in the cells. This allows the data to be sorted and manipulated in various ways while the numerical results in each cell remain intact.

Animals can be ranked by the influence of each individual founder or bloodline as separate analyses (one for each founder). This allows the identification of animals with either very high or very low influences from certain founders. This information can then be used to target DNA sampling, planned conservation mating, or gamete preservation.

APPENDIX 3

A Protocol for Assessing Popular Sires or Dams

This analysis can be done by evaluating the last 20, 50, or however many years are appropriate for the species or breed. The registry database can be searched to count the number of times an animal appears as sire, grandsire, or great grandsire. If the data are not already available, then a database can be constructed with the following columns.

- Identification number.
- Year of birth.
- Name.
- Sire's identification number.
- Dam's identification number.
- Sire's name.
- Dam's name.
- Sire's sire's number.
- Sire's sire's name.
- Sire's dam's number.
- Sire's dam's name.

  (And so on for up to however many generations are desired.)

The data can be filled in automatically using formulas once the identification number, year of birth, name, sire's identification number, and dam's identification number are entered. These data can then be copied and exported as "values only" to get rid of formulas and allow various types of sorting. The database can easily get unwieldy for large populations. If that is the case, the names can be eliminated. The index numbers (usually registration numbers) for sires can then be ranked. However, it is likely to be a bit neater and cleaner to rank based on names because alphabetical sorting usually makes the identification of frequencies easier for the person doing the analysis.

In Microsoft Excel it is possible to sort the various columns. To do this, copy the data set, and then "paste special" as values to eliminate the formulas. Failing to do this leaves an incredible mess as the data sort out and the formulas instruct the program to do a host of illogical and unhelpful things.

Depending on breed and naming protocols, one way to sort is by sires, which can be done by sire registration number. If there are several columns and this one is somewhat to the left of the sheet, it can help the reader's visual recognition to copy the column and put it to the right of the existing columns as an extra column. Leave the original one intact, so this is essentially a duplicate column. The next step is to sum the occurrences of each animal. If you are using Microsoft Excel to do this the formula to use is: =COUNTIF(Q$2:Q$3908,Q2). This is for the data in column Q but gives the general idea. The column can then be filled in automatically and quickly. The sheet can then be saved as "values" to lose the formulas for further sorting.

Similar sheets can be developed for the sire's sire and the dam's sire. If the column of interest is copied and pasted to the right of the main set each time, the formulas will automatically recalculate for whichever data column is of interest.

The final result of this analysis enables the ability to find rare sires or dams, as well as the ability to know which sires and dams are most common or most rare. For example, once the more popular influences are documented it should be possible to search for animals lacking those influences in an effort to capture genetic diversity more adequately. This must always be done with the recognition that some animals that are underrepresented have achieved that status for good reason: unsoundness or defect. But, in many breeds, perfectly sound and typical animals are underrepresented because they are in situations where they are simply overlooked as having excellent potential for the breed and its future. It is these animals that can hold the key to breed survival. This is not to detract in any way from the more widely distributed bloodlines, though, as these have often achieved their popularity for good reasons.

APPENDIX 4

Sample Bylaws

ARTICLE I

TITLE, OBJECTS, LOCATION

SECTION 1. TITLE. The Association shall be known as ____, and shall at all times be operated and conducted as a non-profit corporation in accordance with the laws of the State of _____ for such organizations and by which it shall acquire all such rights as granted to associations of this kind.

SECTION 2. OBJECTS. The purpose of the Association shall be to collect, record, and preserve the pedigrees of _____, to publish a breeding registry to be known as the _____ Herd Book, and to stimulate and regulate any and all other matters such as may pertain to the history, breeding, exhibition, publicity, sale, or improvements of this breed.

SECTION 3. PLACE OF BUSINESS. The principal place of business for the ___ shall be in the state where the current registrar resides, but its members or officers may be residents of any state, territory, or country, and business may be carried on at any place convenient to such members or officials, as may be participating.

ARTICLE II

MEMBERS

SECTION 1. MEMBERS.

A. Membership. Membership is annual, and members are those people paying dues upon joining the Association and renewing their membership by paying dues in January of each year.
B. Members may be individuals, partnerships, or corporations.

C. As a condition of membership in the Association each member shall agree to conform to and abide by the Bylaws, Rules, and Regulations of the Association, and amendments or modifications thereto, which may from time to time be adopted.
D. Application for membership may be made by submitting to the Registrar of the Association an application in the form prescribed by the Board of Directors, accompanied by the established membership fee.
E. All animals shall be registered under a single herd name unless they are owned by a partnership. In the case of a partnership, a partnership agreement shall be placed on file with the current registrar of record at the time of the herd's formation.
F. The Board of Directors shall have the power to accept or reject applications for membership, fix membership fees, and establish Rules and Regulations covering the rights and privileges of members, consistent with the provisions of these Bylaws.
G. Only Active Members shall be entitled to vote on any matter submitted to a vote of the Membership. Each Active Member shall have one vote. Corporations or firms who are Active Members shall designate in writing an individual officer, director, or member of the corporation or firm, who shall exercise on behalf of the corporation or firm, the rights, and privileges of such membership, including the right to vote and hold office. Husband, wife, and children under the age of eighteen are entitled to only one vote, even if each owns animals in his own name. An exception to this rule would be in such cases where spouse or children have purchased separate memberships.
H. Membership in the Association shall cease upon the death, resignation, or expulsion of a member, except as may otherwise be provided in the Rules and Regulations of the Association. Membership is not transferable.
I. The Board of Directors may provide for the issuance of Certificate evidencing membership in the Association.

SECTION 2. ANNUAL MEETINGS. The regular annual meeting of the members may be held at such time and place as may be fixed by the resolution of the Board of Directors for the purpose of electing directors and for the transaction of such other business as may be brought before the meeting.

If an annual meeting is to take place, notice of the meeting shall be given by mailing written notice stating the time and place of such meeting to each member's last known address as it appears on the Association's records not less than thirty (30) days prior to the date of such meeting.

If an annual meeting is not practical or feasible, members may address concerns, questions, or other business via electronic means, regular mail, or telephone to any Board Member to relay on to the rest of the board.

SECTION 3. SPECIAL MEETINGS. The President, or a majority of the Board of Directors, may call special meetings of the members by giving written notice to the membership of the time and place of such meeting at least fifteen (15) days in advance. At a special meeting, the members may transact only such business as is properly specified in the notice of meeting.

SECTION 4. QUORUM AND PROXY. For the purpose of election and the transaction of other business, the quorum shall consist of fifteen (15) or more voting members or ten percent (10%) of the total voting membership present in person, which ever shall be the least. Voting by proxy shall not be permitted.

ARTICLE III

DIRECTORS

SECTION 1. GOVERNMENT. A Board of Directors shall govern the business and property of the Association.

There shall be no less than three nor more than nine directors, as established from time to time by the Board or majority vote of the members at any annual or special meeting.

The initial Board of Directors shall consist of six directors, two of whom are to serve for three-year terms; two of whom are to serve for two-year terms; and two of whom are to serve for one-year terms with such terms to be determined by lot.

Directors elected to succeeding terms will be for a full three-year term. Directors must be Active Members of the Association.

SECTION 2. ELECTION. Elections for members of the Board of Directors may be conducted at the annual meeting or a vote by mail. Members may make nomination suggestions to the Nominating Committee for their review.

No less than thirty (30) days before the membership vote, the Board of Directors shall mail a list of the nominees and their resumes which will not exceed 200 words, to the members eligible to vote at that date. Memberships that have lapsed shall be sent notices of dues, which are due along with the ballot and resumes.

The CPA firm or attorney or a neutral party who will tally the ballots shall be chosen by the Board of Directors.

SECTION 3. GEOGRAPHIC DISTRIBUTION. Directors need not be citizens or residents of the United States of America.

It is declared to be the policy of the Association to have the various areas in which _______ are bred to be fairly represented on the Board of Directors, and it is hereby provided that no more than three Directors may be residents of the same state of the United States of America or residents of the same foreign country. In this instance, the term residence is defined as the state or foreign country in which the headquarters of a particular operation is located. The Headquarters of this Association may not be moved from the boundaries of the United States.

SECTION 4. VACANCY. If a Director, during his term of office, shall die or resign, or shall he disperse his herd and cease to be an active breeder, or shall fail to attend three consecutive meetings, or otherwise fail to perform the duties of a Director, the Board of Directors may, after appropriate notice to such Director, remove him from office and declare a vacancy. The Board of Directors may then fill the vacancy by appointment of a new Director for the unexpired portion of the term.

SECTION 5. RULES AND REGULATIONS. The Board of Directors shall have the power to establish Rules and Regulations for the conduct of the members of the Association and for the conduct of the affairs of the Association consistent with the provisions of these Bylaws.

SECTION 6. COMMITTEES. The Board of Directors may, from time to time appoint standing or special committees which may include nonmembers of the Board of Directors. Standing or special committees appointed by the Board of Directors shall be charged with and limited to such responsibilities as the Board of Directors shall set forth by resolution.

SECTION 7. ANNUAL AND REGULAR MEETINGS. The regular annual meeting of the Board of Directors may be held either in person, via conference call, or other electronic means and no notice shall be required for any such regular meeting of the Board. The Board, by rule, may provide for other regular meetings at stated times and places, of which no notice shall be required.

At an annual meeting, the Board shall proceed to the election of officers of the Association.

SECTION 8. SPECIAL MEETINGS. Special meetings of the Board of Directors shall be held whenever called by direction of the President or by two-thirds (2/3rds) of the Directors in office.

The Secretary shall give notice of each special meeting by mail or telephone to each Director at least ten (10) days before the meeting; but any Director may waive such notice. Unless otherwise indicated in the notice thereof, any and all business may be transacted at a special meeting.

SECTION 9. QUORUM. A majority of the whole number of Directors shall constitute a quorum at any meeting. In the absence of a quorum, a lesser number may adjourn any meeting from time to time, and the meeting may be held as adjourned, without further notice, if a quorum is obtained.

SECTION 10. EXPENSES. When the Directors meet for the transaction of Association business, their expenses incurred for such meetings may be paid from the funds of the Association, as the Directors decide at each meeting.

SECTION 11. ACTION WITHOUT A MEETING. Any action, which may be taken at a meeting of the Directors or of a committee, may be taken without a meeting if consent in writing setting forth the action so taken shall be signed by all of the Directors or all of the members of the committee entitled to vote thereon. Members of the Board of Directors may participate in a meeting of the Board or committee by means of conference telephone or similar communications equipment, by which all persons participating in the meeting can hear each other at the same time. Such participation shall constitute presence in person at the meeting.

ARTICLE IV

OFFICERS

SECTION 1. OFFICERS. The officers of the Association shall consist of the President, a Vice-President, Secretary/Treasurer, and such other officers as the Board of Directors deem necessary.

Officers shall be elected by the Board of Directors at the Board's Annual Meeting, and shall serve for a term of one year or until their successors are elected and qualified.

SECTION 2. PRESIDENT. The President shall be the Chief Executive Officer of the Association, and shall preside at all meetings of the Board of Directors and members; shall be ex-officio member of all committees; shall maintain general supervision of the affairs of the Association; shall see that the Bylaws and Rules and Regulations of the Association are enforced; shall have a vote in the Board of Directors in case of a tie; and shall perform such other duties as may be prescribed by the Board of Directors.

SECTION 3. VICE-PRESIDENT. In the absence of the President, the Vice-President shall have the powers and shall perform the duties of the President, and shall perform such other duties as may be prescribed by the Board of Directors.

SECTION 4. SECRETARY/TREASURER. The Secretary/Treasurer shall keep or cause to be kept exact minutes of the meetings of the Board of Directors of the Association and shall perform such duties as directed by the President and by the Board of Directors. All Secretary/Treasurer records must be turned over to the registrar at the end of each year.

SECTION 5. REGISTRAR. A Registrar shall be employed by the Board of Directors to receive and verify entries for insertion in the Herd Book subject to the Rules and Regulations of the Association; shall keep on file all documents constituting the authority for pedigrees and hold them subject to the inspection of any member of the Association; shall keep and be custodian of the funds and securities of the Association; and, shall deposit, invest, or otherwise dispose of same as the Board of Directors may order; shall sign checks issued by the Association; and, shall perform all other duties properly ordered by the President or the Board of Directors, or which should be pertained to the office of the Registrar.

ARTICLE V

DISCIPLINE, SUSPENSION, EXPULSION

SECTION 1. VIOLATIONS. Whenever any members of the Association or any other person in interest shall represent to the Secretary of the Association in writing stating the facts upon which the complaint is based, that a member of this Association, or any other person who is a holder of a Certificate of Registration issued by this Association, has engaged in misrepresentation or misconduct in connection with the breeding, showing, registration, purchase, or sale of ______, or has willfully violated the Bylaws, Rules, and

Regulations of this Association, the Secretary shall present such charge to the Board of Directors at its next meeting.

SECTION 2. HEARING. Upon receiving a complaint, the Board of Directors shall set a time and place for hearing the charge or charges against the member or holder of a Certificate of Registration. The Board of Directors shall cause a written notice to be mailed to the last known address of the accused person at least thirty (30) days before the date of such hearing. The notice shall state the nature of the charges against the accused.

At the time and place set for the hearing, the accused shall have the opportunity, in person or by counsel, to be heard and to present evidence in their own behalf and to hear and refute the evidence offered against him.

The decision of the Board of Directors shall be final and binding on all parties.

SECTION 3. PENALTIES. If the Board of Directors considers that the charges are sustained, it may suspend or expel such offender if a member of the Association, or impose such other appropriate penalties as it may decide and deprive him of all privileges in the official Record of the Association, including refusal to transfer any Certificate and Registration issued by this Association and cancellation of any registration of an animal standing in the name of the accused person. The Board, in its discretion, may also suspend and hold in abeyance during the pending of any complaint before it, the privileges of membership in the Association if the accused is a member of the Association, or the right to transfer any Certificate of Registration, if the accused is not a member.

ARTICLE VI

MISCELLANEOUS

SECTION 1. ORDER OF BUSINESS. The order of business of an Annual Meeting shall be:

a) Calling the meeting to order by the President.
b) Reading minutes of previous meeting and acting thereon.
c) Annual address of the President.
d) Reports of committees and old business.
e) Election of directors.
f) Unfinished business.
g) New business.

In determining questions not covered by the Articles of Incorporation and Bylaws of this Association, *Robert's Rules of Order* shall be used. The order of business of the Directors' meeting shall be the same as Article VI, Section 1, except that those parts that are not applicable will be omitted.

SECTION 2. FISCAL YEAR. The fiscal year for the Association shall commence on January 1 and end on December 31.

SECTION 3. BONDS. The Registrar or any other employee entrusted with monies of the Association shall be bonded and/or covered by fidelity insurance. Such bonds and/or insurance shall be in an adequate amount as set by the Board of Directors and shall be an expense of the Association.

SECTION 4. AUDIT. It shall be the duty of the Board of Directors to cause to be audited all claims upon the Association and to verify the accounts of the Registrar before they are submitted to the members.

SECTION 5. NOMINATING COMMITTEE. The Board of Directors shall appoint a nominating committee of three members. The nominating committee will evaluate candidates according to guidelines established by the Board of Directors. Such committee shall consider all available candidates for the directorships and offices to be filled at the forth-coming meeting and shall submit a slate of candidates for election. Such submission shall be deemed a nomination of each person named. The committee may recommend one or more than one candidate for each vacancy to be filled.

At an annual meeting of members, nominations may be made by members from the floor.

SECTION 6. PROHIBITION AGAINST POLITICAL ACTIVITIES. The Corporation shall not participate or intervene in (including the publishing or distribution of statements) any political campaign on behalf of any candidate for public office.

SECTION 7. DISTRIBUTION OR DISSOLUTION. In the event of the dissolution of the Corporation, no member shall be entitled to any distribution or division of its remaining property or its proceeds, and the balance of all money and other property received by the Corporation from any source, after the payment of all debts and obligations of the Corporation, shall be used or distributed exclusively for the purposes within the intendment of Section 501c3 of the Internal Revenue Code as the same now exists or as it may be amended from time to time.

ARTICLE VII

AMENDING THE BYLAWS

These Bylaws may be altered or amended by a vote of the majority of the members of the Board of Directors in attendance at any Board meeting and confirmed by a majority vote of the membership voting.

These Bylaws may be amended by a two-thirds (2/3rds) vote of the qualified members voting in person at any annual meeting of the Association.

Proposed Articles of Incorporation or Bylaws changes must be presented in writing to the Board of Directors no less than two (2) months prior to the annual meeting. A proposed change in the Articles of Incorporation and Bylaws when approved by the Board of Directors will be published and forwarded to all members.

Index